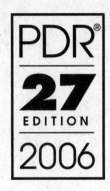

PDR®

for Nonprescription Drugs, Dietary Supplements, and Herbs

THE DEFINITIVE GUIDE TO OTC MEDICATIONS

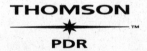

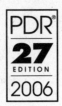

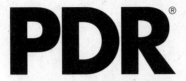

PDR®

for Nonprescription Drugs, Dietary Supplements, and Herbs

THE DEFINITIVE GUIDE TO OTC MEDICATIONS

Senior Vice President, PDR Sales and Marketing:
Dikran N. Barsamian

Vice President, Product Management: William T. Hicks

Vice President, Regulatory Affairs: Mukesh Mehta, RPh

Vice President, PDR Services: Brian Holland

Senior Directors, Pharmaceutical Solutions Sales:
Chantal Corcos, Anthony Sorce

National Solutions Managers: Frank Karkowsky,
Marion Reid, RPh

Senior Solutions Managers: Debra Goldman, Elaine Musco,
Warner Stuart, Suzanne E. Yarrow, RN

Solutions Managers: Eileen Bruno, Cory Coleman,
Marjorie A. Jaxel, Kevin McGlynn, Lois Smith,
Richard Zwickel

Sales Coordinators: Arlene Phayre, Janet Wallendal

Senior Director, Brand and Product Management:
Valerie E. Berger

Associate Product Managers: Michael Casale,
Andrea Colavecchio

Senior Director, Publishing Sales and Marketing:
Michael Bennett

Director, Trade Sales: Bill Gaffney

Associate Director, Marketing: Jennifer M. Fronzaglia

Senior Marketing Manager: Kim Marich

Direct Mail Manager: Lorraine M. Loening

Manager, Marketing Analysis: Dina A. Maeder

Promotion Manager: Linda Levine

Director of Operations: Robert Klein

Director, PDR Operations: Jeffrey D. Schaefer

Director of Finance: Mark S. Ritchin

Director, Client Services: Stephanie Struble

Director, Clinical Content: Thomas Fleming, PharmD

Director, Editorial Services: Bette LaGow

Drug Information Specialists: Michael DeLuca, PharmD,
MBA; Kajal Solanki, PharmD; Greg Tallis, RPh

Project Editors: Neil Chesanow, Harris Fleming

Senior Editor: Lori Murray

Senior Production Editor: Gwynned L. Kelly

Index Editor: Caryn Sobel

Manager, Production Purchasing: Thomas Westburgh

PDR Production Manager: Steven Maher

Production Manager: Gayle Graizzaro

Production Specialist: Christina Klinger

Senior Production Coordinators: Gianna Caradonna,
Yasmin Hernández

Production Coordinator: Nick W. Clark

Format Editor: Michelle G. Auffant

Traffic Assistant: Kim Condon

Production Design Supervisor: Adeline Rich

Senior Electronic Publishing Designer: Livio Udina

Electronic Publishing Designers: Bryan C. Dix,
Carrie Faeth, Monika Popowitz

Production Associate: Joan K. Akerlind

Digital Imaging Manager: Christopher Husted

Digital Imaging Coordinator: Michael Labruyere

ISBN: 1-56363-530-5

Table of Contents

NONPRESCRIPTION DRUG INFORMATION

Provides therapeutic class overviews, drug comparison charts, and product information on hundreds of over-the-counter medications. Entries are arranged alphabetically first by body system or condition, then by indication.

Features clinical monographs of frequently used supplements, including accepted and unproven uses as well as drug interactions and contraindications. Arranged alphabetically by common name.

HERBAL MEDICINE PROFILES...361

Features evidence-based profiles of the most popular herbal supplements, including common uses approved by Commission E, the German government's expert committee on herbal medicines. Arranged alphabetically by common name.

INDEX...378

Foreword

Over-the-counter (OTC) medications play an important role in national healthcare, with consumers buying around 5 billion such products a year. The choices are staggering: More than 100,000 OTC drugs are available, including over 800 active ingredients and 100 therapeutic classes or categories. Factor in the millions of Americans taking prescription medications—not to mention dietary supplements and herbs—and the risk for side effects or drug interactions increases rapidly.

To aid healthcare professionals in providing safe drug management, we've redesigned the format and greatly expanded the information in this latest edition of the *PDR® for Nonprescription Drugs, Dietary Supplements, and Herbs*. The nonprescription drug section is now organized by therapeutic category and indication, allowing you to make faster and more informed decisions. Detailed generic monographs, supplemented with easy-to-ready charts, cover indications, side effects, drug interactions, and dosing information for the most commonly used OTC products. For quick lookups, you'll also find convenient tables at the end of each chapter listing common brand names along with their generic ingredients, strengths, and dosages. In addition, we've included sections containing evidence-based, clinical profiles of dietary supplements and herbal medicines.

PDR® for Nonprescription Drugs, Dietary Supplements, and Herbs is published annually by Thomson PDR. The function of the publisher is the compilation, organization, and distribution of drug information obtained from clinical reviews and manufacturer labeling. During compilation of this information, the publisher has emphasized the necessity of describing drug classes and products comprehensively in order to provide all the facts necessary for sound and intelligent decision making. Descriptions seen here include information made available by clinical reviews and manufacturer labeling. This book lists products that are marketed in compliance with the Code of Federal Regulations labeling requirements for OTC drugs. Please note that information on OTC dietary supplements and herbal remedies marketed under the Dietary Supplement Health and Education Act of 1994 have not been evaluated by the Food and Drug Administration, and that such products are not intended to diagnose, treat, cure, or prevent any disease.

In organizing and presenting the material in *PDR® for Nonprescription Drugs, Dietary Supplements, and Herbs*, the publisher does not warrant or guarantee any of the products described, or perform any independent analysis in connection with any of the product information contained herein. *Physicians' Desk Reference* does not assume, and expressly disclaims, any obligation to obtain and include any information other than that provided by manufacturer labeling. It should be understood that by making this material available, the publisher is not advocating the use of any product described herein, nor is the publisher responsible for misuse of a product due to typographical error. Additional information on any product may be obtained from the manufacturer.

Other Prescribing Aids from *PDR*

For complicated cases and special patient problems, there is no substitute for the in-depth data contained in *Physicians' Desk Reference*. But for those times when you need quick access to critical prescribing information, you may want to consult the **PDR® Monthly Prescribing Guide™**, the essential drug reference designed specifically for use at the point of care. Distilled from the pages of *PDR*, this digest-sized reference presents the key facts on more than 1,500 drug formulations, including therapeutic class, indications and contraindications, warnings and precautions, pregnancy rating, drug interactions and side effects, and adult and pediatric dosages. Each entry also gives the *PDR* page number to turn to for further information. In addition, a full-color insert of pill images allows you to correctly identify each product. Issued monthly, the guide is regularly updated with detailed descriptions of new drugs to receive FDA approval, as well as FDA-approved revisions to existing product information. To learn more about this useful publication and to inquire about subscription rates, call 800-232-7379.

If you prefer to carry drug information with you on a handheld device like a Palm® or Pocket PC, consider **mobilePDR®**. This easy-to-use software allows you to retrieve in an instant concise summaries of the FDA-approved and other manufacturer-supplied labeling for 2,000 of the most frequently prescribed drugs, lets you run automatic interaction checks on multidrug regimens, and even alerts you to significant changes in drug labeling, usually within 24 to 48 hours of announcements. You can look up drugs by brand or generic name, by indication, and by therapeutic class. The drug interaction checker allows you to screen for interactions among as many as 32 drugs. The What's New feature provides daily alerts about drug recalls, labeling changes, new drug introductions, and so on. Our auto-update feature updates the content and the software, so upgrades are easy to manage. mobile*PDR®* works with both the Palm® and Pocket PC operating systems, and it's free for U.S.-based MDs, DOs, dentists, NPs, and PAs in full-time patient practice, as well as for medical students, residents, and other select prescribing allied health professionals. Check it out today at www.pdr.net.

For those who prefer to view drug information on the Internet, **PDR.net** is the best online source for comprehensive FDA-approved and other manufacturer-supplied labeling information, as found in *PDR*. Updated monthly, this incredible resource allows you to look up drugs by brand or generic name, by key word, or by indication, side effect, contraindication, or manufacturer. The drug interaction checker allows you to screen for interactions among as many as 32 different drugs. The site provides an index that can be searched to find comparable drugs, and images of all products are included for easy identification. As an added benefit, *PDR*.net also gives users the option to order drug samples online. Finally, *PDR*.net hosts the download for *mobile*PDR®. At this one website, you get two great *PDR* products in one. Registration for *PDR*.net is free for U.S.-based MDs, DOs, dentists, NPs, and PAs in full-time patient practice, as well as for medical students, residents, and other select prescribing allied health professionals. Visit www.pdr.net today to register.

For more information on these or any other members of the growing family of *PDR* products, please call, toll-free, 1-800-232-7379 or fax 201-722-2680.

How to Use This Book

This new, completely revised edition of *PDR® for Nonprescription Drugs, Dietary Supplements, and Herbs* is organized to help you find the information you need as quickly and easily as possible. Arranged by therapeutic category and indication, you can go directly to the section you need to find the relevant products for a particular condition.

NONPRESCRIPTION DRUG INFORMATION
Each entry in this section includes:

Brief description of the condition
These introductory sections provide a concise yet informative overview of the given condition, including causes, typical presentation, pathogens (if applicable), and available OTC treatments.

Therapeutic class overview
The main generic ingredients of various treatments are covered here, with pharmacology, indications, contraindications, warnings/precautions, adverse reactions, and administration and dosage.

Drug interaction tables
Important and potentially dangerous drug interactions are shown in an easy-to-read table that clearly shows the effects of concomitant administration. Interactions with major clinical significance are indicated with special icons (◆).

Generic ingredient product tables
Quick reference tables listing the brand name and dosage form of available products.

Dosing information comparison tables
These tables offer quick comparisons of the generic ingredients, manufacturers, strengths, and dosing information for common brand-name drugs. Includes pediatric dosing when applicable. The tables are listed alphabetically by brand name. A key to the abbreviations used in these tables is shown on the right-hand side of this page.

DIETARY SUPPLEMENT PROFILES
This section covers the most commonly used dietary supplements. Each monograph in this section includes the supplement's effects, common usage, contraindications, warnings/precautions, drug interactions, food interactions, adverse reactions, and administration and dosage (including pediatric, when available).

HERBAL MEDICINE PROFILES
Like Dietary Supplements, this section describes the most common herbal medicines being used today. Each monograph covers the herb's effects, common usage (including German Commission E accepted usage), contraindications, warnings/precautions, drug interactions, adverse reactions, and administration and dosage (including pediatric, when available).

Key to Drug Administration and General Abbreviations

ac = before meals

bid = twice a day

biw = twice a week

BMS = Bristol-Myers Squibb

cap(s) = capsule(s)

cm = centimeter

d = day(s)

g = gram

GSK = GlaxoSmithKline

h = hour

hs = bedtime

in = inch

J&J = Johnson & Johnson

loz = lozenge

mcg = microgram

mg = milligram

mL = milliliter

oint = ointment

pc = after meals

prn = as needed

q = every

qam = every morning

qd = every day

qh = every hour

qhs = every night or every bedtime

qid = four times a day

qod = every other day

qpm = every night

qw = weekly/every week

supp = suppositories

tab(s) = tablet(s)

tbls = tablespoonful(s)

tid = three times a day

tsps = teaspoonful(s)

yo = years old

NONPRESCRIPTION DRUG INFORMATION

Drowsiness/Lethargy

Drowsiness refers to feeling abnormally sleepy during the day, often with a strong tendency to actually fall asleep in inappropriate situations or at inappropriate times. Common causes include self-imposed short sleep time; medications such as tranquilizers, sleeping pills, and antihistamines; sleep disorders such as sleep apnea or narcolepsy; and other medical conditions such as hypothyroidism, hypercalcemia, and hypo- or hypernatremia. Curing or preventing drowsiness requires treatment of the underlying cause. For occasional mild drowsiness and lethargy, OTC drugs that contain caffeine can be used.

CAFFEINE

PHARMACOLOGY

Central nervous system stimulant—Caffeine stimulates all levels of the central nervous system (CNS), although its cortical effects are milder and of shorter duration than those of amphetamines. In larger doses, caffeine stimulates medullary, vagal, vasomotor, and respiratory centers, promoting bradycardia, vasoconstriction, and increased respiratory rate. This action was previously believed to be due primarily to increased intracellular cyclic 3′,5′-adenosine monophosphate (cyclic AMP) following inhibition of phosphodiesterase, the enzyme that degrades cyclic AMP. More recent studies indicate that caffeine exerts its physiological effects in large part through antagonism of central adenosine receptors.

Analgesia adjunct—Caffeine constricts cerebral vasculature with an accompanying decrease in cerebral blood flow and in the oxygen tension of the brain. It has been suggested that the addition of caffeine to aspirin or aspirin and acetaminophen combinations may help to relieve headache by providing a more rapid onset of action and/or enhanced pain relief with a lower dose of the analgesic. In some patients, caffeine may reduce headache pain by reversing caffeine withdrawal symptoms. Recent studies with ergotamine indicate that the enhancement of effect by the addition of caffeine may be due to improved gastrointestinal absorption of ergotamine when administered with caffeine.

Respiratory stimulant adjunct—Although the exact mechanism of action has not been completely established, caffeine, as other methylxanthines, is believed to act primarily through stimulation of the medullary respiratory center. This action is seen in certain pathophysiologic states, such as in Cheyne-Stokes respiration and in apnea of preterm infants, and when respiration is depressed by certain drugs, such as barbiturates and opioids. Methylxanthines appear to increase the sensitivity of the respiratory center to the stimulatory actions of carbon dioxide, increasing alveolar ventilation, thereby reducing the severity and frequency of apneic episodes.

INDICATIONS

Fatigue or drowsiness (treatment)—Caffeine is used as a mild CNS stimulant to help restore mental alertness or wakefulness when fatigue or drowsiness is experienced.

Apnea, neonatal (treatment adjunct)—Caffeine or citrated caffeine (but not caffeine and sodium benzoate combination) is indicated in the short-term management of neonatal apnea, especially apnea of prematurity, which is characterized by periodic breathing and apneic episodes of more than 15 seconds accompanied by cyanosis and bradycardia, in infants between 28 and 33 weeks' gestational age. Other treatments include increased stimulation (cutaneous, vestibular, or proprioceptive), nasal continuous positive airway pressure (CPAP), increased environmental oxygen, and artificial ventilation. Determination of which therapy is to be undertaken is based upon the assessment of each individual patient's clinical status and therapeutic requirement. Caffeine may be considered a desirable alternative to theophylline when initiating therapy for premature neonatal apnea because some infants are unable to convert theophylline to caffeine, a major metabolite of theophylline in neonates. Caffeine also has a wider therapeutic index than theophylline. Caffeine therapy in the management of apnea is usually required for only a few weeks and rarely for more than a few months, since the apnea usually resolves by about 34 to 36 weeks' gestational age.

Apnea, infant, postoperative (prophylaxis)—Caffeine or citrated caffeine is indicated for the prevention of postoperative apnea in former preterm infants.

Electroconvulsive therapy (ECT) (treatment adjunct)—Caffeine pretreatment is indicated to augment ECT by increasing seizure duration and reducing the need for increases in stimulus intensity.

Caffeine is used in combination with ergotamine to treat *vascular headaches* such as migraine and cluster headaches (histaminic cephalalgia, migrainous neuralgia, Horton's headache).

Caffeine is also used, and has been shown to be effective, as an *analgesic adjunct* in combination with aspirin or acetaminophen and aspirin to enhance pain relief, although it has no analgesic activity of its own. However, caffeine's efficacy as an analgesic adjunct in combination with acetaminophen alone has been questioned.

CONTRAINDICATIONS

Risk-benefit should be considered when the following medical problems exist:

- Anxiety disorders, including agoraphobia and panic attacks—*major clinical significance* (increased risk of anxiety, nervousness, fear, nausea, palpitations, rapid heartbeat, restlessness, and trembling)

- Cardiac disease, severe—*major clinical significance* (high doses not recommended because of increased risk of tachycardia or extrasystoles, which may lead to heart failure)

- Hepatic function impairment—*major clinical significance* (half-life of caffeine may be prolonged, leading to toxic accumulation)

- Hypertension or insomnia—*major clinical significance* (may be potentiated)

- Seizure disorders, in neonates (caution is recommended because seizures have been reported following toxic doses)

- Sensitivity to caffeine or other xanthines

WARNINGS/PRECAUTIONS

Patients sensitive to other xanthines (aminophylline, dyphylline, oxtriphylline, theobromine, theophylline) may be sensitive to caffeine also.

Pregnancy: FDA Category C. Caffeine crosses the placenta and achieves blood and tissue concentrations in the fetus that are similar to maternal concentrations. Heavy caffeine consumption by pregnant women may increase the risk of spontaneous abortion and intrauterine growth retardation. Excessive intake of caffeine by pregnant women has resulted in fetal arrhythmias. It is therefore recommended that pregnant women limit their intake of caffeine to less than 300mg (3 cups of coffee) per day.

Breastfeeding: Use with caution. Caffeine is distributed into breast milk in very small amounts. Although the concentration of caffeine in breast milk is 1% of the mother's plasma concentration, caffeine can accumulate in the infant. It is recommended that nursing mothers limit their intake of caffeine-containing beverages to 1 to 2 cups per day and avoid taking OTC caffeine capsules or tablets.

Drug Interactions for Caffeine

Precipitant Drug	Object Drug	Effect on Object Drug	Description
Barbiturates Primidone	Caffeine	↓	Concurrent use may increase the metabolism of caffeine by induction of hepatic microsomal enzymes, resulting in increased clearance of caffeine; in addition, concurrent use may antagonize the hypnotic or anticonvulsant effects of the barbiturates.
Caffeine	Adenosine	↓	Effects of adenosine are antagonized by caffeine; larger doses of adenosine may be required, or adenosine may be ineffective.
Caffeine	Beta-adrenergic blocking agents (systemic/ophthalmic)	↓	Concurrent use may result in mutual inhibition of therapeutic effects.
Caffeine	Bronchodilators, adrenergic	↑	Concurrent use with caffeine may result in additive CNS stimulation and other additive toxic effects.
Caffeine	♦ Central nervous system (CNS) stimulants	↑	Excessive CNS stimulation causing nervousness, irritability, insomnia, or possibly convulsions or cardiac arrhythmias may occur; close observation is recommended.
Caffeine	Calcium Supplements	↓	Concurrent use with excessive amounts of caffeine may inhibit absorption of calcium.
Caffeine	Lithium	↓	Concurrent use with caffeine increases urinary excretion of lithium, possibly reducing its therapeutic effect.
Cimetidine	Caffeine	↑	Decreased hepatic metabolism of caffeine results in delayed elimination and increased blood concentrations.
Caffeine	Xanthines (aminophylline, dyphylline, oxtriphylline, theobromine, theophylline)	↑	Caffeine may decrease the clearance of theophylline and possibly other xanthines, increasing the potential for additive pharmacodynamic and toxic effects.
Ciprofloxacin Enoxacin Norfloxacin	Caffeine	↑	Hepatic metabolism and clearance of caffeine may be reduced, increasing the risk of caffeine-related CNS stimulation.
Contraceptives, oral	Caffeine	↑	Concurrent use may decrease caffeine metabolism.
Disulfiram	Caffeine	↑	Concurrent use may reduce the elimination rate of caffeine by inhibiting its metabolism; recovering alcoholic patients on disulfiram therapy are best advised to avoid the use of caffeine.
Erythromycin Troleandomycin	Caffeine	↑	Concurrent use may reduce the hepatic clearance of caffeine.
Mexiletine	Caffeine	↑	Concurrent use with caffeine reduces the elimination of caffeine by up to 50% and may increase the potential for adverse effects.
Phenytoin	Caffeine	↓	Concurrent use of phenytoin may increase the clearance of caffeine.
♦ Monoamine oxidase (MAO) inhibitors (furazolidone, procarbazine, selegiline)	Caffeine	↑	Large amounts of caffeine may produce dangerous cardiac arrhythmias or severe hypertension because of the sympathomimetic side effects of caffeine; concurrent use with small amounts of caffeine may produce tachycardia and a mild increase in blood pressure.
Smoking tobacco	Caffeine	↓	Concurrent use of tobacco increases the elimination rate of caffeine.

♦ = Major clinical significance.

ADVERSE REACTIONS

Those indicating need for medical attention: Incidence more frequent

CNS stimulation, excessive (dizziness, fast heartbeat, irritability, nervousness, or severe jitters—in neonates; tremors, trouble in sleeping); *gastrointestinal irritation* (diarrhea, nausea, vomiting); *hyperglycemia* (blurred vision, drowsiness, dry mouth, flushed, dry skin, fruitlike breath odor, increased urination [frequency and volume], ketones in urine, loss of appetite, stomachache, nausea, vomiting, tiredness, troubled breathing [rapid and deep], unconsciousness, unusual thirst)—in neonates; *hypoglycemia* (anxiety, blurred vision, cold sweats, confusion, cool, pale skin, drowsiness, excessive hunger, fast heartbeat, nausea, nervousness, restless sleep, shakiness, unusual tiredness or weakness)—in neonates.

Incidence rare

Necrotizing enterocolitis (abdominal distention; dehydration; diarrhea, bloody; irritability; unusual tiredness or weakness; vomiting)—in neonates.

Those indicating need for medical attention only if they continue or are bothersome: Incidence more frequent

CNS stimulation, mild (nervousness or jitters); gastrointestinal irritation, mild (nausea).

Those indicating possible withdrawal if they occur after medication is abruptly discontinued after prolonged use

Anxiety, dizziness, headache, irritability, muscle tension, nausea, nervousness, stuffy nose, unusual tiredness.

ADMINISTRATION AND DOSAGE

For fatigue or drowsiness:

Adults/Pediatrics ≥12 years of age: 100 to 200mg every 3 to 4 hours prn.

CAFFEINE PRODUCTS	
Brand Name	**Dosage Form**
Vivarin(GSK)	**Tablet:** 200mg
No Doz Maximum Strength(BMS)	**Tablet:** 200mg

DOSING INFORMATION FOR DROWSINESS/LETHARGY PRODUCTS

The following table provides a quick comparison of the ingredients and dosages of common brand-name OTC products. Entries are listed alphabetically by brand name.

BRAND NAME	INGREDIENT/STRENGTH	DOSE
NoDoz caplets (*Bristol-Myers Squibb*)	Caffeine 200 mg	**Adults & Peds ≥12 yo:** 1 tab q3-4h.
Vivarin caplets (*GlaxoSmithKline Consumer Healthcare*)	Caffeine 200 mg	**Adults & Peds ≥12 yo:** 1 tab q3-4h.
Vivarin tablets (*GlaxoSmithKline Consumer Healthcare*)	Caffeine 200 mg	**Adults & Peds ≥12 yo:** 1/2 to 1 tab q3-4h.

Fever

Fever is defined as an elevation in body temperature greater than that normally seen in daily body temperature variations. Normal body temperature varies by person, age, activity, and time of day. The average normal body temperature is 98.6°F (37°C). Body temperature is controlled by the hypothalamus, which has three types of thermosensitive neurons: cold-sensitive, warm-sensitive, and temperature-insensitive. These neurons respond to the temperature in the brain and receive input from thermoreceptors in the skin and spinal cord. Normal body temperature is ordinarily maintained, despite environmental variations, because the thermoregulatory center in the hypothalamus balances the excess heat production derived from metabolic activity in muscle and the liver with heat dissipation from the skin and lungs. Normal daily temperature variation is typically 0.9°F (0.5°C). There are diurnal variations in normal body temperature, with the highest body temperature usually occurring in the evening. Body temperature is often measured orally or rectally; rectal temperatures are generally 0.7°F (0.4°C) higher than oral readings.

During febrile illness, diurnal variations are usually maintained but at higher levels. A fever usually means the body is responding to a viral or bacterial infection. Sometimes heat exhaustion, an extreme sunburn, or certain inflammatory conditions such as temporal arteritis may trigger fever as well. In rare instances, a malignant tumor or some forms of kidney cancer may cause a fever.

Fever can also be a side effect of some medications such as antibiotics and drugs used to treat hypertension or seizures. Some infants and children develop fevers after receiving routine immunizations, such as the diphtheria, tetanus and pertussis (DTaP) or pneumococcal vaccines.

Several medications are available for lowering fever, including aspirin, acetaminophen, and NSAIDs.

ACETAMINOPHEN

Antipyretic—Acetaminophen probably produces antipyresis by acting centrally on the hypothalamic heat-regulating center to produce peripheral vasodilation, resulting in increased blood flow to the skin, sweating, and heat loss. The central action probably involves inhibition of prostaglandin synthesis in the hypothalamus.

For antipyretic use:

Capsules/Granules/Powder/Solution/Suspension/Tablets

Adults/Pediatrics ≥13 years of age: 325 to 500mg every 3 hours; 325 to 650mg every 4 hours; 650 to 1000mg every 6 hours; or 1300mg every 8 hours.

Pediatrics ≤3 months of age: 40mg every 4 hours as needed.

Pediatrics 4 to 12 months of age: 80mg every 4 hours as needed.

Pediatrics 1 to 2 years of age: 120mg every 4 hours as needed.

Pediatrics 2 to 4 years of age: 160mg every 4 hours as needed.

Pediatrics 4 to 6 years of age: 240mg every 4 hours as needed.

Pediatrics 6 to 9 years of age: 320mg every 4 hours as needed.

Pediatrics 9 to 11 years of age: 320mg to 400mg every 4 hours as needed.

Pediatrics 11 to 12 years of age: 320mg to 480mg every 4 hours as needed.

Suppositories

Adults/Pediatrics ≥13 years of age: 325 to 650mg every 4 hours or 650mg every 6 hours as needed.

Pediatrics 2 to 4 years of age: 160mg every 4 hours as needed.

Pediatrics 4 to 6 years of age: 240mg every 4 hours as needed.

Pediatrics 6 to 9 years of age: 320mg every 4 hours as needed.

Pediatrics 9 to 11 years of age: 320mg to 400mg every 4 hours as needed.

Pediatrics 11 to 12 years of age: 320 to 480mg every 4 hours as needed.

For more information, refer to the complete monograph for acetaminophen in "Aches and Pains" under Musculoskeletal System.

ACETAMINOPHEN PRODUCTS	
Brand Name	**Dosage Form**
Anacin Aspirin Free (Insight)	**Tablet:** 500mg
Feverall (Alpharma)	**Suppositories:** 80mg, 120mg, 325mg, 650mg
Tylenol 8 Hour (McNeil)	**Tablet:** 650mg
Tylenol Arthritis (McNeil)	**Tablet:** 650mg
Tylenol Children's (McNeil)	**Suspension:** 160mg/5mL
Tylenol Children's Meltaways (McNeil)	**Tablet:** 80mg
Tylenol Extra Strength (McNeil)	**Capsule:** 500mg **Liquid:** 1000mg/30mL **Tablet:** 500mg
Tylenol Infants' (McNeil)	**Suspension:** 80mg/0.8mL
Tylenol Junior Meltaways (McNeil)	**Tablet:** 160mg
Tylenol Regular Strength (McNeil)	**Tablet:** 325mg

ASPIRIN

Antipyretic—Aspirin may produce antipyresis by acting centrally on the hypothalamic heat-regulating center to produce peripheral vasodilation, resulting in increased cutaneous blood flow, sweating, and heat loss. The central action may involve inhibition of prostaglandin synthesis in the hypothalamus; however, there is some evidence that fevers caused by endogenous pyrogens that do not act via a prostaglandin mechanism may also respond to salicylate therapy.

For antipyretic use:

Suppositories

Adults/Pediatrics ≥12 years of age: 325 to 650mg every 4 hours as needed.

Pediatrics 2 to 4 years of age: 160mg every 4 hours as needed.

Pediatrics 4 to 6 years of age: 240mg every 4 hours as needed.

Pediatrics 6 to 9 years of age: 325mg every 4 hours as needed.

Pediatrics 9 to 11 years of age: 325 to 400mg every 4 hours as needed.

Pediatric 11 to 12 years of age: 325 to 480mg every 4 hours as needed.

Tablets

Adults/Pediatrics ≥12 years of age: 325 to 500mg every 3 hours; 325 to 650mg every 4 hours; or 650 to 1000mg every 6 hours as needed.

Pediatrics 2 to 4 years of age: 160mg every 4 hours as needed.

Pediatrics 4 to 6 years of age: 240mg every 4 hours as needed.

Pediatrics 6 to 9 years of age: 320 to 325mg every 4 hours as needed.

Pediatrics 9 to 11 years of age: 320 to 400mg every 4 hours as needed.

Pediatric 11 to 12 years of age: 320 to 480mg every 4 hours as needed.

For more information, refer to the complete monograph for salicylates in "Aches and Pains" under Musculoskeletal System.

IBUPROFEN

Antipyretic—Ibuprofen probably produces antipyresis by acting centrally on the hypothalamic heat-regulating center to produce peripheral vasodilation, resulting in increased blood flow through the skin, sweating, and heat loss. The central action probably involves reduction of prostaglandin activity in the hypothalamus.

For antipyretic use:

Capsules/Suspension/Tablets

Adults/Pediatrics ≥12 years of age: 200 to 400mg every 4 to 6 hours as needed.

Pediatric 6 months to 12 years of age: 5mg/kg for fevers less than 102.5°F (39.17°C) and 10mg/kg for fevers higher. Dosage may be repeated, if necessary, every 4 to 6 hours.

For more information, refer to the complete monograph for NSAIDs in "Aches and Pains" under Musculoskeletal System.

MAGNESIUM SALICYLATE

Antipyretic: Magnesium salicylate may produce antipyresis by acting centrally on the hypothalamic heat-regulating center to produce peripheral vasodilation, resulting in increased cutaneous blood flow, sweating, and heat loss. The central action may involve inhibition of prostaglandin synthesis in the hypothalamus; however, there is some evidence that fevers caused by endogenous pyrogens that do not act via a prostaglandin mechanism may also respond to salicylate therapy.

ASPIRIN PRODUCTS	
Brand Name	**Dosage Form**
Ascriptin (Novartis)	**Tablet:** 81mg
Aspergum (Schering)	**Gum:** 227mg
Bayer Aspirin Regimen (Bayer)	**Tablet:** 81mg, 325mg
Bayer Children's Aspirin (Bayer)	**Tablet:** 81mg
Bayer Extra Strength (Bayer)	**Tablet:** 500mg
Bayer Genuine Aspirin (Bayer)	**Tablet:** 325mg
Ecotrin (GSK)	**Tablet:** 325mg
Ecotrin Adult Low Strength (GSK)	**Tablet:** 81mg
Ecotrin Maximum Strength (GSK)	**Tablet:** 500mg
Halfprin (Kramer)	**Tablet:** 81mg, 162mg
St. Joseph (McNeil)	**Tablet:** 81mg
BUFFERED ASPIRIN PRODUCTS	
Brand Name	**Dosage Form**
Alka-Seltzer (Bayer)	**Tablet:** 325mg
Alka-Seltzer Extra Strength (Bayer)	**Tablet:** 500mg
Ascriptin (Novartis)	**Tablet:** 325mg
Ascriptin Arthritis Pain (Novartis)	**Tablet:** 325mg
Ascriptin Maximum Strength (Novartis)	**Tablet:** 500mg
Bayer Plus Extra Strength (Bayer)	**Tablet:** 500mg
Bufferin (BMS)	**Tablet:** 325mg
Bufferin Extra Strength (BMS)	**Tablet:** 500mg

For antipyretic use:

Tablets

Adults: 607.4mg every 4 hours as needed, or 934mg every 6 hours as needed.

For more information, refer to the complete monograph for salicylates in "Aches and Pains" under Musculoskeletal System.

NAPROXEN

Antipyretic: Naproxen probably produces antipyresis by acting centrally on the hypothalamic heat-regulating center to produce peripheral vasodilation, resulting in increased blood flow through the skin, sweating, and heat loss. The central action probably involves reduction of prostaglandin activity in the hypothalamus.

For antipyretic use:

Capsules/Tablets

Adults/Pediatrics ≥12 years of age: 200 to 400mg every 4 to 6 hours as needed.

Pediatric 6 months to 12 years of age: 5mg/kg for fevers less than 102.5°F (39.17°C) and 10mg/kg for fevers higher. Dosage may be repeated, if necessary, every 4 to 6 hours.

For more information, refer to the complete monograph for NSAIDs in "Aches and Pains" under Musculoskeletal System.

IBUPROFEN PRODUCTS	
Brand Name	**Dosage Form**
Advil (Wyeth)	**Capsule:** 200mg **Tablet:** 200mg
Advil Children's (Wyeth)	**Tablet:** 50mg
Advil Junior (Wyeth)	**Tablet:** 100mg
Midol Cramp Formula (Bayer)	**Tablet:** 200mg
Motrin IB (McNeil)	**Tablet:** 200mg
Motrin Children's (McNeil)	**Suspension:** 100mg/5mL
Motrin Infants' (McNeil)	**Suspension:** 50mg/1.25mL
Motrin Junior (McNeil)	**Tablet:** 100mg
Motrin Migraine Pain (McNeil)	**Tablet:** 200mg

MAGNESIUM SALICYLATE PRODUCTS	
Brand Name	**Dosage Form**
Doan's Extra Strength (Novartis)	**Tablet:** 500mg
Doan's Regular Strength (Novartis)	**Tablet:** 325mg
Momentum (Medtech)	**Tablet:** 467mg

NAPROXEN PRODUCTS	
Brand Name	**Dosage Form**
Aleve (Bayer)	**Capsule:** 220mg **Tablet:** 220mg
Aleve Arthritis (Bayer)	**Tablet:** 220mg
Midol Extended Relief (Bayer)	**Tablet:** 220mg

DOSING INFORMATION FOR ANTIPYRETIC PRODUCTS

The following table provides a quick comparison of the ingredients and dosages of common brand-name OTC drugs. Products are listed alphabetically by drug category and brand name.

BRAND NAME	GENERIC INGREDIENT/STRENGTH	DOSE
ACETAMINOPHEN		
Anacin Aspirin Free tablets *(Insight Pharmaceuticals)*	Acetaminophen 500mg	**Adults & Peds ≥12 yo:** 2 tabs q6h. **Max:** 8 tabs q24h.
Feverall Childrens' suppositories *(Alpharma)*	Acetaminophen 120mg	**Peds: 3-6 yo:** 1 supp. q4-6h. max 6 supp. q24h.
Feverall Infants' suppositories *(Alpharma)*	Acetaminophen 80mg	**Peds: 3-11 months:** 1 supp. q6h. **12-36 months:** 1 supp. q4h. **Max:** 6 supp. q24h.
Feverall Jr. Strength suppositories *(Alpharma)*	Acetaminophen 120mg	**Peds: 6-12 yo:** 1 supp. q4-6h. **Max:** 6 supp. q24h.
Tylenol 8 Hour caplets *(McNeil Consumer)*	Acetaminophen 650mg	**Adults & Peds ≥12 yo:** 2 tabs q8h prn. **Max:** 6 tabs q24h.

DOSING INFORMATION FOR ANTIPYRETIC PRODUCTS (cont.)

BRAND NAME	GENERIC INGREDIENT/STRENGTH	DOSE
Tylenol 8 Hour geltabs *(McNeil Consumer)*	Acetaminophen 650mg	**Adults & Peds ≥12 yo:** 2 tabs q8h prn. **Max:** 6 tabs q24h.
Tylenol Arthritis caplets *(McNeil Consumer)*	Acetaminophen 650mg	**Adults:** 2 tabs q8h prn. **Max:** 6 tabs q24h.
Tylenol Arthritis geltabs *(McNeil Consumer)*	Acetaminophen 650mg	**Adults:** 2 tabs q8h prn. **Max:** 6 tabs q24h.
Tylenol Children's Meltaways tablets *(McNeil Consumer)*	Acetaminophen 80mg	**Peds: 2-3 yo (24-35 lbs):** 2 tabs. **4-5 yo (36-47 lbs):** 3 tabs. **6-8 yo (48-59 lbs):** 4 tabs. **9-10 yo (60-71 lbs):** 5 tabs. **11 yo (72-95 lbs):** 6 tabs. May repeat q4h. **Max:** 5 doses q24h.
Tylenol Children's suspension *(McNeil Consumer)*	Acetaminophen 160mg/5mL	**Peds: 2-3 yo (24-35 lbs):** 1 tsp (5mL). **4-5 yo (36-47 lbs):** 1.5 tsp (7.5mL). **6-8 yo (48-59 lbs):** 2 tsp (10mL). **9-10 yo (60-71 lbs):** 2.5 tsp (12.5mL). **11 yo (72-95 lbs):** 3 tsp (15mL). May repeat q4h. **Max:** 5 doses q24h.
Tylenol Extra Strength caplets *(McNeil Consumer)*	Acetaminophen 500mg	**Adults & Peds ≥12 yo:** 2 tabs q4-6h prn. **Max:** 8 tabs q24h.
Tylenol Extra Strength Cool caplets *(McNeil Consumer)*	Acetaminophen 500mg	**Adults & Peds ≥12 yo:** 2 tabs q4-6h prn. **Max:** 8 tabs q24h.
Tylenol Extra Strength gelcaps *(McNeil Consumer)*	Acetaminophen 500mg	**Adults & Peds ≥12 yo:** 2 caps q4-6h prn. **Max:** 8 caps q24h.
Tylenol Extra Strength geltabs *(McNeil Consumer)*	Acetaminophen 500mg	**Adults & Peds ≥12 yo:** 2 tabs q4-6h prn. **Max:** 8 tabs q24h.
Tylenol Extra Strength liquid *(McNeil Consumer)*	Acetaminophen 1000mg/30mL	**Adults & Peds ≥12 yo:** 2 tbl (30mL) q4-6h prn. **Max:** 8 tbl (120mL) q24h.
Tylenol Extra Strength tablets *(McNeil Consumer)*	Acetaminophen 500mg	**Adults & Peds ≥12 yo:** 2 tabs q4-6h prn. **Max:** 8 tabs q24h.
Tylenol Infants' suspension *(McNeil Consumer)*	Acetaminophen 80mg/0.8mL	**Peds: 2-3 yo (24-35 lbs):** 1.6 mL q4h prn. **Max:** 5 doses (8mL) q24h.
Tylenol Junior Meltaways tablets *(McNeil Consumer)*	Acetaminophen 160mg	**Peds: 6-8 yo (48-59 lbs):** 2 tabs. **9-10 yo (60-71 lbs):** 2.5 tabs. **11 yo (72-95 lbs):** 3 tabs. **12 yo (≥96 lbs):** 4 tabs. May repeat q4h. **Max:** 5 doses q24h.
Tylenol Regular Strength tablets *(McNeil Consumer)*	Acetaminophen 325mg	**Adults & Peds ≥12 yo:** 2 tabs q4-6h prn. **Max:** 12 tabs q24h. **Peds: 6-11 yo:** 1 tab q4-6h. **Max:** 5 tabs q24h.

NONSTEROIDAL ANTI-INFLAMMATORY DRUGS

Advil Children's Chewables tablets *(Wyeth Consumer Healthcare)*	Ibuprofen 50mg	**Peds: 2-3 yr (24-35 lb):** 2 tabs q6-8h. **4-5 yr (36-47 lb):** 3 tabs q6-8h. **6-8 yr (45-89 lb):** 4 tabs q6-8h. **9-10 yr (60-71 lb):** 5 tabs q6-8h. **11 yr (72-95 lb):** 6 tabs q6-8h. **Max:** 4 doses q24h
Advil Children's suspension *(Wyeth Consumer Healthcare)*	Ibuprofen 100mg/5mL	**Peds: 2-3 yo (24-35 lbs):** 1 tsp (5mL). **4-5 yo (36-47 lbs):** 1.5 tsp (7.5mL). **6-8 yo (48-59 lbs):** 2 tsp (10mL). **9-10 yo (60-71 lbs):** 2.5 tsp (12.5mL). **11 yo (72-95 lbs):** 3 tsp (15mL). May repeat q6-8h. **Max:** 4 doses q24h.
Advil gelcaps *(Wyeth Consumer Healthcare)*	Ibuprofen 200mg	**Adults & Peds ≥12 yo:** 1-2 caps q4-6h. **Max:** 6 caps q24h.
Advil Infants' Drops *(Wyeth Consumer Healthcare)*	Ibuprofen 50mg/1.25mL	**Peds: 6-11 months (12-17 lbs):** 1.25mL. **12-23 months (18-23 lbs):** 1.875mL. May repeat q6-8h. **Max:** 4 doses q24h.
Advil Junior Strength tablets *(Wyeth Consumer Healthcare)*	Ibuprofen 100mg	**Peds: 6-10 yo (48-71 lbs):** 2 tabs. **11 yo (72-95 lbs):** 3 tabs. May repeat q6-8h. **Max:** 4 doses q24h.
Advil liqui-gels *(Wyeth Consumer Healthcare)*	Ibuprofen 200mg	**Adults & Peds ≥12 yo:** 1-2 caps q4-6h. **Max:** 6 caps q24h.

DOSING INFORMATION FOR ANTIPYRETIC PRODUCTS (cont.)

BRAND NAME	GENERIC INGREDIENT/STRENGTH	DOSE
Advil tablets *(Wyeth Consumer Healthcare)*	Ibuprofen 200mg	**Adults & Peds ≥12 yo:** 1-2 tabs q4-6h. **Max:** 6 tabs q24h.
Aleve caplets *(Bayer Healthcare)*	Naproxen Sodium 220mg	**Adults ≥65 yo:** 1 tab q12h. **Max:** 2 tabs q24h. **Adults & Peds ≥12 yo:** 1 tab q8-12h. **Max:** 3 tabs q24h.
Aleve gelcaps *(Bayer Healthcare)*	Naproxen Sodium 220mg	**Adults ≥65 yo:** 1 cap q12h. **Max:** 2 caps q24h. **Adults & Peds ≥12 yo:** 1 cap q8-12h. **Max:** 3 caps q24h.
Aleve tablets *(Bayer Healthcare)*	Naproxen Sodium 220mg	**Adults ≥65 yo:** 1 tab q12h. **Max:** 2 tabs q24h. **Adults & Peds ≥12 yo:** 1 tab q8-12h. **Max:** 3 tabs q24h.
Motrin Children's suspension *(McNeil Consumer)*	Ibuprofen 100mg/5mL	**Peds: 2-3 yo (24-35 lbs):** 1 tsp (5mL). **4-5 yo (36-47 lbs):** 1.5 tsp (7.5mL). **6-8 yo (48-59 lbs):** 2 tsp (10mL). **9-10 yo (60-71 lbs):** 2.5 tsp (12.5mL). **11 yo (72-95 lbs):** 3 tsp (15mL). May repeat q6-8h. **Max:** 4 doses q24h.
Motrin IB caplets *(McNeil Consumer)*	Ibuprofen 200mg	**Adults & Peds ≥12 yo:** 1-2 tabs q4-6h. **Max:** 6 tabs q24h.
Motrin IB gelcaps *(McNeil Consumer)*	Ibuprofen 200mg	**Adults & Peds ≥12 yo:** 1-2 tabs q4-6h. **Max:** 6 tabs q24h.
Motrin IB tablets *(McNeil Consumer)*	Ibuprofen 200mg	**Adults & Peds ≥12 yo:** 1-2 tabs q4-6h. **Max:** 6 tabs q24h.
Motrin Infants' Drops *(McNeil Consumer)*	Ibuprofen 50mg/1.25mL	**Peds: 6-11 months (12-17 lbs):** 1.25mL. **12-23 months (18-23 lbs):** 1.875mL. May repeat q6-8h. **Max:** 4 doses q24h.
Motrin Junior Strength chewable tablets *(McNeil Consumer)*	Ibuprofen 100mg	**Peds: 6-8 yo (48-59 lbs):** 2 tabs. **9-10 yo (60-71 lbs):** 2.5 tabs. **11 yo (72-95 lbs):** 3 tabs. May repeat q6-8h. **Max:** 4 doses q24h.
Nuprin caplets *(Bristol-Myers Squibb)*	Ibuprofen 200mg	**Adults & Peds ≥12 yo:** 1-2 tabs q4-6h. **Max:** 6 tabs q24h.
Nuprin tablets *(Bristol-Myers Squibb)*	Ibuprofen 200mg	**Adults & Peds ≥12 yo:** 1-2 tabs q4-6h. **Max:** 6 tabs q24h.

SALICYLATES

BRAND NAME	GENERIC INGREDIENT/STRENGTH	DOSE
Anacin 81 tablets *(Insight Pharmaceuticals)*	Aspirin 81mg	**Adults & Peds ≥12 yo:** 4-8 tabs q4h. **Max:** 48 tabs q24h.
Aspergum chewable tablets *(Schering-Plough)*	Aspirin 227mg	**Adults & Peds ≥12 yo:** 2 tabs q4h. **Max:** 16 tabs q24h.
Bayer Aspirin Extra Strength caplets *(Bayer Healthcare)*	Aspirin 500mg	**Adults & Peds ≥12 yo:** 1-2 tabs q4-6h. **Max:** 8 tabs q24h.
Bayer Aspirin safety coated caplets *(Bayer Healthcare)*	Aspirin 325mg	**Adults & Peds ≥12 yo:** 1-2 tabs q4h or 3 tabs q6h. **Max:** 12 tabs q24h.
Bayer Children's Aspirin chewable tablets *(Bayer Healthcare)*	Aspirin 81mg	**Adults & Peds ≥12 yo:** 4-8 tabs q4h. **Max:** 48 tabs q24h.
Bayer Low Dose Aspirin tablets *(Bayer Healthcare)*	Aspirin 81mg	**Adults & Peds ≥12 yo:** 4-8 tabs q4h. **Max:** 48 tabs q24h.
Bayer Original Aspirin tablets *(Bayer Healthcare)*	Aspirin 325mg	**Adults & Peds ≥12 yo:** 1-2 tabs q4h or 3 tabs q6h. **Max:** 12 tabs q24h.
Ecotrin Adult Low Strength tablets *(GlaxoSmithKline Consumer Healthcare)*	Aspirin 81mg	**Adults:** 4-8 tabs q4h. **Max:** 48 tabs q24h.
Ecotrin Enteric Low Strength tablets *(GlaxoSmithKline Consumer Healthcare)*	Aspirin 81mg	**Adults:** 4-8 tabs q4h. **Max:** 48 tabs q24h.
Ecotrin Enteric Regular Strength tablets *(GlaxoSmithKline Consumer Healthcare)*	Aspirin 325mg	**Adults & Peds ≥12 yo:** 1-2 tabs q4h. **Max:** 12 tabs q24h.
Ecotrin Maximum Strength tablets *(GlaxoSmithKline Consumer Healthcare)*	Aspirin 500mg	**Adults & Peds ≥12 yo:** 2 tabs q6h. **Max:** 8 tabs q24h.
Ecotrin Regular Strength tablets *(GlaxoSmithKline Consumer Healthcare)*	Aspirin 325mg	**Adults & Peds ≥12 yo:** 1-2 tabs q4h. **Max:** 12 tabs q24h.

DOSING INFORMATION FOR ANTIPYRETIC PRODUCTS (cont.)

BRAND NAME	GENERIC INGREDIENT/STRENGTH	DOSE
Halfprin 162mg tablets *(Kramer Laboratories)*	Aspirin 162mg	**Adults & Peds ≥12 yo:** 2-4 tabs q4h. **Max:** 24 tabs q24h.
Halfprin 81mg tablets *(Kramer Laboratories)*	Aspirin 81mg	**Adults & Peds ≥12 yo:** 4-8 tabs q4h. **Max:** 48 tabs q24h.
St. Joseph Adult Low Strength chewable tablets *(McNeil Consumer)*	Aspirin 81mg	**Adults & Peds ≥12 yo:** 4-8 tabs q4h. **Max:** 48 tabs q24h.
St. Joseph Adult Low Strength tablets *(McNeil Consumer)*	Aspirin 81mg	**Adults & Peds ≥12 yo:** 4-8 tabs q4h. **Max:** 48 tabs q24h.
SALICYLATES, BUFFERED		
Ascriptin Maximum Strength tablets *(Novartis Consumer Health)*	Aspirin Buffered with Maalox/Calcium Carbonate 500mg	**Adults & Peds ≥12 yo:** 2 tabs q4h. **Max:** 8 tabs q24h.
Ascriptin Regular Strength tablets *(Novartis Consumer Health)*	Aspirin Buffered with Maalox/Calcium Carbonate 325mg	**Adults & Peds ≥12 yo:** 2 tabs q4h. **Max:** 12 tabs q24h.
Bayer Extra Strength Plus caplets *(Bayer Healthcare)*	Aspirin Buffered with Calcium Carbonate 500mg	**Adults & Peds ≥12 yo:** 1-2 tabs q4-6h. **Max**: 8 tabs q24h.
Bufferin Extra Strength tablets *(Bristol-Myers Squibb)*	Aspirin Bufferred with Calcium Carbonate/Magnesium Oxide/Magnesium Carbonate 500mg	**Adults & Peds ≥12 yo:** 2 tabs q6h. **Max:** 8 tabs q24h.
Bufferin tablets *(Bristol-Myers Squibb)*	Aspirin Bufferred with Calcium Carbonate/Magnesium Oxide/Magnesium Carbonate 325mg	**Adults & Peds ≥12 yo:** 2 tabs q4h. **Max:** 12 tabs q24h.

Headache/Migraine

A headache is a diffuse pain or discomfort in the head, scalp, or neck. Headaches vary in intensity from mild to moderate to severe. These levels of intensity are rated according to the extent to which the headache interferes with the ability to function. Mild headaches do not interfere with the ability to function; moderate headaches do interfere but do not require bed rest; severe headaches are incapacitating and require bed rest. Headache presents as an acute, subacute, or chronic condition, depending on the length of time it has been present, either intermittently or continuously. The physiologic basis of headache lies in the interaction between the muscular and vascular mechanisms of headache. The most frequent type of headache is the *tension-type* headache. Tension headaches are due to tight, contracted muscles in the shoulders, neck, scalp, and jaw. Tension headaches are often caused by fatigue, lack of sleep, and failure to eat on time. Tension headaches occur most often in the late afternoon.

Migraine is a condition of recurring headaches of moderate to severe intensity that last from 1 to 3 days and tend to be limited to one side of the head. Migraines are often located in the temple or in the back of the head and are typically described as throbbing pain. Pain is also sometimes located in the eye and tends to be sharp and steady. Migraines are usually associated with photophobia and phonophobia, often with nausea, and sometimes also with vomiting. Migraine can also occur with aura; aura symptoms are either visual or somatosensory in nature. The visual disturbances typical of migraine, known as scintillating scotoma, usually start near the center of vision as a small spot surrounded by bright, zigzag lines. *Cluster headache* is a chronic headache condition related to migraine but much less common. The pain of a cluster headache is unilateral and severe—often agonizing—and lasts for one half to 2 hours. The headaches occur once or twice per day and tend to occur at night, waking the patient from sleep 1 to 2 hours after retiring. Several OTC medications are available to treat symptoms of headache, including acetaminophen, aspirin and other salicylates, NSAIDs, and caffeine.

ACETAMINOPHEN

Analgesic—The mechanism of analgesic action has not been fully determined. Acetaminophen may act predominantly by inhibiting prostaglandin synthesis in the central nervous system and, to a lesser extent, through a peripheral action by blocking pain-impulse generation. The peripheral action may also be due to inhibition of prostaglandin synthesis or to inhibition of the synthesis or actions of other substances that sensitize pain receptors to mechanical or chemical stimulation.

Capsule/Granules/Powder/Solution/Suspension/Tablet

For analgesic use:

Adults/Pediatrics ≥13 years of age: 325 to 500mg every 3 hours; 325 to 650mg every 4 hours; 650 to 1000mg every 6 hours; or 1300mg every 8 hours.

Pediatrics ≤3 months of age: 40mg every 4 hours as needed.

Pediatrics 4 to 12 months of age: 80mg every 4 hours as needed.

Pediatrics 1 to 2 years of age: 120mg every 4 hours as needed.

Pediatrics 2 to 4 years of age: 160mg every 4 hours as needed.

Pediatrics 4 to 6 years of age: 240mg every 4 hours as needed.

Pediatrics 6 to 9 years of age: 320mg every 4 hours as needed.

Pediatrics 9 to 11 years of age: 320 to 400mg every 4 hours as needed.

Pediatrics 11 to 12 years of age: 320 to 480mg every 4 hours as needed.

Suppositories

For analgesic use:

Adults/Pediatrics ≥13 years of age: 325 to 650mg every 4 hours or 650mg every 6 hours as needed.

Pediatrics 2 to 4 years of age: 160mg every 4 hours as needed.

Pediatrics 4 to 6 years of age: 240mg every 4 hours as needed.

Pediatrics 6 to 9 years of age: 320mg every 4 hours as needed.

Pediatrics 9 to 11 years of age: 320 to 400mg every 4 hours as needed.

Pediatrics 11 to 12 years of age: 320 to 480mg every 4 hours as needed.

For more information, refer to the complete monograph for acetaminophen in "Aches and Pains" under Musculoskeletal System.

ACETAMINOPHEN PRODUCTS	
Brand Name	**Dosage Form**
Anacin Aspirin Free (Insight)	**Tablet:** 500mg
Feverall (Alpharma)	**Suppositories:** 80mg, 120mg, 325mg, 650mg
Tylenol 8 Hour (McNeil)	**Tablet:** 650mg
Tylenol Arthritis (McNeil)	**Tablet:** 650mg
Tylenol Children's Meltaways (McNeil)	**Tablet:** 80mg
Tylenol Children's (McNeil)	**Suspension:** 160mg/5mL
Tylenol Extra Strength (McNeil)	**Capsule:** 500mg **Liquid:** 1000mg/30mL **Tablet:** 500mg
Tylenol Infants' (McNeil)	**Suspension:** 80mg/0.8mL
Tylenol Junior Meltaways (McNeil)	**Tablet:** 160mg
Tylenol Regular Strength (McNeil)	**Tablet:** 325mg

ASPIRIN

Analgesic—Salicylates produce analgesia through a peripheral action by blocking pain-impulse generation and via a central action, possibly in the hypothalamus. The peripheral action may predominate and probably involves inhibition of the synthesis of prostaglandins, and possibly inhibition of the synthesis and/or actions of other substances, which sensitize pain receptors to mechanical or chemical stimulation.

Suppositories

For analgesic use:

Adults/Pediatrics ≥12 years of age: 325 to 650mg every 4 hours as needed.

Pediatrics 2 to 4 years of age: 160mg every 4 hours as needed.

Pediatrics 4 to 6 years of age: 240mg every 4 hours as needed.

Pediatrics 6 to 9 years of age: 325mg every 4 hours as needed.

Pediatrics 9 to 11 years of age: 325 to 400mg every 4 hours as needed.

Pediatric 11 to 12 years of age: 325 to 480mg every 4 hours as needed.

Tablet

For analgesic use:

Adults/Pediatrics ≥12 years of age: 325 to 500mg every 3 hours; 325 to 650mg every 4 hours; or 650 to 1000mg every 6 hours as needed.

Pediatrics 2 to 4 years of age: 160mg every 4 hours as needed.

Pediatrics 4 to 6 years of age: 240mg every 4 hours as needed.

Pediatrics 6 to 9 years of age: 320 to 325mg every 4 hours as needed.

Pediatrics 9 to 11 years of age: 320 to 400mg every 4 hours as needed.

Pediatric 11 to 12 years of age: 320 to 480mg every 4 hours as needed.

For more information, refer to the complete monograph for salicylates in "Aches and Pains" under Musculoskeletal System.

CAFFEINE

Analgesia adjunct—Caffeine constricts cerebral vasculature, resulting in decreased cerebral blood flow as well as a decrease in the oxygen tension of the brain. It has been suggested that the addition of caffeine to aspirin or aspirin/acetaminophen combinations may help to relieve headache by providing a more rapid onset of action and/or enhanced pain relief with a lower dose of the analgesic. In some patients, caffeine may reduce headache pain by reversing caffeine withdrawal symptoms. Recent studies with ergotamine indicate that the enhanced effect by the addition of caffeine may be due to improved gastrointestinal absorption of ergotamine when administered with caffeine.

For more information, refer to the complete monograph for caffeine in "Drowsiness/Lethargy" under Central Nervous System.

ASPIRIN PRODUCTS	
Brand Name	**Dosage Form**
Aspirin (Novartis)	**Tablet:** 81mg
Aspergum (Schering)	**Gum:** 227mg
Bayer Aspirin Regimen (Bayer)	**Tablet:** 81mg, 325mg
Bayer Children's Aspirin (Bayer)	**Tablet:** 81mg
Bayer Extra Strength (Bayer)	**Tablet:** 500mg
Bayer Genuine Aspirin (Bayer)	**Tablet:** 325mg
Ecotrin (GSK)	**Tablet:** 325mg
Ecotrin Adult Low Strength (GSK)	**Tablet:** 81mg
Ecotrin Maximum Strength (GSK)	**Tablet:** 500mg
Halfprin (Kramer)	**Tablet:** 81mg, 162mg
St. Joseph (McNeil)	**Tablet:** 81mg
BUFFERED ASPIRIN PRODUCTS	
Brand Name	**Dosage Form**
Alka-Seltzer (Bayer)	**Tablet:** 325mg
Alka-Seltzer Extra Strength (Bayer)	**Tablet:** 500mg
Ascriptin (Novartis)	**Tablet:** 325mg
Ascriptin Arthritis Pain (Novartis)	**Tablet:** 325mg
Ascriptin Maximum Strength (Novartis)	**Tablet:** 500mg
Bayer Plus Extra Strength (Bayer)	**Tablet:** 500mg
Bufferin (BMS)	**Tablet:** 325mg
Bufferin Extra Strength (BMS)	**Tablet:** 500mg

IBUPROFEN

Analgesic—Ibuprofen may block pain-impulse generation via a peripheral action that may involve reduction of the activity of prostaglandins, and possibly inhibition of the synthesis or actions of other substances that sensitize pain receptors to mechanical or chemical stimulation. The antibradykinin activity of ibuprofen may also be involved in relief of pain, since bradykinin has been shown to act together with prostaglandins to cause pain.

Capsule/Suspension/Tablet

For analgesic use (mild to moderate pain):

Adults: 200 to 400mg every 4 to 6 hours as needed.

For more information, refer to the complete monograph for NSAIDs in "Aches and Pains" under Musculoskeletal System.

MAGNESIUM SALICYLATE

Analgesic—Salicylates produce analgesia through a peripheral action by blocking pain-impulse generation and via a central action, possibly in the hypothalamus. The peripheral action may predominate and probably involves inhibition of the synthesis of prostaglandins, and possibly inhibition of the synthesis and/or actions of other substances, which sensitize pain receptors to mechanical or chemical stimulation.

Tablets

For analgesic use:

Adults: 607.4mg every 4 hours as needed; or 934mg every 6 hours as needed.

For more information, refer to the complete monograph for salicylates in "Aches and Pains" under Musculoskeletal System.

ACETAMINOPHEN/CAFFEINE PRODUCTS	
Brand Name	**Dosage Form**
Excedrin Tension Headache (BMS)	Tablet: 500mg-65mg

ACETAMINOPHEN/ASPIRIN/CAFFEINE PRODUCTS	
Brand Name	**Dosage Form**
Excedrin Extra Strength (BMS)	Tablet: 250mg-250mg-65mg
Excedrin Migraine (BMS)	Tablet: 250mg-250mg-65mg
Goody's Fast Pain Relief (GSK)	Tablet: 130mg-260mg-16.25mg
Goody's Headache Powders (GSK)	Tablet: 260mg-520mg-32.5mg

ASPIRIN/CAFFEINE PRODUCTS	
Brand Name	**Dosage Form**
Alka-Seltzer Morning Relief (Bayer)	Tablet: 500mg-65mg
Anacin (Wyeth)	Tablet: 400mg-32mg
Anacin Maximum Strength (Wyeth)	Tablet: 500mg-32mg
Bayer Rapid Headache Relief (Bayer)	Tablet: 500mg-65mg

ASPIRIN/CAFFEINE/SALICYLAMIDE PRODUCTS	
Brand Name	**Dosage Form**
BC Powder Original (GSK)	Tablet: 650mg-33.3mg-195mg
BC Powder Arthritis Strength (GSK)	Tablet: 742mg-38mg-222mg

IBUPROFEN PRODUCTS	
Brand Name	**Dosage Form**
Advil (Wyeth)	Capsule: 200mg **Tablet:** 200mg
Advil Children's (Wyeth)	Tablet: 50mg
Advil Junior (Wyeth)	Tablet: 100mg
Midol Cramp Formula (Bayer)	Tablet: 200mg
Motrin IB (McNeil)	Tablet: 200mg
Motrin Children's (McNeil)	Suspension: 100mg/5mL
Motrin Infants' (McNeil)	Suspension: 50mg/1.25mL
Motrin Junior (McNeil)	Tablet: 100mg
Motrin Migraine Pain (McNeil)	Tablet: 200mg

MAGNESIUM SALICYLATE PRODUCTS	
Brand Name	**Dosage Form**
Doan's Extra Strength (Novartis)	Tablet: 500mg
Doan's Regular Strength (Novartis)	Tablet: 325mg
Momentum (Medtech)	Tablet: 467mg

NAPROXEN

Analgesic—Naproxen may block pain-impulse generation via a peripheral action that may involve reduction of the activity of prostaglandins, and possibly inhibition of the synthesis or actions of other substances that sensitize pain receptors to mechanical or chemical stimulation. The antibradykinin activity of naproxen may also be involved in relief of pain, since bradykinin has been shown to act together with prostaglandins to cause pain.

CAPSULE/TABLET

For analgesic use (mild to moderate pain):

Adults: 500mg initially, then 250mg every 6 to 8 hours as needed.

For more information, refer to the complete monograph for NSAIDs in "Aches and Pains" under Musculoskeletal System.

PHENYLEPHRINE

Sympathomimetic amines act on alpha-adrenergic receptors in the mucosa of the respiratory tract to produce vasoconstriction, which temporarily reduces the swelling associated with inflammation of the mucous membranes lining the nasal passages. Decongestant and analgesic combinations are indicated for the temporary relief of nasal and sinus congestion and headache pain caused by sinusitis, common colds, allergy, and hay fever.

PSEUDOEPHEDRINE

Pseudoephedrine acts on alpha-adrenergic receptors in the mucosa of the respiratory tract, producing vasoconstriction. The medication shrinks swollen nasal mucous membranes; reduces tissue hyperemia, edema, and nasal congestion; and increases nasal airway patency. Also, drainage of sinus secretions may be increased and obstructed eustachian ostia may be opened. Decongestant and analgesic combinations are indicated for the temporary relief of nasal and sinus congestion and headache pain caused by sinusitis, common colds, allergy, and hay fever.

For more information, refer to the complete monograph for pseudoephedrine in "Nasal Congestion" under Respiratory System.

NAPROXEN PRODUCTS	
Brand Name	Dosage Form
Aleve (Bayer)	**Capsule:** 220mg **Tablet:** 220mg
Aleve Arthritis (Bayer)	**Tablet:** 220mg
Midol Extended Relief (Bayer)	**Tablet:** 220mg

ACETAMINOPHEN/PHENYLEPHRINE PRODUCTS	
Brand Name	Dosage Form
Excedrin Sinus Headache (BMS)	**Tablet:** 325mg-5mg
ACETAMINOPHEN/PSEUDOEPHEDRINE PRODUCTS	
Brand Name	Dosage Form
Sinutab Sinus (Pfizer)	**Tablet:** 500mg-30mg
Sudafed Sinus Headache (Pfizer)	**Tablet:** 500mg-30mg
NAPROXEN/PSEUDOEPHEDRINE PRODUCTS	
Brand Name	Dosage Form
Aleve Sinus & Headache (BMS)	**Tablet:** 220mg-120mg

DOSING INFORMATION FOR HEADACHE/MIGRAINE PRODUCTS

The following table provides a quick comparison of the ingredients and dosages of common brand-name OTC drugs. Products are listed alphabetically by drug category and brand name.

Brand Name	Ingredient/Strength	Dose
ACETAMINOPHEN		
Anacin Aspirin Free tablets (*Insight Pharmaceuticals*)	Acetaminophen 500mg	**Adults & Peds ≥12 yo:** 2 tabs q6h. **Max:** 8 tabs q24h.
Tylenol 8 Hour caplets (*McNeil Consumer*)	Acetaminophen 650mg	**Adults & Peds ≥12 yo:** 2 tabs q8h prn. **Max:** 6 tabs q24h.
Tylenol 8 Hour geltabs (*McNeil Consumer*)	Acetaminophen 650mg	**Adults & Peds ≥12 yo:** 2 tabs q8h prn. **Max:** 6 tabs q24h.
Tylenol Arthritis caplets (*McNeil Consumer*)	Acetaminophen 650mg	**Adults:** 2 tabs q8h prn. **Max:** 6 tabs q24h.
Tylenol Arthritis geltabs (*McNeil Consumer*)	Acetaminophen 650mg	**Adults:** 2 tabs q8h prn. **Max:** 6 tabs q24h.
Tylenol Children's Meltaways tablets (*McNeil Consumer*)	Acetaminophen 80mg	**Peds: 2-3 yo (24-35 lbs):** 2 tabs. **4-5 yo (36-47 lbs):** 3 tabs. **6-8 yo (48-59 lbs):** 4 tabs. **9-10 yo (60-71 lbs):** 5 tabs. **11 yo (72-95 lbs):** 6 tabs. May repeat q4h. **Max:** 5 doses q24h.
Tylenol Children's suspension (*McNeil Consumer*)	Acetaminophen 160mg/5mL	**Peds: 2-3 yo (24-35 lbs):** 1 tsp (5mL). **4-5 yo (36-47 lbs):** 1.5 tsp (7.5mL). **6-8 yo (48-59 lbs):** 2 tsp (10mL). **9-10 yo (60-71 lbs):** 2.5 tsp (12.5mL). **11 yo (72-95 lbs):** 3 tsp (15mL). May repeat q4h. **Max:** 5 doses q24h.
Tylenol Extra Strength caplets (*McNeil Consumer*)	Acetaminophen 500mg	**Adults & Peds ≥12 yo:** 2 tabs q4-6h prn. **Max:** 8 tabs q24h.
Tylenol Extra Strength Cool caplets (*McNeil Consumer*)	Acetaminophen 500mg	**Adults & Peds ≥12 yo:** 2 tabs q4-6h prn. **Max:** 8 tabs q24h.
Tylenol Extra Strength gelcaps (*McNeil Consumer*)	Acetaminophen 500mg	**Adults & Peds ≥12 yo:** 2 caps q4-6h prn. **Max:** 8 caps q24h.
Tylenol Extra Strength liquid (*McNeil Consumer*)	Acetaminophen 1000mg/30mL	**Adults & Peds ≥12 yo:** 2 tbl (30mL) q4-6h prn. **Max:** 8 tbl (120mL) q24h.
Tylenol Extra Strength tablets (*McNeil Consumer*)	Acetaminophen 500mg	**Adults & Peds ≥12 yo:** 2 tabs q4-6h prn. **Max:** 8 tabs q24h.
Tylenol Infants' suspension (*McNeil Consumer*)	Acetaminophen 80mg/0.8mL	**Peds: 2-3 yo (24-35 lbs):** 1.6 mL q4h prn. **Max:** 5 doses (8mL) q24h.
Tylenol Junior Meltaways tablets (*McNeil Consumer*)	Acetaminophen 160mg	**Peds: 6-8 yo (48-59 lbs):** 2 tabs. **9-10 yo (60-71 lbs):** 2.5 tabs. **11 yo (72-95 lbs):** 3 tabs. **12 yo (≥96 lbs):** 4 tabs. May repeat q4h. **Max:** 5 doses q24h.
Tylenol Regular Strength tablets (*McNeil Consumer*)	Acetaminophen 325mg	**Adults & Peds ≥12 yo:** 2 tabs q4-6h prn. **Max:** 12 tabs q24h. **Peds: 6-11 yo:** 1 tab q4-6h. **Max:** 5 tabs q24h.
ACETAMINOPHEN COMBINATION		
Excedrin Extra Strength caplets (*Bristol-Myers Squibb*)	Acetaminophen/Aspirin/Caffeine 250mg-250mg-65mg	**Adults & Peds ≥12 yo:** 2 tabs q6h. **Max:** 8 tabs q24h.
Excedrin Extra Strength geltabs (*Bristol-Myers Squibb*)	Acetaminophen/Aspirin/Caffeine 250mg-250mg-65mg	**Adults & Peds ≥12 yo:** 2 tabs q6h. **Max:** 8 tabs q24h.
Excedrin Extra Strength tablets (*Bristol-Myers Squibb*)	Acetaminophen/Aspirin/Caffeine 250mg-250mg-65mg	**Adults & Peds ≥12 yo:** 2 tabs q6h. **Max:** 8 tabs q24h.
Excedrin Migraine caplets (*Bristol-Myers Squibb*)	Acetaminophen/Aspirin/Caffeine 250mg-250mg-65mg	**Adults:** 2 tabs prn. **Max:** 2 tabs q24h.
Excedrin Migraine geltabs (*Bristol-Myers Squibb*)	Acetaminophen/Aspirin/Caffeine 250mg-250mg-65mg	**Adults:** 2 tabs prn. **Max:** 2 tabs q24h.
Excedrin Migraine tablets (*Bristol-Myers Squibb*)	Acetaminophen/Aspirin/Caffeine 250mg-250mg-65mg	**Adults:** 2 tabs prn. **Max:** 2 tabs q24h.
Excedrin Quicktabs tablets (*Bristol-Myers Squibb*)	Acetaminophen/Caffeine 500mg-65mg	**Adults & Peds ≥12 yo:** 2 tabs q6h. **Max:** 8 tabs q24h.
Excedrin Sinus Headache caplets (*Bristol-Myers Squibb*)	Acetaminophen/Phenylephrine HCl 325mg-5mg	**Adults & Peds ≥12 yo:** 2 tabs q4h. **Max:** 12 tabs q24h.

DOSING INFORMATION FOR HEADACHE/MIGRAINE PRODUCTS (cont.)

BRAND NAME	INGREDIENT/STRENGTH	DOSE
Excedrin Sinus Headache tablets (Bristol-Myers Squibb)	Acetaminophen/Phenylephrine HCl 325mg-5mg	**Adults & Peds ≥12 yo:** 2 tabs q4h. **Max:** 12 tabs q24h.
Excedrin Tension Headache caplets (Bristol-Myers Squibb)	Acetaminophen/Caffeine 500mg-65mg	**Adults & Peds ≥12 yo:** 2 tabs q6h. **Max:** 8 tabs q24h.
Excedrin Tension Headache geltabs (Bristol-Myers Squibb)	Acetaminophen/Caffeine 500mg-65mg	**Adults & Peds ≥12 yo:** 2 tabs q6h. **Max:** 8 tabs q24h.
Excedrin Tension Headache tablets (Bristol-Myers Squibb)	Acetaminophen/Caffeine 500mg-65mg	**Adults & Peds ≥12 yo:** 2 tabs q6h. **Max:** 8 tabs q24h.
Goody's Headache Powders (GlaxoSmithKline Consumer Healthcare)	Acetaminophen/Aspirin/Caffeine 260mg-520mg-32.5mg	**Adults & Peds ≥12 yo:** 1 powder q4-6h. **Max:** 4 powders q24h.
Tylenol Sinus Maximum Strength gelcaps (McNeil Consumer)	Acetaminophen/Pseudoephedrine HCl 500mg-30mg	**Adults & Peds ≥12 yo:** 2 caps q4-6h. **Max:** 8 caps q24h.
Tylenol Sinus Maximum Strength, caplets (McNeil Consumer)	Acetaminophen/Pseudoephedrine HCl 500mg-30mg	**Adults & Peds ≥12 yo:** 2 caps q4-6h. **Max:** 8 caps q24h.
Vanquish caplets (Bayer Healthcare)	Acetaminophen/Aspirin/Caffeine 194mg-227mg-33mg	**Adults & Peds ≥12 yo:** 2 tabs q6h. **Max:** 8 tabs q24h.
ACETAMINOPHEN/SLEEP AID		
Excedrin PM caplets (Bristol-Myers Squibb)	Acetaminophen/Diphenhydramine 500mg-38mg	**Adults & Peds ≥12 yo:** 2 tabs qhs.
Excedrin PM geltab (Bristol-Myers Squibb)	Acetaminophen/Diphenhydramine citrate 500mg-38 mg	**Adults & Peds ≥12 yo:** 2 tabs qhs.
Excedrin PM tablet (Bristol-Myers Squibb)	Acetaminophen/Diphenhydramine citrate 500mg-38 mg	**Adults & Peds ≥12 yo:** 2 tabs qhs.
Goody's PM Powders (GlaxoSmithKline Consumer Healthcare)	Acetaminophen/Diphenhydramine 1000mg-76mg/dose	**Adults & Peds ≥12 yo:** 1 packet (2 powders) qhs.
Tylenol PM caplets (McNeil Consumer)	Acetaminophen/Diphenhydramine 500mg-25mg	**Adults & Peds ≥12 yo:** 2 tabs qhs.
Tylenol PM gelcaps (McNeil Consumer)	Acetaminophen/Diphenhydramine 500mg-25mg	**Adults & Peds ≥12 yo:** 2 caps qhs.
Tylenol PM geltabs (McNeil Consumer)	Acetaminophen/Diphenhydramine 500mg-25mg	**Adults & Peds ≥12 yo:** 2 tabs qhs.
Tylenol Sinus Night Time caplets (McNeil Consumer)	Acetaminophen/Pseudoephedrine HCl/Doxylamine Succinate 500mg-30mg-6.25mg	**Adults & Peds ≥12 yo:** 2 tabs q4-6h. **Max:** 8 tabs q24h.
NONSTEROIDAL ANTI-INFLAMMATORY DRUGs (NSAIDs)		
Advil caplets (Wyeth Consumer Healtcare)	Ibuprofen 200mg	**Adults & Peds ≥12 yo:** 1-2 tabs q4-6h. **Max:** 6 tabs q24h.
Advil Children's Chewables tablets (Wyeth Consumer Healthcare)	Ibuprofen 50mg	**Peds: 2-3 yr (24-35 lb):** 2 tabs q6-8h. **4-5 (36-47 lb):** 3 tabs q6-8h. **6-8 yr (45-89 lb):** 4 tabs q6-8h. **9-10 yr (60-71 lb):** 5 tabs q6-8h. **11 yr (72-95 lb):** 6 tabs q6-8h. **Max:** 4 doses q24h
Advil Children's suspension (Wyeth Consumer Healthcare)	Ibuprofen 100mg/5mL	**Peds: 2-3 yo (24-35 lbs):** 1 tsp (5mL). **4-5 yo (36-47 lbs):** 1.5 tsp (7.5mL). **6-8 yo (48-59 lbs):** 2 tsp (10mL). **9-10 yo (60-71 lbs):** 2.5 tsp (12.5mL). **11 yo (72-95 lbs):** 3 tsp (15mL). May repeat q6-8h. **Max:** 4 doses q24h.
Advil gelcaps (Wyeth Consumer Healthcare)	Ibuprofen 200mg	**Adults & Peds ≥12 yo:** 1-2 caps q4-6h. **Max:** 6 caps q24h.
Advil Infants' Drops (Wyeth Consumer Healthcare)	Ibuprofen 50mg/1.25mL	**Peds: 6-11 months (12-17 lbs):** 1.25mL. **12-23 months (18-23 lbs):** 1.875mL. May repeat q6-8h. **Max:** 4 doses q24h.
Advil Junior Strength tablets (Wyeth Consumer Healthcare)	Ibuprofen 100mg	**Peds: 6-10 yo (48-71 lbs):** 2 tabs. **11 yo (72-95 lbs):** 3 tabs. May repeat q6-8h. **Max:** 4 doses q24h.
Advil Junior Strength tablets (Wyeth Consumer Healthcare)	Ibuprofen 100mg	**Peds: 6-10 yo (48-71 lbs):** 2 tabs. **11 yo (72-95 lbs):** 3 tabs. May repeat q6-8h. **Max:** 4 doses q24h.

DOSING INFORMATION FOR HEADACHE/MIGRAINE PRODUCTS (cont.)

BRAND NAME	INGREDIENT/STRENGTH	DOSE
Advil liqui-gels *(Wyeth Consumer Healthcare)*	Ibuprofen 200mg	**Adults & Peds ≥12 yo:** 1-2 caps q4-6h. **Max:** 6 caps q24h.
Advil Migraine capsules *(Wyeth Consumer Healthcare)*	Ibuprofen 200mg	**Adults:** 2 caps prn. **Max:** 2 caps q24h.
Advil tablets *(Wyeth Consumer Healthcare)*	Ibuprofen 200mg	**Adults & Peds ≥12 yo:** 1-2 tabs q4-6h. **Max:** 6 tabs q24h.
Aleve caplets *(Bayer Healthcare)*	Naproxen Sodium 220mg	**Adults ≥65 yo:** 1 tab q12h. **Max:** 2 tabs q24h. **Adults & Peds ≥12 yo:** 1 tab q8-12h. **Max:** 3 tabs q24h.
Aleve gelcaps *(Bayer Healthcare)*	Naproxen Sodium 220mg	**Adults ≥65 yo:** 1 cap q12h. **Max:** 2 caps q24h. **Adults & Peds ≥12 yo:** 1 cap q8-12h. **Max:** 3 caps q24h.
Aleve tablets *(Bayer Healthcare)*	Naproxen Sodium 220mg	**Adults ≥65 yo:** 1 tab q12h. **Max:** 2 tabs q24h. **Adults & Peds ≥12 yo:** 1 tab q8-12h. **Max:** 3 tabs q24h.
Motrin Children's suspension *(McNeil Consumer)*	Ibuprofen 100mg/5mL	**Peds: 2-3 yo (24-35 lbs):** 1 tsp (5mL). **4-5 yo (36-47 lbs):** 1.5 tsp (7.5mL). **6-8 yo (48-59 lbs):** 2 tsp (10mL). **9-10 yo (60-71 lbs):** 2.5 tsp (12.5mL). **11 yo (72-95 lbs):** 3 tsp (15mL). May repeat q6-8h. **Max:** 4 doses q24h.
Motrin IB caplets *(McNeil Consumer)*	Ibuprofen 200mg	**Adults & Peds ≥12 yo:** 1-2 tabs q4-6h. **Max:** 6 tabs q24h.
Motrin IB gelcaps *(McNeil Consumer)*	Ibuprofen 200mg	**Adults & Peds ≥12 yo:** 1-2 tabs q4-6h. **Max:** 6 tabs q24h.
Motrin IB tablets *(McNeil Consumer)*	Ibuprofen 200mg	**Adults & Peds ≥12 yo:** 1-2 tabs q4-6h. **Max:** 6 tabs q24h.
Motrin Infants' Drops *(McNeil Consumer)*	Ibuprofen 50mg/1.25mL	**Peds: 6-11 months (12-17 lbs):** 1.25mL. **12-23 months (18-23 lbs):** 1.875mL. May repeat q6-8h. **Max:** 4 doses q24h.
Motrin Junior Strength chewable tablets *(McNeil Consumer)*	Ibuprofen 100mg	**Peds: 6-8 yo (48-59 lbs):** 2 tabs. **9-10 yo (60-71 lbs):** 2.5 tabs. **11 yo (72-95 lbs):** 3 tabs. May repeat q6-8h. **Max:** 4 doses q24h.
Nuprin caplets *(Bristol-Myers Squibb)*	Ibuprofen 200mg	**Adults & Peds ≥12 yo:** 1-2 tabs q4-6h. **Max:** 6 tabs q24h.
Nuprin tablets *(Bristol-Myers Squibb)*	Ibuprofen 200mg	**Adults & Peds ≥12 yo:** 1-2 tabs q4-6h. **Max:** 6 tabs q24h.
Orudis KT tablets *(Wyeth Consumer Healthcare)*	Ketoprofen Magnesium 12.5mg	**Adults:** 1-2 tabs q4-6h. **Max:** 6 tabs q24h.
NSAID COMBINATION		
Aleve Sinus & Headache Caplets *(Bayer Healthcare)*	Naproxen Sodium/Pseudoephedrine HCl 220 mg-120 mg	**Adults & Peds ≥12 yo:** 1 tabs q12h. **Max:** 2 tabs q24h.
Motrin Cold & Sinus Caplets *(McNeil Consumer)*	Ibuprofen/Pseudoephedrine HCl 200mg-30 mg	**Adults & Peds ≥12 yo:** 1-2 tabs q4-6h. **Max:** 6 tabs q24h.
Nuprin Cold and Sinus caplets *(Bristol-Myers Squibb)*	Ibuprofen /Pseudoephedrine HCl 200mg-30 mg	**Adults & Peds ≥12 yo:** 1-2 tabs q4-6h. **Max:** 6 tabs q24h.
SALICYLATES		
Anacin 81 tablets *(Insight Pharmaceuticals)*	Aspirin 81mg	**Adults & Peds ≥12 yo:** 4-8 tabs q4h. **Max:** 48 tabs q24h.
Aspergum chewable tablets *(Schering-Plough)*	Aspirin 227mg	**Adults & Peds ≥12 yo:** 2 tabs q4h. **Max:** 16 tabs q24h.
Bayer Aspirin Extra Strength caplets *(Bayer Healthcare)*	Aspirin 500mg	**Adults & Peds ≥12 yo:** 1-2 tabs q4-6h. **Max:** 8 tabs q24h.
Bayer Aspirin safety coated caplets *(Bayer Healthcare)*	Aspirin 325mg	**Adults & Peds ≥12 yo:** 1-2 tabs q4h or 3 tabs q6h. **Max:** 12 tabs q24h.
Bayer Children's Aspirin chewable tablets *(Bayer Healthcare)*	Aspirin 81mg	**Adults & Peds ≥12 yo:** 4-8 tabs q4h. **Max:** 48 tabs q24h.

DOSING INFORMATION FOR HEADACHE/MIGRAINE PRODUCTS (cont.)

BRAND NAME	INGREDIENT/STRENGTH	DOSE
Bayer Low Dose Aspirin tablets (*Bayer Healthcare*)	Aspirin 81mg	**Adults & Peds ≥12 yo:** 4-8 tabs q4h. **Max:** 48 tabs q24h.
Bayer Original Aspirin tablets (*Bayer Healthcare*)	Aspirin 325mg	**Adults & Peds ≥12 yo:** 1-2 tabs q4h or 3 tabs q6h. **Max:** 12 tabs q24h.
Doan's Extra Strength caplets (*Novartis Consumer Health*)	Magnesium Salicylate Tetrahydrate 580mg	**Adults & Peds ≥12 yo:** 2 tabs q6h. **Max:** 8 tabs q24h.
Doan's Regular Strength caplets (*Novartis Consumer Health*)	Magnesium Salicylate Tetrahydrate 377mg	**Adults & Peds ≥12 yo:** 2 tabs q4h. **Max:** 12 tabs q24h.
Ecotrin Adult Low Strength tablets (*GlaxoSmithKline Consumer Healthcare*)	Aspirin 81mg	**Adults:** 4-8 tabs q4h. **Max:** 48 tabs q24h.
Ecotrin Enteric Low Strength tablets (*GlaxoSmithKline Consumer Healthcare*)	Aspirin 81mg	**Adults:** 4-8 tabs q4h. **Max:** 48 tabs q24h.
Ecotrin Enteric Regular Strength tablets (*GlaxoSmithKline Consumer Healthcare*)	Aspirin 325mg	**Adults & Peds ≥12 yo:** 1-2 tabs q4h. **Max:** 12 tabs q24h.
Ecotrin Maximum Strength tablets (*GlaxoSmithKline Consumer Healthcare*)	Aspirin 500mg	**Adults & Peds ≥12 yo:** 2 tabs q6h. **Max:** 8 tabs q24h.
Ecotrin Regular Strength tablets (*GlaxoSmithKline Consumer Healthcare*)	Aspirin 325mg	**Adults & Peds ≥12 yo:** 1-2 tabs q4h. **Max:** 12 tabs q24h.
Halfprin 162mg tablets (*Kramer Laboratories*)	Aspirin 162mg	**Adults & Peds ≥12 yo:** 2-4 tabs q4h. **Max:** 24 tabs q24h.
Halfprin 81mg tablets (*Kramer Laboratories*)	Aspirin 81mg	**Adults & Peds ≥12 yo:** 4-8 tabs q4h. **Max:** 48 tabs q24h.
St. Joseph Adult Low Strength chewable tablets (*McNeil Consumer*)	Aspirin 81mg	**Adults & Peds ≥12 yo:** 4-8 tabs q4h. **Max:** 48 tabs q24h.
St. Joseph Adult Low Strength tablets (*McNeil Consumer*)	Aspirin 81mg	**Adults & Peds ≥12 yo:** 4-8 tabs q4h. **Max:** 48 tabs q24h.
SALICYLATES, BUFFERED		
Ascriptin Maximum Strength tablets (*Novartis Consumer Health*)	Aspirin Buffered with Maalox/Calcium Carbonate 500mg	**Adults & Peds ≥12 yo:** 2 tabs q4h. **Max:** 8 tabs q24h.
Ascriptin Regular Strength tablets (*Novartis Consumer Health*)	Aspirin Buffered with Maalox/Calcium Carbonate 325mg	**Adults & Peds ≥12 yo:** 2 tabs q4h. **Max:** 12 tabs q24h.
Bayer Extra Strength Plus caplets (*Bayer Healthcare*)	Aspirin Buffered with Calcium Carbonate 500mg	**Adults & Peds ≥12 yo:** 1-2 tabs q4-6h. **Max:** 8 tabs q24h.
Bufferin Extra Strength tablets (*Bristol-Myers Squibb*)	Aspirin Buffered with Calcium Carbonate/Magnesium Oxide/Magnesium Carbonate 500mg	**Adults & Peds ≥12 yo:** 2 tabs q6h. **Max:** 8 tabs q24h.
Bufferin tablets (*Bristol-Myers Squibb*)	Aspirin Buffered with Calcium Carbonate/Magnesium Oxide/Magnesium Carbonate 325mg	**Adults & Peds ≥12 yo:** 2 tabs q4h. **Max:** 12 tabs q24h.
SALICYLATE COMBINATION		
Alka-Seltzer effervescent tablets (*Bayer Healthcare*)	Aspirin/Citric Acid/Sodium Bicarbonate/Sodium 325mg-1000mg-1916mg-567mg	**Adults & Peds ≥12 yo:** 2 tabs q4h. **Max:** 8 tabs q24h.
Alka-Seltzer Extra Strength effervescent tablets (*Bayer Healthcare*)	Aspirin/Citric Acid/Sodium Bicarbonate/Sodium 500mg-1000mg-1985mg-588mg	**Adults & Peds ≥12 yo:** 2 tabs q6h. **Max:** 7 tabs q24h.
Alka-Seltzer Morning Relief effervescent tablets (*Bayer Healthcare*)	Aspirin/Caffeine 500mg-65mg	**Adults & Peds ≥12 yo:** 2 tabs q6h. **Max:** 8 tabs q24h.
Anacin Pain Reliever caplets (*Insight Pharmaceuticals*)	Aspirin/Caffeine 400mg-32mg	**Adults & Peds ≥12 yo:** 2 tabs q6h. **Max:** 8 tabs q24h.
Anacin Extra Strength tablets (*Insight Pharmaceuticals*)	Aspirin/Caffeine 500mg-32mg	**Adults & Peds ≥12 yo:** 2 tabs q6h. **Max:** 8 tabs q24h.
Anacin tablets (*Insight Pharmaceuticals*)	Aspirin/Caffeine 400mg-32mg	**Adults & Peds ≥12 yo:** 2 tabs q6h. **Max:** 8 tabs q24h.
Bayer Back & Body Pain caplets (*Bayer Healthcare*)	Aspirin/Caffeine 500mg-32.5mg	**Adults & Peds ≥12 yo:** 2 tabs q6h. **Max:** 8 tabs q24h.
Bayer Rapid Headache Relief caplets (*Bayer Healthcare*)	Aspirin/Caffeine 500mg-65 mg	**Adults & Peds ≥12 yo:** 2 tabs q6h. **Max:** 8 tabs q24h.

DOSING INFORMATION FOR HEADACHE/MIGRAINE PRODUCTS (cont.)

Brand Name	Ingredient/Strength	Dose
BC Arthritis Strength powders *(GlaxoSmithKline Consumer Healthcare)*	Aspirin/Caffeine/Salicylamide 742mg-38mg-222mg	**Adults & Peds ≥12 yo:** 1 powder q3-4h. **Max:** 4 powders q24h.
BC Original powders *(GlaxoSmithKline Consumer Healthcare)*	Aspirin/Caffeine/Salicylamide 650mg-33.3mg-195mg	**Adults & Peds ≥12 yo:** 1 powder q 3-4 h.
SALICYLATE/SLEEP AID		
Alka-Seltzer PM Pain Reliever & Sleep Aid, effervescent tablets *(Bayer Healthcare)*	Aspirin/Diphenhydramine Citrate 325mg-38 mg	**Adults & Peds ≥12 yo:** 2 tabs qpm.
Bayer Extra Strength Night Time Relief caplets *(Bayer Healthcare)*	Aspirin/Diphenhydramine 500mg-38.3mg	**Adults & Peds ≥12 yo:** 2 tabs qhs.
Doan's Extra Strength PM caplets *(Novartis Consumer Health)*	Magnesium Salicylate Tetrahydrate/ Diphenhydramine 580mg-25mg	**Adults & Peds ≥12 yo:** 2 tabs qhs.

Insomnia

Insomnia is a symptom that can be caused by a variety of pathologic conditions. It is defined as a persistent difficulty falling or staying asleep that impairs daytime functioning. It is the most common sleep complaint and has many manifestations, including trouble falling asleep, frequent awakenings, early morning awakening, insufficient sleep, daytime fatigue or sleepiness, and irritability or lack of concentration. Some of the most common causes of transient or short-term insomnia are change in sleep environment, excessive noise, jet lag, shift work, unpleasant room temperature, withdrawal of CNS depressants, stressful life events, acute medical or surgical illnesses, and ingestion of stimulant medications. Transient insomnia can often be managed by lifestyle modifications such as engaging in regular daytime exercise; avoiding large nighttime meals; avoiding caffeine, alcohol, and tobacco; reducing evening fluid intake; avoiding bright lights, noise, and temperature extremes during the evening; and using relaxation techniques. However, in certain instances medication may be necessary. There are several OTC products available for the treatment of insomnia; most contain antihistamines such as diphenhydramine and doxylamine.

ANTIHISTAMINES

Sedative-hypnotic—Most antihistamines cross the blood-brain barrier and produce sedation due to inhibition of histamine N-methyltransferase and blockage of central histaminergic receptors. Antagonism of other CNS-receptor sites—such as those for serotonin, acetylcholine, and alpha-adrenergic stimulation—may also be involved. Central depression is not significant with cetirizine (low doses), desloratadine, or loratadine because they do not readily cross the blood-brain barrier. Also, they bind preferentially to peripheral H_1-receptors rather than to CNS H_1-receptors.

Insomnia (treatment)—Diphenhydramine and doxylamine are indicated as nighttime sleep aids to help reduce the time to fall asleep in patients having difficulty falling asleep.

Diphenhydramine

For sedative-hypnotic use:

Adults: 50mg 20 to 30 minutes before bedtime if needed.

For more information, refer to the complete monograph for antihistamines in "Allergic Rhinitis" under Respiratory System.

Doxylamine

For sedative-hypnotic use:

Adults: 25mg 30 minutes before bedtime if needed.

For more information, refer to the complete monograph for antihistamines in "Allergic Rhinitis" under Respiratory System.

DIPHENHYDRAMINE PRODUCTS	
Brand Name	**Dosage Form**
Benadryl (Pfizer)	**Capsule:** 25mg **Tablet:** 25mg
Benadryl Allergy (Pfizer)	**Solution:** 12.5mg/5mL **Tablet:** 12.5mg
Benadryl Allergy Fastmelt (Pfizer)	**Tablet:** 19mg
Nytol (GSK)	**Tablet:** 25mg
Nytol Maximum Strength	**Tablet:** 50mg
Simply Sleep (McNeil)	**Tablet:** 25mg
Sominex (GSK)	**Tablet:** 25mg, 50mg
Unisom Maximum Strength Pfizer)	**Tablet:** 50mg

DOXYLAMINE PRODUCTS	
Brand Name	**Dosage Form**
Unisom (Pfizer)	**Tablet:** 25mg

DOSING INFORMATION FOR INSOMNIA PRODUCTS

The following table provides a quick comparison of the ingredients and dosages of common brand-name OTC drugs. Products are listed alphabetically by generic and brand name.

BRAND NAME	GENERIC INGREDIENT/STRENGTH	DOSE
DIPHENHYDRAMINE		
Nytol Quickcaps caplets *(GlaxoSmithKline Consumer Healthcare)*	Diphenhydramine 25mg	**Adults & Peds ≥12 yo:** 2 tabs qpm.
Nytol Quickgels Maximum Strength *(GlaxoSmithKline Consumer Healthcare)*	Diphenhydramine 50mg	**Adults & Peds ≥12 yo:** 1 tabs qpm.
Simply Sleep caplets *(McNeil Consumer)*	Diphenhydramine 25mg	**Adults & Peds ≥12 yo:** 2 tabs qpm.
Sominex tablets *(GlaxoSmithKline Consumer Healthcare)*	Diphenhydramine 25mg	**Adults & Peds ≥12 yo:** 2 tabs qpm.
Sominex Maximum Strength caplets *(GlaxoSmithKline Consumer Healthcare)*	Diphenhydramine 50mg	**Adults & Peds ≥12 yo:** 1 tab qpm.
Unisom Sleepgels *(Pfizer Consumer Healthcare)*	Diphenhydramine 50mg	**Adults & Peds ≥12 yo:** 1 tab qpm.
DIPHENHYDRAMINE COMBINATION		
Alka-Seltzer PM *(Bayer Healthcare)*	Aspirin/Diphenhydramine Citrate 325mg-38 mg	**Adults & Peds ≥12 yo:** 2 tabs qpm.
Bayer Extra Strength Night Time Relief caplets *(Bayer Healthcare)*	Aspirin/Diphenhydramine 500mg-38.3mg	**Adults & Peds ≥12 yo:** 2 tabs qhs.
Doan's Extra Strength PM caplets *(Novartis Consumer Health)*	Magnesium Salicylate Tetrahydrate/ Diphenhydramine 580mg-25mg	**Adults & Peds ≥12 yo:** 2 tabs qhs.
Excedrin PM caplets *(Bristol-Myers Squibb)*	Acetaminophen/Diphenhydramine 500mg-38mg	**Adults & Peds ≥12 yo:** 2 tabs qhs.
Excedrin PM geltabs *(Bristol-Myers Squibb)*	Acetaminophen/Diphenhydramine 500mg-38mg	**Adults & Peds ≥12 yo:** 2 tabs qhs.
Excedrin PM tablets *(Bristol-Myers Squibb)*	Acetaminophen/Diphenhydramine 500mg-38mg	**Adults & Peds ≥12 yo:** 2 tabs qhs.
Goody's PM Powders *(GlaxoSmithKline Consumer Healthcare)*	Acetaminophen/Diphenhydramine 1000mg-76mg/dose	**Adults & Peds ≥12 yo:** 1 packet (2 powders) qhs.
Tylenol PM caplets *(McNeil Consumer)*	Acetaminophen/Diphenhydramine 500mg-25mg	**Adults & Peds ≥12 yo:** 2 tabs qhs.
Tylenol PM gelcaps *(McNeil Consumer)*	Acetaminophen/Diphenhydramine 500mg-25mg	**Adults & Peds ≥12 yo:** 2 caps qhs.
Tylenol PM geltabs *(McNeil Consumer)*	Acetaminophen/Diphenhydramine 500mg-25mg	**Adults & Peds ≥12 yo:** 2 tabs qhs.
DOXYLAMINE		
Unisom Sleeptabs *(Pfizer Consumer Healthcare)*	Doxylamine Succinate 25mg	**Adults & Peds ≥12 yo:** 1 tab 30 min before hs.

Motion Sickness

Motion sickness is a common problem in travelers using any type of transportation, including automobile, train, plane, and particularly boat. The onset can be sudden and progress from a feeling of restlessness to a cold sweat, dizziness, nausea, and vomiting. Motion sickness is more common in women, especially during pregnancy or menstruation. Motion sickness can be minimized by focusing on the horizon or on a distant, stationary object; by minimizing head movement; by avoiding reading; by avoiding spicy food and alcohol; and, if necessary, by lying supine. There are several OTC products available to prevent and minimize motion sickness, including meclizine and antihistamines such as dimenhydrinate and diphenhydramine.

ANTIHISTAMINES

Anti-emetic; antivertigo agent—The mechanism by which some antihistamines exert their anti-emetic, anti-motion sickness, and antivertigo effects is not precisely known but may be related to their central anticholinergic actions. They diminish vestibular stimulation and depress labyrinthine function. An action on the medullary chemoreceptive trigger zone may also be involved in the anti-emetic effect.

Motion sickness (prophylaxis and treatment); *vertigo* (treatment)—Dimenhydrinate and diphenhydramine are indicated for the prevention and treatment of the nausea, vomiting, dizziness, or vertigo related to motion sickness.

Dimenhydrinate

For anti-emetic/antivertigo use:

Adults/Pediatrics ≥12 years of age: 50 to 100mg every 4 to 6 hours.

Pediatrics 2 to 6 years of age: 12.5 to 25mg every 6 to 8 hours as needed; not to exceed 75mg/day.

Pediatrics 6 to 12 years of age: 25 to 50mg every 6 to 8 hours as needed; not to exceed 150mg/day.

For more information, refer to the complete monograph for antihistamines in "Allergic Rhinitis" under Respiratory System.

Diphenhydramine

For anti-emetic/antivertigo use:

Adults: 25 to 50mg every 4 to 6 hours as needed.

Pediatrics: 1 to 1.5mg/kg of body weight every 4 to 6 hours as needed; not to exceed 300mg/day.

For more information, refer to the complete monograph for antihistamines in "Allergic Rhinitis" under Respiratory System.

MECLIZINE

PHARMACOLOGY

Anti-emetic; antivertigo agent—The mechanism by which meclizine exerts its antiemetic, anti-motion sickness, and antivertigo effects is not precisely known but may be related to its central anticholinergic actions. It diminishes vestibular stimulation and depresses labyrinthine function. An action on the medullary chemoreceptive trigger zone may also be involved in the antiemetic effect.

INDICATIONS

Motion sickness (prophylaxis and treatment)—Meclizine is indicated for the prophylaxis and treatment of nausea, vomiting, and dizziness associated with motion sickness.

Vertigo (prophylaxis and treatment)—The US Food and Drug Administration (FDA) has classified meclizine as possibly effective in the management of vertigo associated with diseases affecting the vestibular system, such as labyrinthitis and Ménière's disease. This classification requires the submission of adequate and well-controlled studies to provide substantial evidence of effectiveness.

Nausea and vomiting, radiotherapy-induced (prophylaxis and treatment)—Meclizine is indicated for the prophylaxis and treatment of nausea, vomiting, and dizziness associated with radiotherapy.

DIMENHYDRINATE PRODUCTS	
Brand Name	**Dosage Form**
Dramamine (Pharmacia)	**Tablet:** 50mg

DIPHENHYDRAMINE PRODUCTS	
Brand Name	**Dosage Form**
Benadryl (Pfizer)	**Capsule:** 25mg **Tablet:** 25mg
Benadryl Allergy (Pfizer)	**Solution:** 12.5mg/5mL **Tablet:** 12.5mg
Benadryl Allergy Fastmelt (Pfizer)	**Tablet:** 19mg
Nytol (GSK)	**Tablet:** 25mg
Nytol Maximum Strength (GSK)	**Tablet:** 50mg
Simply Sleep (McNeil)	**Tablet:** 25mg
Sominex (GSK)	**Tablet:** 25mg, 50mg
Unisom Maximum Strength (Pfizer)	**Tablet:** 50mg

CONTRAINDICATIONS

Risk-benefit should be considered when the following medical problems exist:

- Bladder neck obstruction or prostatic hyperplasia, symptomatic (anticholinergic effects of meclizine may precipitate urinary retention).
- Gastroduodenal obstruction (decrease in motility and tone may occur, aggravating obstruction and gastric retention).
- Glaucoma, angle-closure, predisposition to (increased intraocular pressure may precipitate an acute attack of angle-closure glaucoma).
- Pulmonary disease, chronic obstructive (reduction in bronchial secretion may cause inspissation and formation of bronchial plugs).
- Sensitivity to meclizine.

WARNINGS/PRECAUTIONS

Pregnancy: FDA Category B.

Breastfeeding: Use with caution. Meclizine may be distributed into breast milk. Because of its anticholinergic actions, meclizine may inhibit lactation. However, problems in humans have not been documented.

Geriatrics: It is known that geriatric patients exhibit increased sensitivity to anticholinergic agents, which are related pharmacologically to meclizine. Therefore, constipation, dryness of mouth, and urinary retention (especially in males) are more likely to occur in the elderly.

Pediatrics: It is known that pediatric patients exhibit increased sensitivity to anticholinergic agents, which are related pharmacologically to meclizine.

ADVERSE REACTIONS

Those indicating need for medical attention only if they continue or are bothersome: Incidence more frequent

Drowsiness

Incidence less frequent or rare

Blurred vision; dryness of mouth, nose, and throat

ADMINISTRATION AND DOSAGE

For motion sickness (prophylaxis and treatment):

Adults/Pediatrics ≥12 years of age: 25 to 50mg 1 hour before travel. May repeat every 24 hours prn.

For vertigo (prophylaxis and treatment):

Adults/Pediatrics ≥12 years of age: 25 to 100mg qd prn, in divided doses.

Drug Interactions for Meclizine

Precipitant Drug	Object Drug	Effect On Object Drug	Description
♦ Meclizine	Alcohol; CNS depression-producing medications	↑	Concurrent use may potentiate the CNS-depressant effects of either these medications or meclizine.
Meclizine	Anticholinergics	↑	Concurrent use with meclizine may potentiate anticholinergic effects.
Meclizine	Apomorphine	↓	Prior administration of meclizine may decrease the emetic response to apomorphine.

♦ = Major clinical significance; CNS = central nervous system.

MECLIZINE PRODUCTS

Brand Name	Dosage Form
Dramamine II (Pharmacia)	**Tablet:** 25mg
Bonine (Insight)	**Tablet:** 25mg

DOSING INFORMATION FOR MOTION SICKNESS PRODUCTS

The following table provides a quick comparison of the ingredients and dosages of common brand-name OTC drugs.

BRAND NAME	GENERIC INGREDIENT/STRENGTH	DOSE
DIMENHYDRINATE		
Dramamine chewable tablets *(Pharmacia Consumer Healthcare)*	Dimenhydrinate 50mg	**Adults & Peds** ≥12 yo: 1-2 tabs q4-6h. **Max:** 8 tabs q24h. **Peds: 6-12 yo:** 1/2-1 tab q6-8h. **Max:** 3 tabs q24h **Peds: 2-6 yo:** 1/4-1/2 tab q6-8h. **Max:** 1/2-1 tab q24h.
Dramamine tablets *(Pharmacia Consumer Healthcare)*	Dimenhydrinate 50mg	**Adults & Peds** ≥12 yo: 1-2 tabs q4-6h. **Max:** 8 tabs q24h. **Peds: 6-12 yo:** 1/2-1 tab q6-8h. **Max:** 3 tabs q24h **Peds: 2-6 yo:** 1/4-1/2 tab q6-8h. **Max:** 1/2-1 tab q24h.
MECLIZINE		
Bonine chewable tablets *(Pfizer Consumer Healthcare)*	Meclizine HCl 25mg	**Adults & Peds** ≥12 yo: Take 1-2 tabs qd as directed.
Dramamine Less Drowsy Formula *(Pharmacia Consumer Healthcare)*	Meclizine HCl 25mg	**Adults & Peds** ≥12 yo: Take 1-2 tabs qd as directed.

Smoking Cessation

Tobacco is the agent most responsible for avoidable illness and death in the United States. Millions of Americans consume this toxic material daily. Cigarette smoking is the single most important cause of cancer mortality and is a significant contributor to cardiovascular disease-related deaths, cerebrovascular disease, and gastric and duodenal ulcers. Tobacco use is driven by nicotine dependence and should be treated essentially like any other addiction. The causes of tobacco abuse are multifactorial, involving various neuropharmacologic, genetic, psychosocial, and environmental factors. Over 4000 substances have been identified in cigarette smoke, including some that are pharmacologically active, antigenic, cytotoxic, mutagenic, or carcinogenic. Nicotine is a highly toxic alkaloid that is both a ganglionic stimulant and a depressant. Many of its complex effects are mediated by catecholamine release. Nicotine produces a withdrawal syndrome that begins within a few hours of abstinence, peaks within the first week, and continues for several weeks. The clinical manifestations of the withdrawal syndrome include dysphoria, insomnia, irritability, anxiety, difficulty concentrating, restlessness, slowed heart rate, and increased appetite. Several dosage forms of nicotine have been developed for OTC use to help prevent the symptoms of withdrawal and aid in smoking cessation.

NICOTINE

PHARMACOLOGY

Smoking cessation adjunct—Nicotine acts as an agonist at the nicotinic cholinergic receptors at the autonomic ganglia, in the adrenal medulla, at neuromuscular junctions, and in the brain. Nicotine's positive reinforcing properties are believed to be the result of the release of neurotransmitters including acetylcholine, beta-endorphin, dopamine, norepinephrine, serotonin, and others that mediate pleasure, arousal, elevated mood, appetite, and other desirable psychological states. When the gum is chewed, nicotine is displaced from polacrilex by alkaline saliva.

INDICATIONS

Nicotine dependence (treatment adjunct)—Nicotine replacement therapy products (eg, chewing gum, lozenges, transdermal systems) are indicated as temporary aids for the cigarette smoker who wants to give up smoking. They serve as alternative sources of nicotine and provide relief of nicotine withdrawal symptoms in nicotine-dependent individuals who are acutely withdrawing from cigarette smoking.

—It is recommended that nicotine replacement therapy be used in conjunction with comprehensive behavior modification programs that include education, counseling, and psychological support.

—Generally, smokers who have a strong physical nicotine dependence are more likely to benefit from the use of these nicotine products. Smoking withdrawal effects such as irritability, drowsiness, fatigue, headache, and nicotine craving are lessened with their use.

CONTRAINDICATIONS

Except under special circumstances, this medication should not be used when the following medical problems exist:

- Angina pectoris, severe; cardiac arrhythmias, life-threatening; cerebrovascular accident, recent—*Major clinical significance*.

- Post-myocardial infarction—*Major clinical significance* (may be exacerbated by action on the heart of catecholamines released from adrenal medulla).

Risk-benefit should be considered when the following medical problems exist:

- Angina pectoris; cardiac arrhythmias; diabetes, type 1.

- Hypertension—*Major clinical significance*.

- Hyperthyroidism; myocardial infarction, history of; pheochromocytoma.

- Vasospastic diseases, such as Buerger's disease and Prinzmetal's (or variant) angina (increases in blood pressure, heart rate, and plasma glucose concentrations may result from effects of nicotine-induced catecholamine release; risk of progression to malignant hypertension in patients with accelerated hypertension).

- Peptic ulcer disease, active (nicotine delays healing; caution is recommended).

- Sensitivity to nicotine or to any component of the product.

For the chewing gum only (in addition to the above):

- Dental problems; temporomandibular (TMJ) joint disorder (injury to teeth or aggravation of TMJ may result from mechanical effects of chewing gum).

- Esophagitis, history of; inflammation of mouth or throat (may be exacerbated).

For the transdermal systems only (in addition to the above):

- Skin diseases, such as atopic or eczematous dermatitis (transdermal systems may be irritating).

WARNINGS/PRECAUTIONS

Pregnancy: Nicotine chewing gum—FDA Category C. Nicotine transdermal systems—FDA Category D.

Breastfeeding: Not recommended for use in nursing women (nicotine is distributed into and accumulates in breast milk).

Pediatrics: Small amounts of nicotine can cause serious harm in children. Even nicotine transdermal systems that have been used still contain enough nicotine to cause toxicity in children.

Dental: When used over an extended period of time, nicotine gum may cause severe occlusal stress because its viscosity is heavier than that of ordinary chewing gum. Nicotine gum can cause loosening of inlays or fillings, can stick to dentures, and can cause damage to oral mucosa and natural teeth. The use of hard sugarless candy between doses of gum is recommended to help provide oral stimulation required by some patients. Also, some TMJ joint dysfunction and pain have been associated with excessive chewing.

Drug Interactions for Nicotine

Precipitant Drug	Object Drug	Effect on Object Drug	Description
Nicotine	Acetaminophen ♦ Bronchodilators, xanthine-derivative, except dyphylline; caffeine; imipramine; oxazepam; pentazocine ♦ Propoxyphene ♦ Propranolol, and possibly other beta-adrenergic blocking agents	↑	Smoking cessation may increase therapeutic effects of these agents by decreasing metabolism, thereby increasing serum concentrations; a decrease in dosage may be necessary.
Nicotine	♦ Alpha-adrenergic blocking agents, such as labetalol and prazosin	↑	Smoking cessation may increase the therapeutic effects of these agents as a result of the decrease in circulating catecholamines; a decrease in dosage may be necessary.
Nicotine	♦ Insulin	↑	Smoking cessation and concurrent therapy with nicotine chewing gum, transdermal systems, or other smoking deterrents, such as lobeline sulfate and silver acetate, may increase the therapeutic effects of insulin by increasing absorption, thereby increasing serum concentrations; a decrease in insulin dosage may be necessary when a patient with diabetes who is taking insulin suddenly stops smoking.
Nicotine	♦ Sympathomimetic agents, such as isoproterenol and phenylephrine	↓	Smoking cessation may decrease the therapeutic effects of these agents as a result of the decrease in circulating catecholamines; an increase in dosage may be necessary.

♦ = Major clinical significance.

ADVERSE REACTIONS

Those indicating need for medical attention: Incidence more frequent

For chewing gum only

Injury or irritation to mouth, teeth, or dental work. (Note: Nicotine gum is stickier and of heavier viscosity than ordinary gum, making it harder to chew.)

Incidence less frequent

For all nicotine replacement products

Hypertension

Incidence rare

For all nicotine replacement products

Fast or irregular heartbeat; hypersensitivity reactions, local or generalized, including edema, erythema, pruritus, rash, or urticaria.

(Note: If fast or irregular heartbeat or hypersensitivity reactions occur, use of nicotine replacement products should be discontinued. Further exposure in patients who have experienced a hypersensitivity reaction could result in serious allergic reactions to all forms of nicotine, including cigarettes.)

Those indicating need for medical attention only if they continue or are bothersome:

Incidence more frequent

For all nicotine replacement products

Headache, mild; increased appetite

For chewing gum only

Belching (may be minimized by modifying chewing technique), increased watering of mouth, mild; jaw muscle ache; sore mouth or throat.

For transdermal systems only

Erythema, pruritus, and/or burning at site of application (redness, itching, and/or burning)—usually subsides within 24 hours. (Note: If erythema, pruritus, or burning at site of application is severe or persists, use of transdermal systems should be discontinued.)

Incidence less frequent or rare

For all nicotine replacement products

Change in sense of taste; coughing; increased dizziness or lightheadedness, mild; drowsiness; dryness of mouth; dysmenorrhea; gastrointestinal effects (such as abdominal or stomach pain, constipation, diarrhea, flatulence, mild indigestion, loss of appetite, and nausea or vomiting); muscle or joint pain; sweating, increased; trouble in sleeping or abnormal dreams; unusual irritability or nervousness. (Note: If trouble in sleeping or abnormal dreams occur when the transdermal system is worn for 24 hours, it should be taken off at bedtime [after approximately 16 hours] and replaced upon arising the next day.)

For chewing gum only

Hiccups; hoarseness

For lozenge only

Heartburn (pain in the chest below the breastbone, belching, feeling of indigestion); hiccups

ADMINISTRATION AND DOSAGE

General Dosing Information

The necessity of immediate cessation of smoking upon initiation of therapy must be emphasized. Continued smoking while using nicotine replacement products may cause adverse effects as a result of peak nicotine concentrations higher than those found after smoking alone.

For chewing gum only:

When there is an urge to smoke, one piece of gum is chewed very slowly and intermittently (chewing it several times, then "parking" it between the cheek and gums; chewing again after the tingling sensation subsides) for about 30 minutes until most of the nicotine is released. The amount of nicotine released depends on the rate of chewing and the amount of time the saliva is in contact with the resin. No liquids, especially acidic beverages, should be consumed within 15 minutes before or while chewing a piece of gum because a decrease in the pH of the mouth may interfere with the absorption of the nicotine.

The use of nicotine polacrilex for longer than 6 months may be an indication that this medication is being used as a substitute source of nicotine to maintain nicotine dependence. However, while the use of nicotine replacement products is preferable to a return to smoking, these products should be continued beyond 6 months only if the patient believes that discontinuation of replacement therapy will definitely result in an immediate resumption of smoking.

For lozenge only:

Avoid eating or drinking for 15 minutes before using the lozenge. Effectiveness of the lozenge may be reduced by some beverages. Suck on the lozenge slowly until it dissolves. Do not chew it or bite it like a hard candy. Do not swallow the lozenge. Stop using the lozenge after 12 weeks. Patients should talk to their healthcare professional if they still feel the need to use the lozenge. Do not continue to smoke, chew tobacco, or use snuff or any other product containing nicotine (e.g., nicotine gum or patch).

For transdermal systems only:

If a patient is unable to stop smoking by the fourth week of therapy, treatment should be discontinued, as the patient is unlikely to quit on that attempt. It is recommended that the nicotine transdermal system be removed during, and a new system applied following, strenuous exercise. If the patch is left on, nicotine plasma concentrations may be increased as a result of increased absorption of nicotine from the skin depot, increased skin temperature, and increased cutaneous vasodilation and perfusion. The use of nicotine transdermal systems for longer than 12 weeks in patients who have stopped smoking has not been evaluated and is not recommended. Most manufacturers supply supportive instructional materials and provide telephone information accessible by patients.

Nicotine Polacrilex Gum

Adults:

Patients smoking fewer than 25 cigarettes a day, use the 2-mg strength.

Patients smoking 25 or more cigarettes a day, use the 4mg strength. Weeks 1 to 6—Oral, one piece of chewing gum every 1 to 2 hours.

Weeks 7 to 9—Oral, one piece of chewing gum every 2 to 4 hours.

Weeks 10 to 12—Oral, one piece of chewing gum every 4 to 8 hours.

Note: Patients should use at least 9 pieces of chewing gum daily during the first 6 weeks of therapy.

Maximum: 24 pieces of chewing gum a day.

Nicotine Polacrilex Lozenges

Adults:

Patients who smoke their first cigarette within 30 minutes of waking up should take/use the 4mg strength.

Patients who smoke their first cigarette after 30 minutes of waking up should take/use the 2mg strength.

Weeks 1 to 6—Oral, suck one lozenge every 1 to 2 hours.

Weeks 7 to 9—Oral, suck one lozenge every 2 to 4 hours.

Weeks 10 to 12—Oral, suck one lozenge every 4 to 8 hours.

Maximum: 20 lozenges a day.

Nicotine Transdermal System

Adults:

Patients weighing more than 100lb (45 kg), smoking more than 10 cigarettes a day, and without cardiovascular disease:

16-hour system: Topical, to intact skin:

Nicotrol: One 15mg system applied for 16 hours per day for 6 weeks. Alternatively, one 15mg system applied for 16 hours per day for 8 weeks. Patients who have successfully abstained from smoking for 8 weeks should have their dosage reduced to one 10mg system applied for 16 hours per day for 2 weeks. The dosage should be further reduced to one 5mg system applied for 16 hours per day for 2 weeks.

24-hour system: Topical, to intact skin:

Habitrol: Initially, one 21mg system per day for 3 to 8 weeks. Patients who have successfully abstained from smoking should have their dosage reduced to one 14mg system per day for the next 2 to 4 weeks. The dosage should be further reduced to one 7mg system per day for the following 2 to 4 weeks.

Nicoderm, NicoDerm CQ, or generic: Initially, one 21mg system per day for 6 weeks. Patients who have successfully abstained from smoking should have their dosage reduced to one 14mg system per day for 2 weeks. The dosage should be further reduced to one 7mg system per day for 2 weeks.

Patients weighing less than 100lb (45 kg), smoking fewer than 10 cigarettes a day, or with cardiovascular disease:

16-hour system: Topical, to intact skin:

Nicotrol: One 15mg system applied for 16 hours per day for 6 weeks.

24-hour system: Topical, to intact skin:

Habitrol: Initially, one 14mg system per day for 4 to 8 weeks. Patients who have successfully abstained from smoking should have their dosage reduced to one 7mg system per day for the next 2 to 4 weeks.

Nicoderm, NicoDerm CQ, or generic: Initially, one 14-mg system per day for 6 weeks. Patients who have successfully abstained from smoking should have their dosage reduced to one 7mg system per day for 2 to 4 weeks.

NICOTINE PRODUCTS	
Brand Name	**Dosage Form**
Commit (GSK)	**Lozenge:** 2mg, 4mg
Habitrol (Southwood)	**Patch:** 7mg/24hr, 14mg/24hr, 21mg/24hr
Nicoderm CQ (GSK)	**Patch:** 7mg/24hr, 14mg/24hr, 21mg/24hr
Nicoderm CQ Clear (GSK)	**Patch:** 7mg/24hr, 14mg/24hr, 21mg/24hr
Nicorette (GSK)	**Gum:** 2mg,4mg
Nicotrol	**Patch:** 15mg/16hr

DOSING INFORMATION FOR SMOKING CESSATION PRODUCTS

The following table provides a quick comparison of the ingredients and dosages of common brand-name OTC drugs. Products are listed alphabetically by brand name.

BRAND NAME	GENERIC INGREDIENT/STRENGTH	DOSE
Commit Stop Smoking 2mg lozenges (*GlaxoSmithKline Consumer Healthcare*)	Nicotine Polacrilex 2mg	**Adults:** If smoking first cigarettte more then 30 minutes after waking up use 2mg lozenge. **Weeks 1 to 6:** 1 lozenge q1-2h. **Weeks 7 to 9:** 1 lozenge q2-4h. **Weeks 10 to 12:** 1 lozenge q4-8h. **Max:** 5 lozenges/6 hours; 20 lozenges/day. Stop using at the end of 12 weeks.
Commit Stop Smoking 4mg lozenges (*GlaxoSmithKline Consumer Healthcare*)	Nicotine Polacrilex 4mg	**Adults:** If smoking first cigarettte within 30 minutes after waking up use 4mg lozenge. **Weeks 1 to 6:** o 1 lozenge q1-2h. **Weeks 7 to 9:** 1 lozenge q2-4h. **Weeks 10 to 12:** 1 lozenge q4-8h. **Max:** 5 lozenges/6 hours; 20 lozenges/day. Stop using at the end of 12 weeks.
NicoDerm CQ Step 1 clear patch (*GlaxoSmithKline Consumer Healthcare*)	Nicotine 21mg	**Adults:** If smoking more then 10 cigarettes/day. **Step 1-Weeks 1 to 6:** Apply one 21mg patch/day. **Step 2-Weeks 7 to 8:** Apply one 14mg patch/day. **Step 3-Weeks 9 to 10:** Apply one 7mg patch/day.
NicoDerm CQ Step 2 clear patch (*GlaxoSmithKline Consumer Healthcare*)	Nicotine 14mg	**Adults:** If smoking less than 10 cigarettes/day. **Step 2-Weeks 1 to 6:** Apply one 14mg patch/day. **Step 3-Weeks 7 to 8:** Apply one 7mg patch/day.
NicoDerm CQ Step 3 clear patch (*GlaxoSmithKline Consumer Healthcare*)	Nicotine 7mg	**Adults:** Apply 1 patch qd weeks 9 to 10 if smoking >10 cigarettes/day or weeks 7 to 8 if smoking ≤10 cigarettes/day.
Nicorette 2mg, Original/Mint/Orange gum (*GlaxoSmithKline Consumer Healthcare*)	Nicotine Polacrilex 2mg	**Adults:** If smoking <25 cigarettes/day use 2mg gum. **Weeks 1 to 6:** 1 piece q1-2h. **Weeks 7 to 9:** 1 piece q2-4h. **Weeks 10 to 12:** 1 piece q4-8h. **Max:** 24 pieces/day.
Nicorette 4mg, Original/Mint/Orange gum (*GlaxoSmithKline Consumer Healthcare*)	Nicotine Polacrilex 4mg	**Adults:** If smoking ≥25 cigarettes/day use 4mg gum. **Weeks 1 to 6:** 1 piece q1-2h. **Weeks 7 to 9:** 1 piece q2-4h. **Weeks 10 to 12:** 1 piece q4-8h. **Max:** 24 pieces/day.
Nicotrol Step 1 transdermal system (*Pfizer Consumer Healthcare*)	Nicotine 15mg/16hr	**Adults:** If smoking more then 10 cigarettes/day. **Step 1-Weeks 1 to 6:** Apply one 15mg patch/day. **Step 2-Weeks 7 to 8:** Apply one 10mg patch/day. **Step 3-Weeks 9 to 10:** Apply one 7mg patch/day.
Nicotrol Step 2 transdermal system (*Pfizer Consumer Healthcare*)	Nicotine 10mg/16hr	**Adults:** If smoking more then 10 cigarettes/day. **Step 1-Weeks 1 to 6:** Apply one 15mg patch/day. **Step 2-Weeks 7 to 8:** Apply one 10mg patch/day. **Step 3-Weeks 9 to 10:** Apply one 7mg patch/day.
Nicotrol Step 3 transdermal system (*Pfizer Consumer Healthcare*)	Nicotine 5mg/16hr	**Adults:** If smoking more then 10 cigarettes/day. **Step 1-Weeks 1 to 6:** Apply one 15mg patch/day. **Step 2-Weeks 7 to 8:** Apply one 10mg patch/day. **Step 3-Weeks 9 to 10:** Apply one 7mg patch/day.

Weight Management

Obesity is a chronic, relapsing disease characterized by an excessive accumulation of body fat. The exact pathophysiology of obesity is unknown, although genetic, environmental, metabolic, and behavioral factors are all likely to play important parts in its development. Obesity can be viewed as a disease of energy imbalance. When energy stored exceeds energy expended, body mass accrues in the form of both fat and nonfat tissues. Current societal pressures expose individuals to high-calorie, high-fat fast foods, while improvements in technology promote sedentary behavior. Thus, modern life fosters the development of obesity. Above a body mass index (BMI) of 25 kg/m^2, morbidity for a number of health conditions increases as the BMI increases. Higher morbidity in association with overweight and obesity has been observed for hypertension, type 2 diabetes, coronary heart disease, stroke, gallbladder disease, osteoarthritis, sleep apnea and respiratory problems, and specific cancers (endometrial, breast, prostate, colon). Obesity is associated with complications of pregnancy, menstrual irregularities, hirsutism, stress incontinence, and psychological disorders such as depression.

Lifestyle modification is the primary therapeutic modality in the management of overweight and obese patients. For optimal weight loss success, a combination of low-calorie dieting, increased physical activity, and behavior therapy is recommended. This combination should be tried for approximately 6 months before considering pharmacotherapy. The general goals of weight loss and management are to reduce body weight by about 10% initially and then to maintain a lower body weight over the long term. If this is not possible, at a minimum the therapeutic goal is to prevent further weight gain. The rationale for this initial goal is that moderate weight loss of 10% of the initial body weight can significantly decrease the severity of obesity-associated risk factors. It also can set the stage for further weight loss. Clinical studies have shown that an average weight loss of approximately 8% of the initial body weight can be achieved in 6 months. However, at about that point the body adjusts to the lower caloric intake, and patients find it increasingly difficult to continue losing weight on the same diet and exercise regimen. Generally, after losing 10% of their body weight, patients will reach a plateau and stop losing weight, probably due to the bodily defense mechanisms that protect against starvation. When motivated patients stop losing weight, they should be encouraged to start the maintenance phase and try to avoid gaining weight. Otherwise, if patients expect to continue to lose weight and don't, frustration and a sense of failure are likely to lead to relapse and weight gain. It is healthier to maintain a moderate weight loss over a prolonged period than to regain after a marked weight loss. Further weight loss can be considered after this initial goal is achieved and maintained for 6 months.

Initial treatment, known as the weight-reduction phase, should provide 500 to 1000 kcal d less than the estimated normal maintenance requirement diet. A 500 to 1000 kcal/d energy deficit typically results in a loss of 1 to 2 lb per week. For most women, such a diet contains 1000 to 1200 kcal/d; for most men, 1200 to 1600 kcal/d. Eating-behavior modification is essential. In grossly obese, sedentary patients especially, non-weight-bearing exercise such as bicycling and swimming should be considered before weight-bearing exercise. Walking is a good weight-bearing exercise. A multidisciplinary approach to weight loss is recommended. Optimally, such an approach includes a hypocaloric diet, behavior modification to change eating behaviors, both aerobic and anaerobic exercise, and social support.

Except for the greater limitation on total daily caloric intake, the same diet should be used that would be used for healthy people who are not obese: a low-fat, high complex-carbohydrate, high-fiber diet. Intake of a wide variety of predominantly unprocessed foods and limitation of foods that provide large amounts of calories without other nutrients, such as fat, sucrose, and alcohol, is recommended. There is no proven advantage to special diets that restrict carbohydrates, advocate large amounts of protein or fats, or recommend ingestion of foods one at a time. An increase in physical activity, both aerobic and anaerobic, is an important component of weight loss therapy because it leads to increased expenditure of energy. Increased physical activity may also inhibit food intake in overweight patients. Physical activity can be helpful in maintaining a desirable weight. Exercise also reduces the risk of coronary heart disease. Aerobic exercise directly increases the daily energy expenditure and is particularly useful for long-term weight maintenance. Anaerobic exercise preserves lean body mass and buffers the decrease in basal energy expenditure seen with caloric restriction. Increased physical activity alone can create a caloric deficit and contribute to weight loss. However, efforts to achieve weight loss through physical activity alone generally produce an average 2% to 3% decrease in body weight or BMI. Even so, increased physical activity is a useful adjunct to low-calorie diets in promoting weight reduction. There are also several OTC drugs available to help aid weight reduction when used in combination with diet and exercise. Many of these products contain a combination of vitamins, minerals, and herbs to help increase energy and reduce appetite.

DOSING INFORMATION FOR WEIGHT MANAGEMENT PRODUCTS

The following table provides a quick comparison of the ingredients and dosages of common brand-name OTC drugs. Products are listed alphabetically by brand name.

BRAND NAME	INGREDIENT/STRENGTH	DOSE
1-EZ Diet Appetite Suppressant capsules *(Maximum International)*	Gelatin, Magnesium Stearate, Silicon Dioxide	**Adults:** Take 2 caps with meals bid.
1-EZ Diet Fat & Carb Blocker capsules *(Maximum International)*	Gelatin, Magnesium Stearate, Silicon Dioxide	**Adults:** Take 2 caps with meals bid.
Applied Nutrition Diet System 6 capsules *(Omni Nutraceuticals)*	Vitamin C, Vitamin E, Thiamin (B1), Riboflavin (B2), Niacin (B3), Vitamin B12, Pantothenic acid, Selenium, Chromium, Garcinia Cambogia Extract, Kola Nut Extract, L-Carnitine, L-Tyrosine, Green Tea Extract, Choline, Inositol, Cayenne Powder, Ginger Root Powder, Spirulina, Bioperine Complex, Proprietary Xendrol Blend	**Adults:** Take 2 caps with meals tid.
Applied Nutrition Diet System 6, Carbo Binding Diet Program caplets *(Omni Nutraceuticals)*	Calcium Carbonate, Microcrystalline Cellulose, Stearic Acid, Croscarmellose Sodium, Magnesium Stearate, Silicon Dioxide, Hydroxypropyl Methylcellulose, Polyethylene Glycol	**Adults:** Take 1-2 caps with meals bid.
Applied Nutrition Diet System 6, Fat Binding Diet Program capsules *(Applied Nutrition)*	Gelatin, Silica, Magnesium Stearate	**Adults:** Take 1-2 caps with meals bid.
Applied Nutrition Green Tea Diet capsules *(Applied Nutrition)*	Gelatin, Glycerin, Vegetable Oil, Water, Lecithin, Beeswax, Sodium Copper Chlorophyllin	**Adults:** Take 1-2 caps with meals qd.
Applied Nutrition The New Grapefruit Diet capsules *(Applied Nutrition)*	Gelatin, Silica, Magnesium Stearate	**Adults:** Take 1-2 caps with meals tid.
Aqua-Ban Maximum Strength Diuretic tablets *(Blairex Laboratories)*	Pamabrom 50mg	**Adults:** Take 1 tab with meals qid. **Max:** 4 tabs q24h.
Atkins Essential Oils Vita-Nutrient Supplement Formula softgels *(Atkins Nutritional)*	Flaxseed Oil, Borage Seed Oil, Fish Oil	**Adults:** Take 1-2 caps with meals qd.
BioMD Nutraceuticals Metabolism T3 capsules *(BioMD Nutraceuticals)*	Calcium Phosphate, Gum Guggle Extract, L-Tyrosine, Garcinia Cambogia, Dipotassium Phosphate, Sodium Phosphate, Disodium Phosphate, Phosphatidyl Choline	**Adults:** Take 2 caps with meal tid.
Biotest Hot-Rox capsules *(Biotest Laboratories)*	Gelatin, Cellulose, Magnesium Stearate, FD&C Red 40, FD&C Yellow 6, Titanium Dioxide	**Adults:** Take 1-2 caps with meals bid. **Max:** 4 caps q24h.
Bodyonics Pinnacle Estrolean Fat Burner Supreme capsules *(Bodyonics)*	Apple Extract, Pomegranite Extract, Sea Vegetable Extract, Plant Based Enzymes, Herbal Metabogenics, Herbal Modulators	**Adults:** Take 2 caps with meal qam.
Bodyonics Pinnacle SugarEase capsules *(Bodyonics)*	Banabalean leaves, Promolin fenugreek extract seeds, Dang Shen, Bai Zhu, Fu Ling, Gan Cao, Sheng Jiang, Da Zao, Yerba Mate Extract, Cocoa extract, tyramine, Citrus Naringinean, Natural Caffeine	**Adults:** Take 1 cap with meal tid.
Carb Cutter Original Formula tablets *(Health & Nutrition Systems)*	Dicalcium Phosphate, Stearic Acid, Magnesium Stearate, Silica, Pharmaceutical Glaze	**Adults:** Take 1-2 tabs with meals bid.
Carb Cutter Phase 2 Starch Neutralizer tablets *(Health & Nutrition Systems)*	Dicalcium Phosphate, Microcrystalline Cellulose, Croscarmellose Sodium, Stearic Acid, Magnesium Stearate, Silica, Pharmaceutical Glaze	**Adults:** Take 1-2 tabs with meals bid.
Chroma Slim Apple Cider Vinegar caplets *(Richardson Labs)*	Microcrystalline Cellulose, Maltodextrin, Dicalcium Phosphate, Crospovidone, Modified Food Starch, Hydroxypropyl Methylcellulose, Calcium Silicate, Silica, Magnesium Stearate, PEG	**Adults:** Take 2 caps with meals bid.

DOSING INFORMATION FOR WEIGHT MANAGEMENT PRODUCTS (cont.)

Brand Name	Ingredient/Strength	Dose
Chroma Slim Chitosan-C with Chromium Picolinate capsules *(Richardson Labs)*	Dicalcium Phosophate, Calcium Carbonate, Microcrystalline Cellulose, Croscarmellose Sodium, Stearic Acid, Sodium Lauryl Sulfate, Magnesium Stearate, Silica, Hydroxypropyl Methylcellulose, Hydroxypropylcellulose, PEG, Natural Peppermint Flavor, Carnuba Wax	**Adults:** Take 2 caps with meals bid.
CortiLess Anti-Stress Weight Loss Supplement capsules *(Diet a Day)*	Gelatin, Cellulose, Magnesium Stearate, Silica	**Adults:** Take 1 cap with meals bid. **Max:** 6 caps q24h.
Cortislim Cortisol Control Weight Loss Formula capsules *(Window Rock Enterprises)*	Microcrystalline Cellulose, Gelatin, Magnesium Stearate, Water, Silicon Dioxide	**Adults:** Take 2 caps with meals bid-tid. **Max:** 6 caps q24h.
CSE Naturally hGH chewable tablets *(Biomed Comm)*	Homeopathic Recombinant Human Growth Hormone (HrhGH) 6C + 100C + 200C (Anti-Aging)	**Adults:** Chew 1 tab with meals tid.
Dexatrim Max Maximum Weight Loss Power, Epheda Free caplets *(Chattem)*	Thiamin (B1), Riboflavin (B2), Niacin (B3), Vitamin B6, Vitamin B12, Pantothenic acid, Chromium, Green Tea Leaf Extract, Asian Ginseng Standardized Extract	**Adults:** Take 1-2 tabs qd.
Dexatrim Natural Green Tea Formula caplets *(Chattem)*	Calcium, Chromium, Microcrystalline Cellulose, Croscarmellose Sodium, Stearic Acid, Silica, Magnesium Stearate, Hypromellose, Hydroxypropyl Cellulose, PEG 400, Titanium Dioxide, Riboflavin, Caramel (245-8)	**Adults:** Take 1 cap with meal tid.
Dexatrim Results Advanced Appetite Control Formula caplets *(Chattem)*	Dicalcium Phosphate, Microcrystalline Cellulose, Croscarmellose Sodium, Stearic Acid, Magnesium Stearate, Silica, Coating ingredients: (mono- and diglycerides, Hypromellose, Hydroxypropylcellulose, PEG-400), Carnuba Wax (224-175)	**Adults:** Take 1 cap with meals tid. **Max:** 3 caps q24h.
Diet Lean Weight Loss Multivitamin tablets *(Naturade)*	Vitamin A, Vitamin C, Vitamin D, Vitamin E, Vitamin K, Thiamin (B1), Riboflavin (B2), Niacin (B3), Vitamin B6, Folate, Folic Acid, Folacin, Vitamin B12, Pantothenic acid, Calcium, Iron, Magnesium, Zinc, Selenium, Copper, Manganese, Chromium, EGCG	**Adults:** Take 1 tab with meal qd.
Diurex Long Acting Water capsules *(Alva-Amco Pharmacal)*	Caffeine Anhydrous, Acetaminophen, Potassium Salicylate	**Adults:** Take 1 cap qam after breakfast.
EAS CLA capsules *(EAS)*	Gelatin, Water, Glycerin	**Adults:** Take 2 caps with meals tid.
EAS Lean DynamX, Orange Cream powder *(EAS)*	Calcium, Chromium, Conjugated Linoleic Acid, Calcium B-hydroxy B-methylbutyrate, Mate, L-Carnitine, L-Tartrate	**Adults:** Mix 1 tsp with 8 ounces of water bid-tid.
EAS Lean DynamX, Raspberry Tea powder *(EAS)*	Calcium, Chromium, Conjugated Linoleic Acid, Calcium B-hydroxy B-methylbutyrate, Mate, L-Carnitine L-Tartrate	**Adults:** Mix 1 tsp with 8 ounces of water bid-tid.
Estrin-D capsules *(Covaxil Laboratories)*	Vitamin B6, Magnesium, Estrin-D Blend	**Adults:** Take 2 caps with meals qd. **Max:** 6 caps q24h.
Health and Nutrition Systems Eat Less Dietary Supplement capsules *(Health & Nutrition Systems International)*	Galactomannan, Cellulose, Glucomannan, Apple Pectin, Beet Fiber, Citrus Pectin, Oat Fiber	**Adults:** Take 1-2 caps with meals bid.
Hydroxycut Advanced Weight Loss Formula, Ephedra-Free capsules *(Muscletech R&D)*	Gelatin, Magnesium Stearate, Silica, Cellulose	**Adults:** Take 3 caps with meals tid. **Max:** 4 caps q24h.
Hydroxycut Fat Loss Support Formula, Caffeine-Free capsules *(MuscleTech R&D)*	Gelatin, Magnesium Stearate, Silica, Cellulose	**Adults:** Take 3 caps with meals tid. **Max:** 9 caps q24h.
Isatori Lean System 7 Triple Action Fat-Loss Formula with 7-Keto capsules *(Isatori Global Technologies)*	Gelatin, Rice Flour, Magnesium Stearate, Titanium Dioxide	**Adults:** Take 3 caps with meals bid. **Max:** 6 caps q24h.
Metab-O-Fx Ephedra Free caplets *(Richardson Labs)*	Guarana Extract, Caffeine, Black Tea Extract, Rutin, EGCG, Ginger Extract	**Adults:** Take 1 tab with meal bid-tid. **Max:** 3 tabs q24h.

DOSING INFORMATION FOR WEIGHT MANAGEMENT PRODUCTS (cont.)

Brand Name	Ingredient/Strength	Dose
Metabolife Ephedra Free Dietary Supplement tablets (Metabolife International)	Maltodextrin, Modified Cellulose, Caffeine, Dicalcium Phosophate, Stearic Acid, Sodium Bicarbonate, Dextrin, Silica, Citric Acid, Sodium Copper Chlorophyllin, Dextrose, Lecithin, Sodium Carboxymethylcellulose, Sodium Citrate	**Adults:** Take 2 tabs with meals tid.
Metabolife Ultra caplets (Metabolife International)	Modified Cellulose, Maltodextrin, Caffeine, Dicalcium Phosophate, Stearic Acid, Dextrin, Dextrose, Lecithin, Sodium Carboxymethylcellulose, Magnesium Stearate, Sodium Citrate, Each Caplet Contains 54 mg Caffeine, 6.6 mg Synephrine	**Adults:** Take 2-3 caps with meals bid-tid. **Max:** 6 caps q24h.
Metabolife Ultra Caffeine Free caplets (Metabolife International)	Thiamin (B1), Riboflavin (B2), Niacin (B3), Vitamin B6, Pantothenic acid, Calcium, Chromium, Potassium	**Adults:** Take 2 tabs with meals tid. **Max:** 6 tabs q24h.
MHP TakeOff, Hi-Energy Fat Burner capsules (Maximum Human Performance)	Citrus Aurantium Extract, Guarana Seed Extract and Green Tea Leaf Extract, L-Tyrosine, Triple-Ginseng Concentrate, Adrenal Support Blend, Ginkgo Biloba Leaf Extract	**Adults:** Take 1-2 caps with meal prn.
MHP Thyro-Slim A.M./P.M. tablets (Maximum Human Performance)	Dicalcium Phosphate, Microcrystalline Cellulose, Hydroxypropyl Methylcellulose, Methylcellulose, Stearic Acid, Vegetable Stearin, Silica, Magnesium Stearate, Hydroxypropyl Cellulose, Polyethylene Glycol, Croscarmellose Sodium	**Adults:** Take 2 tabs with meals bid.
Natrol Carb Intercept with Phase 2 Starch Neutralizer capsules (Pharmachem Laboratories)	Silica, Magnesium Stearate, Gelatin	**Adults:** Take 2 caps with meals tid.
Natrol Chitosan 500mg capsules (Natrol)	Chitosan, Gelatin	**Adults:** Take 3 caps with meals qd. **Max:** 6 caps q24h.
Natrol CitriMax Balance tablets (Natrol)	Vitamin B6, Magnesium, Chromium, Vanadium, Hydroxycitric Acid (HCA) Extract, Green Tea Extract, Gymnerna Sylvestre Extract, Bitter Orange Extract	**Adults:** Take 2 tabs with meals tid.
Natrol Green Tea 500mg capsules (Natrol)	Gelatin, Magnesium Stearate, Rice Powder, Silica	**Adults:** Take 1 cap with meals qd.
Natural Balance Fat Magnet capsules (Natural Balance)	Gelatin, Starch, Microcrystalline Cellulose	**Adults:** Take 2 caps with meals bid.
Nature Made High Potency Chromium Picolinate, 200mcg, tablets (Nature Made Nutritional Products)	Dibasic Calcium Phosphate, Cellulose, Magnesium Stearate, Chromium Picolinate, Croscarmellose Sodium	**Adults:** Take 1 tab with meals qd.
Nature's Bounty Super Green Tea Diet capsules (US Nutrition)	Gelatin, Vegetable Magnesium Stearate, Silica	**Adults:** Take 1 cap with meals bid.
Nature's Bounty Xtreme Lean Zn-3 Ephedra Free capsules (Zoller Laboratories)	Yerba Mate, Ilex paraguatensis, Guarana, Paulinia cupana, Damiana, Turnera aphrodisiacal, Schizonepeta, Nepeta tenuifolia, Green Tea Extract, Camellia sinensis, White Pepper, Piper nigrum, Tibet-seng™, Rhodiola crenulata, Panax Ginseng, Maca Root, Lepidium meyenii, Cocoa Nut, Theobroma cacao, Kola Nut, Cola acuminata, Thea Sinensis Complex	**Adults:** Take 1 cap with meals tid.
Nunaturals LevelRight, For Blood Sugar Management capsules (NuNaturals)	Gymenema Sylvestre Extract, Fenugreek Extract, Bitter Melon Extract, Siberian Ginseng Extract, Alpha Lipoic Acid, Cinnamon Bark Extract, Banaba Leaf Extract, Biotin, Chromium Polynicotinate, Chromium Picolinate, Vanadium	**Adults:** Take 1 cap with meals tid.

DOSING INFORMATION FOR WEIGHT MANAGEMENT PRODUCTS (cont.)

Brand Name	Ingredient/Strength	Dose
One-A-Day Weight Smart Dietary Supplement tablets (Bayer Healthcare)	Calcium Carbonate, Cellulose, Magnesium Oxide, Green Tea Extract, Ascorbic Acid, Ferrous Fumarate, Acacia, dl-Alpha Tocopherol Acetate, Niacinamide, Croscarmellose Sodium, Zinc Oxide, Dextrin, d-Calcium Pantothenate, Dicalcium Phosphate, Caffeine Powder, Silicon Dioxide, Hypromellose, Magnesium Stearate, Titanium Dioxide, Gelatin, Corn Starch, Crospovidone, Glucose, Manganese Sulfate, Calcium Silicate, Cupric Sulfate, Polyethylene Glycol, Pyridoxine, Hydrochloride, Riboflavin, Dextrose, Thiamine Mononitrate, Lecithin, Beta Carotene, Chromium Chloride, Resin, FD&C Blue 1 Lake, Folic Acid, Sodium Selenate, Phytonadione, Tricalcium Phosphate, Cholecalciferol, Cyanocobalamin	**Adults:** Take 1 tab with meals qd.
OraLabs Cheat & Lean Fat Blocker capsules (OraLabs)	Chromium, Chitosan	**Adults:** Take 3 caps with meal bid.
PatentLean Effective And Trusted Fat And Weight Loss Supplement (PatentHEALTH)	3-Acetyl-7-Oxo-Dehydroepiandrosterone, Magnesium Stearate, Maltodextrin, Gelatin, FD&C Blue 1, FD&C Red 3, Titanium Dioxide	**Adults:** Take 1 cap with meals bid. **Max:** 2 caps q24h.
Prolab BCAA Plus capsules (Natrol)	Vitamin C, Vitamin B6, L-Leucine, L-Isoleucine, L-Valine	**Adults:** Take 6 caps after workout.
Prolab Enhanced CLA softgels (Pro Lab Nutrition)	Sunflower Oil, Safflower Oil, Gelatin, Purified Water, Glycerin, Carob	**Adults:** Take 3 caps with meals qd.
Relora Anti-Anxiety & Stress Relief, 250mg capsules (Solanova)	Snow White Filler, Magnesium Stearate, Silicon Dioxide, Gelatin, Glycerin, Purified Water	**Adults:** Take 1 cap with meals tid.
Slim Form patch (Long Life Services)	Marine Algae (Fucus Vesiculosus), Mannitol, Chlorides, Potassium, Sodium, Magnesium, Amino Acids, Calcium, Glucose, Phosphate, Fucose	**Adults:** Apply patch as directed.
Stacker 2 Ephedra Free capsules (NVE Pharmaceuticals)	Dextrose, Stearic Acid, Magnesium Stearate, Titanium Dioxide, FD&C Yellow 5, FD&C Blue 1, FD&C Red 3, FD&C Yellow 6	**Adults:** Use as directed. **Max:** 3 caps tid.
Tetrazene KGM-90 Rapid Weight Loss Catalyst capsules (BioQuest Pharmaceuticals)	Magnesium Stearate, Gelatin, Water	**Adults:** Take 2 caps with meals tid. **Max:** 6 caps q24h.
Thermogenics Plus Stimulant-Free capsules (SilverSage)	Proprietary Blend	**Adults:** Take 2 caps tid.
ThyroStart with Thydrazine, Thyroid Support capsules (SilverSage)	Rice Flour	**Adults:** Take 2 caps with meals tid.
Twinlab GTF Chromium, 200mcg tablets (Twin Laboratories)	Brewers Yeast, Cellulose, Stearic Acid, Croscarmellose Sodium, Magnesium Stearate, Silica	**Adults:** Take 1 tab qd.
Twinlab Mega L-Carnitine 500mg tablets (Twin Laboratories)	Cellulose, Calcium Phosphate, Vegetable Oil (Palm Olein, Soy, Coconut and High Oleic Sunflower Oils), Povidone, Croscarmellose Sodium, Silica, Magnesium Stearate, Polyethylene Glycol, Water	**Adults:** Take 1-4 tabs with meals qd.
Twinlab Metabolift, Ephedra Free Formula capsules (Twin Laboratories)	Guarana Seed Extract, Citrus Aurantium Fruit Extract, Proprietary Thermogenic and Metabolic Blend, St. John's Wort Extract, L-Phenylalanine, Green Tea Leaf Extract, Quercetin Dihydrate, Citrus Bioflavonoid Complex, Ginger Root, Cayenne Fruit	**Adults:** Take 2 caps with meals tid. **Max:** 6 caps q24h.
Ultra Diet Pep tablets (Natural Balance)	Microcrystalline Cellulose, Modified Cellulose Gum, Silicon Dioxide, Stearic Acid, Magnesium Stearate	**Adults:** Take 1 tab with meals bid.

DOSING INFORMATION FOR WEIGHT MANAGEMENT PRODUCTS (cont.)

Brand Name	Ingredient/Strength	Dose
Xenadrine NRG 8 Hour Power tablets *(Cytodyne)*	Calcium Phosphate, Cellulose, Sorbitol, Gamma Cyclodextrin, Cephalins, Xanthan, Inulin, Magnesium Stearate, Natural Protective Coating Utilized	**Adults:** Take 3 tabs qd. **Max:** 12 caps q24h.
XtremeLean Advanced Formula, Ephedra Free capsules *(Nature's Bounty)*	Gelatin, Vegetable Magnesium Stearate, Silica	**Adults:** Take 2 caps with meals bid.
Zantrex 3, Ephedrine Free capsules *(Zoller Laboratories)*	Rice Flour	**Adults:** Take 2 caps with meals qd. **Max:** 6 cap q24h.

Acne

The pathogenesis of acne includes several factors: (1) abnormal keratinization of the sebaceous follicles of the face, chest, and back that leads to the filling of the follicle with keratin, sebum, and bacteria; (2) increased bacterial colonization by the anaerobe *Propionibacterium acnes*, a ubiquitous organism that thrives on sebum; (3) excessive immune response to the bacterial colonization, possibly genetically determined, producing inflammation; and (4) hormonal influences, especially those of androgens that enhance sebum production at the time of puberty. Although there appears to be a genetic predisposition to severe acne, other factors modify disease expression, and the severity of disease in a specific individual cannot be accurately predicted based on the family history of acne. Other, secondary influences on acne may include external application of comedogenic agents, such as oils or greases; seasonal changes; and stress. To date, there is no credible evidence that any food causes acne; thus, diet is unlikely to be a pathogenic factor.

The basic types of acne lesion are comedones, inflammatory lesions, and scars. *Closed comedones* are the primary acne lesions, caused by the filling of sebaceous follicles with keratin, sebum, and bacteria. When the opening of a closed comedone is large, pigment and oxidized lipids accumulate at the surface and the lesion then becomes an *open comedone*, or blackhead. When the follicular wall has been ruptured and comedonal lesions become inflamed, papules are created. A *papule* with an accumulation of polymorphonuclear leukocytes at the surface is a *pustule*, or whitehead. When a large (>5 mm) follicle or more than one adjacent follicle is involved with extensive inflammation, *nodules* are formed. When inflammation extends into the collagen-filled dermis, there is potential for scarring in all types of inflammatory lesions, especially nodules. *Acne scars* are of three types: (1) postinflammatory hyperpigmentation consisting of melanin or increased vascularization, which eventually resolve over 6 to 18 months after healing of an inflammatory acne lesion; (2) depressions in the skin, including the classic small "ice-pick" scars resulting from damage to dermal collagen; and (3) in certain individuals, keloid formation, especially on the shoulders, chest, and jawline. There are many OTC medications available, in many dosage forms (creams, gels, lotions, cleansers, soaps) to treat acne, most of which contain keratolytics such as benzoyl peroxide or salicylic acid.

BENZOYL PEROXIDE

PHARMACOLOGY

Benzoyl peroxide slowly releases active oxygen.

Acne vulgaris—Benzoyl peroxide has antibacterial action against *Propionibacterium acnes* in the treatment of acne vulgaris. It also improves both inflammatory and noninflammatory lesions of acne. The medication also has some keratolytic effect, which produces comedo lysis, as well as drying and desquamative actions that contribute to its efficacy.

Decubital or stasis ulcers—Benzoyl peroxide stimulates epithelial cell proliferation and the production of granulation tissue in the treatment of decubital or stasis ulcers.

INDICATIONS

Acne vulgaris (treatment)—Indicated for the topical treatment of mild to moderate acne vulgaris. In more severe acne, benzoyl peroxide may be indicated as an adjunct in therapeutic regimens including oral and topical antibiotics, retinoic acid preparations, and sulfur/salicylic acid-containing preparations.

Ulcer, decubital (treatment); *ulcer, stasis* (treatment)—Benzoyl peroxide, usually in a 20% strength, is used as an oxidizing agent in the treatment of decubital or stasis ulcers.

CONTRAINDICATIONS

Risk-benefit should be considered when the following medical problems exist:

- Dermatitis, seborrheic
- Eczema
- Inflammation of skin, acute, or denuded skin, including sunburn—*major clinical significance* (irritation may be increased; benzoyl peroxide should be discontinued until the skin is less sensitive)
- Sensitivity to benzoyl peroxide or parabens

WARNINGS/PRECAUTIONS

Pregnancy: FDA Category C. This medicine may be systemically absorbed. Studies have not been done in humans or animals.

Breastfeeding: It is not known whether benzoyl peroxide is distributed into breast milk. Problems in humans have not been documented; however, benzoyl peroxide may be systemically absorbed.

ADVERSE REACTIONS

Those indicating need for medical attention: Incidence less frequent or rare

Allergic contact dermatitis (burning, blistering, crusting, itching, severe redness, or swelling of skin); irritant effect (painful irritation of skin); skin rash.

Those indicating need for medical attention only if they continue or are bothersome: Incidence less frequent

Dryness or peeling of skin—may occur after a few days; feeling of warmth, mild stinging, or redness of skin.

ADMINISTRATION AND DOSAGE

General Dosing Information

This medication contains an oxidizing agent that may bleach hair and colored fabrics.

For treatment of acne:

Benzoyl peroxide should not be applied to acutely inflamed, denuded, or highly sensitive skin, unless otherwise directed by physician as in treating an ulceration. Therapy may be initiated with the 2.5% or 5% cream, gel, or lotion, then changed to the 10% strength after 3 to 4 weeks, if needed, or sooner if tolerance to the lower strengths has been determined. After treatment with benzoyl peroxide for approximately 8 to 12 weeks, maximum lesion reduction may be expected. Continued prophylactic use of benzoyl peroxide is usually required to maintain optimal thera-peutic response. In fair-skinned patients or under excessively dry atmospheric conditions, it is recommended that therapy be initi-ated with one application daily and gradually increased up to 2 to 4 times a day (depending on the dosage form) as tolerated.

For treatment of decubital or stasis ulcers:

A protective ointment should be applied to a wide area bordering the ulcer to decrease the possibility of irritant dermatosis of the surrounding skin. Ulcers should be treated by applying a sterile dressing of terry cloth moistened with normal saline and satu-rated with 20% lotion to the clean and surgically debrided ulcer. Occlude the dressed area with a plastic film and apply an abdominal dressing pad overall and tape firmly in place. Change the dressing every 8 hours in large ulcers and every 12 hours in small ulcers. For maximal therapeutic efficacy, the lotion dress-ing should be kept moist and as close to 37°C (98.6°F) as possi-ble: the plastic film is used to retain moisture and the abdominal dressing pad is used to increase the local temperature through its insulating effect. Exuberant granulation tissue may be kept below the epidermal level with cauterization by a silver nitrate stick to facilitate ingrowth of epithelium. Severe ulcers may be treated by packing with surgical gauze saturated with 20% lotion to facilitate good contact with the walls of the cavity and then occluding. Large amounts of serous exudate appearing on the ulcer surface is a normal response to benzoyl peroxide therapy. Two weeks may pass before progress is visible in large chronic ulcers.

For acne vulgaris:

Bar

Adults/Pediatrics ≥12 years of age: Use 2 or 3 times a day.

Cream/Gel/Lotion

Adults/Pediatrics ≥12 years of age: Apply to affected area 1 or 2 times a day.

Facial mask

Adults/Pediatrics ≥12 years of age: Apply once a week to once a day.

Stick

Adults/Pediatrics ≥12 years of age: Apply to affected area 1 to 3 times a day.

SALICYLIC ACID

Salicylic acid facilitates desquamation by solubilizing the inter-cellular cement that binds scales in the stratum corneum, thereby loosening the keratin. This keratolytic effect may provide an antifungal action because removal of the stratum corneum sup-presses fungal growth; it also aids in the penetration of other antifungal agents. Salicylic acid also has a mild antiseptic action.

Acne vulgaris (treatment)—Salicylic acid gel, lotion, ointment, pads, soap, and topical solution are indicated as peeling and dry-ing agents in the treatment of acne vulgaris.

Gel 0.5% to 5%

Adults/Pediatrics: Apply to affected area once a day.

Drug Interactions for Benzoyl Peroxide

Precipitant Drug	Object Drug	Effect On Object Drug	Description
Acne products, topical (resorcinol, salicylic acid, sulfur) Alcohol-containing products, topical (after-shave lotions, astringents) Cosmetic or soaps w/strong drying effect Hair removal products Isotretinoin Soaps or cleansers, abrasive	Benzoyl peroxide	↑	Concurrent use with benzoyl peroxide on the same area of the skin may cause a cumulative irritant or drying effect, especially with the application of peeling, desquamating, or abrasive agents, resulting in excessive irritation of the skin. If irritation occurs, the strength or dose of benzoyl peroxide may need to be reduced or application temporarily discontinued until the skin is less sensitive.
Benzoyl peroxide	Antibiotics, topical (clindamycin, erthyromycin); retinoids, topical (adapalene, tretinoin)	↓	Although these medications are used in a treatment regimen w/benzoyl peroxide for therapeutic effect, their use on the same area of the skin at the same time is not recommended. The oxidizing action of benzoyl peroxide degrades antibiotics over time. A physical incompatibility between the use of the medications and benzoyl peroxide or a change in pH may reduce their efficacy if used simultaneously. When used together for clinical effect, it is recommended that these medications and benzoyl peroxide be used at different times of the day, to minimize possible skin irritation, unless otherwise directed.

Lotion 1% to 2%

Adults/Pediatrics: Apply to affected area 1 to 3 times a day.

Ointment 2% to 6%

Adults/Pediatrics: Apply to affected area once a day.

Pads 0.5% to 2%

Adults/Pediatrics: Apply to affected area 1 to 3 times a day.

Soap 2% to 3.5%

Adults/Pediatrics: Apply to affected area once a day.

Solution 0.5% to 2%

Adults/Pediatrics: Apply to affected area one to three times a day.

For more information, refer to complete monograph for salicylic acid in "Calluses, Corns, and Warts" under Dermatological Conditions.

SALICYLIC ACID/SULFUR

Salicylic acid—*See above.*

Sulfur has germicidal, fungicidal, parasiticidal, and keratolytic actions. Its germicidal activity may be the result of its conver-sion to pentathionic acid by epidermal cells or by certain microorganisms.

Acne vulgaris or oily skin (treatment)—Salicylic acid and sulfur combinations (bar or cleansing lotion) are indicated for the treatment of acne and oily skin.

Bar

Adults/Pediatrics: Apply to affected area 2 or 3 times a day.

Cleasing lotion

Adults/Pediatrics: Apply to the affected area 1 to 3 times a day. Massage lather into wet skin for 1 minute, then rinse.

For more information, refer to complete monograph for salicylic acid/sulfur in "Calluses, Corns, and Warts" under Dermatological Conditions.

BENZOYL PEROXIDE PRODUCTS

Brand Name	Dosage Form
Clearasil Tinted Acne Treatment (Boots)	**Cream:** 10%
Clearasil Vanishing Acne Treatment (Boots)	**Cream:** 10%
Neutrogena Acne Mask (Neutrogena)	**Cream:** 5%
Neutrogena On-The-Spot Acne (Neutrogena)	**Cream:** 2.5%
Oxy Balance Spot Treatment (GSK)	**Gel:** 5%
Oxy 10 Balance Spot Treatment (GSK)	**Gel:** 10%
Oxy 10 Balance Medicated Face Wash (GSK)	**Liquid:** 10%
Panoxyl Aqua Gel (Stiefel)	**Gel:** 10%
Panoxyl Bar 5 (Stiefel)	**Soap:** 5%
Panoxyl Bar 10 (Stiefel)	**Soap:** 10%

SALICYLIC ACID PRODUCTS

Brand Name	Dosage Form
Neutrogena Acne Wash (Neutrogena)	**Liquid:** 2%
Neutrogena Clear Pore (Neutrogena)	**Gel:** 2%
Oxy Balance Deep Pore Cleansing (GSK)	**Gel:** 2%
	Pads: 0.50%
Stri-dex Body Focus (Blistex)	**Gel:** 2%
Stri-dex Clear Cycle (Blistex)	**Soap:** 2%
Stri-dex Essential Care (Blistex)	**Pads:** 1%
Stri-dex Facewipes To Go (Blistex)	**Pads:** 0.50%
Stri-dex Fruit Therapy (Blistex)	**Cream:** 2%
Stri-dex Maximum Strength (Blistex)	**Pads:** 2%
Stri-dex Sensitive Skin (Blistex)	**Pads:** 0.50%
Stri-dex Super Scrub (Blistex)	**Pads:** 2%

SALICYLIC ACID/SULFUR PRODUCTS

Brand Name	Dosage Form
Pernox Scrub Cleanser (Westwood-Squibb)	**Cream:** 1.5%-2%
SAStid (Stiefel)	**Soap:** 3%-10%

SULFUR

PHARMACOLOGY

Sulfur has germicidal, fungicidal, parasiticidal, and keratolytic actions. Its germicidal activity may be the result of its conversion to pentathionic acid by epidermal cells or by certain microorganisms.

INDICATIONS

Acne vulgaris (treatment)—Sulfur (cream, lotion, ointment, and bar soap) is indicated as an aid in the treatment of acne vulgaris.

Dermatitis, seborrheic (treatment)—Sulfur ointment is indicated for the treatment of seborrheic dermatitis.

Scabies (treatment)—Sulfur ointment is indicated for the treatment of scabies, especially in infants less than 2 months of age and in pregnant and nursing women.

Rosacea (treatment)—Sulfur (cream, lotion, ointment, and bar soap) is used in strengths of up to 15% to treat rosacea.

CONTRAINDICATIONS

Risk-benefit should be considered when the following medical problem exists:

● Sensitivity to sulfur.

WARNINGS/PRECAUTIONS

Pregnancy: Problems in humans have not been documented.

Breastfeeding: Problems in humans have not been documented.

ADVERSE REACTIONS

Those indicating need for medical attention:

Skin irritation not present before therapy.

Those indicating need for medical attention only if they continue or are bothersome:

Redness and peeling of skin—may occur after a few days.

ADMINISTRATION AND DOSAGE

General Dosing Information

Before the ointment is applied, the affected areas should be washed with soap and water and then dried thoroughly.

For acne:

Cream/Ointment/Bar soap

Adults/Pediatrics: Apply to affected area as needed.

Lotion

Adults/Pediatrics: Apply to affected area 2 or 3 times a day.

For seborrheic dermatitis:

Ointment

Adults/Pediatrics: Apply to affected area 1 or 2 times a day.

Drug Interactions for Sulfur

Precipitant Drug	Object Drug	Effect On Object Drug	Description
Alcohol-containing preparations, topical (e.g., after-shave lotions, astringents, perfumed toiletries, shaving creams/lotions)	Sulfur	↑	Concurrent use with sulfur may cause a cumulative irritant or drying effect, especially with the application of peeling, desquamating, or abrasive agents, resulting in excessive irritation of the skin
Abrasive or medicated soaps/cleansers			
Acne preparations or preparations containing a peeling agent (e.g., benzoyl peroxide, resorcinol, salicylic acid, tretinoin, other topical agents)			
Cosmetics/soaps with a strong drying effect			
Isotretinoin			
Medicated cosmetics/cover-ups			
Mercury compounds, topical	Sulfur	↔	Concurrent use with sulfur may result in a chemical reaction releasing hydrogen sulfide, which has a foul odor, may be irritating, and may stain the skin black.

SULFUR PRODUCTS	
Brand Name	**Dosage Form**
Sulfoam (Doak)	Shampoo: 2%
Sulpho-Lac (Doak)	Cream: 5%
Sulpho-Lac Soap (Doak)	Liquid: 5%

DOSING INFORMATION FOR ACNE PRODUCTS

The following table provides a quick comparison of the ingredients and dosages of common brand-name OTC drugs. Products are listed alphabetically by generic ingredient and brand name.

BRAND NAME	GENERIC INGREDIENT/STRENGTH	DOSE
BENZOYL PEROXIDE		
Clean & Clear Continuous Control Acne Cleanser *(Johnson & Johnson/Merck Consumer)*	Benzoyl Peroxide 10%	**Adults & Peds:** Use bid.
Clean & Clear Persa-Gel 10, Maximum Strength *(Johnson & Johnson/Merck Consumer)*	Benzoyl Peroxide 10%	**Adults & Peds:** Use qd-tid.
Clearasil Maximum Strength Acne Treatment vanishing cream *(Boots Healthcare)*	Benzoyl Peroxide 10%	**Adults & Peds:** Use qd-tid.
Clearasil Total Control Acne Crisis Clear Up *(Boots Healthcare)*	Benzoyl Peroxide 10%	**Adults & Peds:** Use qd-tid.
Clearasil Ultra Acne Treatment tinted cream *(Boots Healthcare)*	Benzoyl Peroxide 10%	**Adults & Peds:** Use tid.
Clearasil Ultra Acne Treatment vanishing cream *(Boots Healthcare)*	Benzoyl Peroxide 10%	**Adults & Peds:** Use tid.
Neutrogena Clear Pore Cleanser Mask *(Neutrogena)*	Benzoyl Peroxide 3.5%	**Adults & Peds:** Use biw-tiw.
Neutrogena On-the-Spot Acne Treatment vanishing cream *(Neutrogena)*	Benzoyl Peroxide 2.5%	**Adults & Peds:** Apply qd initially, then bid-tid.
Oxy 10 Balance Oil-Free Maximum Strength Acne Wash *(GlaxoSmithKline Consumer Healthcare)*	Benzoyl Peroxide 10%	**Adults & Peds:** Use qd-tid.
Oxy Balance Acne Treatment for Sensitive Skin vanishing cream *(GlaxoSmithKline Consumer Healthcare)*	Benzoyl Peroxide 5%	**Adults & Peds:** Use qd-tid.
Oxy Balance Maximum Acne Treatment tinted lotion *(GlaxoSmithKline Consumer Healthcare)*	Benzoyl Peroxide 10%	**Adults & Peds:** Use qd-tid.
PanOxyl Aqua Gel Maximum Strength gel *(Stiefel)*	Benzoyl Peroxide 10%	**Adults & Peds:** Apply qd initially, then bid-tid.
PanOxyl Bar 10% Maximum Strength *(Stiefel)*	Benzoyl Peroxide 10%	**Adults & Peds:** Use qd initially, then bid-tid.
PanOxyl Bar 5% *(Stiefel)*	Benzoyl Peroxide 5%	**Adults & Peds:** Use qd initially, then bid-tid.
ZAPZYT Maximum Strength Acne Treatment gel *(Waltman Pharmaceuticals)*	Benzoyl Peroxide 10%	**Adults & Peds:** Use qd-tid.
ZAPZYT Treatment Bar *(Waltman Pharmaceuticals)*	Benzoyl Peroxide 10%	**Adults & Peds:** Use qd-tid.
SALICYLIC ACID		
Aveeno Clear Complexion Foaming Cleanser *(Johnson & Johnson/Merck Consumer)*	Salicylic Acid 0.5%	**Adults & Peds:** Use daily.
Aveeno Correcting Treatment, Clear Complexion *(Johnson & Johnson/Merck Consumer)*	Salicylic Acid 1%	**Adults & Peds:** Use qd-tid.
Biore Blemish Fighting Cleansing Cloths *(Kao Brands Company)*	Salicylic Acid 0.5%	**Adults & Peds:** Use qd-tid.
Biore Blemish Fighting Ice Cleanser *(Kao Brands Company)*	Salicylic Acid 2%	**Adults & Peds:** Use qd.
Bye Bye Blemish Acne Lemon Scrub *(Beauty Beat)*	Salicylic Acid 1%	**Adults & Peds:** Use qd-bid.
Bye Bye Blemish Drying Lotion *(Beauty Beat)*	Salicylic Acid 2%	**Adults & Peds:** Apply pm.
Bye Bye Blemish Purifying Acne Mask *(Beauty Beat)*	Salicylic Acid 0.5%	**Adults & Peds:** Use qd.

DOSING INFORMATION FOR ACNE PRODUCTS (cont.)

Brand Name	Generic Ingredient/Strength	Dose
Clean & Clear Advantage Acne Cleanser (Johnson & Johnson/Merck Consumer)	Salicylic Acid 2%	**Adults & Peds:** Use qd.
Clean & Clear Advantage Daily Cleansing Pads (Johnson & Johnson/Merck Consumer)	Salicylic Acid 2%	**Adults & Peds:** Use qd.
Clean & Clear Blackhead Clearing Astringent (Johnson & Johnson/Merck Consumer)	Salicylic Acid 1%	**Adults & Peds:** Use qd.
Clean & Clear Blackhead Clearing Daily Cleansing Pads (Johnson & Johnson/Merck Consumer)	Salicylic Acid 1%	**Adults & Peds:** Use qd.
Clean & Clear Blackhead Clearing Scrub (Johnson & Johnson/Merck Consumer)	Salicylic Acid 2%	**Adults & Peds:** Use qd.
Clean & Clear Clear Advantage Daily Acne Clearing lotion (Johnson & Johnson/Merck Consumer)	Salicylic Acid 1%	**Adults & Peds:** Use qd.
Clean & Clear Continuous Control Acne Wash, Oil Free (Johnson & Johnson/Merck Consumer)	Salicylic Acid 2%	**Adults & Peds:** Use qd.
Clean & Clear Facial Cleansing Bar, Blackhead Clearing (Johnson & Johnson/ Merck Consumer)	Salicylic Acid 0.5%	**Adults & Peds:** Use qd.
Clean & Clear Oil-Free Dual Action Moisturizer lotion (Johnson & Johnson/ Merck Consumer)	Salicylic Acid 0.5%	**Adults & Peds:** Use qd-tid.
Clearasil 3 in 1 Acne Defense Cleanser (Boots Healthcare)	Salicylic Acid 2%	**Adults & Peds:** Use qd-tid.
Clearasil Acne Fighting Cleansing Wipes (Boots Healthcare)	Salicylic Acid 2%	**Adults & Peds:** Use qd.
Clearasil Acne Fighting Facial Moisturizer (Boots Healthcare)	Salicylic Acid 2%	**Adults & Peds:** Use qd-tid.
Clearasil Acne Fighting Foaming Cleanser (Boots Healthcare)	Salicylic Acid 2%	**Adults & Peds:** Use bid-tid.
Clearasil Blackhead Clearing Pads with Targeted Action (Boots Healthcare)	Salicylic Acid 2%	**Adults & Peds:** Use qd-tid.
Clearasil Blackhead Clearing Scrub (Boots Healthcare)	Salicylic Acid 2.0%	**Adults & Peds:** Use qd.
Clearasil Icewash, Acne Gel Cleanser (Boots Healthcare)	Salicylic Acid 2%	**Adults & Peds:** Use qd.
Clearasil Maximum Strength Pore Cleansing Pads (Boots Healthcare)	Salicylic Acid 2%	**Adults & Peds:** Use qd-tid.
Clearasil Oil Control Acne Wash (Boots Healthcare)	Salicylic Acid 2%	**Adults & Peds:** Use qd.
Clearasil Overnight Acne Defense Gel (Boots Healthcare)	Salicylic Acid 2%	**Adults & Peds:** Use qd-tid.
Clearasil Total Control Daily Skin Perfecting Treatment (Boot Healthcare)	Salicylic Acid 0.5%	**Adults & Peds:** Use qd.
Clearasil Total Control Deep Pore Cream Cleanser (Boots Healthcare)	Salicylic Acid 2%	**Adults & Peds:** Use qd.
Clearasil Ultra Acne Clearing Scrub (Boots Healthcare)	Salicylic Acid (2%)	**Adults & Peds:** Use qd.
Clearasil Ultra Deep Pore Cleansing Pads (Boots Healthcare)	Salicylic Acid (2%)	**Adults & Peds:** Use qd-tid.
L'Oreal Pure Zone Pore Unclogging Scrub Cleanser (L'Oreal)	Salicylic Acid 1%	**Adults & Peds:** Use bid.
L'Oreal Pure Zone Skin Clearing Foaming Cleanser (L'Oreal)	Salicylic Acid 2%	**Adults & Peds:** Use bid.

DOSING INFORMATION FOR ACNE PRODUCTS (cont.)

Brand Name	Generic Ingredient/Strength	Dose
Neutrogena Clear Pore Treatment—Night Time *(Neutrogena)*	Salicylic Acid 1%	**Adults & Peds:** Use qd.
Neutrogena Advanced Solutions Acne Mark Fading Peel with CelluZyme *(Neutrogena)*	Salicylic Acid 2.0%	**Adults & Peds:** Use qw-tiw.
Neutrogena Blackhead Eliminating Astringent *(Neutrogena)*	Salicylic Acid 0.5%	**Adults & Peds:** Use qd-tid.
Neutrogena Blackhead Eliminating Daily Scrub *(Neutrogena)*	Salicylic Acid 2%	**Adults & Peds:** Use prn.
Neutrogena Blackhead Eliminating Treatment Mask *(Neutrogena)*	Salicylic Acid 0.5%	**Adults & Peds:** Use biw-tiw.
Neutrogena Body Clear Body Scrub *(Neutrogena)*	Salicylic Acid 2%	**Adults:** Use qd.
Neutrogena Body Clear Body Wash *(Neutrogena)*	Salicylic Acid 2%	**Adults:** Use qd.
Neutrogena Clear Pore Oil-Controlling Astringent *(Neutrogena)*	Salicylic Acid 2%	**Adults & Peds:** Use qd-tid.
Neutrogena Maximum Strength Oil Controlling Pads *(Neutrogena)*	Salicylic Acid 2%	**Adults & Peds:** Use qd-tid.
Neutrogena Multi-Vitamin Acne Treatment *(Neutrogena)*	Salicylic Acid 1.5%	**Adults & Peds:** Use prn.
Neutrogena Oil Free Acne Wash Cleansing Cloths *(Neutrogena)*	Salicylic Acid 2.0%	**Adults & Peds:** Use qd.
Neutrogena Oil Free Acne Wash Cream Cleanser *(Neutrogena)*	Salicylic Acid 2%	**Adults & Peds:** Use bid.
Neutrogena Rapid Clear Acne Defense Lotion *(Neutrogena)*	Salicylic Acid 2%	**Adults & Peds:** Use qd-tid.
Neutrogena Rapid Clear Acne Eliminating Gel *(Neutrogena)*	Salicylic Acid 2%	**Adults & Peds:** Use qd-tid.
Neutrogena Skin Clearing Face Wash *(Neutrogena)*	Salicylic Acid 1.5%	**Adults & Peds:** Use bid.
Neutrogena Skin Clearing Moisturizer *(Neutrogena)*	Salicylic Acid 2%	**Adults & Peds:** Use prn.
Noxzema Continuous Clarifying Toner *(Procter & Gamble)*	Salicylic Acid 1%	**Adults & Peds:** Use qd-tid.
Noxzema Continuous Clean Deep Foaming Cleanser *(Procter & Gamble)*	Salicylic Acid 2%	**Adults & Peds:** Use qd.
Noxzema Triple Clean Pads *(Procter & Gamble)*	Salicylic Acid 2%	**Adults & Peds:** Use qd-tid.
Olay Daily Facials Clarity Daily Scrub *(Procter & Gamble)*	Salicylic Acid 2%	**Adults & Peds:** Apply qd.
Olay Daily Facials Clarity, Purifying Toner *(Procter & Gamble)*	Salicylic Acid 2%	**Adults & Peds:** Apply qd-tid.
Oxy Balance Daily Cleansing Pads, Sensitive Skin *(GlaxoSmithKline Consumer Healthcare)*	Salicylic Acid 0.5%	**Adults & Peds:** Use qd-tid.
Oxy Balance Deep Pore Cleansing Pads, Gentle *(GlaxoSmithKline Consumer Healthcare)*	Salicylic Acid 0.5%	**Adults & Peds:** Use qd-tid.
Oxy Deep Pore Acne Medicated Cleansing Pads, Maximum Strength *(GlaxoSmithKline Consumer Healthcare)*	Salicylic Acid 2%	**Adults & Peds:** Use qd-tid.
Phisoderm Clear Confidence Body Wash *(Chattem)*	Salicylic Acid 2%	**Adults & Peds:** Use qd.
Phisoderm Clear Confidence Facial Wash *(Chattem)*	Salicylic Acid 2%	**Adults & Peds:** Use qd.
St. Ives Medicated Apricot Scrub *(St. Ives Laboratories)*	Salicylic Acid 2%	**Adults & Peds:** Use qd.

DOSING INFORMATION FOR ACNE PRODUCTS (cont.)

Brand Name	Generic Ingredient/Strength	Dose
Stridex Facewipes to Go with Acne Medication *(Blistex)*	Salicylic Acid 0.5%	**Adults & Peds:** Use qd-tid.
Stridex Triple Action Acne Pads Maximum Strength, Alcohol Free *(Blistex)*	Salicylic Acid 2%	**Adults & Peds:** Use qd-tid.
Stridex Triple Action Acne Pads with Salicylic Acid, Super Scrub *(Blistex)*	Salicylic Acid 2.0%	**Adults & Peds:** Use qd-tid.
Stridex Triple Action Medicated Acne Pads, Sensitive Skin *(Blistex)*	Salicylic Acid 0.5%	**Adults & Peds:** Use qd-tid.
ZAPZYT Acne Wash Treatment For Face & Body *(Waltman Pharmaceuticals)*	Salicylic Acid 2%	**Adults & Peds:** Use bid.
ZAPZYT Pore Treatment Gel *(Waltman Pharmceuticals)*	Salicylic Acid 2%	**Adults & Peds:** Use qd-tid.

Alopecia

The hair follicle cycle includes phases of growth (anagen), involution (catagen), and rest (telogen). Normally, up to 90% of the hair follicles in the scalp are growing (anagen), less than 1% are undergoing involution (catagen), and up to 10% are resting (telogen). The duration of anagen determines the length of hair, and the volume of the hair bulb determines the diameter. The average growth rate of terminal scalp hairs is approximately 1 cm per month (1 inch every 2.5 months), and the average duration of anagen ranges from 2 to 7 years. Growth rates and hair cycles can be affected by age, genetic factors, gender, race, and season. The average telogen phase on the scalp lasts about 100 days, after which the hairs are shed; up to 100 telogen hairs may be shed from the scalp daily. Because hair cycles are asynchronous, hair shedding may be diffuse and often goes unnoticed until about 50% of the scalp hair is lost.

Both genes and hormones play a role in the pathophysiology of male androgenetic alopecia (male pattern alopecia). This male pattern alopecia appears to be inherited in either an autosomal dominant and/or polygenic manner. The expression of the disease is influenced by androgens and in particular dihydrotestosterone (DHT). Testosterone is converted to DHT by the enzyme 5-alpha-reductase, which has two isoenzymes (Type I and Type II). DHT is elevated in balding scalp skin, causing the miniaturization of hair follicles in genetically predisposed individuals, with resultant miniaturized hair fibers. On the scalp this process may be perceived as thinning or balding. Patients with genetic absence of Type II 5-alpha-reductase do not develop male androgenetic alopecia, supporting the importance of DHT in the development of male androgenetic alopecia.

Female pattern alopecia has been described in four categories: early-onset with androgen excess; early-onset without androgen excess; late-onset/postmenopausal with androgen excess; and late-onset/postmenopausal without androgen excess. Results of biochemical studies on scalp skin biopsy specimens from balding females suggest that aromatase levels are elevated in frontal scalp skin specimens as compared to biopsy samples from the balding area. Thus, it has been postulated that this enzyme may be "protective" and prevent the development of the type of balding seen in males. Most women with alopecia do not have any signs or symptoms of hyperandrogenism, and serum testosterone and DHT levels are usually normal. Affected women may develop their balding patterns in puberty or in the perimenopausal or menopausal periods. Women who develop balding in puberty will frequently have a positive family history for pattern baldness in both male and female family members. Women who develop pattern alopecia in the menopausal and perimenopausal periods frequently complain of diffuse hair shedding, corresponding changes in hair density, and even changes in hair texture. Increased androgen metabolism in the hair follicle has been implicated in the pathogenesis of female pattern alopecia.

Currently, minoxidil is the only FDA-approved OTC medication indicated for the treatment of hair loss in both men and women.

MINOXIDIL

PHARMACOLOGY

Topical minoxidil stimulates hair growth in some persons with alopecia androgenetica. Its mechanism of action has not been established, but possible explanations include increased cutaneous blood flow as a result of vasodilation, stimulation of resting hair follicles (telogen phase) into active growth (anagen phase), and stimulation of hair follicle cells.

INDICATIONS

Alopecia androgenetica (treatment)—Minoxidil topical solution is indicated for treatment of alopecia androgenetica (also called male-pattern baldness in men) in both adult males and females for the 2% strength and in adult males only for the 5% strength. Alopecia androgenetica is expressed in males as baldness of the vertex of the scalp and/or as frontal hair recession. In females, it is expressed as diffuse hair loss or thinning in the frontoparietal areas. Topical minoxidil is less likely to be effective in men with predominantly frontal hair loss than in patients with the other forms of alopecia androgenetica.

CONTRAINDICATIONS

Risk-benefit should be considered when the following medical problems exist

- Allergy to minoxidil or propylene glycol
- Cardiovascular disease or hypertension (Patients with these conditions were excluded from the clinical trials of topical minoxidil because of the potential that adverse systemic effects could occur for the rare patient who might receive significant systemic absorption from its use. Although their deaths were not attributable to topical minoxidil treatment, unexplained sudden death occurred in two patients with underlying undetected, untreated cardiovascular conditions who used topical minoxidil.)
- Skin irritation or abrasion, including scalp psoriasis or severe sunburn (systemic absorption may be increased)

WARNINGS/PRECAUTIONS

Pregnancy: Adequate and well-controlled studies in humans have not been done.

Breastfeeding: Orally administered minoxidil is distributed into breast milk. It is not known whether topical minoxidil is distributed into breast milk. However, because of the potential for adverse effects, topical minoxidil should not be administered to women who are nursing.

ADVERSE REACTIONS

Those indicating need for medical attention: Incidence less frequent

Contact dermatitis (itching or skin rash).

Incidence rare:

Allergic reaction (reddened skin, skin rash, facial swelling); alopecia, increased (increased hair loss); burning of scalp; folliculitis (acne, inflammation or soreness at root of hair)—at site of application.

Signs and symptoms of systemic absorption: Rare

Chest pain; fast or irregular heartbeat; headache; hypotension — usually not symptomatic; lightheadedness; neuritis (numbness or tingling of hands, feet, or face); reflex hypertension; sexual dysfunction (decrease of sexual ability or desire); sodium and water retention (swelling of face, hands, feet, or lower legs; rapid weight gain); vasodilation (flushing, headache); visual disturbances, including decreased visual acuity (blurred vision or other changes in vision).

ADMINISTRATION AND DOSAGE

General Dosing Information

If systemic effects occur, topical minoxidil should be discontinued and the patient should be seen by a physician. Females are advised not to use the 5% solution because it does not work any better in females than the 2% solution and has caused excessive or unusual facial hair growth in females. Minoxidil will not work in males or females who experience hair loss caused by endocrine or nutritional problems or caused by skin damage that can occur from scarring, burns, or severe hair-grooming methods, such as hair loss from ponytails or corn rowing. Minoxidil will not work for sudden or patchy hair loss.

If dermatologic reactions occur, discontinuation of topical minoxidil therapy should be considered. Patients should not apply minoxidil if skin is red, infected, irritated, or painful. Hair loss may continue for 2 weeks after initiation of minoxidil therapy, but if it continues past 2 weeks, patients should notify their physician. If hair growth has not improved in 4 months of therapy, patients should reconsider continuing the use of topical minoxidil. Patients should be instructed about proper administration of topical minoxidil, including the avoidance of inhaling the spray mist. In the event of accidental contact with sensitive areas (eye, abraded skin, mucous membranes), the sensitive area that is burning or irritated should be washed with copious amounts of cool water. Application should be restricted to the thinning or balding area of the scalp, and hands should be washed afterwards to avoid inadvertent application of minoxidil to inappropriate areas of the body. Waiting 2 to 4 hours for minoxidil to dry before going to bed is also recommended to avoid wiping the medication on other areas of the body and to avoid rubbing it off inadvertently onto bed linens. Minoxidil may stain bed linens, hats, or clothing if it has not fully dried.

Topical minoxidil should be applied to the dry skin of the scalp. A hairdryer should not be used after application, as it might interfere with the efficacy of minoxidil. At least 4 hours should be allowed after minoxidil application before shampooing. Hair colorings, hair permanents, and hair relaxers may be used with topical minoxidil. However, to avoid skin irritation, patients should wash minoxidil from the scalp first before having hair treatments; avoid using minoxidil 24 hours before and 24 hours after having chemical treatments; and avoid making up missed doses by using more minoxidil when treatment is reinitiated.

Solution

Adults/Pediatrics up to 65 years old: Apply 1 mL to the scalp 2 times a day.

Drug Interactions for Minoxidil

Precipitent Drug	Object Drug	Effect on Object Drug	Description
◆ Corticosteroids, topicals ◆ Petrolatum, topicals ◆ Retinoids, topicals	Minoxidil	↑	Concurrent use is not recommended. Using these drugs on the same area may enhance cutaneous absorption of topical minoxidil because of increased stratum corneum permeability.

◆ = Major clinical significance

MINOXIDIL PRODUCTS

Brand Name	Dosage Form
Rogaine for Men (Pharmacia)	Solution: 2%
Rogaine for Men Extra Strength(Pharmacia)	Solution: 5%
Rogaine for Women(Pharmacia)	Solution: 2%

DOSING INFORMATION FOR ALOPECIA PRODUCTS

The following table provides a quick comparison of the ingredients and dosages of common brand-name OTC drugs. Products are listed alphabetically by brand name.

BRAND NAME	GENERIC INGREDIENT/STRENGTH	DOSE
Men's Rogaine Extra Strength Hair Regrowth Treatment, Ocean Rush liquid *(Pfizer Consumer Healthcare)*	Minoxidil 5%	**Adults:** Apply bid.
Men's Rogaine Extra Strength Hair Regrowth Treatment, Ocean Rush liquid *(Pfizer Consumer Healthcare)*	Minoxidil 5%	**Adults:** Apply bid.
Men's Rogaine Regular Strength Hair Regrowth Treatment, Ocean Rush liquid *(Pfizer Consumer Healthcare)*	Minoxidil 2%	**Adults:** Apply bid.
Women's Rogaine Hair Regrowth Treatment *(Pfizer Consumer Healthcare)*	Minoxidil 2%	**Adults:** Apply bid.
Women's Rogaine Hair Regrowth Treatment, Spring bloom liquid *(Pfizer Consumer Healthcare)*	Minoxidil 2%	**Adults:** Apply bid.

Athlete's Foot and Jock Itch

Athlete's foot (tinea pedis) refers to dermatophytosis of the plantar surface or the toe webs. There are three common recognized patterns: (1) interdigital; (2) inflammatory or vesicular; and (3) chronic hyperkeratotic (also called moccasin foot). The *interdigital* variety is the most common, and the patient typically presents with macerated, fissured, scaling, interdigital lesions usually involving the web space of the fourth and fifth toes. In the *vesicular* variety of tinea pedis, there are painful pruritic vesicles or bullous lesions on the instep. Infection may be disabling, and this variety has historically been a particular problem in the military. The dermatophytic reaction can be associated with the vesicular variety. When this reaction occurs, the patient may have an eczematous-appearing rash on one or both hands that may resemble dishidrotic eczema on the palms or sides of fingers. This rash is considered a hypersensitivity reaction to the fungal foot infection. The *hyperkeratotic* variety of tinea pedis is characterized by dry, scaly, hyperkeratotic changes on the plantar surface of one or both feet. Fungal nail disease generally is present, and the patient also may have palmar infection (tinea manuum). Chronic infections that are recalcitrant to therapy typically occur.

Jock itch (tinea cruris) refers to dermatophytosis of the inguinal region, including the gluteal folds, the crural folds, and the proximal medial thighs. Intense pruritus is common, hence the lay term "jock itch." Adult men are more commonly infected than women. Risk factors include maceration and occlusion. The scrotal skin appears immune to infection by dermatophytes, although candidiasis and erythrasma occur in this region. Women are more likely to present with cutaneous candidiasis in the genital and inguinal areas than with dermatophytosis.

There are currently several OTC antifungals available in different dosage forms (creams, powders, sprays) to treat athlete's foot and jock itch, including undecylenic acid, tolnaftate, miconazole, clotrimazole, terbinafine, and butenafine.

BUTENAFINE

PHARMACOLOGY

Butenafine is fungicidal and inhibits the epoxidation of squalene. This action blocks the biosynthesis of ergosterol, an important component of fungal cell membranes.

INDICATIONS

Tinea pedis (treatment); *tinea corporis* (treatment); *tinea cruris* (treatment)—Butenafine is indicated in the treatment of interdigital tinea pedis (athlete's foot), tinea corporis (ringworm), or tinea cruris (jock itch) due to *Epidermophyton floccosum*, *Trichophyton mentagrophytes*, *T rubrum*, or *T tonsurans*.

Tinea (pityriasis) versicolor (treatment)—Butenafine is indicated in the treatment of tinea (pityriasis) versicolor due to *Malassezia furfur*.

CONTRAINDICATIONS

Risk-benefit should be considered when the following medical problem exists:

• Sensitivity to butenafine or allylamines.

WARNINGS/PRECAUTIONS

Patients sensitive to allylamine antifungal agents may also be sensitive to butenafine.

Pregnancy: FDA Category B. Adequate and well-controlled studies in humans have not been done.

Breastfeeding: It is not known whether butenafine is distributed into breast milk. Problems in humans have not been documented.

ADVERSE REACTIONS

Those indicating need for medical attention: Incidence rare

Contact dermatitis (rash); hypersensitivity (blistering, burning, itching, oozing, stinging, swelling, or other signs of skin irritation not present before use of this medicine); redness.

ADMINISTRATION AND DOSAGE

For tinea pedis, interdigital:

Adults/Pediatrics ≥12 years of age: Apply to affected skin and surrounding areas, once a day for 4 weeks or twice a day for 7 days.

For tinea corporis/tinea cruris/tinea (pityriasis) versicolor:

Adults/Pediatrics ≥12 years of age: Apply to affected skin and surrounding areas, once a day for 2 weeks.

CLOTRIMAZOLE

PHARMACOLOGY

Clotrimazole belongs to the class of drugs known as azole antifungals. These drugs are fungistatic and may be fungicidal, depending on concentration. Their exact mechanism of action is unknown. Azoles inhibit biosynthesis of ergosterol or other sterols, damaging the fungal cell membrane and altering its permeability. As a result, loss of essential intracellular elements may occur.

Azoles also inhibit biosynthesis of triglycerides and phospholipids by fungi. In addition, azoles inhibit oxidative and peroxidative enzyme activity, resulting in intracellular buildup of toxic concentrations of hydrogen peroxide, which may contribute to deterioration of subcellular organelles and cellular necrosis. In *Candida albicans*, azoles inhibit transformation of blastospores into invasive mycelial form.

INDICATIONS

Candidiasis, cutaneous (treatment)—Topical clotrimazole is indicated in the treatment of cutaneous candidiasis (moniliasis) caused by *Candida albicans*.

BUTENAFINE PRODUCTS	
Brand Name	**Dosage Form**
Lotrimin Ultra (Schering)	**Cream:** 1%
Mentax (Mylan Bertek)	**Cream:** 1%

Tinea corporis (treatment); *tinea cruris* (treatment); *tinea pedis* (treatment)—Topical clotrimazole is indicated in the treatment of tinea corporis (ringworm of the body), tinea cruris (ringworm of the groin, or "jock itch"), and tinea pedis (ringworm of the foot, or "athlete's foot") caused by *Trichophyton rubrum, T mentagrophytes, Epidermophyton floccosum,* and *Microsporum canis.*

Tinea (pityriasis) versicolor (treatment)—Topical clotrimazole is indicated in the treatment of tinea versicolor (pityriasis versicolor, or "sun fungus") caused by *Malassezia furfur.*

Paronychia (treatment); *tinea barbae* (treatment); *tinea capitis* (treatment)—Topical clotrimazole is used in the treatment of paronychia, tinea barbae (ringworm of the beard, or "barber's itch"), and tinea capitis.

CONTRAINDICATIONS

Risk-benefit should be considered when the following medical problem exists:

- Sensitivity to clotrimazole.

WARNINGS/PRECAUTIONS

Pregnancy: FDA Category B. Adequate and well-controlled studies in humans have not been done during the first trimester. Studies in humans given intravaginal clotrimazole during the second and third trimesters have not shown that clotrimazole causes adverse effects on the fetus.

Breastfeeding: It is not known whether clotrimazole, applied topically, is distributed into breast milk. However, problems in humans have not been documented.

ADVERSE REACTIONS

Those indicating need for medical attention:

Hypersensitivity (skin rash, hives, blistering, burning, itching, peeling, redness, stinging, swelling, or other sign of skin irritation not present before therapy).

ADMINISTRATION AND DOSAGE

General Dosing Information

Use of topical antifungals may lead to skin sensitization, resulting in hypersensitivity reactions with subsequent topical use of the medication. Improvement of condition, with relief of pruritus, usually occurs within the first week of therapy. When this medication is used in the treatment of candidiasis, occlusive dressings should be avoided since they provide conditions that favor growth of yeast and release of its irritating endotoxin.

Cream/Lotion/Topical solution

Adults/Pediatrics: Apply to affected area of skin and surrounding areas, 2 times a day, morning and evening.

MICONAZOLE

PHARMACOLOGY

Miconazole belongs to the class of drugs known as azole antifungals. These drugs are fungistatic and may be fungicidal, depending on concentration. Their exact mechanism of action is unknown. Azoles inhibit biosynthesis of ergosterol or other sterols, damaging the fungal cell membrane and altering its permeability. As a result, loss of essential intracellular elements may occur.

Azoles also inhibit biosynthesis of triglycerides and phospholipids by fungi. In addition, azoles inhibit oxidative and peroxidative enzyme activity, resulting in intracellular buildup of toxic concentrations of hydrogen peroxide, which may contribute to deterioration of subcellular organelles and cellular necrosis. In *Candida albicans,* azoles inhibit transformation of blastospores into invasive mycelial form.

INDICATIONS

Candidiasis, cutaneous (treatment)—Miconazole is indicated in the topical treatment of cutaneous candidiasis caused by *Candida albicans.*

Tinea corporis (treatment); *tinea cruris* (treatment); *tinea pedis* (treatment)—Miconazole is indicated in the topical treatment of tinea corporis (ringworm of the body), tinea cruris (ringworm of the groin, or "jock itch"), and tinea pedis (ringworm of the foot, or "athlete's foot") caused by *Trichophyton rubrum, T mentagrophytes,* and *Epidermophyton.*

Tinea versicolor (treatment)—Miconazole is indicated in the topical treatment of tinea versicolor (pityriasis versicolor, or "sun fungus") caused by *Malassezia furfur.*

Paronychia (treatment); *tinea barbae* (treatment); *tinea capitis* (treatment)—Miconazole is used in the topical treatment of paronychia, tinea barbae (ringworm of the beard, or "barber's itch"), and tinea capitis.

CONTRAINDICATIONS

Risk-benefit should be considered when the following medical problem exists:

- Sensitivity to topical miconazole

WARNINGS/PRECAUTIONS

Pregnancy: Problems in humans have not been documented.

Breastfeeding: Problems in humans have not been documented.

CLOTRIMAZOLE PRODUCTS	
Brand Name	**Dosage Form**
Cruex (Novartis)	**Cream**: 1%
Lotrimin (Schering-Plough)	**Cream**: 1% **Lotion**: 1% **Solution**: 1%
Lotrimin AF (Schering-Plough)	**Cream**: 1% **Lotion**: 1% **Solution**: 1%

MICONAZOLE PRODUCTS	
Brand Name	**Dosage Form**
Baza Antifungal (Coloplast)	**Cream**: 2%
Desenex (Novartis)	**Powder**: 2% **Spray**: 2%
Lotrimin AF (Schering)	**Powder**: 2% **Spray**: 2%
Micatin (Pharmacia)	**Cream**: 2% **Powder**: 2% **Spray**: 2%
Neosporin AF (Pfizer)	**Cream**: 2% **Powder**: 2% **Spray**: 2%
Zeasorb AF (Stiefil)	**Lotion**: 2% **Powder**: 2%

ADVERSE REACTIONS

Those indicating need for medical attention:

Blistering, burning, redness, skin rash, or other sign of skin irritation not present before therapy.

ADMINISTRATION AND DOSAGE

General Dosing Information

Use of topical antifungals may lead to skin sensitization, resulting in hypersensitivity reactions with subsequent topical or systemic use of the medication. The lotion is preferred for use on intertriginous areas; if the cream is used, it should be used sparingly and massaged in well to avoid maceration effects. When this medication is used in the treatment of candidiasis, occlusive dressings should be avoided since they provide conditions that favor growth of yeast and release of its irritating endotoxin. To reduce the possibility of recurrence, *Candida* infections, tinea cruris, and tinea corporis should be treated for 2 weeks and tinea pedis for 1 month.

Aersol powder/Aerosol solution/Powder

For tinea corporis/tinea cruris/tinea pedis:

Adults/Pediatrics: Apply to affected area 2 times a day, morning and evening.

Cream/Lotion

For candidiasis, cutaneous/tinea corporis/tinea cruris/tinea pedis:

Adults/Pediatrics: Apply to affected area 2 times a day, morning and evening.

For tinea versicolor:

Adults/Pediatrics: Apply to affected area once a day.

TERBINAFINE

PHARMACOLOGY

Terbinafine is fungistatic and interferes with membrane synthesis and growth; it may also be fungicidal. Terbinafine inhibits squalene epoxidase (a key enzyme in sterol biosynthesis in fungi), which results in a deficiency in ergosterol and a corresponding increase in squalene within the fungal cell, causing fungal cell death.

INDICATIONS

Tinea corporis (treatment), *tinea cruris* (treatment), *tinea pedis, interdigital* (treatment), and *tinea pedis, plantar* (treatment)—Terbinafine is indicated as a primary agent in the topical treatment of tinea corporis (ringworm of the body), tinea cruris (ringworm of the groin, or "jock itch"), interdigital tinea pedis (ringworm of the foot, or "athlete's foot") caused by *Trichophyton rubrum*, *T mentagrophytes*, or *Epidermophyton floccosum*, and plantar tinea pedis (moccasin-type) caused by *T mentagrophytes* or *T rubrum*.

Tinea versicolor (treatment)—Terbinafine cream and solution are indicated for the topical treatment of tinea versicolor due to *Malassezia furfur*.

Candidiasis, cutaneous (treatment)—Terbinafine cream is indicated for the topical treatment of yeast infections of the skin, principally those caused by the genus *Candida*, (eg, *C albicans*).

CONTRAINDICATIONS

Risk-benefit should be considered when the following medical problem exists:

- Onychomycosis (patients with onychomycosis are less likely to have a favorable response to terbinafine therapy for plantar tinea pedis).

WARNINGS/PRECAUTIONS

Patients sensitive to the oral form of terbinafine may be sensitive to the topical form also.

Pregnancy: FDA Category B. Adequate and well-controlled studies in humans have not been done.

Breastfeeding: Terbinafine is distributed into breast milk after oral administration. However, it is not known whether terbinafine is distributed into breast milk after topical administration. Breastfeeding women should avoid applying topical terbinafine to the breasts.

ADVERSE REACTIONS

Those indicating need for medical attention: Incidence rare

- Dryness, redness, itching, burning, peeling, rash, stinging, tingling, or other signs of skin irritation not present before use of this medicine.

ADMINISTRATION AND DOSAGE

General Dosing Information

For cream dosage form:

Improvement is gradual. In many patients treated with shorter durations of therapy (1-2 weeks), improvement may continue during the 2 to 6 weeks after completion of therapy. Patients should not be considered therapeutic failures until after the 2- to 6-week observation period. The patient's diagnosis should be reviewed if a successful outcome is not achieved by the end of the 6-week post-therapy period. A gauze strip may be placed over the cream if intertriginous infections are present.

For solution dosage form:

Relief of signs and symptoms usually begins within the 1-week treatment period. Continued improvement may occur over a period of 2 to 7 weeks after therapy has been completed.

Cream

For tinea corporis/tinea cruris:

Adults/Pediatrics ≥12 years of age: Apply to affected area and surrounding areas, 1 or 2 times a day. Treatment should be continued for at least 1 week *and* until there is significant improvement in the clinical signs and symptoms of the disease. Treatment should not be continued beyond 4 weeks.

For tinea pedis, interdigital:

Adults/Pediatrics ≥12 years of age: Apply to affected area and surrounding areas 2 times a day. Treatment should be continued

TERBINAFINE PRODUCTS	
Brand Name	**Dosage Form**
Lamisil AT Athlete's Foot (Novartis)	**Cream**: 1% **Spray**: 1%
Lamisil AT Jock Itch (Novartis)	**Cream**: 1% **Spray**: 1%
Lamisil AT for Women (Novartis)	**Cream**: 1%

for at least 1 week *and* until there is significant improvement in the clinical signs and symptoms of the disease. Treatment should not be continued beyond 4 weeks.

For tinea pedis, plantar:

Adults/Pediatrics ≥12 years of age: Apply to affected area and surrounding areas 2 times a day. Treatment should be continued for 2 weeks. Treatment may be affected by the presence of onychomycosis. Patients with a toenail infection may be less likely to respond favorably to terbinafine therapy.

For tinea versicolor:

Adults: Apply to affected area and surrounding areas 1 or 2 times a day for 2 weeks.

For cutaneous candidiasis:

Adults: Apply to affected area and surrounding areas, one or two times a day for two weeks.

Solution

For tinea corporis/tinea cruris:

Adults: Apply to affected area and surrounding areas once a day for 1 week. Treatment should be continued for at least 1 week *even though* symptoms of the disease may have improved.

For tinea pedis/tinea versicolor:

Adults: Apply to affected area and surrounding areas 2 times a day for 2 weeks. Treatment should be continued for at least 1 week *even though* symptoms of the disease may have improved.

TOLNAFTATE

PHARMACOLOGY

Tolnaftate is fungicidal but the exact mechanism of action is unknown. However, it has been reported to distort the hyphae and stunt mycelial growth in susceptible organisms.

INDICATIONS

Tinea capitis (treatment)—Tolnaftate is indicated in the topical treatment of tinea capitis.

Tinea corporis (treatment), *tinea cruris* (treatment), *tinea manuum* (treatment), and *tinea pedis* (treatment)—Tolnaftate is indicated in the topical treatment of tinea corporis (ringworm of the body), tinea cruris (ringworm of the groin, or "jock itch"), tinea manuum, and tinea pedis (ringworm of the foot, or "athlete's foot") caused by *Trichophyton rubrum, T mentagrophytes, T tonsurans, Microsporum canis, M audouini,* and *Epidermophyton floccosum.*

Tinea versicolor (treatment)—Tolnaftate is indicated in the topical treatment of tinea versicolor (pityriasis versicolor, or "sun fungus") caused by *Malassezia furfur.*

Tinea barbae (treatment)—Tolnaftate is used in the topical treatment of tinea barbae (ringworm of the beard, or "barber's itch").

WARNINGS/PRECAUTIONS

Pregnancy: Problems in humans have not been documented.

Breastfeeding: It is not known whether topical tolnaftate is distributed into breast milk. However, problems in humans have not been documented.

ADVERSE REACTIONS

Those indicating need for medical attention:

Hypersensitivity (skin irritation not present before therapy).

ADMINISTRATION AND DOSAGE

General Dosing Information

Therapy for a period of 2 to 3 weeks is usually sufficient; however, treatment for 4 to 6 weeks may be necessary, especially if thickening of the skin has occurred. The medication should be continued for 2 weeks after symptoms have disappeared. Tolnaftate may be used concurrently with an oral antifungal agent, such as griseofulvin, in the treatment of onychomycosis or chronic infections of the scalp, palms, or skin. The powder and powder aerosol forms are recommended for adjunctive use in fungal infections of intertriginous or other naturally moist skin areas in which drying may enhance the therapeutic response. They may also be used alone in the treatment of mild infections that respond to antifungal powder in conjunction with measures that promote skin hygiene. Following complete remission of the infection, the powder or powder aerosol may be continued as part of a daily personal hygiene program to help prevent reinfection.

Aerosol powder/Aerosol solution/Cream/Gel/Powder/Solution

Adults/Pediatrics ≥2 years of age: Apply to affected area 2 times a day.

UNDECYLENIC ACID

PHARMACOLOGY

Compound undecylenic acid has a fungistatic action. The zinc present in the zinc undecylenate component provides a beneficial astringent action, which aids in reducing rawness and irritation.

INDICATIONS

Compound undecylenic acid has been used for the topical treatment of tinea cruris, tinea pedis, and other tinea infections. However, in the opinion of US Pharmacopeia (USP) medical experts, it has been superseded by newer and more effective topical antifungal agents.

TOLNAFTATE PRODUCTS	
Brand Name	**Dosage Form**
Tinactin (Schering)	**Cream**: 1% **Powder**: 1% **Solution**: 1% **Spray**: 1%
Tinactin Jock Itch (Schering)	**Cream**: 1% **Powder**: 1%
Absorbine JR. Antifungal (W. F. Young)	**Cream**: 1%

CALCIUM UNDECYLENATE & UNDECYLENIC ACID PRODUCTS	
Brand Name	**Dosage Form**
Caldesene (Heritage)	**Powder**: 10%
Cruex (Novartis)	**Powder**: 10%
Elon Dual Defense (Dartmouth)	**Tincture**: 25%
Sanafitil (Tarmac)	**Spray**: 10%

WARNINGS/PRECAUTIONS

Pregnancy: Problems in humans have not been documented.

Breastfeeding: It is not known whether topical compound undecylenic acid is distributed into breast milk. However, problems in humans have not been documented.

ADVERSE REACTIONS

Those indicating need for medical attention:

Hypersensitivity (skin irritation not present before therapy).

ADMINISTRATION AND DOSAGE

General Dosing Information

Use of topical antifungals may lead to skin sensitization, resulting in hypersensitivity reactions with subsequent topical use of the medication. Before application of this medication, the affected and surrounding areas should be cleansed and thoroughly dried. The medication should be continued for 2 weeks after symptoms have disappeared. For persistent fungal infection, the ointment is used for nighttime application and the powder for daytime application to relieve burning and itching. Following complete remission of the infection, the powder or aerosol powder may be continued as part of a daily personal hygiene program to prevent reinfection.

Aerosol foam/Aerosol powder/Cream/Ointment/Powder/Solution

Adults/Pediatrics ≥2 years of age: Apply to affected area 2 times a day.

DOSING INFORMATION FOR ANTIFUNGAL PRODUCTS

The following table provides a quick comparison of the ingredients and dosages of common brand-name OTC drugs. Products are listed alphabetically by generic ingredient and brand name.

BRAND NAME	GENERIC INGREDIENT/STRENGTH	DOSE
BUTENAFINE		
Lotrimin Ultra Antifungal cream (*Schering-Plough*)	Butenafine Hydrochloride 1%	**Adults & Peds ≥12 yo:** Use bid.
CLOTRIMAZOLE		
Clearly Confident Triple Action Toenail & Foot Treatment (*Gandeden Biotech*)	Clortrimazole 1%	**Adults:** Apply to affected area qd.
FungiCure Anti-Fungal Liquid Spray (*Alva-Amco Pharmacal*)	Clotrimazole 1%	**Adults & Peds:** Use bid.
Lotrimin AF Antifungal Athlete's Foot cream (*Schering-Plough*)	Clotrimazole 1%	**Adults & Peds ≥2 yo:** Use bid.
Lotrimin AF Antifungal Athlete's Foot topical solution (*Schering-Plough*)	Clotrimazole 1%	**Adults & Peds ≥2 yo:** Use bid.
Swabplus Foot Care Athlete's Foot Relief Swabs (*Swabplus*)	Clotrimazole 1%	**Adults & Peds:** Use bid.
MICONAZOLE		
Desenex Antifungal liquid spray (*Novartis Consumer Health*)	Miconazole Nitrate 2%	**Adults:** Apply to affected area bid.
Desenex Antifungal powder (*Novartis Consumer Health*)	Miconazole Nitrate 2%	**Adults:** Apply to affected area bid.
Desenex Antifungal spray powder (*Novartis Consumer Health*)	Miconazole Nitrate 2%	**Adults:** Apply to affected area bid.
DiabetAid Antifungal Foot Bath tablets (*Del Pharmaceuticals*)	Miconazole Nitrate 2%	**Adults & Peds ≥2yo:** Use prn.
Diabet-X Antifungal Skin Treatment cream (*Del Pharmaceuticals*)	Miconazole Nitrate 2%	**Adults & Peds ≥2yo:** Use prn.
Lotrimin AF Antifungal Aerosol liquid spray (*Schering-Plough*)	Miconazole Nitrate 2%	**Adults & Peds ≥2 yo:** Use bid.
Lotrimin AF Antifungal Jock Itch aerosol powder spray (*Schering-Plough*)	Miconazole Nitrate 2%	**Adults & Peds ≥2 yo:** Use bid.
Lotrimin AF Antifungal powder (*Schering-Plough*)	Miconazole Nitrate 2%	**Adults & Peds ≥2 yo:** Use bid.
Micatin Antifungal liquid spray (*Pfizer Consumer Healthcare*)	Miconazole Nitrate 2%	**Adults & Peds ≥12 yo:** Use bid.
Micatin Antifungal Spray Powder (*Pfizer Consumer Healthcare*)	Miconazole Nitrate 2%	**Adults & Peds ≥12 yo:** Use bid.
Micatin Athlete's Foot cream (*Pfizer Consumer Healthcare*)	Miconazole nitrate 2%	**Adults:** Apply to affected area bid. **Max:** 2 weeks.
Micatin Athlete's Foot spray liquid (*Pfizer Consumer Healthcare*)	Miconazole nitrate 2%	**Adults:** Apply to affected area bid. **Max:** 2 weeks.

DOSING INFORMATION FOR ANTIFUNGAL PRODUCTS (cont.)

Brand Name	Generic Ingredient/Strength	Dose
Micatin Athlete's Foot spray powder (Pfizer Consumer Healthcare)	Miconazole nitrate 2%	**Adults:** Apply to affected area bid. **Max:** 2 weeks.
Micatin Jock Itch Spray powder (Pfizer Consumer Healthcare)	Miconazole nitrate 2%	**Adults:** Apply to affected area bid. **Max:** 2 weeks.
Neosporin AF Antifungal cream (Pfizer Consumer Healthcare)	Miconazole Nitrate 2%	**Adults & Peds ≥12 yo:** Use bid.
Neosporin AF Athlete's Foot Spray liquid (Pfizer Consumer Healthcare)	Miconazole Nitrate 2%	**Adults & Peds ≥12 yo:** Use bid.
Neosporin AF Athlete's Foot, Spray powder (Pfizer Consumer Healthcare)	Miconazole Nitrate 2%	**Adults & Peds ≥12 yo:** Use bid.
Zeasorb Super Absorbent Antifungal powder (Steifel Laboratories)	Miconazole Nitrate 2%	**Adults & Peds:** Use bid.
TERBINAFINE		
Lamisil AT Athlete's Foot cream (Novartis Consumer Health)	Terbinafine Hydrochloride 1%	**Adults & Peds ≥12 yo:** Use bid.
Lamisil AT Athlete's Foot Spray Pump (Novartis Consumer Health)	Terbinafine Hydrochloride 1%	**Adults & Peds ≥12 yo:** Use bid.
Lamisil AT for Women cream (Novartis Consumer Health)	Terbinafine Hydrochloride 1%	**Adults & Peds ≥12 yo:** Use bid.
Lamisil AT Jock Itch cream (Novartis Consumer Health)	Terbinafine Hydrochloride 1%	**Adults & Peds ≥12 yo:** Use bid.
Lamisil AT Jock Itch Spray Pump (Novartis Consumer Health)	Terbinafine Hydrochloride 1%	**Adults & Peds ≥12 yo:** Use bid.
TOLNAFTATE		
Aftate Antifungal Liquid Spray for Athlete's Foot (Schering-Plough)	Tolnaftate 1%	**Adults:** Apply to affected area qd-bid.
FungiCure Anti-Fungal Gel (Alva-Amco Pharmacal)	Tolnaflate 1%	**Adults & Peds:** Use bid.
Gold Bond Antifungal Foot Swabs (Chattem)	Tolnaftate 1%	**Adults & Peds:** Use bid.
Miracle of Aloe Miracle Anti-Fungal (Ontel Products)	Tolnaftate 1%	**Adults & Peds ≥12 yo:** Use bid.
Swabplus Foot Care Fungus Relief Swabs (Swabplus)	Tolnaftate 1%	**Adults & Peds:** Use bid.
Tinactin Antifungal Aerosol Deodorant Powder Spray (Schering-Plough)	Tolnaftate 1%	**Adults & Peds:** Use bid.
Tinactin Antifungal Aerosol liquid spray (Schering-Plough)	Tolnaftate 1%	**Adults & Peds:** Use bid.
Tinactin Antifungal Aerosol powder spray (Schering-Plough)	Tolnaftate 1%	**Adults & Peds:** Use bid.
Tinactin Antifungal cream (Schering-Plough)	Tolnaftate 1%	**Adults & Peds:** Use bid.
Tinactin Antifungal Foot powder (Schering-Plough)	Tolnaftate 1%	**Adults & Peds:** Use bid.
Tinactin Antifungal Jock Itch powder spray (Schering-Plough)	Tolnaftate 1%	**Adults & Peds:** Use bid.
UNDECYLENIC ACID		
Fungi Nail Anti-fungal Solution (Kramer Laboratories)	Undecylenic Acid 25%	**Adults & Peds:** Use bid.
FungiCure Anti-fungal Liquid (Alva-Amco Pharmacal)	Undecylenic Acid 10%	**Adults & Peds:** Use bid.
Tineacide Antifungal cream (Blaine Labs)	Undecylenic Acid 10%	**Adults & Peds ≥12 yo:** Use bid.

Bacterial Infections

Damage to the skin can lead to bacterial infections and the development of an abscess. A skin abscess is a collection of pus and infected material in or on the skin. Skin abscesses are fairly common and usually follow a bacterial infection, often staphylococcus. Bacterial infections and skin abscesses usually develop after a minor wound, injury, or as a complication of folliculitis or boils. Nonprescription topical antibiotics are useful for preventing or treating minor skin infections involving the epidermis or papillary dermis. There are several OTC topical antibiotics available, most of which contain combinations of bacitracin, neomycin, and polymyxin B.

BACITRACIN

PHARMACOLOGY

Bacitracin, a polypeptide antibiotic, is usually bactericidal against gram-positive organisms. It acts within the bacterial cell membrane and interferes with bacterial cell wall synthesis by binding to and inhibiting the dephosphorylation of a membrane-bound lipid pyrophosphate. Pyrophosphate is the precursor of a carrier molecule, undecaprenyl phosphate, which is involved in peptidoglycan polymerization.

INDICATIONS

Skin infections, bacterial, minor (prophylaxis)—Topical bacitracin combination is indicated in the prophylaxis of superficial skin infections caused by susceptible organisms in minor abrasions, burns, and cuts.

CONTRAINDICATIONS

Risk-benefit should be considered when the following medical problem exists:

* Sensitivity to bacitracin

WARNINGS/PRECAUTIONS

Pregnancy: Problems in humans have not been documented.

Breastfeeding: Problems in humans have not been documented.

ADVERSE REACTIONS

Those indicating need for medical attention: Incidence more frequent

Hypersensitivity (itching, rash, redness, swelling, or other sign of irritation not present before therapy).

ADMINISTRATION AND DOSAGE

General Dosing Information

Use of topical antibacterials may lead to skin sensitization, resulting in hypersensitivity reactions with subsequent topical or systemic use of the medication. The treated area(s) may be covered with gauze dressing if desired.

Ointment:

Adults/Pediatrics: Apply to affected area 2 to 5 times a day.

NEOMYCIN

PHARMACOLOGY

Neomycin is actively transported across the bacterial cell membrane, binds to a specific receptor protein on the 30 S subunit of bacterial ribosomes, and interferes with an initiation complex between messenger RNA (mRNA) and the 30 S subunit, inhibiting protein synthesis. DNA may be misread, thus producing nonfunctional proteins; polyribosomes are split apart and are unable to synthesize protein.

INDICATIONS

Skin infections, bacterial, minor (prophylaxis)—Topical neomycin is indicated in the prophylaxis of superficial infections in minor abrasions, burns, and cuts.

Skin infections, bacterial, minor (treatment); *ulcer, dermal* (treatment)—Topical neomycin is used in the treatment of minor bacterial skin infections and dermal ulcer.

CONTRAINDICATIONS

Risk-benefit should be considered when the following medical problem exists:

* Sensitivity to aminoglycosides.

WARNINGS/PRECAUTIONS

Patients sensitive to one aminoglycoside may be sensitive to other aminoglycosides also.

Pregnancy: Problems in humans have not been documented.

Breastfeeding: It is not known whether topical neomycin is distributed into breast milk. However, problems in humans have not been documented.

ADVERSE REACTIONS

Those indicating need for medical attention: Incidence more frequent

Contact dermatitis (itching, rash, redness, swelling, or other sign of skin irritation not present before therapy).

Incidence rare:

Ototoxicity (loss of hearing).

ADMINISTRATION AND DOSAGE

General Dosing Information

Use of topical antibacterials may lead to skin sensitization, resulting in hypersensitivity reactions with subsequent topical or systemic use of the medication. The treated area(s) may be covered with a gauze dressing if desired. Nephrotoxicity and moderate to severe ototoxicity may occur, especially if renal function is impaired and systemic nephrotoxic and/or ototoxic drugs are given concurrently.

BACITRACIN PRODUCTS	
Brand Name	**Dosage Form**
Bacitracin (Various)	**Ointment:** 500U/g

Cream/Ointment

Adults/Pediatrics >2 years of age: Apply to affected area 1 to 3 times a day.

NEOMYCIN/POLYMYXIN B

PHARMACOLOGY

Neomycin is actively transported across the bacterial cell membrane, binds to a specific receptor protein on the 30 S subunit of bacterial ribosomes, and interferes with an initiation complex between messenger RNA (mRNA) and the 30 S subunit, inhibiting protein synthesis. RNA may be misread, thus producing nonfunctional proteins. Polyribosomes are split apart and are unable to synthesize protein.

Polymyxin B is bactericidal and active against *Pseudomonas aeruginosa* and other gram-negative bacteria. It is a surface-active basic polypeptide that binds to anionic phospholipid sites in bacterial cytoplasmic membranes, disrupts membrane structure, and alters membrane permeability to allow leakage of intracellular contents.

INDICATIONS

Skin infections, bacterial, minor (prophylaxis)—Neomycin and polymyxin B combination is indicated in the topical prophylaxis of superficial skin infections caused by susceptible organisms in minor abrasions, burns, and cuts.

Ulcer, dermal (treatment)—Neomycin and polymyxin B combination is used in the topical treatment of dermal ulcer.

CONTRAINDICATIONS

Risk-benefit should be considered when the following medical problem exists:

● Sensitivity to neomycin, polymyxin B, other aminoglycosides or polymyxins, or parabens.

WARNINGS/PRECAUTIONS

Patients sensitive to other aminoglycosides or polymyxins may be sensitive to this medication also.

Pregnancy: Problems in humans have not been documented.

Breastfeeding: Problems in humans have not been documented.

DRUG INTERACTIONS

Aminoglycosides, other: Concurrent topical and systemic use with neomycin or related drugs is not recommended since hypersensitivity reactions may occur more frequently; if significant systemic absorption occurs, hearing loss may also result, may progress to deafness even after discontinuation of the drug, and may be permanent.

ADVERSE REACTIONS

Those indicating need for medical attention: Incidence more frequent

Hypersensitivity (itching, pain, skin rash, swelling, redness, or other sign of skin irritation not present before therapy).

Incidence rare:

Ototoxicity (loss of hearing).

ADMINISTRATION AND DOSAGE

General Dosing Information

Neomycin and polymyxin B combination should not be used in the eyes. This medication should not be used on extensive areas of the body or for more than 1 week unless directed by a physician. Ototoxicity and nephrotoxicity have been reported. Toxicity may also be increased when this medication is used in the treatment of leg ulcers, decubitus ulcers, and otitis externa. This medication should not be used on deep wounds, puncture wounds, animal bites, serious burns, or raw areas without checking with a physician or pharmacist. Prolonged use of neomycin-containing preparations increases the possibility of allergic reactions. If redness, irritation, swelling, or pain occurs, treatment with neomycin and polymyxin B combination should be discontinued. The treated area(s) may be covered with a gauze dressing if desired. Use of topical antibacterials may lead to skin sensitization, resulting in hypersensitivity reactions with subsequent topical or systemic use of the medication.

Cream

Adults/Pediatrics ≥2 years of age: Apply to affected area 1 to 3 times a day.

NEOMYCIN/POLYMYXIN B/BACITRACIN

PHARMACOLOGY

Neomycin is actively transported across the bacterial cell membrane, binds to a specific receptor protein on the 30 S subunit of bacterial ribosomes, and interferes with an initiation complex between messenger RNA (mRNA) and the 30 S subunit, inhibiting protein synthesis. DNA may be misread, thus producing nonfunctional proteins; polyribosomes are split apart and are unable to synthesize protein.

NEOMYCIN/POLYMYXIN B/PRAMOXINE PRODUCTS	
Brand Name	**Dosage Form**
Neosporin Plus Pain Relief (Pfizer)	**Cream:** 3.5mg-10,000U-10mg

NEOMYCIN/POLYMYXIN B/BACITRACIN PRODUCTS	
Brand Name	**Dosage Form**
Neosporin (Pfizer)	**Ointment:** 3.5g-5000U-400U
Neosporin Neo to Go (Pfizer)	**Ointment:** 3.5g-5000U-400U

NEOMYCIN/POLYMYXIN B/BACITRACIN/PRAMOXINE PRODUCTS	
Brand Name	**Dosage Form**
Neosporin Plus Pain Relief (Pfizer)	**Ointment:** 3.5g-10,000U-500U-10mg

Polymyxin B is bactericidal and active against *Pseudomonas aeruginosa* and other gram-negative bacteria. It is a surface-active basic polypeptide that binds to anionic phospholipid sites in bacterial cytoplasmic membranes, disrupts membrane structure, and alters membrane permeability to allow leakage of intracellular contents. Its action is antagonized by calcium and magnesium.

Bacitracin, a polypeptide antibiotic, is usually bactericidal against gram-positive organisms. It acts within the bacterial cell membrane and interferes with bacterial cell wall synthesis by binding to and inhibiting the dephosphorylation of a membrane-bound lipid pyrophosphate. Pyrophosphate is the precursor of a carrier molecule, undecaprenyl phosphate, which is involved in peptidoglycan polymerization.

INDICATIONS

Skin infections, bacterial, minor (prophylaxis)—Topical neomycin, polymyxin B, and bacitracin combination is indicated in the prophylaxis of superficial skin infections caused by susceptible organisms in minor abrasions, burns, and cuts.

Skin infections, bacterial, minor (treatment); *ulcer, dermal* (treatment)—Topical neomycin, polymyxin B, and bacitracin combination is used in the treatment of minor bacterial skin infections and dermal ulcer.

CONTRAINDICATIONS

Risk-benefit should be considered when the following medical problem exists:

- Sensitivity to neomycin, polymyxin B, or bacitracin.

WARNINGS/PRECAUTIONS

Patients sensitive to one aminoglycoside or polymyxin may be sensitive to other aminoglycosides or polymyxins also.

Pregnancy: Problems in humans have not been documented.

Breastfeeding: Problems in humans have not been documented.

DRUG INTERACTIONS

Aminoglycosides, other: Concurrent topical and systemic use with neomycin or related drugs is not recommended since hypersensitivity reactions may occur more frequently during concurrent use; if significant systemic absorption occurs, hearing loss may also result, may progress to deafness even after discontinuation of the drug, and may be permanent.

ADVERSE REACTIONS

Those indicating need for medical attention: Incidence more frequent

Hypersensitivity (itching, rash, redness, swelling, or other sign of irritation not present before therapy).

Incidence rare:

Ototoxicity (loss of hearing).

ADMINISTRATION AND DOSAGE

General Dosing Information

Use of topical antibacterials may lead to skin sensitization, resulting in hypersensitivity reactions with subsequent topical or systemic use of the medication. The treated area(s) may be covered with a gauze dressing if desired. Nephrotoxicity and moderate to severe ototoxicity may occur, especially if renal function is impaired and systemic nephrotoxic and/or ototoxic drugs are given concurrently. Neomycin, polymyxin B, and bacitracin ointment is available in a petrolatum base that helps retain moisture and may be useful in treating infections on dry or scaling skin. It is also available in a base containing polyethylene glycols, liquid and white petrolatum, and glyceride wax that is miscible with tissue exudates and skin oils and waxes and may be used on weeping, exudative lesions.

Ointment

Adults/Pediatrics: Apply to affected area 2 to 5 times a day.

DOSING INFORMATION FOR ANTIBACTERIAL PRODUCTS

The following table provides a quick comparison of the ingredients and dosages of common brand-name OTC drugs. Products are listed alphabetically by brand name.

BRAND NAME	INGREDIENT/STRENGTH	DOSE
Bacitracin ointment *(Various)*	Bacitracin 500 U	**Adults & Peds:** Apply to affected area qd-tid.
Neosporin ointment *(Pfizer Consumer Healthcare)*	Neomycin/polymyxin B/bacitracin 3.5mg-5,000 U-400 U	**Adults & Peds:** Apply to affected area qd-tid.
Neosporin Plus Pain Relief cream *(Pfizer Consumer Healthcare)*	Neomycin/polymyxin B/pramoxine 3.5mg-10,000 U-10mg	**Adults & Peds:** Apply to affected area qd-tid.
Neosporin Plus Pain Relief ointment *(Pfizer Consumer Healthcare)*	Neomycin/polymyxin B/bacitracin/pramoxine 3.5mg-10,000 U-500 U-10mg	**Adults & Peds:** Apply to affected area qd-tid.
Neosporin To Go ointment *(Pfizer Consumer Healthcare)*	Neomycin/polymyxin B/bacitracin 3.5mg-5,000 U-400 U	**Adults & Peds:** Apply to affected area qd-tid.
Polysporin ointment *(Pfizer Consumer Healthcare)*	Neomycin/polymyxin B/bacitracin 3.5mg-5,000 U-400 U	**Adults & Peds:** Apply to affected area qd-tid.
Neosporin To Go ointment *(Pfizer Consumer Healthcare)*	Polymyxin B/Bacitracin 10,000 U-500 U	**Adults & Peds:** Apply to affected area qd-tid.

Blisters

Blisters represent discrete accumulations of fluid, histologically residing either within the epidermis or immediately below it in the basement membrane zone. Clinically, they are sharply marginated, elevated lesions that contain clear fluid. Blisters are termed *vesicles* if they are less than 1cm in diameter. Lesions larger than 1cm are known as *bullae*. Clinically, the level of skin involved is reflected in the resultant blisters. Intraepidermal blisters tend to have thin roofs that rupture easily, leading to erosions. Subepidermal blisters tend to be thick walled and remain intact. Prevention of traumatic blisters can often be accomplished by eliminating the source of friction or trauma. Adequate hygiene and wound care are recommended for treating blisters. OTC topical antibiotics can be used to prevent possible bacterial infection. Most products contain different combinations of bacitracin, neomycin, and polymyxin B.

NEOMYCIN/POLYMYXIN B/BACITRACIN

Neomycin is actively transported across the bacterial cell membrane, binds to a specific receptor protein on the 30 S subunit of bacterial ribosomes, and interferes with an initiation complex between mRNA (messenger RNA) and the 30 S subunit, inhibiting protein synthesis. DNA may be misread, thus producing nonfunctional proteins; polyribosomes are split and are unable to synthesize protein.

Polymyxin B is bactericidal and active against *Pseudomonas aeruginosa* and other gram-negative bacteria. It is a surface-active basic polypeptide that binds to anionic phospholipid sites in bacterial cytoplasmic membranes, disrupts membrane structure, and alters membrane permeability to allow leakage of intracellular contents. Its action is antagonized by calcium and magnesium.

Bacitracin, a polypeptide antibiotic, is usually bactericidal against gram-positive organisms. It acts within the bacterial cell membrane and interferes with bacterial cell wall synthesis by binding to and inhibiting the dephosphorylation of a membrane-bound lipid pyrophosphate. Pyrophosphate is the precursor of a carrier molecule, undecaprenyl phosphate, which is involved in peptidoglycan polymerization.

Skin infections, bacterial, minor (prophylaxis)—Topical neomycin, polymyxin B, and bacitracin combination is indicated in the prophylaxis of superficial skin infections caused by susceptible organisms in minor abrasions, burns, and cuts.

Cream

Adults/Pediatrics ≥2 year of age: Apply to affected area 1 to 3 times a day.

Ointment

Adults/Pediatrics: Apply to affected area 2 to 5 times a day.

For more information, refer to the complete monographs for bacitracin; neomycin; neomycin/polymyxin B; and neomycin/polymyxin B/bacitracin in "Bacterial Infections" under Dermatological Conditions.

NEOMYCIN/POLYMYXIN B/PRAMOXINE PRODUCTS	
Brand Name	**Dosage Form**
Neosporin Plus Pain Relief (Pfizer)	**Cream:** 3.5mg-10,000 U-10mg
BACITRACIN PRODUCTS	
Brand Name	**Dosage Form**
Bacitracin (Various)	**Ointment:** 500 U/g
NEOMYCIN/POLYMYXIN B/BACITRACIN PRODUCTS	
Brand Name	**Dosage Form**
Neosporin (Pfizer)	**Ointment:** 3.5g-5,000 U-400 U
Neosporin Neo to Go (Pfizer)	**Ointment:** 3.5g-5,000 U-400 U
NEOMYCIN/POLYMYXIN B/BACITRACIN/PRAMOXINE PRODUCTS	
Brand Name	**Dosage Form**
Neosporin Plus Pain Relief (Pfizer)	**Ointment:** 3.5g-10,000 U-500 U-10mg

DOSING INFORMATION FOR BLISTER PRODUCTS

The following table provides a quick comparison of the ingredients and dosages of common brand-name OTC drugs. Products are listed alphabetically by brand name.

BRAND NAME	GENERIC INGREDIENT/STRENGTH	DOSE
Bacitracin ointment *(Various)*	Bacitracin 500 U	**Adults & Peds:** Apply to affected area qd-tid.
Neosporin ointment *(Pfizer Consumer Healthcare)*	Neomycin/polymyxin B/bacitracin 3.5mg-5,000 U-400 U	**Adults & Peds:** Apply to affected area qd-tid.
Neosporin Plus Pain Relief cream *(Pfizer Consumer Healthcare)*	Neomycin/polymyxin B/pramoxine 3.5mg-10,000 U-10mg	**Adults & Peds:** Apply to affected area qd-tid.
Neosporin Plus Pain Relief ointment *(Pfizer Consumer Healthcare)*	Neomycin/polymyxin B/bacitracin/pramoxine 3.5mg-10,000 U-500 U-10mg	**Adults & Peds:** Apply to affected area qd-tid.
Neosporin To Go ointment *(Pfizer Consumer Healthcare)*	Neomycin/polymyxin B/bacitracin 3.5mg-5,000 U-400 U	**Adults & Peds:** Apply to affected area qd-tid.
Neosporin To Go ointment *(Pfizer Consumer Healthcare)*	Neomycin/polymyxin B/bacitracin 3.5mg-5,000 U-400 U	**Adults & Peds:** Apply to affected area qd-tid.
Neosporin To Go ointment *(Pfizer Consumer Healthcare)*	Neomycin/polymyxin B/bacitracin 3.5mg-5,000 U-400 U	**Adults & Peds:** Apply to affected area qd-tid.
Neosporin To Go ointment *(Pfizer Consumer Healthcare)*	Neomycin/polymyxin B/bacitracin 3.5mg-5,000 U-400 U	**Adults & Peds:** Apply to affected area qd-tid.
Polysporin ointment *(Pfizer Consumer Healthcare)*	Polymyxin B/Bacitracin 10,000 U-500 U	**Adults & Peds:** Apply to affected area qd-tid.

Burns

A burn is skin damage due to intense heat or another physical stimulus, such as chemicals or electricity. There are three levels of burns: *first-degree* burns affect only the outer layer of the skin and cause pain, redness, and swelling; *second-degree* (partial thickness) burns affect both the outer and underlying layer of skin and cause pain, redness, swelling, and blistering; and *third-degree* (full thickness) burns extend into deeper tissues and cause white or blackened, charred skin that may be numb. Thermal burns are the most common types and often occur due to hot metals, scalding liquids, steam, or flames coming into contact with the skin. Burn symptoms include blisters, pain, peeling skin, red skin, swelling, and white or charred skin. Minor burns can be treated with cool water, sterile bandages, or clean dressings, and OTC medications such as aspirin, acetaminophen, NSAIDs, topical antibiotics, topical anesthetics, topical corticosteroids, and moisturizers.

NEOMYCIN/POLYMYXIN B/BACITRACIN

Neomycin is actively transported across the bacterial cell membrane, binds to a specific receptor protein on the 30 S subunit of bacterial ribosomes, and interferes with an initiation complex between mRNA (messenger RNA) and the 30 S subunit, inhibiting protein synthesis. DNA may be misread, thus producing non-functional proteins; polyribosomes are split apart and are unable to synthesize protein.

Polymyxin B is bactericidal and active against *Pseudomonas aeruginosa* and other gram-negative bacteria. It is a surface-active basic polypeptide that binds to anionic phospholipid sites in bacterial cytoplasmic membranes, disrupts membrane structure, and alters membrane permeability to allow leakage of intracellular contents. Its action is antagonized by calcium and magnesium.

Bacitracin, a polypeptide antibiotic, is usually bactericidal against gram-positive organisms. It acts within the bacterial cell membrane and interferes with bacterial cell wall synthesis by binding to and inhibiting the dephosphorylation of a membrane-bound lipid pyrophosphate. Pyrophosphate is the precursor of a carrier molecule, undecaprenyl phosphate, which is involved in peptidoglycan polymerization.

Skin infections, bacterial, minor (prophylaxis)—Topical neomycin, polymyxin B, and bacitracin combination is indicated in the prophylaxis of superficial skin infections caused by susceptible organisms in minor abrasions, burns, and cuts.

Cream

Adults/Pediatrics ≥2 year of age: Apply to affected area 1 to 3 times a day.

Ointment

Adults/Pediatrics: Apply to affected area 2 to 5 times a day.

For more information, refer to the complete monographs for bacitracin; neomycin; neomycin/polymyxin B; and neomycin/polymyxin B/bacitracin in "Bacterial Infections" under Dermatological Conditions.

TOPICAL ANESTHETICS

PHARMACOLOGY

Local anesthetics block both the initiation and the conduction of nerve impulses by decreasing the neuronal membrane's permeability to sodium ions. This reversibly stabilizes the membrane and inhibits depolarization, resulting in the failure of a propagated action potential and subsequent conduction blockade.

INDICATIONS

Skin disorders, minor (treatment)—Topical anesthetics are indicated to relieve pain, pruritus, and inflammation associated with minor skin disorders (burns, minor, including sunburn; bites [or stings], insect; dermatitis, contact, including poison ivy, poison oak, and poison sumac; wounds, minor, such as cuts and scratches).

NEOMYCIN/POLYMYXIN B/PRAMOXINE PRODUCTS	
Brand Name	**Dosage Form**
Neosporin Plus Pain Relief (Pfizer)	**Cream:** 3.5mg-10,000 U-10mg
BACITRACIN PRODUCTS	
Brand Name	**Dosage Form**
Bacitracin (Various)	**Ointment:** 500 U/g
NEOMYCIN/POLYMYXIN B/BACITRACIN PRODUCTS	
Brand Name	**Dosage Form**
Neosporin (Pfizer)	**Ointment:** 3.5g-5,000 U-400 U
Neosporin Neo to Go (Pfizer)	**Ointment:** 3.5g-5,000 U-400 U
NEOMYCIN/POLYMYXIN B/BACITRACIN/PRAMOXINE PRODUCTS	
Brand Name	**Dosage Form**
Neosporin Plus Pain Relief (Pfizer)	**Ointment:** 3.5g-10,000 U-500 U-10mg

CONTRAINDICATIONS

Risk-benefit should be considered when the following medical problems exist:

- Local infection at the site of application (infection may alter the pH at the treatment site, leading to decrease or loss of local anesthetic effect).

- Sensitivity to the topical anesthetic being considered for use or to chemically related anesthetics and, for the ester derivatives, to para-aminobenzoic acid (PABA), parabens, or paraphenylenediamine, or sensitivity to other ingredients in the formulation.

- Skin disorders, severe or extensive, especially if the skin is abraded or broken (increased absorption of anesthetic).

WARNINGS/PRECAUTIONS

Cross-sensitivity and/or related problems: Patients sensitive to one ester-derivative local anesthetic (especially a PABA derivative) may also be sensitive to other ester derivatives. Patients sensitive to PABA, parabens, or paraphenylenediamine (a hair dye) may also be sensitive to PABA-derivative topical anesthetics. Patients sensitive to one amide derivative may rarely be sensitive to other amide derivatives also. Cross-sensitivity between amide derivatives and ester derivatives, or between amides or esters and the chemically unrelated pramoxine, has not been reported.

Pregnancy—Lidocaine: FDA Category B. *Tetracaine:* FDA Category C. *For benzocaine, butamben, dibucaine, and pramoxine:* Studies in animals and humans have not been done. Problems with topical anesthetics have not been documented in humans.

Breastfeeding: Problems in humans have not been documented.

Pediatrics: Benzocaine should be used with caution in infants and young children because increased absorption through the skin (with excessive use) may result in methemoglobinemia. Benzocaine-containing topical formulations should not be used in children younger than 2 years of age unless prescribed by a physician.

Other topical anesthetics—No information is available on the relationship of age to the effects of these medications in pediatric patients following application to the skin. However, it is recommended that a physician be consulted before any topical local anesthetic is used in children younger than 2 years of age.

ADVERSE REACTIONS

Those indicating need for medical attention: Incidence less frequent

Angioedema (large, hivelike swellings on skin, mouth, or throat); dermatitis, contact (skin rash, redness, itching, or hives; burning, stinging, swelling, or tenderness not present before therapy)

ADMINISTRATION AND DOSAGE

Benzocaine/Dibucaine/Pramoxine/Tetracaine

Adults/Pediatrics ≥*2 years of age:* Apply to the affected area 3 or 4 times a day as needed.

Butamben

Adults: Apply to the affected area 3 or 4 times a day as needed.

Lidocaine

Adults: Apply to the affected area 3 or 4 times a day as needed.

Pediatrics: Dosage must be individualized, depending on the child's age, weight, and physical condition, up to a maximum of 4.5mg/kg of body weight.

Drug Interactions for Topical Anesthetics

Precipitant Drug	Object Drug	Effect On Object Drug	Description
Cholinesterase inhibitors (eg, antimyasthenics; cyclophosphamide; demecarium; echothiophate; insecticides, neurotoxic; isoflurophate; thiotepa)	Ester derivatives Anesthetics	↑	These agents may inhibit metabolism of ester derivatives; absorption of significant quantities of ester derivatives in patients receiving a cholinesterase inhibitor may lead to increased risk of toxicity.
Beta-adrenergic blocking agents	Lidocaine	↑	Concurrent use may slow metabolism of lidocaine because of decreased hepatic blood flow, leading to increased risk of lidocaine toxicity if large quantities are absorbed.
Cimetidine	Lidocaine	↑	Cimetidine inhibits hepatic metabolism of lidocaine; concurrent use may lead to lidocaine toxicity if large quantities are absorbed.
Lidocaine	Antiarrhythmic agents (eg, mexiletine; tocainide; lidocaine, systemic or parenteral-local)	↑	Risk of cardiotoxicity associated with additive cardiac effects, and, with systemic or parenteral-local lidocaine, the risk of overdose may be increased in patients receiving these medications if large quantities of topically applied lidocaine are absorbed.
Topical anesthetics	Sulfonamides	↓	Metabolites of PABA-derivative topical anesthetics may antagonize antibacterial activity of sulfonamides, especially if the anesthetics are absorbed in significant quantities over prolonged periods of time

BENZOCAINE PRODUCTS	
Brand Name	**Dosage Form**
Solarcaine (Schering)	**Spray:** 20%
BENZOCAINE/BENZETHONIUM CHLORIDE PRODUCTS	
Brand Name	**Dosage Form**
Lanacane Anti-itch (Combe)	**Cream:** 6%-0.2%
Lanacane First-Aid (Combe)	**Cream:** 20%-0.2%
Lanacane Maximum Strength (Combe)	**Cream:** 20%-0.2%
BENZOCAINE/CHLOROXYLENOL PRODUCTS	
Brand Name	**Dosage Form**
Foille Medicated First Aid (Blistex)	**Ointment:** 5%-0.1%
	Spray: 5%-0.1%
DIBUCAINE PRODUCTS	
Brand Name	**Dosage Form**
Nupercainal (Novartis)	**Cream:** 0.5% **Ointment:** 1%
LIDOCAINE PRODUCTS	
Brand Name	**Dosage Form**
Solarcaine Aloe Extract (Schering)	**Gel:** 0.5% **Spray:** 0.5%
PRAMOXINE PRODUCTS	
Brand Name	**Dosage Form**
Sarna Sensitive (Stiefel)	**Lotion:** 1%
PRAMOXINE/MENTHOL PRODUCTS	
Brand Name	**Dosage Form**
Gold Bond Medicated Anti-itch Maximum Strength (Chattem)	**Cream:** 1%-1%

DOSING INFORMATION FOR TOPICAL ANESTHETIC/ANTIBIOTIC PRODUCTS

The following table provides a quick comparison of the ingredients and dosages of common brand-name OTC drugs. Products are listed alphabetically by drug category and brand name.

BRAND NAME	GENERIC INGREDIENT/STRENGTH	DOSE
ANESTHETICS		
Lanacane Maximum Strength cream *(Combe)*	Benzocaine/Benzethonium Chloride 20%-0.2%	**Adults & Peds ≥2 yo:** Apply to clean dry affected area qd-tid.
Lanacane Maximum Strength spray *(Combe)*	Benzocaine/Benzethonium Chloride 20%-0.2%	**Adults & Peds ≥2 yo:** Apply to clean dry affected area qd-tid.
Lanacane Original Formula cream *(Combe)*	Benzocaine/Benzethonium Chloride 6%-0.2%	**Adults & Peds ≥2 yo:** Apply to clean dry affected area qd-tid.
Solarcaine Aloe Extra Burn Relief gel *(Schering-Plough)*	Lidocaine HCl 0.5%	**Adults & Peds ≥2 yo:** Apply to clean dry affected area tid-qid.
Solarcaine Aloe Extra Burn Relief spray *(Schering-Plough)*	Lidocaine 0.5%	**Adults & Peds ≥2 yo:** Apply to clean dry affected area tid-qid.
Tender's Afterburn Aloe gel *(Tender Corporation)*	Lidocaine 0.5%	**Adults & Peds ≥2 yo:** Apply to clean dry affected area tid-qid.
Water-Jel Burn Jel *(Water-Jel Technologies)*	Lidocaine HCl 2.0%	**Adults & Peds ≥2 yo:** Apply to clean dry affected area tid-qid.
ANTIBIOTICS		
Bacitracin ointment *(Various)*	Bacitracin 500 U	**Adults & Peds:** Apply to affected area qd-tid.
Neosporin ointment *(Pfizer Consumer Healthcare)*	Neomycin/polymyxin B/bacitracin 3.5mg-5,000 U-400 U	**Adults & Peds:** Apply to affected area qd-tid.
Neosporin Plus Pain Relief cream *(Pfizer Consumer Healthcare)*	Neomycin/polymyxin B/pramoxine 3.5mg-10,000 U-10mg	**Adults & Peds:** Apply to affected area qd-tid.
Neosporin Plus Pain Relief ointment *(Pfizer Consumer Healthcare)*	Neomycin/polymyxin B/bacitracin/pramoxine 3.5mg-10,000 U-500 U-10mg	**Adults & Peds:** Apply to affected area qd-tid.
Neosporin To Go ointment *(Pfizer Consumer Healthcare)*	Neomycin/polymyxin B/bacitracin 3.5mg-5,000 U-400 U	**Adults & Peds:** Apply to affected area qd-tid.
Polysporin ointment *(Pfizer Consumer Healthcare)*	Polymyxin B/Bacitracin 10,000 U-500 U	**Adults & Peds:** Apply to affected area qd-tid.

Calluses, Corns, and Warts

Calluses and corns are thickened epidermal layers of skin caused by chronic, repeated pressure, friction, or trauma. A corn refers to thickened skin on the top or side of a toe that's usually due to shoes that do not fit properly. A callus refers to thickened skin on the hands or the soles of the feet. Corns and calluses can be prevented and treated by preventing friction, pressure, and trauma to vulnerable areas. There are also corn pads, pumice stones and files, and one OTC keratolytic medication (salicylic acid) available to treat corns and calluses.

Warts are extremely common and can persist for years. The various clinical types include the common wart (*verruca vulgaris*), plantar wart (*verruca plantaris*), flat wart (*verruca plana*), and genital wart (*condyloma acuminatum*). Common warts and plantar warts can often be treated with OTC agents. Common warts can occur on almost any area of the body, most often in children, but also in any age group. In children, however, one half of all warts will regress spontaneously in 1 year, and two thirds of all warts will clear in 2 years without therapy. For treatment, one may use keratolytic acid paintings that are available OTC under a variety of names. Typical preparations contain 17% salicylic acid and should be applied twice daily. Plantar warts, appearing on the soles of the feet, are particularly recalcitrant to therapy. They occur most frequently on weight-bearing prominences and at times are extremely painful. They must be differentiated from calluses that have increased skin lines and from hard corns. Dark dots that represent thrombosed blood vessels usually are present in plantar warts. The differential diagnosis includes verrucous carcinoma and amelanotic melanoma that also can occur on the sole. Plantar warts may be treated with the same modalities used for common warts. There are several OTC dosage forms of salicylic acid available to treat warts.

SALICYLIC ACID

PHARMACOLOGY

Salicylic acid facilitates desquamation by solubilizing the intercellular cement that binds scales in the stratum corneum, thereby loosening the keratin. This keratolytic effect may provide an antifungal action because removal of the stratum corneum suppresses fungal growth; it also aids in the penetration of other antifungal agents. Salicylic acid also has a mild antiseptic action.

INDICATIONS

Acne vulgaris (treatment)—Salicylic acid gel, lotion, ointment, pads, soap, and topical solution are indicated as peeling and drying agents in the treatment of acne vulgaris.

Dandruff (treatment); *dermatitis, seborrheic* (treatment); *dermatitis, seborrheic, of scalp* (treatment)—Salicylic acid lotion and shampoo are indicated to help control scaling of the scalp associated with dandruff and seborrheic dermatitis. Salicylic acid ointment is indicated in the treatment of seborrheic dermatitis.

Psoriasis (treatment)—Salicylic acid gel and ointment are indicated as adjuncts in the treatment of psoriasis.

Hyperkeratotic skin disorders (treatment)—Salicylic acid is indicated as a topical aid in the removal of excessive keratin in hyperkeratotic skin disorders, including verrucae and the various ichthyoses (vulgaris, sex-linked, and lamellar); keratosis palmaris and keratosis plantaris; keratosis pilaris; and pityriasis rubra pilaris. It is also indicated as a topical aid in the removal of excessive keratin on dorsal and plantar hyperkeratotic lesions. Salicylic acid cream, plaster, and topical solution are indicated to treat corns and calluses. Salicylic acid gel, ointment, plaster, and topical solution are indicated to treat common warts; the gel, plaster, and topical solution are indicated to treat plantar warts.

CONTRAINDICATIONS

Except under special circumstances, this medication should not be used when the following medical problems exist:

- Hypersensitivity to salicylic acid or any other component of the product—*major clinical significance.*

- Influenza in children and adolescents—*major clinical significance.*

- Varicella in children and adolescents—*major clinical significance* (should not be used due to potential risk of developing Reye's syndrome unless directed by a physician).

Risk-benefit should be considered when the following medical problems exist:

- Hepatic impairment—*major clinical significance.*

- Renal impairment—*major clinical significance* (prolonged use over large areas could result in salicylism; area to be treated should be limited and patient monitored closely for signs of salicylate toxicity).

For 25% and 60% cream, 25% to 60% ointment, 12% to 50% plaster, 12% to 26% gel, and 5% to 27% topical solution:

- Diabetes mellitus or peripheral vascular disease (acute inflammation or ulceration may occur, especially on the extremities).

- Inflammation, irritation, or infection of the skin.

WARNINGS/PRECAUTIONS

Pregnancy: FDA Category C. No data are available regarding potential reproductive effects of salicylic acid. Studies in humans have not been done; however, salicylic acid may be systemically absorbed. There is concern regarding the possibility of the premature closure of the ductus arteriosis. Salicylic acid should be used during pregnancy only if the potential benefit justifies the potential risk to the fetus.

Breastfeeding: Problems in humans have not been documented; however, salicylic acid may be systemically absorbed. Because of the potential for serious adverse reactions in nursing infants, a decision should be made whether to discontinue nursing or to discontinue the drug, taking into account the importance of the drug to the mother.

Pediatrics: Young children may be at increased risk of toxicity because of increased absorption of salicylic acid through the skin and the increased ratio of total body surface area to treated area. In addition, young children may have a lower threshold for skin irritation from salicylic acid. Salicylic acid should not be applied to large areas of the body, for prolonged periods of time, or under occlusion to substantial areas. Salicylic acid should not be used in children younger than 2 years of age.

Geriatrics: Elderly patients are more likely to have age-related peripheral vascular disease and therefore may be more prone to acute inflammation or ulceration of the extremities when they are treated with the 25% or 60% cream, 12% to 17% gel, 25%

Drug Interactions for Salicylic Acid

Precipitant Drug	Object Drug	Effect On Object Drug	Description
Abrasive/medicated soaps/cleansers Acne preparations (eg, benzoyl peroxide, resorcinol, sulfur, tretinoin, other topical agents) Alcohol-containing preparations, topical (e.g., after-shave lotions, astringents, perfumed toiletries having creams/lotions) Cosmetics/soaps with strong drying effect IsotretinoinMedicated cosmetics	Salicylic acid	↑	Concurrent use with salicylic acid may cause a cumulative irritant or drying effect, especially with the application of peeling, desquamating, or abrasive agents, resulting in excessive irritation of the skin.
Acidifying agents	Salicylic acid	↑	May increase plasma salicylate level by altering renal tubular reabsorption.
Alkalizing agents	Salicylic acid	↓	May decrease plasma salicylate levels by altering renal tubular reabsorption.
Corticosteroids	Salicylic acid	↓	May decrease plasma salicylate level by altering renal tubular reabsorption; tapering doses of steroids may promote salicylism.
Salicylic acid	Anticoagulants, oral	↑	May increase bleeding due to competition for binding to serum albumin.
Salicylic acid	Heparin	↑	Salicylate may decrease platelet adhesiveness and interfere with hemostasis in heparin-treated patients.
Salicylic acid	Methotrexate	↑	Decreases tubular reabsorption; clinical toxicity from methotrexate can result.
Salicylic acid	Pyrazinamide	↔	May inhibit pyrazinamide-induced hyperuricemia.
Salicylic acid	Sulfonylureas	↑	May potentiate hypoglycemia due to competition for binding to serum albumin.
Salicylic acid	Uricosuric agents (e.g., phenylbutazone, probenemide, sulfinpyrazone)	↓	Concomitant use may inhibit effect of these drugs.

to 60% ointment, 12% to 50% plaster, and 5% to 27% topical solution.

ADVERSE REACTIONS

Those indicating need for medical attention: Incidence less frequent or rare

Skin irritation, moderate to severe, not present before therapy; skin ulceration or erosion—especially when using medication with a high percentage of salicylic acid.

Erythema (flushing, redness of skin; unusually warm skin)— from use on open skin lesions.

Salicylism (ringing or buzzing in ears; hearing loss; confusion, severe; diarrhea; stomach pain; headache; dizziness; lightheadedness; severe drowsiness; fast or deep breathing; nausea; vomiting)—from use on open skin lesions.

Scaling (dryness and peeling of skin)— from use on open skin lesions.

Those indicating need for medical attention only if they continue or are bothersome: Incidence more frequent

Skin irritation, mild, not present before therapy; stinging.

ADMINISTRATION AND DOSAGE

General Dosing Information

In young children, use is not recommended on large areas of the body, for prolonged periods of time, or under occlusion to sizable areas of the body.

For the stronger strengths of salicylic acid, such as the 25% and 60% cream, 25% and 60% ointment, 12% to 50% plaster, 12% to 26% gel, and 5% to 27% topical solution:

These products are not recommended for use on irritated, inflamed, or infected skin; on facial, genital, nasal, or oral warts; on warts with hair growing from them; on moles; or on birthmarks. In addition, these products are not recommended for use on patients with diabetes mellitus or impaired blood circulation.

For the gel dosage form:

Before application of the gel, wet packs should be applied to the affected areas for at least 5 minutes in order to enhance its effect. The method of use usually preferred is application of the gel to the affected area with an occlusive dressing at night.

For the 25% to 60% creams and ointments:

Application of these creams or ointments should be made only by a physician. Caution should be used to avoid getting these creams or ointments on skin surrounding the area being treated. Following application of these creams or ointments, an occlusive dressing is applied.

For the 12% to 50% plaster dosage form:

The affected area should be washed and dried. Warts may be soaked in warm water for 5 minutes before drying. The plaster should be cut to fit the wart, corn, or callus.

For corns and calluses: Application should be repeated every 48 hours as needed for up to 14 days until the corn or callus is removed. The corn or callus may be soaked in warm water for 5 minutes to aid in removal.

For warts: Depending on the product, the plaster should either be applied every 48 hours or be applied at bedtime, left in place for at least 8 hours, removed in the morning, and the application repeated every 24 hours. In either case, application should be repeated for up to 12 weeks until the wart is removed.

For the 5% to 27% topical solution dosage form for treatment of warts, corns, or calluses:

The affected areas should be washed and dried. Warts may be soaked in warm water for 5 minutes before drying. Medication should be applied one drop at a time to completely cover the wart, corn, or callus. Procedure should be repeated once or twice daily for up to 14 days for corns or calluses or up to 12 weeks for warts, until the wart, corn, or callus is removed. Corns and calluses may be soaked in water for 5 minutes to aid in removal.

Cream 2%-10%

Adults/Pediatrics: Apply to affected area daily.

Gel 0.5%-17%

Adults/Pediatrics: Apply to affected area once daily.

Lotion 1%-2%

Adults/Pediatrics: Apply to affected area 1 to 3 times a day.

Pads 0.5%-2%

Adults/Pediatrics: Apply to affected area 1 to 3 times a day.

Shampoo

Adults/Pediatrics: Apply to the scalp 1 to 2 times a week.

Soap

Adults/Pediatrics: Apply to affected area daily.

Topical Solution 0.5%-17%

Adults/Pediatrics: Apply to affected area 1 to 3 times a day.

SALICYLIC ACID PRODUCTS (ACNE)

Brand Name	Dosage Form
Neutrogena Acne Wash (Neutrogena)	Liquid: 2%
Neutrogena Clear Pore (Neutrogena)	Gel: 2%
Oxy Balance Deep Pore Cleansing (GSK)	Gel: 2% Pads: 0.50%
Stri-dex Body Focus (Blistex)	Gel: 2%
Stri-dex Clear Cycle (Blistex)	Soap: 2%
Stri-dex Essential Care (Blistex)	Pads: 1%
Stri-dex Facewipes To Go (Blistex)	Pads: 0.50%
Stri-dex Fruit Therapy (Blistex)	Cream: 2%
Stri-dex Maximum Strength (Blistex)	Pads: 2%
Stri-dex Sensitive Skin (Blistex)	Pads: 0.50%
Stri-dex Super Scrub (Blistex)	Pads: 2%

SALICYLIC ACID PRODUCTS (CALLUSES/CORNS/WARTS)

Brand Name	Dosage Form
Compound W (Medtech)	Gel: 17% Liquid: 17%
Compound W One Step Wart Remover (Medtech)	Pads: 40%
Duofilm (Schering)	Liquid: 17% Patch: 17%
Duoplant (Schering)	Gel: 17%
Mediplast (Beiersdorf)	Pads: 40%
Occlusal-HP (Medicis)	Liquid: 17%
Wart-off Maximum Strength (Pfizer)	Liquid: 17%

SALICYLIC ACID PRODUCTS (PSORIASIS/SEBORRHEIC DERMATITIS)

Brand Name	Dosage Form
Dermarest Psoriasis (Del)	Shampoo: 3%
Dermarest Psoriasis Medicated Moisturizer (Del)	Lotion: 2%
Dermarest Psoriasis Skin Treatment (Del)	Gel: 3%
Dermarest Psoriasis Scalp Treatment (Del)	Gel: 3%
Neutrogena Healthy Scalp (Neutrogena)	Shampoo: 1.80%
Neutrogena T/Sal Maximum Strength (Neutrogena)	Liquid: 3%

DOSING INFORMATION FOR CALLUS/CORN/WART PRODUCTS

The following table provides a quick comparison of the ingredients and dosages of common brand-name OTC drugs. Products are listed alphabetically by brand name.

Brand Name	Generic Ingredient/Strength	Dose
Band-Aid Corn Remover, Medicated Regular Cushions *(Johnson & Johnson/Merck Consumer)*	Salicylic Acid 40%	**Adults:** Use as directed.
Compound W One Step Pads *(Medtech Products)*	Salicylic Acid 40%	**Adults:** Apply to affected area qod.
Compound W Wart Remover gel *(Medtech Products)*	Salicylic Acid 17%	**Adults:** Apply to affected area qd-bid.
Curad Mediplast Corn, Callus & Wart Remover pads *(Beiersdorf)*	Salicylic Acid 40%	**Adults:** Apply to affected area qod.
Dr. Scholl's Clear Away One Step Plantar Wart Remover pads *(Schering-Plough)*	Salicylic Acid 40%	**Adults:** Apply to affected area qod.
Dr. Scholl's Clear Away Wart Remover pads & discs *(Schering-Plough)*	Salicylic Acid 40%	**Adults:** Apply to affected area qod.
Dr. Scholl's Corn Removers pads *(Schering-Plough)*	Salicylic Acid 40%	**Adults:** Apply to affected area qod.
Dr. Scholl's Liquid Corn & Callus Remover *(Schering-Plough)*	Salicylic Acid 12.6%	**Adults:** Apply qd-bid.
Dr. Scholl's One Step Corn Removers *(Schering-Plough)*	Salicylic Acid 40%	**Adults:** Apply to affected area qod.
Dr. Scholl's One Step Corn Removers *(Schering-Plough)*	Salicylic Acid 17%	**Adults:** Apply to affected area qod.
Duofilm *(Schering-Plough)*	Salicylic Acid 17%	**Adults:** Apply qd-bid.
Wart-Off Maximum Strength Painless Wart Remover liquid *(Pfizer Consumer Healthcare)*	Salicylic Acid 17%	**Adults:** Apply qd-bid.

Contact Dermatitis

Eczema is the most common dermatologic complaint. Eczema presents as small bubbles dispersed in a red, edematous area of skin. The bubbles can vary in size from 1 or 2 mm in diameter (<10mm are *vesicles*) to several centimeters (≥10mm are *bullae*). While eczema is usually very pruritic (itchy), the pruritus sometimes subsides over time. By far the most common cause of eczematous rashes is *contact dermatitis (CD)*, a spectrum of inflammatory reactions induced by exposure to an external agent. This inflammation is most commonly recognized as a dermatitis (eczema) and less often as hives (urticaria), acne, hypo- or hyperpigmentation, or phototoxic or photoallergic reactions. It is estimated that there are more than 85,000 chemicals in the environment worldwide; most of them, when in contact with the skin, can induce an *irritant contact dermatitis (ICD)*. About 3,000 of these can elicit an *allergic contact dermatitis (ACD)*. The identification and subsequent avoidance of the relevant agent are the primary management goals for patients with CD.

A broad spectrum of adverse cutaneous reactions can occur when an external agent comes in contact with skin. The most common of these adverse reactions are nonimmunologic irritations. This ICD is a polymorphous lesion that may involve chemical irritation or physical abrasion or damage. Cytotoxic agents that can produce ICD include industrial or household chemicals, medications, detergents, solvents, alcohol, creams, ointments, lotions, and powders. Environmental factors that may contribute to ICD include washing, overhydration, improper drying, perspiration, and temperature extremes. These irritant (non-immunologic) reactions begin with direct damage to the epidermal keratinocytes, resulting in the release of proinflammatory mediators. These mediators produce further tissue damage and activate underlying inflammatory cells (i.e., mast cells or T cells), which then release other proinflammatory mediators that perpetuate the cellular damage. The inflammatory response is dose and time dependent. The clinical presentation of ICD is essentially restricted to the skin site directly in contact with the offending agent. The evolution and resolution of ICD are less predictable than that of ACD.

ACD is recognized as the prototypical antigen-induced Type IV, or delayed hypersensitivity, immunologic reaction. The clinical presentation of ACD is described as *acute, subacute,* or *chronic*. The inciting agent must have a haptenic structure (i.e., an incomplete, low-molecular-weight antigen) and must be in solution (usually sweat) in order to encounter a dendritic, antigen-presenting cell (usually a Langerhans cell) in the epidermis, which subsequently delivers the antigen to the draining lymph node. In the lymph node, the antigen/hapten is presented to a nonsensitized T-helper (Th0) cell, which then produces a clone of specifically sensitized Th1 cells that subsequently enter the circulatory system. Some of the sensitized Th1 cells possess "homing" surface receptors that draw them to the antigen entry site in the epidermis. The residual antigen will, upon contact with sensitized Th1 cells, indirectly cause the release of proinflammatory mediators that result in eczema. Once the patient is sensitized, 24 to 48 hours typically elapse from the subsequent contact until the initial clinical reaction; however, subsequent reactions to the same agent will occur in half the time (an anamnestic response). The allergenicity of a hapten is significantly influenced by the thickness and integrity of the skin surface:

thinner sites such as the eyelids, earlobes, and genital skin are most vulnerable, while thicker skin sites such as the palms and soles are more resistant. The exposure pattern determines the appearance of the dermatitis. Episodic exposure, as in rhus dermatitis, usually presents as a very pruritic, linear, vesiculobullous rash. Protracted exposure—for example, to nickel in jewelry or environmental agents—presents as a thickened (lichenified), scaly, red plaque. Rhus dermatitis—that is, exposure to plants of the genus *Rhus (Toxicodendron)*, namely poison ivy, poison oak, and poison sumac—is the most common cause of allergic skin reactions in the United States. More than 85% of individuals will develop ACD if exposed to these plants. There are many OTC products available to treat contact dermatitis, including emollients, topical corticosteroids, topical anesthetics, and antihistamines.

ANTIHISTAMINES

Antihistaminic (H_1-receptor)—Antihistamines used in the treatment of allergy act by competing with histamine for H_1-receptor sites on effector cells. They thereby prevent, but do not reverse, responses mediated by histamine alone. Antihistamines antagonize, in varying degrees, most of the pharmacological effects of histamine, including urticaria and pruritus. Also, the anticholinergic actions of most antihistamines provide a drying effect on the nasal mucosa.

Pruritus (treatment); *urticaria* (treatment); *angioedema* (treatment); *dermatographism* (treatment); *transfusion reactions, urticarial* (treatment)—Antihistamines are indicated for the symptomatic treatment of pruritus associated with allergic reactions and of mild, uncomplicated allergic skin manifestations of urticaria and angioedema, in dermatographism, and in urticaria associated with transfusions.

Brompheniramine

Capsules/Elixir/Tablets

Adults/Pediatrics ≥12 years of age: 4mg every 4 to 6 hours as needed.

Pediatrics 2 to 6 years of age: 1mg every 4 to 6 hours as needed.

Pediatrics 6 to 12 years of age: 2mg every 4 to 6 hours as needed.

Chlorpheniramine

Capsules, extended-release/Tablets, extended-release

Adults/Pediatrics ≥12 years of age: 8 to 12mg every 8 to 12 hours as needed.

Syrup/Tablets

Adults/Pediatrics ≥12 years of age: 4mg every 4 to 6 hours as needed.

Pediatrics 6 to 12 years of age: 2mg 3 or 4 times a day as needed. Max: 12mg per day.

Clemastine

Syrup/Tablets

Adults/Pediatrics ≥12 years of age: 1.34mg 2 times a day; or 2.68mg 1 to 3 times a day as needed.

Pediatrics 6 to 12 years of age: 0.67mg to 1.34mg 2 times a day; not to exceed 4.02mg/day.

Diphenhydramine

Capsules

Adults/Pediatrics ≥12 years of age: 25 to 50mg every 4 to 6 hours as needed.

Pediatrics up to 6 years of age: 6.25 to 12.5mg every 4 to 6 hours.

Pediatrics 6 to 12 years of age: 12.5 to 25mg every 4 to 6 hours; not to exceed 150mg/day.

Elixir/Tablets

Adults/Pediatrics ≥12 years of age: 25 to 50mg every 4 to 6 hours as needed.

Pediatrics: 1.25mg/kg of body weight or 37.5mg/m^2 of body surface, every 4 to 6 hours; not to exceed 300mg/day.

Pediatrics weighing up to 9.1kg: 6.25 to 12.5mg every 4 to 6 hours.

Pediatrics weighing 9.1kg and over: 12.5 to 25mg every 4 to 6 hours.

Loratadine

Syrup

Adults/Pediatrics ≥6 years of age: 10mg once a day.

Pediatrics 2 to 6 years of age: 5mg once a day.

For more information, refer to the complete monograph for antihistamines in "Allergic Rhinitis" under Respiratory System.

TOPICAL ANESTHETICS

Local anesthetics block both the initiation and conduction of nerve impulses by decreasing the neuronal membrane's permeability to sodium ions. This reversibly stabilizes the membrane and inhibits depolarization, resulting in the failure of a propagated action potential and subsequent conduction blockade.

Skin disorders, minor (treatment)—Topical anesthetics are indicated to relieve pain, pruritus, and inflammation associated with minor skin disorders, including:

- Burns, minor, including sunburn
- Bites (or stings), insect
- Dermatitis, contact (including poison ivy, poison oak, or poison sumac)
- Wounds, minor, such as cuts and scratches

Benzocaine/Dibucaine/Pramoxine/Tetracaine *(See products on next page)*

Adults/Pediatrics ≥2 years of age: Apply to the affected area 3 or 4 times a day as needed.

Lidocaine *(See products on next page)*

Adults: Apply to the affected area 3 or 4 times a day as needed.

Pediatrics: Dosage must be individualized, depending on the child's age, weight, and physical condition, up to a maximum of 4.5 mg per kg of body weight.

For more information, refer to the complete monograph for topical anesthetics in "Burns" under Dermatological Conditions.

BROMPHENIRAMINE PRODUCTS	
Brand Name	**Dosage Form**
Dimetapp Allergy (Wyeth)	**Capsule:** 4mg **Tablet:** 4mg
Dimetapp Allergy Children's (Wyeth)	**Elixir:** 2mg/5mL
Dimetane Extentabs (Wyeth)	**Tablet:** 12mg

CHLORPHENIRAMINE PRODUCTS	
Brand Name	**Dosage Form**
Chlor-Trimeton (Schering)	**Syrup:** 2mg/5mL **Tablet:** 4mg,8mg,12mg
Efidac 24 (Novartis)	**Tablet:** 16mg

CLEMASTINE PRODUCTS	
Brand Name	**Dosage Form**
Tavist-1 (Novartis)	**Tablet:** 1.34mg

DIPHENHYDRAMINE PRODUCTS	
Brand Name	**Dosage Form**
Benadryl (Pfizer)	**Capsule:** 25mg **Tablet:** 25mg
Benadryl Allergy (Pfizer)	**Solution:** 12.5mg/5mL **Tablet:** 12.5mg
Benadryl Allergy Fastmelt (Pfizer)	**Tablet:** 19mg

LORATADINE PRODUCTS	
Brand Name	**Dosage Form**
Alavert (Wyeth)	**Tablet:** 10mg
Claritin (Schering)	**Solution:** 5mg/5mL
	Tablet: 10mg
Claritin Hives Relief (Schering)	**Tablet:** 10mg
Claritin RediTabs(Schering)	**Tablet:** 10mg

TOPICAL ANTIHISTAMINES

PHARMACOLOGY

Antihistaminic (H_1-receptor)—Antihistamines used in the treatment of allergy act by competing with histamine for H_1-receptor sites on effector cells. They thereby prevent, but do not reverse, responses mediated by histamine alone. Antihistamines antagonize, in varying degrees, most of the pharmacological effects of histamine, including urticaria and pruritus.

INDICATIONS

Pruritus (treatment)—Antihistamines are indicated for the symptomatic treatment of pruritus and pain associated with insect bites, minor burns, sunburn, minor skin irritations, minor cuts, scrapes, and rashes due to poison ivy, poison oak, and poison sumac.

WARNINGS/PRECAUTIONS

Patients sensitive to one of the antihistamines may be sensitive to others. Do not use on chicken pox or measles; with any other product containing diphenhydramine, even one, take orally; or on large areas of the body, including large areas of poison ivy, sunburn, or broken, blistered or, oozing skin. Avoid contact with eyes.

ADVERSE REACTIONS

Those indicating need for medical attention: Only if they continue or are bothersome

Incidence rare (only if significant systemic absorption):

Drowsiness; dryness of mouth, nose, or throat.

ADMINISTRATION AND DOSAGE

Diphenhydramine

Cream/Gel

Adults/Pediatrics ≥ 2 years of age: Apply to affected area not more than 3 to 4 times daily.

TOPICAL CORTICOSTEROIDS

PHARMACOLOGY

Corticosteroids diffuse across cell membranes and complex with specific cytoplasmic receptors. These complexes then enter the cell nucleus, bind to DNA (chromatin), and stimulate transcription of messenger RNA (mRNA) and subsequent protein synthesis of various inhibitory enzymes responsible for the anti-inflammatory effects of topical corticosteroids. These

BENZOCAINE PRODUCTS	
Brand Name	**Dosage Form**
Solarcaine (Schering)	**Spray:** 20%

BENZOCAINE/BENZETHONIUM CHLORIDE PRODUCTS	
Brand Name	**Dosage Form**
Lanacane Anti-Itch (Combe)	**Cream:** 6%-0.2%
Lanacane First-Aid (Combe)	**Cream:** 20%-0.2%
Lanacane Maximum Strength (Combe)	**Cream:** 20%-0.2%

BENZOCAINE/CHLOROXYLENOL PRODUCTS	
Brand Name	**Dosage Form**
Foille Medicated First Aid (Blistex)	**Ointment:** 5%-0.1% **Spray:** 5%-0.1%

DIBUCAINE PRODUCTS	
Brand Name	**Dosage Form**
Nupercainal (Novartis)	**Cream:** 0.50% **Ointment:** 1%

LIDOCAINE PRODUCTS	
Brand Name	**Dosage Form**
Solarcaine Aloe Extract (Schering)	**Gel:** 0.5% **Spray:** 0.50%

PRAMOXINE PRODUCTS	
Brand Name	**Dosage Form**
Sarna Sensitive (Stiefel)	**Lotion:** 1%

PRAMOXINE/MENTHOL PRODUCTS	
Brand Name	**Dosage Form**
Gold Bond Medicated Anti-Itch Maximum Strength (Chattem)	**Cream:** 1%-1%

DIPHENHYDRAMINE PRODUCTS	
Brand Name	**Dosage Form**
Benadryl Itch Relief Stick Extra Strength (Pfizer)	**Stick:** 2%
Benadryl Itch Stopping Cream Original (Pfizer)	**Cream:** 1%
Benadryl Itch Stopping Cream Extra Strength (Pfizer)	**Cream:** 2%
Benadryl Itch Stopping Gel Extra Strength (Pfizer)	**Gel:** 2%
Benadryl Itch Stopping Spray Extra Strength (Pfizer)	**Spray:** 2%

anti-inflammatory effects include inhibition of early processes such as edema, fibrin deposition, capillary dilatation, movement of phagocytes into the area, and phagocytic activities. Later processes, such as capillary production, collagen deposition, and keloid formation, are also inhibited by corticosteroids. The overall actions of topical corticosteroids are catabolic.

Factors that increase the clinical efficacy and potential for adverse effects of topical corticosteroids include enhancement of pharmacologic activity of the compound by altering molecular structure, increasing stratum corneum penetration of the compound, and increasing bioavailability of the compound from the vehicle. The pharmacologic activity of topical corticosteroids is increased by several changes in molecular structure. Addition of a 9-alpha-fluorine atom increases the anti-inflammatory glucocorticoid activity, but simultaneously increases undesired mineralocorticoid activity. Mineralocorticoid activity is diminished by addition of a 16-hydroxy or 16-methyl group. Substitution or masking of 16- or 17-hydroxy groups with longer side chains such as acetonide, propionate, or valerate increases lipophilicity and subsequently stratum corneum penetration.

Dental paste in dental dosage forms acts as an adhesive vehicle for application of corticosteroids to oral mucosa. The vehicle also reduces pain by serving as a protective covering.

The following table lists a potency rank of low, medium, high, or very high for topical corticosteroid preparations. Products with **low potency** have a modest anti-inflammatory effect and are safest for chronic application. They are also the safest products for use on the face and intertriginous areas, with occlusion, and in infants and young children.

Products with **medium potency** are used for moderate inflammatory dermatoses, including chronic conditions such as hand eczema and atopic eczema. They may be used on the face and intertriginous areas for a limited duration.

High potency preparations are used for more severe inflammatory dermatoses, including lichen simplex chronicus and psoriasis. They may be used for an intermediate duration, or for longer periods in areas with thickened skin due to chronic conditions. High potency preparations may also be used on the face and intertriginous areas but only for a short time.

Very high potency products are used primarily as an alternative to systemic corticosteroid therapy when local areas are involved. They are used for conditions marked by thick, chronic lesions caused by psoriasis, lichen simplex chronicus, discoid lupus erythematosus, and other severe skin disorders. There is a high likelihood of skin atrophy with the use of very high potency preparations. They should be used for only a short time and on small surface areas. Occlusive dressings should not be used with these products.

INDICATIONS

Topical corticosteroids are indicated to provide symptomatic relief of inflammation and/or pruritus associated with acute and chronic corticosteroid-responsive disorders. The location of the skin lesion to be treated should be considered in selecting a formulation. In areas with thinner skin, such as facial, eye, and intertriginous areas, low-potency corticosteroid preparations are preferred for long-term therapy. Low- to medium-potency products may be used on the ears, trunk, arms, legs, and scalp. Medium- to very high-potency formulations may be required for treatment of dermatologic disorders in areas with thicker skin, such as the palms and soles. Lotion, aerosol, and gel formulations are cosmetically better suited for hairy areas.

The type of lesion to be treated should also be considered in product selection. For dry, scaly, cracked, thickened, or hardened skin, ointments of medium potency are often used. Medium-potency lotions, aerosols, or creams are preferred in treating moister, weeping lesions or areas or in treating conditions with intense inflammation. High- to very high-potency ointments may be required to treat hyperkeratotic or thick skin lesions.

Dermatitis, atopic, mild to moderate; dermatitis, contact; dermatitis, nummular, mild; dermatitis, seborrheic, facial and intertriginous areas; dermatoses, other forms of, mild to moderate; dermatoses, inflammatory, other, mild to moderate; intertrigo; lichen planus, facial and intertriginous areas; lupus erythematosus, discoid, facial and intertriginous areas; polymorphous light eruption; pruritus, anogenital; pruritus senilis; psoriasis, facial and intertriginous areas; xerosis, inflammatory phase—Topical corticosteroids of low to medium potency are indicated in the treatment of corticosteroid-responsive dermatologic disorders. Occlusive dressings may also be required for chronic or severe cases of lichen simplex chronicus, psoriasis, eczema, atopic dermatitis, or chronic hand eczema. The more potent topical corticosteroids and/or occlusive dressings may be required for conditions such as discoid lupus erythematosus, lichen planus, granuloma annulare, psoriatic plaques, and psoriasis affecting the palms, soles, elbows, or knees.

Alopecia areata; dermatitis, atopic, moderate to severe; dermatitis, exfoliative, generalized; dermatitis, nummular, moderate to severe; dermatitis, other forms of, moderate to severe; dermatoses, inflammatory, other, moderate to severe; granuloma annulare; keloids, reduction of associated itching; lichen planus; lichen simplex chronicus; lichen striatus; lupus erythematosus, discoid and subacute cutaneous; myxedema, pretibial; necrobiosis lipoidica diabeticorum; pemphigoid; pemphigus; pityriasis rosea; psoriasis; sarcoidosis; sunburn—Topical corticosteroids of medium to very high potency are indicated in the treatment of corticosteroid-responsive dermatologic disorders. Systemic therapy with, or intralesional injection of, a corticosteroid may be required for some of the disorders, as determined by the type and severity of the condition or inadequate response to topical therapy. Occlusive dressings may also be required for conditions such as discoid lupus erythematosus, bullous disorders, lichen planus, granuloma annulare, psoriatic plaques, and psoriasis affecting the palms, soles, elbows, or knees.

Oral lesions, inflammatory or ulcerative (treatment)—Hydrocortisone acetate and triamcinolone acetonide dental pastes are indicated for adjunctive treatment and temporary relief of symptoms associated with nonherpetic oral inflammatory and ulcerative lesions, including recurrent aphthous stomatitis. Formulations of high potency gels and very high potency ointments are also used in the treatment of aphthous stomatitis. These agents are also used to treat other gingival disorders, such as desquamative gingivitis and oral lichen planus, when the diagnosis has been confirmed by biopsy testing. Gel formulations of high potency corticosteroids and dental triamcinolone are used in the treatment of lichen planus of the mucous membranes. Other topical corticosteroids are also used to treat gingival disorders.

Phimosis—Topical corticosteroids are indicated for the treatment of phimosis in boys.

Potency Rankings of Topical Corticosteroids

Generic Name	Dosage Form(s)	Strength (%)	Potency Ranking
Alclometasone dipropionate			
	Cream	0.05	Low
	Ointment	0.05	Low
Amcinonide			
	Cream	0.1	High
	Lotion	0.1	High
	Ointment	0.1	High
Beclomethasone dipropionate			
	Cream	0.025	Medium
	Lotion	0.025	Medium
	Ointment	0.025	Medium
Betamethasone benzoate			
	Cream	0.025	Medium
	Gel	0.025	Medium
	Lotion	0.025	Medium
Betamethasone dipropionate			
	Cream		
	Diprolene AF	0.05	Very high
	Others	0.05	High
	Gel		
	Diprolene	0.05	Very high
	Lotion		
	Diprolene	0.05	Very high
	Others	0.05	High
	Ointment		
	Diprolene	0.05	Very high
	Others	0.05	High
	Topical aerosol	0.1	High
Betamethasone valerate			
	Cream	0.01	Medium
	Cream	0.05	Medium
	Cream	0.1	Medium
	Foam	0.12	Medium
	Lotion	0.05	Medium
	Lotion	0.1	Medium
	Ointment	0.05	Medium
	Ointment	0.1	Medium
Clobetasol propionate			
	Cream	0.05	Very high
	Ointment	0.05	Very high
	Solution	0.05	Very high
Clobetasone butyrate			
	Cream	0.05	Medium
	Ointment	0.05	Medium

Potency Rankings of Topical Corticosteroids (cont.)

Generic Name	Dosage Form(s)	Strength (%)	Potency Ranking
Clocortolone pivalate			
	Cream	0.1	Low
Desonide			
	Cream	0.05	Low
	Lotion	0.05	Low
	Ointment	0.05	Low
Desoximetasone			
	Cream	0.05	Medium
	Cream	0.25	High
	Gel	0.05	High
	Ointment	0.25	High
Dexamethasone			
	Gel	0.1	Low
	Topical aerosol	0.01	Low
	Topical aerosol	0.04	Low
Dexamethasone sodium phosphate			
	Cream	0.1(phosphate)	Low
Diflorasone diacetate			
	Cream	0.05	High
	Ointment		
	Psorcon	0.05	Very high
	Others	0.05	High
Diflucortolone valerate			
	Cream	0.1	Medium
	Ointment	0.1	Medium
Flumethasone pivalate			
	Cream	0.03	Low
	Ointment	0.03	Low
Fluocinolone acetonide			
	Cream	0.01	Medium
	Cream	0.025	Medium
	Cream	0.2	High
	Ointment	0.01	Medium
	Ointment	0.025	Medium
	Topical solution	0.01	Medium
Fluocinonide			
	Cream	0.01	High
	Cream	0.05	High
	Gel	0.05	High
	Ointment	0.01	High
	Ointment	0.05	High
	Topical solution	0.05	High

Potency Rankings of Topical Corticosteroids (cont.)

Generic Name	Dosage Form(s)	Strength (%)	Potency Ranking
Flurandrenolide			
	Cream	0.0125	Low
	Cream	0.025	Medium
	Cream	0.05	Medium
	Lotion	0.05	Medium
	Ointment	0.0125	Low
	Ointment	0.025	Medium
	Ointment	0.05	Medium
	Tape	4 mcg/cm	Medium
Fluticasone propionate			
	Cream	0.05	Medium
	Ointment	0.005	Medium
Halcinonide			
	Cream	0.025	High
	Cream	0.1	High
	Ointment	0.1	High
	Topical solution	0.1	High
Halobetasol propionate			
	Cream	0.05	Very high
	Ointment	0.05	Very high
Hydrocortisone			
	Cream	0.25	Low
	Cream	0.5	Low
	Cream	1	Low
	Cream	2.5	Low
	Lotion	0.25	Low
	Lotion	0.5	Low
	Lotion	1	Low
	Lotion	2	Low
	Lotion	2.5	Low
	Ointment	0.5	Low
	Ointment	1	Low
	Ointment	2.5	Low
	Topical aerosol solution	0.5	Low
	Topical spray solution	0.5	Low
	Topical solution	1	Low
	Topical solution	2.5	Low

Potency Rankings of Topical Corticosteroids (cont.)

Generic Name	Dosage Form(s)	Strength (%)	Potency Ranking
Hydrocortisone acetate			
	Cream	0.1	Low
	Cream	0.5	Low
	Cream	1	Low
	Lotion	0.5	Low
	Ointment	0.5	Low
	Ointment	1	Low
	Topical aerosol foam	1	Low
Hydrocortisone butyrate			
	Cream	0.1	Medium
	Ointment	0.1	Medium
Hydrocortisone valerate			
	Cream	0.2	Medium
	Ointment	0.2	Medium
Mometasone furoate			
	Cream	0.1	Medium
	Lotion	0.1	Medium
	Ointment	0.1	Medium
Triamcinolone acetonide			
	Cream	0.025	Medium
	Cream	0.1	Medium
	Cream	0.5	High
	Lotion	0.025	Medium
	Lotion	0.1	Medium
	Ointment	0.025	Medium
	Ointment	0.1	Medium
	Ointment	0.5	High
	Topical aerosol	0.015	Medium

CONTRAINDICATIONS

Except under special circumstances, this medication should not be used when the following medical problem exists:

- Hypersensitivity to the topical corticosteroid prescribed or to any of its components or to any other corticosteroid—*major clinical significance.*

Risk-benefit should be considered when the following medical problems exist:

- Infection at treatment site (may be exacerbated if no appropriate antimicrobial agent is used concurrently).
- Skin atrophy, preexisting (may be exacerbated due to atrophigenic properties of corticosteroids).
- For use in the oral cavity: herpes simplex at treatment site (may be transmitted to other sites, including the eye).
- With long-term use of more potent formulations or if substantial absorption occurs: cataracts (corticosteroids may promote progression of cataracts, especially with the use of high- to very high-potency products in periorbital area); diabetes mellitus (loss of control of diabetes may occur due to possible elevations in blood glucose); glaucoma (intraocular pressure may be increased, especially with the use of high- to very high-potency products in periorbital area); tuberculosis (may be exacerbated or reactivated; appropriate antitubercular chemotherapy or prophylaxis should be administered concurrently).

WARNINGS/PRECAUTIONS

Mutagenicity:

Betamethasone—Betamethasone was found to be genotoxic in the in vitro human peripheral blood lymphocyte chromosome aberration assay with metabolic activation and in the in vivo mouse bone marrow micronucleus assay.

Fluocinonide—Fluocinonide revealed no evidence of mutagenic or clastogenic potential based on the Ames test and an in vitro chromosomal aberration assay in human lymphocytes. However, fluocinonide was positive for clastogenic potential when tested in the in vivo mouse bone marrow micronucleus assay.

Fluticasone—No mutagenicity was shown with fluticasone propionate in the Ames test, *Escherichia coli* fluctuation test, *Saccharomyces cerevisiae* gene conversion test, or Chinese hamster ovarian cell assay. Fluticasone was not clastogenic in mouse micronucleus or cultured human lymphocyte tests.

Halobetasol—Halobetasol propionate was not found to be genotoxic in the Ames/ Salmonella assay, sister chromatid exchange test in Chinese hamster somatic cells, chromosome aberration studies of germinal and somatic cells of rodents, and a mammalian spot test to determine point mutations. It was found to be mutagenic in a Chinese hamster micronucleus test, and in a mouse lymphoma gene mutation assay in vitro.

Hydrocortisone and prednisolone—Studies on mutagenicity with hydrocortisone and prednisolone yielded negative results.

Mometasone—No mutagenicity was shown with mometasone in the Ames test, mouse lymphoma assay, and a micronucleus test.

Pregnancy: FDA Category C. Topical corticosteroids, especially the more potent ones, should not be used extensively, in large amounts, or for protracted periods in pregnant patients or in patients who are planning to become pregnant. Adequate and well-controlled studies in humans have not been done. Studies in animals have shown that topical corticosteroids are systemically absorbed and may cause fetal abnormalities, especially when used in large amounts, with occlusive dressings, for prolonged periods of time, or if the more potent agents are used.

Breastfeeding: It is not known whether topical corticosteroids are distributed into breast milk. However, problems in humans have not been documented. Systemic corticosteroids are distributed into breast milk and may cause unwanted effects, such as growth suppression, in the infant. Topical corticosteroids should not be applied to the breasts prior to nursing.

Pediatrics: Children and adolescents have a large skin surface area to body weight ratio and less developed, thinner skin, which may result in absorption of greater amounts of topical corticosteroids compared with older patients. Absorption is also greater in premature infants than in full-term newborns, due to inadequate development of the stratum corneum. Adrenal suppression, Cushing's syndrome, intracranial hypertension, and growth retardation due to the systemic absorption of topical corticosteroids have been documented in children. Therefore, special care must be exercised when these agents are used in children and growing adolescents, especially if factors that increase absorption are involved. It is recommended that only low-potency, unfluorinated topical corticosteroids that have a free 17-hydroxyl group be used in children or growing adolescents unless there is a demonstrated need for one of the other topical corticosteroids. Generally, pediatric therapy continuing for longer than 2 weeks and consisting of doses in excess of one daily application (with medium- or high-potency corticosteroids) or two daily applications (with low-potency corticosteroids) should be evaluated carefully by the physician. This is especially important if medication is applied to more than 5% to 10% of the body surface or if an occlusive dressing is used. A tight-fitting diaper or one covered with plastic pants may constitute an occlusive dressing.

Geriatrics: Although appropriate studies with topical corticosteroids have not been performed in the geriatric population, geriatrics-specific problems are not expected to limit the usefulness of topical corticosteroids in the elderly. However, elderly patients may be more likely to have preexisting skin atrophy secondary to aging. Purpura and skin lacerations that may raise the skin and subcutaneous tissue from deep fascia may be more likely to occur with the use of topical corticosteroids in geriatric patients. Therefore, topical corticosteroids should be used infrequently, for brief periods, or under close medical supervision in patients with evidence of preexisting skin atrophy. Use of lower-

potency topical corticosteroids may also be necessary in some patients.

ADVERSE REACTIONS

Those indicating need for medical attention: Incidence less frequent or rare

Allergic contact dermatitis (burning and itching of skin; apparent chronic therapeutic failure)—may also be caused by vehicle ingredients.

Folliculitis, furunculosis, pustules, pyoderma, vesiculation (painful, red or itchy, pus-containing blisters in hair follicles)—more frequent with occlusion or use of ointments in intertriginous areas.

Hyperesthesia (increased skin sensitivity).

Numbness in fingers.

Purpura (blood-containing blisters on skin).

Skin atrophy (thinning of skin with easy bruising, especially when used on facial or intertriginous areas).

Skin infection, secondary—more frequent with occlusion.

Stripping of epidermal layer—for tape dosage forms.

Telangiectasia (raised, dark red, wartlike spots on skin, especially when used on the face).

Incidence rare—with prolonged use or other factors that increase absorption

Acneiform eruptions (acne or oily skin, especially when used on the face).

Cataracts, posterior subcapsular (gradual blurring or loss of vision)—reported with use of systemic corticosteroids; caution is advised with use of high- and very high-potency topical corticosteroids in periorbital area.

Cushing's syndrome (backache; filling or rounding out of the face; irritability; menstrual irregularities; mental depression; in men—unusual decrease in sexual desire or ability; unusual tiredness or weakness).

Dermatitis, perioral (irritation of skin around mouth).

Ecchymosis (unusual bruising).

Edema (increased blood pressure; rapid weight gain; swelling of feet or lower legs). Gastric ulcer (loss of appetite; nausea; stomach bloating, burning, cramping, or pain; vomiting; weight loss).

Glaucoma, secondary (eye pain; gradual decrease in vision; nausea; vomiting)—with use of high- and very high-potency topical corticosteroids in periorbital area.

Hirsutism or hypertrichosis (unusual increase in hair growth, especially on the face). Hypertension.

Hypokalemic syndrome (irregular heartbeat; loss of appetite; muscle cramps or pain; nausea; severe weakness of extremities and trunk; vomiting).

Hypopigmentation (lightened skin color) or other changes in skin pigmentation.

Infection, aggravation of miliaria rubra (burning and itching of skin with pinhead-sized red blisters).

Protein depletion (muscle weakness).

Skin laceration (tearing of skin).

Skin maceration (softening of skin).

Striae (reddish purple lines on arms, face, legs, trunk, or groin).

Subcutaneous tissue atrophy.

Unusual loss of hair, especially on the scalp.

Those indicating need for medical attention only if they continue or are bothersome:

Incidence less frequent or rare

Burning, dryness, irritation, itching, or redness of skin, mild and transient.

Increased redness or scaling of skin lesions, mild and transient.

Skin rash, minor and transient.

Those not indicating need for medical attention:

Stinging, mild and temporary—when foam, gel, lotion, solution, or aerosol form of medication is applied.

ADMINISTRATION AND DOSAGE

General Dosing Information

For topical dosage forms:

To minimize the possibility of significant systemic absorption of corticosteroids during long-term therapy, treatment may be interrupted periodically, small amounts of the preparation may be applied, or one area of the body may be treated at a time. Occlusion, whether by oleaginous ointment, a thin film of polyethylene, dermatologic patch, or tape, promotes increased hydration of the stratum corneum and increased absorption. Rarely, body temperature may be elevated if large areas are covered with an occlusive dressing; occlusive dressings should not be used if body temperature is elevated. Use of intermittent rather than continuous occlusion may decrease the risk of side effects. Generally, occlusive dressings should be changed every 24 hours or more frequently. Very high-potency topical corticosteroid formulations should not be used with occlusive dressings.

Rarely, gradual withdrawal of therapy or supplemental systemic corticosteroid therapy may be required to avoid symptoms of steroid withdrawal. Gradual withdrawal of therapy by decreasing the frequency of application or by using products of decreasing potency may also be necessary to avoid a rebound flare-up of certain conditions such as psoriasis. Tachyphylaxis may also result from continual usage.

Certain topical corticosteroids may be used as adjunctive therapy to antimicrobial agents for controlling inflammation, erythema, and pruritus associated with bacterial or fungal skin infections. If symptomatic relief is not noted within a few days to 1 week, the topical corticosteroid should be discontinued until the infection is controlled.

Hydrocortisone (only available OTC topical corticosteroid)

Cream/Lotion/Ointment

Adults: Apply to affected area 1 to 4 times a day.

Pediatrics ≥2 years of age: 0.25%-0.05%: Apply to affected area 1 to 4 times a day. 1%: Apply to affected area 1 to 2 times a day.

Topical Solution

Adults: Apply to affected area 1 to 4 times a day.

Pediatrics ≥2 years of age: Apply to affected area 1 to 2 times a day.

HYDROCORTISONE PRODUCTS (DERMATITIS)

Brand Name	Dosage Form
Aveeno Anti-itch (J & J)	**Cream:** 1%
Caldecort (Novartis)	**Cream:** 1% **Spray:** 0.50%
Caldecort Light (Novartis)	**Cream:** 1%
Cortaid Intensive Therapy (Pharmacia)	**Cream:** 1%
Cortaid Maximum Strength (Pharmacia)	**Cream:** 1%
	Ointment: 1% **Stick:** 1%
Cortaid Sensitive Skin w/aloe (Pharmacia)	**Cream:** 0.05%
Cortixaine (UCB)	**Cream:** 0.05%
Cortizone-5(Pfizer)	**Ointment:** 0.50%
Cortizone-10 (Pfizer)	**Cream:** 1% **Ointment:** 1%
Cortizone-10 Plus (Pfizer)	**Cream:** 1%
Cortizone 10 QuickShot(Pfizer)	**Spray:** 1%
Dermarest Dricort (Del)	**Cream:** 1%
Dermarest Eczema Medicated (Del)	**Lotion:** 1%
Gynecort Anti-itch (Combe)	**Cream:** 1%
Hytone (Dermik)	**Lotion:** 1%
Ivy Soothe (Enviroderm)	**Cream:** 1%
Ivy State Dual Action Poison Ivy	**Gel:** 1%
Exfoliant and Treatment (Tec)	
Lanacort (Combe)	**Cream:** 1%
Massengill Medicated Towelettes (GSK)	**Pads:** 0.50%
Neutrogena T/Scalp (Neutrogena)	**Liquid:** 1%
Nupercainal HC 1% (Novartis)	**Cream:** 1%
Scalpicin (Combe)	**Liquid:** 1%

HYDROCORTISONE PRODUCTS (HEMORRHOIDS)

Brand Name	Dosage Form
Anusol HC-1 (Pfizer)	**Ointment:** 1%
Preparation H Cortisone (Wyeth)	**Cream:** 1%

DOSING INFORMATION FOR CONTACT DERMATITIS PRODUCTS

The following table provides a quick comparison of the ingredients and dosages of common brand-name OTC drugs. Products are listed alphabetically by drug category and brand name.

BRAND NAME	GENERIC INGREDIENT/STRENGTH	DOSE
ANTIHISTAMINE		
Benadryl Extra Strength Gel Pump *(Pfizer Consumer Healthcare)*	Diphenhydramine HCl 2%	**Adults & Peds ≥12 yo:** Apply to affected area tid-qid.
ANTIHISTAMINE COMBINATION		
Benadryl Extra Strength Cream *(Pfizer Consumer Healthcare)*	Diphenhydramine HCl/Zinc Acetate 2%-0.1%	**Adults & Peds ≥12 yo:** Apply to affected area tid-qid.
Benadryl Extra Strength Spray *(Pfizer Consumer Healthcare)*	Diphenhydramine HCl/Zinc Acetate 2%-0.1%	**Adults & Peds ≥12 yo:** Apply to affected area tid-qid.
Benadryl Itch Relief Stick *(Pfizer Consumer Healthcare)*	Diphenhydramine HCl/Zinc Acetate 2%-0.1%	**Adults & Peds ≥2 yo:** Apply to affected area tid-qid.
Benadryl Original Cream *(Pfizer Consumer Healthcare)*	Diphenhydramine HCl/Zinc Acetate 1%-0.1%	**Adults & Peds ≥2 yo:** Apply to affected area tid-qid.
CalaGel Anti-Itch Gel *(Tec Laboratories)*	Diphenhydramine HCl/Zinc Acetate/ Benzenthonium Chloride 1.8%-0.21%-15%	**Adults & Peds ≥2 yo:** Apply to affected area qd-tid.
Ivarest Anti-Itch Cream *(Blistex)*	Diphenhydramine HCl/Calamine 2%-14%	**Adults & Peds ≥2 yo:** Apply to affrected area tid-qid.

DOSING INFORMATION FOR CONTACT DERMATITIS PRODUCTS (cont.)

BRAND NAME	GENERIC INGREDIENT/STRENGTH	DOSE
ASTRINGENT		
Bomeboro Powder Packets *(Bayer Healthcare)*	Aluminum Acetate/Aluminum Sulfate 938mg-1191mg	**Adults & Peds:** Dissolve 1-2 packets and apply to affected area for 15-30 min. tid.
Ivy-Dry Super Lotion Extra Strength *(Ivy Corporation)*	Zinc Acetate/Benzyl Alcohol 2%-10%	**Adults & Peds ≥6 yo:** Apply to affected area qd-tid.
ASTRINGENT COMBINATION		
Aveeno Anti-Itch Cream *(Johnson & Johnson Consumer)*	Calamine/Pramoxine HCl/Camphor 3%-1%-0.47%	**Adults & Peds ≥2 yo:** Apply to affected area qd-qid.
Aveeno Anti-Itch Lotion *(Johnson & Johnson Consumer)*	Calamine/Pramoxine HCl/Camphor 3%-1%-0.47%	**Adults & Peds ≥2 yo:** Apply to affected area qd-qid.
Caladryl Clear Lotion *(Pfizer Consumer Healthcare)*	Zinc Acetate/Pramoxine HCl 0.1%-1%	**Adults & Peds ≥2 yo:** Apply to affected area tid-qid.
Caladryl Lotion *(Pfizer Consumer Healthcare)*	Calamine/Pramoxine HCl 8%-1%	**Adults & Peds ≥2 yo:** Apply to affected area tid-qid.
Calamine lotion *(Various)*	Calamine/Zinc Oxide 6.971%-6.971%	**Adults & Peds:** Apply to affected area prn.
CLEANSER		
Ivy-Dry Scrub *(Ivy Corporation)*	Polyethylene, sodium lauryl sulfoacetate, cetearyl alcohol, nonoxynol-9, camellia sinensis oil, phenoxyethanol, methylparaben, propylparaben, triethanolamine, carbomer, erythorbic acid, aloe barbadensis extract, tocopheryl acetate extract, tetrasodium EDTA	**Adults & Peds:** Wash affected area prn.
IvyStat! Gel/Exfoliant *(Tec Laboratories)*	Hydrocortisone 1% (gel), Cocamidopropylsultaine, PEG-4 laurate, cocamide DEA, polyethylene beads, sodium chloride, benzethonium chloride (cleanser)	**Adults & Peds ≥2 yo:** Apply to affected area tid-qid.
CORTICOSTEROID		
Aveeno Anti-Itch Cream 1% *(Johnson & Johnson Consumer)*	Hydrocortisone 1%	**Adults & Peds ≥2 yo:** Apply to affected area tid-qid.
Cortaid Intensive Therapy Cooling Spray *(Pharmacia Consumer Healthcare)*	Hydrocortisone 1%	**Adults & Peds ≥2 yo:** Apply to affected area tid-qid.
Cortaid Intensive Therapy Moisturizing Cream *(Pharmacia Consumer Healthcare)*	Hydrocortisone 1%	**Adults & Peds ≥2 yo:** Apply to affected area tid-qid.
Cortaid Maximum Strength Cream *(Pharmacia Consumer Healthcare)*	Hydrocortisone 1%	**Adults & Peds ≥2 yo:** Apply to affected area tid-qid.
Cortizone-10 Cream *(Pfizer Consumer Healthcare)*	Hydrocortisone 1%	**Adults & Peds ≥2 yo:** Apply to affected area tid-qid.
Cortizone-10 Maximum Strength Anti-Itch Ointment *(Pfizer Consumer Healthcare)*	Hydrocortisone 1%	**Adults & Peds ≥2 yo:** Apply to affected area tid-qid.
Cortizone-10 Ointment *(Pfizer Consumer Healthcare)*	Hydrocortisone 1%	**Adults & Peds ≥2 yo:** Apply to affected area tid-qid.
Cortizone-10 Plus Maximum Strength Cream *(Pfizer Consumer Healthcare)*	Hydrocortisone 1%	**Adults & Peds ≥2 yo:** Apply to affected area tid-qid.
Cortizone-10 Quick Shot Spray *(Pfizer Consumer Healthcare)*	Hydrocortisone 1%	**Adults & Peds ≥2 yo:** Apply to affected area tid-qid.
Dermarest Eczema Lotion *(Del Laboratories)*	Hydrocortisone 1%	**Adults & Peds ≥2 yo:** Apply to affected area tid-qid.
COUNTERIRRITANT		
Gold Bond First Aid Quick Spray *(Chattem)*	Menthol/Benzethonium Chloride 1%-0.13%	**Adults & Peds ≥2 yo:** Apply to affected area tid-qid.
Gold Bond Medicated Maximum Strength Anti-Itch Cream *(Chattem)*	Menthol/Pramoxine HCl 1%-1%	**Adults & Peds ≥2 yo:** Apply to affected area tid-qid.
Ivy Block Lotion *(Enviroderm Pharmaceuticals)*	Bentoquatam 5%	**Adults & Peds ≥6 yo:** Apply q4h for continued protection.
LOCAL ANESTHETIC		
Solarcaine Aloe Extra Burn Relief Gel *(Schering-Plough)*	Lidocaine HCl 0.5%	**Adults & Peds ≥2 yo:** Apply to affected area tid-qid.

DOSING INFORMATION FOR CONTACT DERMATITIS PRODUCTS (cont.)

Brand Name	Generic Ingredient/Strength	Dose
Solarcaine Aloe Extra Spray *(Schering-Plough)*	Lidocaine 0.5%	**Adults & Peds ≥2 yo:** Apply to affected area tid-qid.
Solarcaine First Aid Medicated Spray *(Schering-Plough)*	Benzocaine/Triclosan 20%-0.13%	**Adults & Peds ≥2 yo:** Apply to affected area qd-tid.
LOCAL ANESTHETIC COMBINATION		
Bactine First Aid Liquid *(Bayer Healthcare)*	Lidocaine HCl/Benzalkonium Cl 2.5%-0.13%	**Adults & Peds ≥2 yo:** Apply to affected area qd-tid.
Bactine Pain Relieving Cleansing Spray *(Bayer Healthcare)*	Lidocaine HCl/Benzalkonium Cl 2.5%-0.13%	**Adults & Peds ≥2 yo:** Apply to affected area qd-tid.
Lanacane Maximum Strength Cream *(Combe)*	Benzocaine/Benzethonium Chloride 20%-0.2%	**Adults & Peds ≥2 yo:** Apply to affected area qd-tid.
Lanacane Maximum Strength Spray *(Combe)*	Benzocaine/Benzethonium Chloride/Ethanol 20%-0.2%-36%	**Adults & Peds ≥2 yo:** Apply to affected area qd-tid.
Lanacane Original Formula Cream *(Combe)*	Benzocaine/Benzethonium Chloride 6%-0.2%	**Adults & Peds ≥2 yo:** Apply to affected area qd-tid.
SKIN PROTECTANT		
Aveeno Itch Relief Lotion *(Johnson & Johnson Consumer)*	Dimethicone, Allantoin	**Adults & Peds ≥2 yo:** Apply to affected area tid-qid.
Aveeno Skin Relief Moisturizing Cream *(Johnson & Johnson Consumer)*	Dimethicone 2.5%	**Adults & Peds:** Apply to affected area prn.
Dermarest Poison Ivy Mousse *(Del Laboratories)*	Kaolin 5%	**Adults & Peds:** Apply to affected area prn.
SKIN PROTECTANT COMBINATION		
Gold Bond Extra Strength Medicated Body Lotion *(Chattem)*	Dimethicone/Menthol 5%-0.5%	**Adults & Peds:** Apply to affected area prn.
Gold Bond Medicated Body Lotion *(Chattem)*	Dimethicone/Menthol 5%-0.15%	**Adults & Peds:** Apply to affected area prn.
Gold Bond Medicated Extra Strength Powder *(Chattem)*	Zinc Oxide/Menthol 5%-0.8%	**Adults & Peds ≥2 yo:** Apply to affected area tid-qid.
Vaseline Intensive Care Lotion Advanced Healing *(Kendall)*	Dimethicone 1%-White Petrolatum	**Adults & Peds:** Apply to affected area prn.

Dandruff

Dandruff is characterized as a noninflammatory condition of the scalp that results in the production of white skin flakes that can be dry or greasy and vary in size. While dandruff is commonly confined to the scalp, itchy flaking may also appear on the eyebrows or around the hairline, ears, or nose. Dandruff is the result of hyperproliferation of skin cells that grow and die off too fast. Dandruff carries no health risk and is classified as a cosmetic problem only. There are a number of medicated shampoos available OTC to treat dandruff; most include pyrithione zinc, selenium sulfide, ketoconazole, or coal tar.

COAL TAR

Coal tar suppresses hyperplastic skin associated with some proliferative disorders. Although there is no confirmed evidence explaining its pharmacologic effects, its actions in humans have been reported as antiseptic, antipruritic, antiparasitic, antifungal, antibacterial, keratoplastic, and antiacantholic. Vasoconstrictive activity has also been reported.

Dandruff (treatment)—Indicated for the relief of itching, burning, and other symptoms associated with generalized persistent dermatoses, such as psoriasis, eczema, atopic dermatitis, and seborrheic dermatitis, and for the control of dandruff.

Coal tar preparations are also used in conjunction with ultraviolet (UV) light or sunlight, under the supervision of a physician, in the treatment of psoriasis or other conditions responding to this combined therapy.

Shampoo

Adults: Apply to scalp once a week to once a day.

For more information, refer to the complete monograph for coal tar in "Psoriasis" under Dermatological Conditions.

KETOCONAZOLE

PHARMACOLOGY

Ketoconazole belongs to the class of drugs known as azole antifungals. These drugs are fungistatic and may be fungicidal, depending on concentration. Their exact mechanism of action is unknown. Azoles inhibit biosynthesis of ergosterol or other sterols, damaging the fungal cell membrane and altering its permeability. As a result, loss of essential intracellular elements may occur.

Azoles also inhibit biosynthesis of triglycerides and phospholipids by fungi. In addition, azoles inhibit oxidative and peroxidative enzyme activity, resulting in intracellular buildup of toxic concentrations of hydrogen peroxide, which may contribute to deterioration of subcellular organelles and cellular necrosis. In *Candida albicans,* azoles inhibit transformation of blastospores into invasive mycelial form.

INDICATIONS

Tinea corporis (treatment); *tinea cruris* (treatment)—Ketoconazole cream is indicated as a primary agent in the topical treatment of tinea corporis (ringworm of the body) and tinea cruris (ringworm of the groin, or "jock itch") caused by *Trichophyton rubrum, T mentagrophytes*, and *Epidermophyton floccosum.*

Tinea pedis (treatment)—Ketoconazole cream is indicated as a primary agent in the topical treatment of tinea pedis ("athlete's foot").

Pityriasis versicolor (treatment)—Ketoconazole cream and ketoconazole 2% shampoo are indicated as primary agents in the topical treatment of pityriasis versicolor (tinea versicolor, or "sun fungus") caused by *Malassezia furfur.*

COAL TAR PRODUCTS	
Brand Name	**Dosage Form**
Denorex Therapeutic Protection (Wyeth)	**Shampoo:** 2.5%
Denorex Therapeutic Protection 2-in-1 (Wyeth)	**Shampoo:** 2.5%
Doak Tar (Doak)	**Shampoo:** 0.5%
Ionil-T (Healthpoint)	**Shampoo:** 1%
Ionil-T Plus (Healthpoint)	**Shampoo:** 2%
MG 217 (Triton)	**Ointment:** 2% **Shampoo:** 3%
Neutrogena T/Gel Extra Strength (Neutrogena)	**Shampoo:** 1%
Neutrogena T/Gel Original Formula (Neutrogena)	**Shampoo:** 0.5%
Neutrogena T/Gel Stubborn Itch (Neutrogena)	**Shampoo:** 0.5%
Pentrax (Medicis)	**Shampoo:** 0.5%
Polytar (Stiefel)	**Shampoo:** 0.5% **Soap:** 0.5%
Psoriasin (Alva-Amco)	**Gel:** 1.25% **Liquid:** 0.66%
Tegrin (GSK)	**Cream:** 0.8% **Shampoo:** 1.1%

KETOCONAZOLE PRODUCTS	
Brand Name	**Dosage Form**
Nizoral A-D (McNeil)	**Shampoo:** 1%

Candidiasis, cutaneous (treatment)—Ketoconazole cream is indicated as a primary agent in the topical treatment of cutaneous candidiasis caused by *Candida* species.

Dermatitis, seborrheic (treatment); *dermatitis, seborrheic* (prophylaxis)—Ketoconazole cream and ketoconazole 2% shampoo are indicated in the treatment of seborrheic dermatitis. Ketoconazole 2% shampoo is indicated in the prophylaxis of seborrheic dermatitis.

Dandruff (treatment); *dandruff* (prophylaxis)—Ketoconazole shampoo 1% and ketoconazole shampoo 2% are indicated in the treatment and prophylaxis of the flaking, scaling, and itching associated with dandruff.

Paronychia (treatment); *tinea barbae* (treatment); *tinea capitis* (treatment)—Ketoconazole cream is used as a primary agent in the topical treatment of paronychia. Ketoconazole cream is used as a secondary agent in the topical treatment of tinea barbae (ringworm of the beard, or "barber's itch") and tinea capitis (ringworm of the scalp).

CONTRAINDICATIONS

Risk-benefit should be considered when the following medical problems exist:

- Sensitivity to topical ketoconazole.
- Sensitivity to sulfites present in ketoconazole cream.

WARNINGS/PRECAUTIONS

Persons sensitive to miconazole or other imidazoles may also be sensitive to ketoconazole.

Pregnancy: FDA Category C. Ketoconazole crosses the placenta. Adequate and well-controlled studies in humans have not been done.

Breastfeeding: It is not known whether ketoconazole cream, applied topically on a regular basis, is absorbed systemically in sufficient amounts to be distributed into breast milk in detectable quantities. However, no systemic absorption was detected following a single application of ketoconazole cream to the chest, back, and arms of healthy volunteers. In addition, ketoconazole shampoo was not detected in plasma after chronic shampooing. Therefore, topical ketoconazole is unlikely to be distributed into breast milk in significant amounts or to cause adverse effects in the nursing infant.

ADVERSE REACTIONS

Those indicating need for medical attention (cream or shampoo): Incidence less frequent

Itching, stinging, or irritation not present before therapy.

For the cream—Incidence rare:

Contact dermatitis(skin rash).

Those indicating need for medical attention only if they continue or are bothersome:

For the shampoo—Incidence less frequent:

Dry skin; dryness or oiliness of the hair and scalp.

For the shampoo—Incidence rare:

Increase in normal hair loss.

ADMINISTRATION AND DOSAGE

General Dosing Information

Prolonged use of topical ketoconazole may rarely lead to skin sensitization, resulting in hypersensitivity reactions with subsequent topical or systemic use of the medication. Tinea versicolor may cause hyper- or hypopigmented patches on the body. Treatment of the infection may not result in normalization of the pigment for several months.

Cream (only available as prescription)

To reduce the possibility of recurrence of infection, tinea corporis and tinea cruris should be treated for at least 2 to 4 weeks. Candida and pityriasis versicolor should be treated for at least 2 to 3 weeks. Seborrheic dermatitis should be treated for at least 4 weeks or until clinical clearing occurs. Tinea pedis should be treated for approximately 4 to 6 weeks.

Shampoo 1% (only dosage form available OTC)

For dandruff:

Adults: Use twice a week for 2 to 4 weeks. Leave in place for 3 to 5 minutes before rinsing. *Prophylaxis*: Use once a week every 1 or 2 weeks.

PYRITHIONE ZINC

PHARMACOLOGY

Pyrithione zinc may act by an antimitotic action, resulting in a reduction in the turnover of epidermal cells. It also has bacteriostatic and fungistatic activity, but it is not known if this action contributes to the antiseborrheic effects of the drug.

INDICATIONS

Dandruff (treatment); *dermatitis, seborrheic* (treatment)—Depending on the formulation, pyrithione zinc is indicated to help control dandruff and seborrheic dermatitis of the scalp and/or seborrheic dermatitis of the body, face, and scalp.

PYRITHIONE ZINC PRODUCTS	
Brand Name	**Dosage Form**
DermaZinc (Dermalogix)	**Cream**: 0.25% **Shampoo**: 2% **Spray**: 0.25%
Denorex (Wyeth)	**Shampoo**: 2%
DHS Zinc Shampoo (Person & Covey)	**Shampoo**: 2%
Head & Shoulders Dandruff Conditioner (Procter & Gamble)	**Shampoo**: 0.5%
Head & Shoulders Dandruff Shampoo (Procter & Gamble)	**Shampoo**: 1%
Head & Shoulders Soothing Lotion (Procter & Gamble)	**Lotion**: 0.1%
Neutrogena Triple Moisture Active Soothing Shampoo (Neutrogena)	**Shampoo**: 0.5%
Pert Plus Dandruff Control (Procter & Gamble)	**Shampoo**: 1%
Selsun Blue Dandruff Conditioner (Chattem)	**Shampoo**: 0.75%
Zincon (Medtech)	**Shampoo**: 1%
ZNP (Stiefel)	**Soap**: 2%

CONTRAINDICATIONS

Risk-benefit should be considered when the following medical problems exist:

- Sensitivity to pyrithione zinc.

WARNINGS/PRECAUTIONS

Pregnancy: Problems in humans have not been documented.

Breastfeeding: Problems in humans have not been documented.

ADVERSE REACTIONS

Those indicating need for medical attention: Incidence more frequent

Irritation of skin.

ADMINISTRATION AND DOSAGE

General Dosing Information

The scalp and hair should be wetted with lukewarm water and enough shampoo massaged into the scalp to work up a lather; then the scalp and hair should be rinsed. Application should be repeated, then the scalp and hair rinsed thoroughly.

For dandruff/seborrheic dermatitis:

Bar

Adults/Pediatrics: Apply to affected areas of body, face, or scalp once a day for at least 2 times a week. Lather, massage into affected skin or scalp, rinse, and repeat.

Cream/Lotion

Adults/Pediatrics: Apply to affected areas of body, face, or scalp 1 to 3 times a day.

Shampoo

Adults/Pediatrics: Apply to scalp once a day for at least 2 times a week. Apply after wetting hair, leave on scalp for several minutes or massage vigorously, then rinse. May be used once a day if needed.

SELENIUM SULFIDE

PHARMACOLOGY

Selenium sulfide may act by an antimitotic action, resulting in a reduction in the turnover of epidermal cells. It also has local irritant, antibacterial, and mild antifungal activity, which may contribute to its effectiveness.

INDICATIONS

Dandruff (treatment); *dermatitis, seborrheic, of scalp* (treatment)—Selenium sulfide is indicated for the treatment of dandruff or seborrheic dermatitis of the scalp.

Tinea versicolor (treatment)—Selenium sulfide is indicated for the treatment of tinea versicolor.

CONTRAINDICATIONS

Risk-benefit should be considered when the following medical problems exist:

- Inflammation or exudation of skin, acute (an increase in absorption may occur).
- Sensitivity to selenium sulfide.

WARNINGS/PRECAUTIONS

Pregnancy: FDA Category C. It is recommended that selenium sulfide not be used for the treatment of tinea versicolor in pregnant women.

Breastfeeding: Problems in humans have not been documented.

ADVERSE REACTIONS

Those indicating need for medical attention: Incidence less frequent or rare

Skin irritation.

Those indicating need for medical attention only if they continue or are bothersome:Incidence more frequent

Unusual dryness or oiliness of hair or scalp.

Incidence less frequent

Increase in normal hair loss.

ADMINISTRATION AND DOSAGE

General Dosing Information

Selenium sulfide should not be used when acute inflammation or exudate is present, because an increase in absorption may occur. Discoloration of the hair may occur following use of selenium sulfide, especially if used on hair that is light, blond, or gray or has been chemically treated (ie, bleached, tinted, or permanent-waved). The discoloration may be minimized or avoided by thoroughly rinsing the hair for at least 5 minutes after treatment.

For dandruff/seborrheic dermatitis:

Lotion/Shampoo

Adults/Pediatrics: Apply to scalp 2 times a week for 2 weeks and then at less frequent intervals of once a week or once every 2 or more weeks.

For tinea versicolor:

Lotion (2.5%)

Adults/Pediatrics: Apply to body once a day for 7 days.

SELENIUM SULFIDE PRODUCTS	
Brand Name	**Dosage Form**
Head & Shoulders Intensive Treatment (Procter & Gamble)	**Shampoo:** 1%
Selsun Blue Dandruff (Chattem)	**Shampoo:** 1%

DOSING INFORMATION FOR DANDRUFF PRODUCTS

The following table provides a quick comparison of the ingredients and dosages of common brand-name OTC drugs. Products are listed alphabetically by generic ingredient and brand name.

BRAND NAME	GENERIC INGREDIENT/STRENGTH	DOSE
COAL TAR		
Denorex Dandruff Shampoo + Conditioner, Therapeutic (*Medtech Products*)	Coal Tar 2.5%	**Adults & Peds:** Use biw.
DHS Tar Dermatological Hair & Scalp Shampoo (*Person & Covey*)	Coal Tar 0.5%	**Adults & Peds:** Use biw.
Ionil T Therapeutic Coal Tar Shampoo (*Healthpoint*)	Coal Tar 5%	**Adults & Peds:** Use biw.
Neutrogena T-Gel Original Shampoo (*Neutrogena*)	Coal Tar 0.5%	**Adults & Peds:** Use biw.
Neutrogena T-Gel Shampoo, Extra Strength (*Neutrogena*)	Coal Tar 1%	**Adults & Peds:** Use biw.
Neutrogena T-Gel Shampoo, Stubborn Itch Control (*Neutrogena*)	Coal Tar 0.5%	**Adults & Peds:** Use biw.
KETOCONAZOLE		
Nizoral Anti-Dandruff Shampoo (*McNeil Consumer*)	Ketoconazole 1%	**Adults & Peds ≥12:** Use q3-4d prn.
PYRITHIONE ZINC		
Denorex Dandruff Shampoo, Daily Protection (*Medtech Products*)	Pyrithione zinc 2%	**Adults & Peds:** Use biw.
Garnier Fructis Fortifying Shampoo, Anti-Dandruff (*Garnier*)	Pyrithione zinc 1%	**Adults & Peds:** Use biw.
Head & Shoulders Dandruff Conditioner, Dry Scalp Care (*Procter & Gamble*)	Pyrithione zinc 1%	**Adults & Peds:** Use biw.
Head & Shoulders Dandruff Conditioner, Extra Fullness (*Procter & Gamble*)	Pyrithione zinc 0.5%	**Adults & Peds:** Use biw.
Head & Shoulders Dandruff Shampoo Plus Conditioner, Smooth & Silky (*Procter & Gamble*)	Pyrithione zinc 1%	**Adults & Peds:** Use biw.
Head & Shoulders Dandruff Shampoo, Citrus Breeze (*Procter & Gamble*)	Pyrithione zinc 1%	**Adults & Peds:** Use biw.
Head & Shoulders Dandruff Shampoo, Classic Clean (*Procter & Gamble*)	Pyrithione zinc 1%	**Adults & Peds:** Use biw.
Head & Shoulders Dandruff Shampoo, Dry Scalp Care (*Procter & Gamble*)	Pyrithione zinc 1%	**Adults & Peds:** Use biw.
Head & Shoulders Dandruff Shampoo, Extra Volume (*Procter & Gamble*)	Pyrithione zinc 1%	**Adults & Peds:** Use biw.
Head & Shoulders Dandruff Shampoo, Refresh (*Procter & Gamble*)	Pyrithione zinc 1%	**Adults & Peds:** Use biw.
Head & Shoulders Dandruff Shampoo, Sensitive Care (*Procter & Gamble*)	Pyrithione zinc 1%	**Adults & Peds:** Use biw.
L'Oreal VIVE for Men Shampoo, Thickening Anti-Dandruff (*L'Oreal*)	Pyrithione zinc 1%	**Adults & Peds:** Use biw.
Neutrogena T-Gel Daily Control Dandruff Shampoo (*Neutrogena*)	Pyrithione zinc 1%	**Adults & Peds:** Use biw.
Nexxus Dandarrest Dandruff Control Shampoo (*Nexxus Products*)	Pyrithione zinc 1.1%	**Adults & Peds:** Use biw.
Pantene Pro-V Shampoo + Conditioner, Anti-Dandruff (*Procter & Gamble*)	Pyrithione zinc 1%	**Adults & Peds:** Use biw.
Pert Plus Shampoo Plus Conditioner, Dandruff Control (*Procter & Gamble*)	Pyrithione zinc 1%	**Adults & Peds:** Use biw.
Selsun Blue Dandruff Conditioner (*Ross Products*)	Pyrithione zinc 0.75%	**Adults & Peds:** Use biw.
Suave for Men 2 in 1 Shampoo/Conditioner, Dandruff (*Suave*)	Pyrithione zinc 0.5%	**Adults & Peds:** Use biw.

DOSING INFORMATION FOR DANDRUFF PRODUCTS (cont.)

BRAND NAME	GENERIC INGREDIENT/STRENGTH	DOSE
SALICYLIC ACID		
Denorex Dandruff Shampoo, Extra Strength *(Medtech Products)*	Salicylic Acid 3%	**Adults & Peds:** Use biw.
Neutrogena T/Sal Shampoo, Scalp Build-up Control *(Neutrogena)*	Salicylic Acid 3.0%	**Adults & Peds:** Use biw.
Scalpicin Anti-Itch Liquid Scalp Treatment *(Combe)*	Salicylic Acid 3.0%	**Adults:** Apply to affected area qd-qid.
SELENIUM SULFIDE		
Head & Shoulders Dandruff Shampoo, Intensive Treatment *(Procter & Gamble)*	Selenium Sulfide 1%	**Adults & Peds:** Use biw.
Selsun Blue Dandruff Shampoo, Medicated Treatment *(Ross Products)*	Selenium Sulfide 1%	**Adults & Peds:** Use biw.
Selsun Blue Dandruff Shampoo Plus Conditioner *(Ross Products)*	Selenium Sulfide 1%	**Adults & Peds:** Use biw.
Selsun Blue Dandruff Shampoo, Balanced Treatment *(Ross Products)*	Selenium Sulfide 1%	**Adults & Peds:** Use biw.
Selsun Blue Dandruff Shampoo, Moisturizing Treatment *(Chattem)*	Selenium Sulfide 1%	**Adults & Peds:** Use biw.
SULFUR/SALICYLIC ACID		
Sebulex Medicated Dandruff Shampoo *(Westwood-Squibb)*	Sulfur/Salicylic Acid 2%-2%	**Adults & Peds** $\geq$**12:** Use qd.

Diaper Rash

Diaper rash is form of dermatitis defined as an acute, inflammatory reaction of the skin characterized by reddish, puffy, and perhaps slightly warmer skin in the diaper region. Diaper rash is caused by a local environmental irritant such as prolonged exposure to urine or feces, tight-fitting diapers, or bacterial or fungal infection, or it may result from the use of certain products such as disposable wipes, disposable diapers, and detergents. The recommended approach to treating diaper rash is prevention, which can be accomplished by changing diapers often, rinsing the baby's skin with water after each diaper change, and avoiding tight-fitting diapers and products known to cause or suspected of causing irritation. A wide variety of topical OTC products are available for the treatment of diaper rash; most contain a combination of white petrolatum, zinc oxide, and/or dimethicone.

DOSING INFORMATION FOR DIAPER RASH PRODUCTS

The following table provides a quick comparison of the ingredients and dosages of common brand-name OTC drugs. Products are listed alphabetically by brand name.

BRAND NAME	GENERIC INGREDIENT/STRENGTH	DOSE
WHITE PETROLATUM		
Balmex Extra Protective Clear Ointment *(Johnson & Johnson/Merck Cosumer)*	White Petrolatum 51%	**Peds:** Apply prn.
Vaseline Baby, Baby Fresh Scent *(Chesebrough Ponds)*	White Petrolatum	**Peds:** Apply prn.
Vaseline Petroleum Jelly *(Chesebrough Ponds)*	White Petrolatum	**Peds:** Apply prn.
ZINC OXIDE		
Balmex Diaper Rash Ointment with Aloe & Vitamin E *(Johnson & Johnson/Merck Consumer)*	Zinc Oxide 11.3%	**Peds:** Apply prn.
Boudreaux's Butt Paste, Diaper Rash Ointment *(George Boudreaux P.D.)*	Zinc Oxide 16%	**Peds:** Apply prn.
California Baby Diaper Rash Cream *(California Baby)*	Zinc Oxide 12%	**Peds:** Apply prn.
Canus Li'l Goat's Milk Ointment *(Canus)*	Zinc Oxide 40%	**Peds:** Apply prn.
Desitin Diaper Rash Ointment, Creamy, Fresh Scent *(Pfizer Consumer Healthcare)*	Zinc Oxide 10%	**Peds:** Apply prn.
Desitin Diaper Rash Ointment, Hypoallergenic *(Pfizer Consumer Healthcare)*	Zinc Oxide 40%	**Peds:** Apply prn.
Huggies Diaper Rash Cream *(Kimberly-Clark)*	Zinc Oxide 10%	**Peds:** Apply prn.
Johnson's Baby Diaper Rash Cream with Zinc Oxide *(Johnson & Johnson/Merck Consumer)*	Zinc Oxide 13%	**Peds:** Apply prn.
Mustela Bebe Vitamin Barrier Cream *(Pharmascience Laboratories)*	Zinc Oxide 10%	**Peds:** Apply prn.
Mustela Dermo-Pediatrics, Stelactiv Diaper Rash Cream *(Expanscience Laboratoires)*	Zinc Oxide 10%	**Peds:** Apply prn.
COMBINATION PRODUCTS		
A+D Original Ointment, Diaper Rash and All-Purpose Skincare Formula *(Schering-Plough)*	Petrolatum/Lanolin 53.4%-15.5%	**Peds:** Apply prn.
A+D Zinc Oxide Diaper Rash Cream with Aloe *(Schering-Plough)*	Dimethicone/Zinc Oxide 1%-10%	**Peds:** Apply prn.
Aveeno Baby Diaper Rash Cream *(Johnson & Johnson/Merck Consumer)*	Zinc Oxide/Dimethicone 13%-5%	**Peds:** Apply prn.

Dry Skin

Dry skin is a common condition that happens more often in winter when the cold air outside and the heated air inside cause low humidity. It develops because the skin loses moisture, leading to cracking, peeling, scaling, and flaking of the skin. Dry skin is most common on the arms, lower legs, sides of the abdomen, and thighs. It can cause the skin to feel and look rough and may cause pruritus that can be intense.

Dry skin is usually the result of environmental factors such as low humidity, central heating or air conditioning, bathing too frequently or for too long, and harsh soaps and/or detergents. The best treatment for dry skin is prevention, which can be accomplished by avoiding the environmental factors that cause it. Such practices as keeping baths and showers short, using warm—not hot—water, using mild cleansers and as little soap as possible, and patting the skin dry instead of rubbing it can prevent dry skin from developing. Using a humidifier and drinking plenty of water throughout the day can also be helpful. There are many OTC products available to help relieve symptoms and moisturize the skin.

DOSING INFORMATION FOR DRY SKIN PRODUCTS

The following table provides a quick comparison of the ingredients and dosages of common brand-name OTC drugs. Products are listed alphabetically by brand name.

BRAND NAME	INGREDIENT/STRENGTH	DOSE
EMOLLIENT		
AmLactin Moisturizing Cream (Upsher-Smith)	Lactic acid, ammonium hydroxide, light mineral oil, glyceryl stearate, PEG-100 stearate, glycerin, propylene glycol, magnesium aluminum silicate, laureth 4, polyoxyl 40 stearate, cetyl alcohol, methylcellulose, methyl and propylparabens	**Adults & Peds:** Apply to affected area bid.
AmLactin Moisturizing Lotion (Upsher-Smith)	Lactic acid, ammonium hydroxide, light mineral oil, glyceryl stearate, PEG-100 stearate, glycerin, propylene glycol, magnesium aluminum silicate, laureth 4, polyoxyl 40 stearate, cetyl alcohol, methylcellulose, methyl and propylparabens	**Adults & Peds:** Apply to affected area bid.
AmLactin XL Moisturizing Lotion Ultraplex Formulation (Upsher-Smith)	Ammonium lactate, potassium lactate, sodium lactate, emulsifyin wax, light mineral oil, white petrolatum, glycerin, propylene glycol, stearic acid, xanthum gum, methyl and propylparabens	**Adults & Peds:** Apply to affected area bid.
Aquaphor Baby Healing Ointment (Beiersdorf)	Petrolatum, mineral oil, cerein, lanolin alcohol	**Adults & Peds:** Apply to affected area prn.
Aquaphor Original Ointment (Beiersdorf)	Petrolatum, mineral oil, cerein, lanolin alcohol	**Adults & Peds:** Apply to affected area prn.
Aveeno Baby Moisture Soothing Relief Cream (Johnson & Johnson Consumer)	Glycerin, petrolatum, mineral oil, cetyl alcohol, dimethicone, avena sativa kernel flour, carbomer, sodium hydroxide, ceteareth-6, hydrolyzed milk protein, hydrolyzed oats, hydrolyzed soy protein, PEG-25 soya sterol, tetrasodium EDTA, methylparaben, citric acid, sodium citrate, benzalkonium chloride, benzaldehyde, butylene glycol, butylparaben, ethylparaben, ethyl alcohol, isobutylparaben, phenoxyethanol, propylparaben, stearyl alcohol	**Adults & Peds:** Apply to affected area prn.
Aveeno Bath Moisturizing Packets (Johnson & Johnson Consumer)	Colloidal Oatmeal 43%	**Adults & Peds:** Bathe in 1 packet for 15-20 min. qd-bid.
Aveeno Daily Baby Lotion (Johnson & Johnson Consumer)	Dimethicone 1.2%	**Peds:** Apply prn.
Aveeno Daily Moisturizer, Ultra-Calming SPF 15 (Johnson & Johnson Consumer)	Avobenzone/Octinoxate/Octisalate 3%-7.5%-2.%	**Adults:** Use qd.

DOSING INFORMATION FOR DRY SKIN PRODUCTS (cont.)

BRAND NAME	INGREDIENT/STRENGTH	DOSE
Aveeno Daily Moisturizing Lotion (Johnson & Johnson Consumer)	Dimethicone 1.25%	**Adults:** Use prn.
Aveeno Intense Relief Hand Cream (Johnson & Johnson Consumer)	Glycerin, distearyldimonium chloride, petrolatum, isopropyl palmitate, cetyl alcohol, aluminum starch octenylsuccinate, dimethicone, avena sativa kernel flour, benzyl alcohol, sodium chloride	**Adults & Peds:** Apply to affected area prn.
Aveeno Moisturizing Bar for Dry Skin (Johnson & Johnson Consumer)	Oat flour, cetearyl alcohol, stearic acid, sodium cocoyl isethionate, water, disodium lauryl sulfosuccinate, glycerin, hydrogenated vegetable oil, titanium dioxide, citric acid, sodium trideceth sulfate, hydrogenated castor oil	**Adults & Peds:** Wash face daily.
Aveeno Moisturizing Lotion, Skin Relief (Johnson & Johnson Consumer)	Dimethicone 1.25%	**Adults & Peds ≥2 yo:** Use daily.
Aveeno Positively Smooth Facial Moisturizer (Johnson & Johnson Consumer)	C12-15 alkyl benzoate, cetearyl alcohol, bis-phenylpropyl dimethicone, glycine, soja seed extract, butylene glycol, arachidyl alcohol, glycine soja protein, dimethicone, glycerin, panthenol, polyacrylamide, phenoxyethanol, cetearyl glucoside, behenyl alcohol, benzyl alcohol, C13-14 isoparaffin, DMDM hydantoin, arachidyl glucoside, disodium EDTA, methylparaben, laureth 7, BHT, ethylparaben, butylparaben, propylparaben, isobutylparaben, fragrance, iodopropynyl butylcarbamate	**Adults:** Use prn.
Aveeno Positively Smooth Moisturizing Lotion (Johnson & Johnson Consumer)	Glycerin, emulsifying wax, isononanoate, gylcine soja seed extract, propylene glycol isoceteth-3 acetate, dimethicone, cyclomethicone, polyacrylamide, stearic acid, panthenyl ethyl ether, tocopheryl acetate, panthenol, phenoxyethanol, C13-14 isoparaffin, dimethicone copolyol, benzyl alcohol, DMDM hydantoin, glyceryl laurate, laureth 7, methylparaben, cetearyl alcohol, tetrasodium EDTA, butylparaben, ethylparaben, BHT, propylparaben, isobutylparaben, fragrance, iodopropyl butylcarbamate	**Adults:** Use prn.
Aveeno Positively Smooth Moisturizing Pads (Johnson & Johnson Consumer)	Cocamidopropyl betaine, decyl glucoside, glycerin, disodium lauroamphodiacetate, PEG-16 soy sterol, polysorbate 20, PPG-2 hydroxyethyl cocamide, phenoxyethanol, tetrasodium EDTA, butylene glycol, sodium coco PG-dimonium chloride phosphate, sodium citrate, glycine soja protein, citric acid, PEG-14M, methylparaben, butylparaben, ethylparaben, isobutylparaben, propylparaben, fragrance	**Adults:** Use daily.
Aveeno Radiant Skin Daily Moisturizer with SPF 15 (Johnson & Johnson Consumer)	Octinoxate (octyl methoxycinnamate)/ Avobenzone 3%/Octisalate (octyl salicylate) 7.5%-3%-2%	**Adults:** Use prn.

DOSING INFORMATION FOR DRY SKIN PRODUCTS (cont.)

Brand Name	Ingredient/Strength	Dose
Aveeno Skin Relief Body Wash, Fragrance Free (Johnson & Johnson Consumer)	Glycerin, cocamidopropyl betaine, sodium laureth sulfate, decyl glucoside, oat Flour, glycol stearate, sodium lauroampho-PG-acetate phosphate, guar hydroxypropyltrimonium chloride, hydroxypropyltrimonium hydrolyzed wheat protein, PEG 20 glycerides, hydroxypropyltrimonium hydrolyzed wheat starch, PEG 150 pentaerythrityl tetrastearate, PEG 120 methyl glucose trioleate, tetrasodium EDTA, PEG-6 caprylic/capric glyceride, quaternium 15, coriandum sativum extract, elettaria cardamomum seed extract, conmiphora myhrrha extract	**Adults:** Use prn.
Carmol-10 Lotion (Doak)	Urea 10%	**Adults & Peds:** Apply to affected area qd-bid.
Carmol-20 Cream (Doak)	Urea 20%	**Adults & Peds:** Apply to affected area qd-bid.
Cetaphil Daily Facial Moisturizer SPF 15 (Galderma Laboratories)	Avobenzone 3%, Octocrylene 10%, Diisopropyl adipate, cyclomethicone, glyceryl stearate, PEG-100 stearate, glycerin, polymethyl methacrylate, phenoxyethanol, benzyl alcohol, acrylates/C10-30 alkyl acrylate crosspolymer, tocopheryl acetate, carbomer 940, disodium EDTA, triethanolamine	**Adults & Peds:** Apply to affected area prn.
Cetaphil Moisturizing Cream (Galderma Laboratories)	Glyceryl polymethacrylate, propylene glycol; petrolatum, dicaprylyl ether, PEG-5 glyceryl stearate, glycerin, dimethicone, dimethiconol, cetyl alcohol, sweet almond oil, acrylates/C10-30 alkylacrylate crosspolymer, tocopheryl acetate, phenoxyethanol, benzyl alcohol, disodium EDTA, sodium hydroxide, lactic acid	**Adults & Peds:** Apply to affected area prn.
Cetaphil Moisturizing Lotion (Galderma Laboratories)	Glycerin, hydrogenated polyisobutene, cetearyl alcohol, ceteareth-20, macadamia nut oil, dimethicone, tocopheryl acetate, stearoxytrimethylsilane, stearyl alcohol, panthenol, farnesol, benzyl alcohol, phenoxyethanol, acrylates/C10-30 alkyl acrylate crosspolymer, sodium hydroxide, Citric Acid	**Adults & Peds:** Apply to affected area prn.
Cetaphil Therapeutic Hand Cream (Galderma Laboratories)	Glycerin, cetearyl alcohol, oleth-2, PEG-2 stearate, butyrospermum parkii, ethylhexyl methoxycinnamate, dimethicone, stearyl alcohol, glyceryl stearate, PEG-100 stearate, methylparaben, tocopherol, arginine PCA, chlorhexidine digluconate	**Adults & Peds:** Apply to affected area prn.
Corn Huskers Lotion (Pfizer Consumer Healthcare)	Glycerin, SD alcohol 40, sodium calcium aginate, oleyl sarcosine, methylparaben, guar gum, triethanolamine, calcium sulfate, calcium chloride, fumaric acid, boric acid	**Adults & Peds:** Apply to affected area prn.
Eucerin Creme Original (Beiersdorf)	Petrolatum, mineral oil, ceresin, lanolin Alcohol, methylchloroisothiazolinone, methylisothiazolinone	**Adults & Peds:** Apply to affected area prn.
Eucerin Dry Skin Therapy Calming Crème (Beiersdorf)	Glycerin, cetyl palmitate, mineral oil, caprylic/capric triglyceride, octyldodecanol, cetyl alcohol, glyceryl stearate, colloidal oatmeal, dimethicone, PEG-40 stearate, phenoxyethanol, DMDM hydantoin	**Adults:** Apply to affected area prn.

DOSING INFORMATION FOR DRY SKIN PRODUCTS (cont.)

Brand Name	Ingredient/Strength	Dose
Eucerin Dry Skin Therapy Plus Intensive Repair Lotion *(Beiersdorf)*	Mineral oil, PEG-7 hydrogenated castor oil, isohexadecane, sodium lactate, urea, glycerin, isopropyl palmitate, panthenol, microcrystalline wax, magnesium sulfate, lanolin alcohol, bisabolol, methylchloroisothiazolinone, methylisothiazolinone	**Adults:** Apply to affected area prn.
Eucerin Gentle Hydrating Cleanser *(Beiersdorf)*	Sodium laureth sulfate, cocamidopropyl betaine, disodium cocoamphodiacetate, glycol distearate, PEG-7 glyceryl cocoate, PEG-5 lanolate, cocamide MEA, laureth 10, citric acid, PEG-120 methyl glucose dioleate, lanolin alcohol, imidazolidinyl urea	**Adults:** Use on affected area qd.
Eucerin Hand Creme Extensive Repair *(Beiersdorf)*	Glycerin, urea, glyceryl stearate, stearyl alcohol, dicaprylyl ether, sodium lactate, dimethicone, PEG-40 stearate, cyclopentasiloxane, cyclohexasiloxane, aluminum starch octenylsuccinate, lactic aid, xanthan gum, phenoxyethanol, methylparaben, propylparaben	**Adults & Peds:** Apply to affected area qd.
Eucerin Lotion Daily Replenishing *(Beiersdorf)*	Sunflower seed oil, petrolatum, glycerin, glyceryl stearate SE; octyldodecanol, caprylic/capric triglyceride, stearic acid, dimethicone, cetearyl alcohol, lanolin alcohol, panthenol, tocopheryl acetate, cholesterol, carbomer, disodium EDTA, sodium hydroxide, Phenoxyethanol, methylparaben, ethylparaben, propylparaben, butylparaben, BHT	**Adults & Peds:** Apply to affected area qd.
Eucerin Lotion Original *(Beiersdorf)*	Mineral oil, isopropyl myristate, PEG-40 sorbitan peroleate, glyceryl lanolate, sorbitol, propylene glycol, cetyl palmitate, magnesium sulfate, aluminum stearate, lanolin alcohol, BHT, methylchloroisothiazolinone, methylisothiazolinone	**Adults & Peds:** Apply to affected area prn.
Eucerin Lotion Plus Intensive Repair *(Beiersdorf)*	Mineral oil, PEG-7 hydrogenated castor oil, isohexadecane, sodium lactate, urea, glycerin, isopropyl palmitate, panthenol, microcrystalline wax, magnesium sulfate, lanolin alcohol, bisabolol, methylchloroisothiazolinone, methylisothiazolinone	**Adults & Peds:** Apply to affected area prn.
Eucerin Redness Relief Daily Perfecting Lotion *(Beiersdorf)*	Octinoxate, octisalate, titanium dioxide, glycerin, dimethicone, olyglyceryl-3 methylglucose distearate, butyrospermum parkii, lauroyl lysine, squalane, alcohol Denat., sorbitan stearate, phenoxyethanol, butylene glycol, magnesium aluminum silicate, glycyrrhiza inflata root extract, xanthan gum, methylparaben, Propylparaben, Ethylparaben, iodopropynyl butylcarbamate, trimethoxycaprylylsilane, chromium oxide greens, chromium hydroxide green, ultramarines	**Adults & Peds:** Apply to affected area prn.
Eucerin Redness Relief Soothing Cleanser *(Beiersdorf)*	Glycerin, sodium laureth sulfate, carbomer, phenoxyethanol, PEG-40 hydrogenated castor oil, sodium methyl cocoyl taurate, PEG-7 glyceryl cocoate, decyl glucoside, glycyrrhiza inflata root extract, xanthan gum, sodium hydroxide, methylparaben, butylparaben, ethylparaben, isobutylparaben, propylparaben, benzophenone-4	**Adults & Peds:** Apply to affected area qam and qpm.

DOSING INFORMATION FOR DRY SKIN PRODUCTS (cont.)

BRAND NAME	INGREDIENT/STRENGTH	DOSE
Eucerin Redness Relief Soothing Night Creme *(Beiersdorf)*	Glycerin, panthenol, caprylic/capric triglyceride, dicaprylyl carbonate, octyldodecanol, C12-15 alkyl benzoate, dimethicone, squalane, tapioca starch, cetearyl alcohol, glyceryl stearate citrate, myristyl myristate, butylene glycol, benzyl alcohol, glycyrrhiza inflata root extract, carbomer, phenoxyethanol, ammonium acryloyldimethyltaurate/VP copolymer, sodium hydroxide, methylparaben, propylparaben, iodopropynyl butylcarbamate	**Adults & Peds:** Apply to affected area qpm.
Gold Bond Ultimate Healing Skin Therapy Lotion *(Chattem)*	Glycerin, dimethicone, petrolatum, jojoba esters, cetyl alcohol, aloe barbadensis leaf juice, stearyl alcohol, distearyldimonium chloride, cetearyl alcohol, steareth-21, steareth-2, propylene glycol, chamomilla recutita flower extract, polysorbate 60, stearamidopropyl PG-dimonium chloride phosphate, methyl gluceth 20, tocopheryl acetate, magnesium ascorbyl phosphate, hydrolyzed collagen, hydrolyzed elastin, retinyl palmitate, hydrolyzed ojoba esters, glyceryl stearate, dipotassium EDTA, fragrance, triethanolamine, diazolidinyl urea, methylparaben, propylparaben	**Adults & Peds:** Apply to affected area prn.
Gold Bond Ultimate Healing Skin Therapy Powder *(Chattem)*	Corn Starch, sodium bicarbonate, silica, fragrance, ascrobyl palmitate, aloe barbadensis leaf extract, lavandula angustifolia extract, chamomilla recutita flower extract, rosmarinus officinalis leaf extract, acacia farnesiana extract, tocopheryl acetate, retinyl palmitate, polyoxymethylene urea, Isopropyl myristate, benzethonium chloride	**Adults & Peds:** Apply to affected area prn.
Keri Moisture Therapy Advance Extra Dry Skin Lotion *(Bristol-Myers Squibb)*	Glycerin, stearic acid, hydrogenated polyisobutene, petrolatum, cetyl alcohol, aloe barbadensis gel, tocopheryl acetate, cyclopentasiloxane, dimethicone copolyol, glyceryl stearate, PEG-100 stearate, dimethicone, carbomer, methylparaben, PEG-5 soya sterol, magnesium aluminum silicate, propylparaben, phenoxyethanol, disodium EDTA, diazolidinyl urea, sodium hydroxide,	**Adults & Peds:** Apply to affected area prn.
Keri Moisture Therapy Lotion, Sensitive Skin *(Bristol-Myer Squibb)*	Glycerin, stearic acid, hydrogenated polyisobutene, petrolatum, cetyl alcohol, aloe barbadensis gel, tocopheryl acetate, cyclopentasiloxane, dimethicone copolyol, glyceryl stearate, PEG-100 Stearate, dimethicone, carborner, methylparaben, PEG-5 soya sterol, magnesium aluminum silicate, propylparaben, phenoxyethanol, disodium EDTA, diazolidinyl urea, sodium hydroxide	**Adults:** Apply to skin prn.
Keri Original Formula Lotion *(Bristol-Myers Squibb)*	Mineral oil, propylene glycol, PEG-40 stearate, glyceryl stearate/PEG-100 stearate, PEG-4 dilaurate, laureth-4, lanolin oil, methylparaben, carbomer, propylparaben, fragrance, triethanolamine, dioctyl sodium sulfosuccinate, quaternium-15	**Adults & Peds:** Apply to affected area prn.

DOSING INFORMATION FOR DRY SKIN PRODUCTS (cont.)

BRAND NAME	INGREDIENT/STRENGTH	DOSE
Keri Shea Butter Moisture Therapy Lotion *(Bristol-Myers Squibb)*	Mineral oil, glycerin, butyrospermum parkii, PEG-40 stearate, glyceryl stearate, PEG-100 stearate, PEG-4 dilaurate, laureth 4, aloe barbadensis leaf juice, helianthus annuus seed oil, tocopheryl Acetate, carbomer, methylparaben, propylparaben, DMDM hydantoin, iodopropynyl butylcarbamate, sodium hydroxide, sodium EDTA	**Adults & Peds:** Apply to affected area prn.
Lac-Hydrin Five Lotion *(Westwood-Squibb)*	Lactic acid, ammonium hydroxide, glycerin, petrolatum, squalane, steareth-2, POE-21-stearyl ether, propylene glycol dioctanoate, cetyl alcohol, dimethicone, methylchloroisothiazoline, methylisothiazolinone	**Adults & Peds:** Apply to affected area bid.
Lubriderm Advanced Therapy Lotion *(Pfizer Consumer Healthcare)*	Cetyl alcohol, glycerin, mineral oil, cyclomethicone, propylene glycol dicaprylate/dicaprate, PEG-40 stearate, isopropyl isostearate, emulsifying wax, lecithin, carbomer, diazolidinyl urea, titanium dioxide, sodium benzoate, BHT, PPG-3 myristyl ether citrate, disodium EDTA, retinyl palmitate, tocopheryl acetate, sodium pyruvate, fragrance, sodium hydroxide, xanthan gum, iodopropynyl butylcarbamate	**Adults & Peds:** Apply to affected area prn.
Lubriderm Daily Moisture Fragrance Free Lotion *(Pfizer Consumer Healthcare)*	Mineral Oil, petrolatum, sorbitol solution, stearic acid, lanolin, lanolin alcohol, cetyl alcohol, glyceryl stearate/PEG-100 stearate, triethanolamine, dimethicone, propylene glycol, microcrystalline wax, PPG-3 myristyl ether citrate, disodium EDTA, methylparaben, ethylparaben, propylparaben, xanthan gum, butylparaben, methyldibromo glutaronitrile	**Adults & Peds:** Apply to affected area prn.
Lubriderm Daily Moisture Lotion *(Pfizer Consumer Healthcare)*	Mineral oil, petrolatum, sorbitol solution, stearic acid, lanolin, lanolin alcohol, cetyl alcohol, glyceryl stearate/PEG-100 stearate, triethanolamine; Dimethicone; Propylene Glycol; microcrystalline wax, PPG-3 myristyl ether citrate, disodium EDTA, methylparaben, ethylparaben, propylparaben, xanthan gum, butylparaben, methyldibromo glutaronitrile	**Adults & Peds:** Apply to affected area prn.
Lubriderm Sensitive Skin Lotion *(Pfizer Consumer Healthcare)*	Butylene glycol, mineral oil, petrolatum, glycerin, cetyl alcohol, propylene glycol dicaprylate/dicaprate, PEG-40 stearate, C11-13 isoparaffin, glyceryl stearate, PPG-3 myristyl ether citrate, emulsifying wax, dimethicone, DMDM hydantoin, methylparaben, carbomer 940, ethylparaben, propylparaben, titanium dioxide, disodium EDTA, sodium hydroxide, butylparaben, xanthan gum	**Adults & Peds:** Apply to affected area prn.
Lubriderm Skin Nourishing Premium Oat Extract Lotion *(Pfizer Consumer Healthcare)*	Caprylic/capric triglycerides, glycerin, glyceryl stearate SE, petrolatum, camellia oleifera seed oil, castor oil, cocoa butter, cetyl alcohol, wax, brassica alba seed extract, oat kernel extract, cassia angustifolia seed polysaccharide, glyceryl stearate, PEG 100 stearate, diazolidinyl urea, xanthan gum, disodium EDTA, iodopropynyl butylcarbamate, soybean oil	**Adults & Peds:** Apply to affected area prn.
Lubriderm Daily UV Moisturizer Lotion, SPF 15 *(Pfizer Consumer Healthcare)*	Octyl Methoxycinnamate/Octyl Salicylate/Oxybenzone 7.5%-4%-3%	**Adults & Peds >6 mo:** Apply to skin prn

DOSING INFORMATION FOR DRY SKIN PRODUCTS (cont.)

Brand Name	Ingredient/Strength	Dose
Lubriderm Lotion, Skin Therapy - Fresh Scent *(Pfizer Consumer Healthcare)*	Mineral oil, petrolatum, sorbitol solution, stearic acid, lanolin, lanolin alcohol, cetyl alcohol, glyceryl stearate, PEG-100 stearate, triethanolamine, dimethicone, propylene glycol, tri (PPG-3 myristyl ether) citrate, disodium EDTA, methylparaben, ethylparaben, propylparaben, fragrance, xanthan gum, butylparaben, methyldibromo glutaronitrile	**Adults:** Apply to skin prn.
Lubriderm Skin Nourishing Moisturizing Lotion with Shea and Cocoa Butters *(Pfizer Consumer Healthcare)*	Glycerin, cetyl alcohol, glyceryl stearate SE, petrolatum, emulsifying wax, caprylic/capric triglyceride, castor oil, octyldodecanol, shea butter, cocoa butter, dimethicone, tocopheryl acetate, diazolidinyl urea, xanthan gum, disodium EDTA, fragrance, iodopropynyl butylcarbamate	**Adults:** Apply to skin prn.
Neutrogena Body Moisturizer Cream *(Neutrogena)*	Glycerin, emulsifying wax, octyl isononanoate, dimethicone, propylene glycol isoceteth-3 acetate, cyclomethicone, stearic acid, aloe extract, matricaria extract, tocopheryl acetate, dimethicone copolyol, acrylates/C10-30 alkyl acrylate crosspolymer, cetearyl alcohol, sodium cetearyl sulfate, sodium sulfate, hydrogenated lanolin, glyceryl laurate, tetrasodium EDTA, triethanolamine, BHT, geranium, dipropylene glycol, propylene glycol, methylparaben, ethylparaben, propylparaben, diazolidinyl urea, benzalkonium chloride	**Adults & Peds:** Apply to affected area prn.
Neutrogena Fragrance-Free Body Moisturizer Cream *(Neutrogena)*	Glycerin, emulsifying wax, octyl isononanoate, dimethicone, propylene glycol isoceteth-3 acetate, cyclomethicone, stearic acid, aloe extract, matricaria extract, tocopheryl acetate, dimethicone copolyol, acrylates/C10-30 alkyl acrylate crosspolymer, cetearyl alcohol, sodium cetearyl sulfate, sodium sulfate, hydrogenated lanolin, glyceryl laurate, tetrasodium EDTA, triethanolamine, BHT, geranium, dipropylene glycol, propylene glycol, methylparaben, ethylparaben, propylparaben, diazolidinyl urea, benzalkonium chloride	**Adults & Peds:** Apply to affected area prn.
Neutrogena Moisture for Sensitive Skin *(Neutrogena)*	Glycerin, octyl palmitate, dimethicone, petrolatum, cyclomethicone, soy sterol, isopropyl isostearate, cetyl alcohol, PEG-10 soya sterol, glyceryl stearate, PEG-100 stearate, C 12-1 5 alkyl benzoate, carbomer, tetrasodium EDTA, odium hydroxide, diazolidinyl urea, ethylparaben, methylparaben, propylparaben.	
Neutrogena Norwegian Formula Body/Hand Cream *(Neutrogena)*	Glycerin, cetearyl alcohol, stearic acid, sodium cetearyl sulfate, methylparaben, propylparaben, dilauryl thiodipropionate, sodium sulfate	**Adults & Peds:** Apply to affected area qd.
Nivea Body Creamy Conditioning Oil, Very Dry, Flaky Skin *(Beiersdorf)*	Mineral oil, isopropyl myristate, PEG-40 sorbitan peroleate, glyceryl lanolate, sorbitol, propylene glycol, cetyl palmitate, magnesium sulfate, aluminum stearate, lanolin alcohol, fragrance, BHT, methylchloroisothiazolinone, methylisothiazolinone	**Adults:** Apply to damp skin prn.

DOSING INFORMATION FOR DRY SKIN PRODUCTS (cont.)

Brand Name	Ingredient/Strength	Dose
Nivea Body Original Lotion, Dry Skin (Beiersdorf)	Mineral Oil, glycerin, isopropyl palmitate, glyceryl stearate SE, cetearyl alcohol, tocopheryl acetate, isopropyl myristate, simethicone, fragrance, carbomer, hydroxypropyl methylcellulose, Sodium hydroxide, methylchloroisothiazolinone, methylisothiazolinone	**Adults:** Apply to damp skin prn.
Nivea Body Original Skin Oil, Extremely Dry, Chapped Skin (Beiersdorf)	Mineral oil, triple purified water, lanolin, petrolatum, glyceryl lanolate, lanolin alcohol, fragrance, sodium borate, methylchloroisothiazolinone, methylisothiazolinone	**Adults:** Apply to affected area prn.
Nivea Body Sheer Moisture Lotion, Normal to Dry Skin (Beiersdorf)	Mineral oil, caprylic/capric triglycerides, SD alcohol 40B, glycerin, glyceryl stearate citrate, cetearyl alcohol, dimethicone, tocopheryl acetate, panthenol, lanolin alcohol, fragrance, carbomer, sodium hydroxide, methylchloroisothiazolinone, methylisothiazolinone	**Adults:** Apply to damp skin prn.
Nivea Creme (Beiersdorf)	Mineral oil, petrolatum, glycerin, isohexadecane, microcrystalline wax, lanolin alcohol, paraffin, panthenol, magnesium sulfate, decyl oleate, octyldodecanol, aluminum stearate, methylchloroisothiazolinone, methylisothiazolinone, citric acid, magnesium stearate	**Adults & Peds:** Apply to affected area prn.
Nivea Extra-Enriched Lotion (Beiersdorf)	Mineral oil, isohexadecane, PEG-40 sorbitan peroleate, polyglyceryl-3 diisostearate, glycerin, petrolatum, isopropyl palmitate, cetyl palmitate, tocopheryl acetate (Vitamin E), glyceryl lanolate, lanolin alcohol, magnesium sulfate, aluminum stearate, phenoxyethanol, methyldibromo glutaronitrile	**Adults & Peds:** Apply to damp skin after shower or bath.
Pacquin Plus Hand & Body Cream (Pfizer Consumer Healthcare)	Glycerin, stearic acid, potassium stearate, carbomer, cetyl alcohol, cetyl esters wax, diisopropyl sebacate, lanolin, myristyl lactate, sodium stearate, methyl and propylparabens	**Adults & Peds:** Apply to affected area qd.
Vaseline Dual Action Petroleum Jelly Cream (Kendall)	Petrolatum, glycerin, potassium lactate, stearic acid, butylene glycol, glycol stearate, PEG-100 stearate, caprylic/capric triglyceride, lactic acid, dimethicone, helianthus annuus seed pil or glycine Soja (Soybean) oil, glyceryl stearate, tocopheryl acetate, tocopheryl acetate, fragrance, cetyl alcohol, xanthan gum, glycine soja sterols, ethylhexyl methoxyethylcellulose, stearamide AMP, lecithin, methylparaben, DMDM hydantoin, disodium EDTA	**Adults & Peds:** Apply to affected area prn.
Vaseline Intensive Care Advanced Healing Fragrance Free (Kendall)	White petrolatum, glycerin, stearic acid, glycol stearate, helianthus annuus seed oil, glycine soja sterol, lecithin, tocopheryl acetate, retinyl palmitate, urea, collagen amino scids, sodium stearoyl lactate, mineral water, sodium PCA, potassium lactate, lactic acid, cetyl alcohol, glyceryl stearate, magnesium aluminum silicate, carbomer, stearamide AMP, ethylene brassylate, trolamine, corn oil, disodium EDTA, methylparaben, DMDM hydantoin, BHT, titanium dioxide	**Adults & Peds:** Apply to affected area prn.

DOSING INFORMATION FOR DRY SKIN PRODUCTS (cont.)

Brand Name	Ingredient/Strength	Dose
Vaseline Intensive Care Firming & Radiance Age-Defying Lotion (Kendall)	Octinoxate (1.25%)	**Adults & Peds:** Apply to affected area prn.
Vaseline Intensive Care Healthy Body Complexion Nourishing Body Lotion (Kendall)	Glycerin, dimethicone, potassium lactate, stearic acid, sodium hydroxypropyl starch phosphate, mineral oil, glycol stearate, lactic acid, glycine soja sterol, lecithin, petrolatum, tocopheryl acetate, retinyl palmitate, helianthus annuus seed acid, sodium PCA, sodium stearoyl lactate, urea, collagen amino acids, mineral water, glyceryl stearate, cetyl alcohol, magnesium aluminum silicate, fragrance, stearamide AMP, ethylhexyl methoxycinnamate, corn oil, methylparaben, DMDM hydantoin, disodium EDTA, xanthan gum, BHT	**Adults & Peds:** Apply to affected area prn.
Vaseline Intensive Care Healthy Hand & Nail Lotion (Kendall)	Potassium lactate, sodium hydroxypropyl starch phosphate, glycerin, stearic acid, mineral oil, dimethicone, lactic acid, glycol stearate, PEG 100 stearate, keratin, glycine soja sterol, lecithin, tocopheryl acetate, retinyl palmitate, healianthus annuus seed oil, sodium PCA, sodium stearoyl Lactate, Urea, collagen amino acids, ethylhexyl methoxycinnamate, petrolatum, mineral water, cetyl alcohol, stearamide AMP, cyclomethicone, magnesium aluminum silicate, glyceryl stearate, fragrance, xanthan gum, corn Oil, BHT, disodium EDTA, methylparaben, DMDM hydantoin	**Adults & Peds:** Apply to affected area prn.
Vaseline Intensive Care Lotion Aloe and Naturals (Kendall)	Glycerin, stearic acid, aloe barbadensis leaf juice glycol stearate, helianthus annuus, seed oil, glycine soja sterols, lecithin, panthenol, tocopheryl acetate, retinyl palmitate, sucumis sativus extract, urea, collagen amino acids, sodium stearoyl lactate, mineral water, sodium PCA, potassium lactate, lactic acid, petrolatum, dimethicone, glyceryl stearate, cetyl alcohol, methyl palmitate, magnesium aluminum silicate, eucalyptus globulus oil; lavandula angustifolia oil, citrus aurantium dulcis oil, carbomer, stearamide AMP, triethanolamine, corn oil, butylene glycol, methylparaben, DMDM hydantoin; disodium EDTA, BHT, titanium dioxide	**Adults & Peds:** Apply to affected area prn.
Vaseline Intensive Care Lotion Total Moisture (Kendall)	Glycerin, stearic acid, glycol stearate, petrolatum, helianthus annuus seed oil, glycine soja sterols, lecithin, tocopheryl acetate, retinyl palmitate, urea, collagen amino acids, sodium stearoyl lactylate, mineral water, sodium PCA, potassium lactate, lactic acid, dimethicone, avena sativa kernel flour; keratin, glyceryl stearate, cetyl alcohol, magnesium aluminum silicate, fragrance, carbomer, stearamide AMP, triethanolamine, corn oil, methylparaben, DMDM hydantoin, iodopropynyl butylcarbamate, disodium EDTA, BHT, propylene glycol, titanium dioxide	**Adults & Peds:** Apply to affected area prn.

DOSING INFORMATION FOR DRY SKIN PRODUCTS (cont.)

Brand Name	Ingredient/Strength	Dose
Vaseline Intensive Care Lotion Total Moisture *(Kendall)*	Glycerin, stearic acid, glycol stearate, petrolatum, helianthus annuus seed oil, glycine soja sterols, lecithin, tocopheryl acetate, retinyl palmitate, urea, collagen amino acids, sodium stearoyl lactylate, mineral water, sodium PCA, potassium lactate, lactic acid, dimethicone, avena sativa kernel flour; keratin, glyceryl stearate, cetyl alcohol, magnesium aluminum silicate, fragrance, carbomer, stearamide AMP, triethanolamine, corn oil, methylparaben, DMDM hydantoin, iodopropynyl butylcarbamate, disodium EDTA, BHT, propylene glycol, titanium dioxide	**Adults & Peds:** Apply to affected area prn.
Vaseline Intensive Care Nightly Renewal Light Body Lotion *(Kendall)*	Glycerin, isopropyl myristate, dimethicone, cyclopentasiloxane, stearic acid, tapioca starch, glycol stearate, helianthus annuus seed oil, glycine oja soil, glycine soja sterol (Soybean), vitis vinefera seed extract, lavandula angustifolia extract, lecithin, tocopheryl acetate, retinyl palmitate, urea, collagen amino acids, sodium PCA, potassium lactate, lactic acid, cetyl alcohol, glyceryl stearate, magnesium Aluminum silicate, carbomer, methyl methacrylate crosspolymer, fragrance	**Adults & Peds:** Apply to affected area prn.
Vaseline Jelly *(Kendall)*	White petrolatum	**Adults & Peds:** Apply to affected area prn.
Vaseline Petroleum Jelly Cream Deep Moisture *(Kendall)*	White petrolatum 10%	**Adults & Peds:** Apply to affected area prn.
Vaseline Soothing Moisture, Moisturizing Cream w/ Cocoa Butter *(Kendall)*	Petrolatum, caprylic/capric triglyceride, stearic acid, glycerin, sodium hydroxypropyl starch phosphate, glycol stearate, PEG-100 stearate, cocoa butter, cyclomethicone, glyceryl stearate, cetyl alcohol, tocopheryl acetate, acrylates/C10-30 alkyl acrylate crosspolymer, fragrance, stearamide AMP, potassium hydroxide, DMDM hydantoin, disodium EDTA, iodopropyl butylcarbamate, titanium dioxide	**Adults & Peds:** Apply to affected area prn.

Folliculitis, Furuncles, and Carbuncles

Folliculitis is an inflammation of the hair follicles, usually caused by *Staphylococcus aureus*. Other causes of sporadic infection include *Pseudomonas aeruginosa* ("hot-tub folliculitis") and various gram-negative bacteria, fungi, and viruses. Folliculitis may be clinically classified by depth of involvement. Superficial folliculitis (Bockhart's impetigo) is confined to the upper portion of the hair follicle. Affected patients have small, dome-shaped, follicle-centered pustules. Lesions may or may not be tender or pruritic. Commonly affected areas include the scalp, beard area, back, axillae, buttocks, and extremities. These lesions heal without any residual scarring. Deep folliculitis involves the entire hair follicle. The lesions are characterized by painful, tender, swollen, erythematous papules that often form larger pustules. Scarring is common. Deep folliculitis classically involves the beard area (sycosis barbae). Because deep folliculitis and furunculosis are frequently clinically indistinguishable, many experts often use the terms interchangeably.

Noninfectious folliculitis is typically caused by mineral oils, tar products, and cutting oils that obstruct the pilosebaceous unit; the resulting inflammation is typically sterile. Eosinophilic folliculitis, a rare disorder of unknown etiology, presents as an intensely pruritic folliculitis involving the head, neck, trunk, and proximal extremities. It is associated with advanced HIV infection (CD4+ T lymphocyte count <100 cells/µL) and is characterized histopathologically by infiltration of eosinophils around the hair follicles. Secondary *S aureus* infection frequently complicates noninfectious folliculitis. Predisposing factors for folliculitis include occlusive skin coverings (clothing, plastic, prostheses, plaster); prolonged sitting or lying; residence in a hot, humid climate; chronic systemic antibiotic or topical corticosteroid use; and preexisting dermatoses. Shaving or extracting hair with wax or depilatories may also facilitate follicular inflammation. Folliculitis is a common dermatologic problem that may affect men and women of any age. However, certain populations are at higher risk for developing infectious folliculitis, including people who have diabetes mellitus, immunosuppressed persons, and chronic staphylococcal carriers.

A furuncle (also known as a boil) is a red, tender nodule resulting from deep-seated infection around a hair follicle. Any hair-bearing area may be affected, although regions that are subject to friction, perspiration, and maceration are especially vulnerable. Such regions include the face, neck, axillae, groin, and buttocks. A furuncle typically begins as a superficial infection within a hair follicle (folliculitis) and progresses to involve the entire hair follicle and adjacent subcutaneous tissue. Furuncles may occur as single or multiple lesions that tend to enlarge and become fluctuant after several days. Resolution occurs after rupture of the lesion and the discharge of pus and necrotic material. Although lesions usually resolve spontaneously, furunculosis may be a chronic and recurrent problem.

A carbuncle is a coalescence of furuncles that develop in close proximity to each other. It is a more extensive and infiltrative lesion than a furuncle and may be associated with systemic symptoms such as fever and malaise. Carbuncles are typically very painful indurated lesions with a predilection for the nape of the neck, thighs, and back—areas where the poor distensibility of overlying skin promotes the lateral spread of infection. As the carbuncle evolves, pustules develop on its surface that subsequently discharge pus from adjacent hair follicles. With spontaneous drainage of the lesion, the center of the lesion may necrose, leaving an irregular and sometimes sizable crater. Large lesions often result in a significant scar.

Furuncles and carbuncles are most commonly caused by *S aureus*, but other infectious agents may be involved, especially in immunocompromised patients. Although not completely understood, evidence indicates that the pathogenesis of staphylococcal skin infection involves virulence factors produced by the microorganism (eg, coagulase, hemolysin, leukocidin, exfoliatin, alpha toxin) combined with a breakdown in the integrity of the skin or of the host immune system. Furuncles typically evolve from staphylococcal folliculitis, and carbuncles typically evolve from coalescing furuncles. A variety of factors may predispose patients to furuncles, including preexisting skin disorders, diabetes mellitus, blood dyscrasias, congestive heart failure, immunologic deficiencies (including defects in bactericidal capability and cellular chemotaxis), hyper-IgE syndrome (Job's syndrome), obesity, poor hygiene, and treatment with corticosteroids or cytotoxic agents. However, most furuncles occur in patients without an apparent predisposing factor.

Superficial bacterial folliculitis may resolve without treatment. However, resolution may be hastened by local skin care, such as the use of antibacterial soaps or an antiseptic skin cleanser. Prevention and treatment of furuncles and carbuncles, like folliculitis, often just require good skin care and hygiene. Application of a warm, moist compress to the affected area for 15 minutes several times a day promotes localization and drainage of infection and helps relieve pain and discomfort. Prescription antibiotics may be necessary to treat folliculitis, furuncles, and carbuncles.

Fungal Infections

Dermatophytoses are caused by a closely related group of organisms that are similar in morphology, pathogenicity, and physiology and have a special affinity for the keratinized tissues of the hair, skin, and nails. The dermatophytes encompass only three genera—*Epidermophyton, Microsporum,* and *Trichophyton*—but are collectively the largest group of fungi that cause cutaneous diseases. They are also referred to as ringworms because of the characteristic ring that develops on the infected skin. Diseases produced by these organisms are prefaced by the adjective "tinea" and are named according to the body part infected (e.g., tinea capitis affects scalp hair follicles, tinea pedis affects the plantar surface, tinea cruris affects the groin, tinea manuum affects the palmar surface, tinea unguium affects the nails, tinea barbae affects the beard region, and tinea corporis affects the glabrous skin). Although the causative organisms are closely related, the various dermatophytoses produce protean manifestations and can resemble numerous cutaneous diseases.

Tinea corporis infects the glabrous skin of the trunk, extremities, and face and occurs in all ages, ethnic backgrounds, and nationalities. It is most common in warm, humid climates. Predisposing factors include contact with animals (especially kittens, cattle, and horses), crowded living conditions, participation in contact sports and the use of gymnasiums, and a variety of systemic disorders including diabetes mellitus and HIV infection. Contact with infected animals is a common cause. Kittens particularly are a problem, and large epidemics have resulted from a single infected animal. Typical lesions of tinea corporis are pruritic, oval, annular (ringlike), erythematous, scaly patches that may have a slightly elevated border. However, the presentation of tinea corporis is quite variable and can mimic many other dermatoses. It should be stressed that not all annular dermatoses are tinea corporis. The diagnosis is especially challenging if blistering or pustular lesions occur. Scratching may lead to lichenification and the appearance of a neurodermatitis (eczematous response). Occasionally, this lichenified presentation may mimic psoriasis.

The terms tinea unguium and onychomycosis are often used interchangeably; however, the former specifies dermatophytic infection of the nail unit, whereas onychomycosis encompasses all forms of fungal infection that cause nail disease. Onychomycosis is responsible for approximately 50% of dystrophic nails and occurs in an estimated 15% to 20% of people aged 40 to 60 years. Toenails are involved more often than fingernails. The most common presentation is the distal subungual variety, manifested by subungual debris and thickening with associated onycholysis and thickening of the nail plate. However, there are other presentations of fungal nail disease, including white superficial onychomycosis and candidiasis in nails. It is important to stress that not all patients with dystrophic nails have fungal disease. For example, psoriasis and lichen planus can mimic onychomycosis and can be differentiated by a culture.

Tinea capitis, or dermatophytosis of the scalp hair follicles, occurs mostly in children. Currently, there is an epidemic of *Trichophyton tonsurans* infection in urban areas of the United States. Many infected children are African-American or Hispanic, and infection is often recalcitrant to griseofulvin therapy. There are inflammatory and noninflammatory varieties of tinea capitis. With the inflammatory variety, the clinical picture varies from a few pustules in the scalp to widespread abscesses or kerions. Alopecia and tender cervical lymphadenopathy generally are associated. If untreated, a permanent scarring alopecia may result. The noninflammatory variety may resemble alopecia areata and present with oval, generally scaly patches of alopecia. Prominent cervical adenopathy, the presence of scale, and the lack of exclamation-point hairs in patches of alopecia point to a diagnosis of tinea capitis.

There are several OTC antifungals available in different dosage forms (creams, powders, sprays) to treat dermatophytoses, including undecylenic acid, tolnaftate, miconazole, clotrimazole, ketoconazole, terbinafine, and butenafine.

For information on tinea pedis and tinea cruris, see "Athlete's Foot and Jock Itch" under Dermatological Conditions.

BUTENAFINE

Butenafine is fungicidal and inhibits the epoxidation of squalene. This action blocks the biosynthesis of ergosterol, an important component of fungal cell membranes.

Tinea pedis (treatment); *tinea corporis* (treatment); *tinea cruris* (treatment)—Butenafine is indicated in the treatment of interdigital tinea pedis (athlete's foot), tinea corporis (ringworm), and tinea cruris (jock itch) due to *Epidermophyton floccosum, Trichophyton mentagrophytes, T rubrum,* or *T tonsurans.*

Tinea (pityriasis) versicolor (treatment)—Butenafine is indicated in the treatment of tinea (pityriasis) versicolor due to *Malassezia furfur.*

For tinea pedis, interdigital:

Adults/Pediatrics >12 years of age: Apply to affected skin and surrounding areas, once a day for 4 weeks or twice a day for 7 days.

For tinea corporis/tinea cruris/tinea (pityriasis) versicolar:

Adults/Pediatrics >12 years of age: Apply to affected skin and surrounding areas, once a day for 2 weeks.

For more information, refer to the complete monograph for butenafine in "Athlete's Foot and Jock Itch" under Dermatological Conditions.

BUTENAFINE PRODUCTS	
Brand Name	**Dosage Form**
Lotrimin Ultra (Schering)	**Cream:** 1%
Mentax (Mylan Bertek)	**Cream:** 1%

CLOTRIMAZOLE

Clotrimazole is fungistatic and may be fungicidal, depending on concentration. It inhibits biosynthesis of ergosterol or other sterols, damaging the fungal cell wall membrane and altering its permeability. As a result, loss of essential intracellular elements may occur.

Clotrimazole also inhibits biosynthesis of triglycerides and phospholipids by fungi. In addition, it inhibits oxidative and peroxidative enzyme activity, resulting in intracellular buildup of toxic concentrations of hydrogen peroxide, which may contribute to deterioration of subcellular organelles and cellular necrosis. In *Candida albicans*, clotrimazole inhibits transformation of blastospores into invasive mycelial form.

Candidiasis, cutaneous (treatment)—Topical clotrimazole is indicated in the treatment of cutaneous candidiasis (moniliasis) caused by *C albicans*.

Tinea corporis (treatment), *tinea cruris* (treatment), and *tinea pedis* (treatment)—Topical clotrimazole is indicated in the treatment of tinea corporis (ringworm of the body), tinea cruris (ringworm of the groin, or "jock itch"), and tinea pedis (ringworm of the foot, or "athlete's foot") caused by *Trichophyton rubrum*, *T mentagrophytes*, *Epidermophyton floccosum*, and *Microsporum canis*.

Tinea versicolor (treatment)—Topical clotrimazole is indicated in the treatment of tinea versicolor (pityriasis versicolor, or "sun fungus") caused by *Malassezia furfur*.

Paronychia (treatment), *tinea barbae* (treatment), or *tinea capitis* (treatment)—Topical clotrimazole is used in the treatment of paronychia, tinea barbae, and tinea capitis.

Cream/Lotion/Topical solution

Adults/Pediatrics: Apply to affected area of skin and surrounding areas 2 times a day, morning and evening.

For more information, refer to the complete monograph for clotrimazole in "Athlete's Foot and Jock Itch" under Dermatological Conditions.

MICONAZOLE

Miconazole is fungistatic and may be fungicidal, depending on concentration. It inhibits biosynthesis of ergosterol or other sterols, damaging the fungal cell wall membrane and altering its permeability. As a result, loss of essential intracellular elements may occur.

Miconazole also inhibits biosynthesis of triglycerides and phospholipids by fungi. In addition, it inhibits oxidative and peroxidative enzyme activity, resulting in intracellular buildup of toxic concentrations of hydrogen peroxide, which may contribute to deterioration of subcellular organelles and cellular necrosis. In *Candida albicans*, miconazole inhibits transformation of blastospores into invasive mycelial form.

Candidiasis, cutaneous (treatment)—Miconazole is indicated in the topical treatment of cutaneous candidiasis caused by *C albicans*.

Tinea corporis (treatment), *tinea cruris* (treatment), and *tinea pedis* (treatment)—Miconazole is indicated in the topical treatment of tinea corporis (ringworm of the body), tinea cruris (ringworm of the groin, or "jock itch"), and tinea pedis (ringworm of the foot, or athlete's foot) caused by *Trichophyton rubrum*, *T mentagrophytes*, and *Epidermophyton floccosum*.

Tinea versicolor (treatment)—Miconazole is indicated in the topical treatment of tinea versicolor (pityriasis versicolor, or "sun fungus") caused by *Malassezia furfur* (also called *Pityrosporon orbiculare*).

Paronychia (treatment), *tinea barbae* (treatment), and *tinea capitis* (treatment)—Miconazole is used in the topical treatment of paronychia, tinea barbae, and tinea capitis.

Aersol powder/Aerosol solution/Powder

For tinea corporis/tinea cruris/tinea pedis:

Adults/Pediatrics: Apply to affected area 2 times a day, morning and evening.

Cream/Lotion

For candidiasis, cutaneous/tinea corporis/tinea cruris/tine pedis:

Adults/Pediatrics: Apply to affected area two times a day, morning and evening.

For tinea versicolor:

Adults/Pediatrics: Apply to affected area once a day.

For more information, refer to the complete monograph for miconazole in "Athlete's Foot and Jock Itch" under Dermatological Conditions.

CLOTRIMAZOLE PRODUCTS	
Brand Name	**Dosage Form**
Cruex (Novartis)	**Cream:** 1%
Lotrimin (Schering)	**Cream:** 1% **Lotion:** 1% **Solution:** 1%
Lotrimin AF (Schering)	**Cream:** 1% **Lotion:** 1% **Solution:** 1%

MICONAZOLE PRODUCTS	
Brand Name	**Dosage Form**
Baza Antifungal (Coloplast)	**Cream:** 2%
Desenex (Novartis)	**Powder:** 2% **Spray:** 2%
Lotrimin AF (Schering)	**Powder:** 2% **Spray:** 2%
Micatin (Pharmacia)	**Cream:** 2% **Powder:** 2% **Spray:** 2%
Neosporin AF (Pfizer)	**Cream:** 2% **Powder:** 2% **Spray:** 2%
Zeasorb AF (Stiefil)	**Lotion:** 2% **Powder:** 2%

TERBINAFINE

Terbinafine is fungistatic and interferes with membrane synthesis and growth; it may also be fungicidal. Terbinafine inhibits squalene epoxidase (a key enzyme in sterol biosynthesis in fungi), which results in a deficiency in ergosterol and a corresponding increase in squalene within the fungal cell, causing fungal cell death.

Tinea corporis (treatment), *tinea cruris* (treatment), *tinea pedis, interdigital* (treatment), and *tinea pedis, plantar* (treatment)—Terbinafine is indicated as a primary agent in the topical treatment of tinea corporis (ringworm of the body), tinea cruris (ringworm of the groin, or "jock itch"), interdigital tinea pedis (ringworm of the foot, or "athlete's foot") caused by *Trichophyton rubrum*, *T mentagrophytes*, or *Epidermophyton floccosum*, and plantar tinea pedis (moccasin-type) caused by *T mentagrophytes* or *T rubrum*.

Tinea versicolor (treatment)—Terbinafine cream and solution are indicated for the topical treatment of tinea versicolor due to *Malassezia furfur*.

Candidiasis, cutaneous (treatment)—Terbinafine cream is indicated for the topical treatment of yeast infections of the skin, principally those caused by the genus *Candida*, (e.g., C *albicans*).

Cream

For tinea corporis/tinea cruris:

Adults/Pediatrics ≥12 years of age: Apply to affected area and surrounding areas, 1 or 2 times a day. Treatment should be continued for at least 1 week *and* until there is significant improvement in the clinical signs and symptoms of the disease. Treatment should not be continued beyond 4 weeks.

For tinea pedis, interdigital:

Adults/Pediatrics ≥12 years of age: Apply to affected area and surrounding areas 2 times a day. Treatment should be continued for at least 1 week *and* until there is significant improvement in the clinical signs and symptoms of the disease. Treatment should not be continued beyond 4 weeks.

For tinea pedis, plantar:

Adults/Pediatrics ≥12 years of age: Apply to affected area and surrounding areas 2 times a day. Treatment should be continued for 2 weeks. Treatment may be affected by the presence of onychomycosis. Patients with a toenail infection may be less likely to respond favorably to terbinafine therapy.

For tinea versicolor:

Adults: Apply to affected area and surrounding areas 1 or 2 times a day for 2 weeks.

For cutaneous candidiasis:

Adults: Apply to affected area and surrounding areas, one or two times a day for two weeks.

Solution

For tinea corporis/tinea cruris:

Adults: Apply to affected area and surrounding areas once a day for 1 week. Treatment should be continued for at least 1 week *even though* symptoms of the disease may have improved.

For tinea pedis/tinea versicolor:

Adults: Apply to affected area and surrounding areas 2 times a day for 2 weeks. Treatment should be continued for at least 1 week *even though* symptoms of the disease may have improved.

For more information, refer to the complete monograph for terbinafine in "Athlete's Foot and Jock Itch" under Dermatological Conditions.

TOLNAFTATE

Tolnaftate is fungicidal but the exact mechanism of action is unknown. However, it has been reported to distort the hyphae and stunt mycelial growth in susceptible organisms.

Tinea capitis (treatment)—Tolnaftate is indicated in the topical treatment of tinea capitis.

Tinea corporis (treatment), *tinea cruris* (treatment), *tinea manuum* (treatment), and *tinea pedis* (treatment)—Tolnaftate is indicated in the topical treatment of tinea corporis (ringworm of the body), tinea cruris (ringworm of the groin, or "jock itch"), tinea manuum, and tinea pedis (ringworm of the foot, or "athlete's foot") caused by *Trichophyton rubrum*, *T mentagrophytes*, *T tonsurans*, *Microsporum canis*, *M audouini*, and *Epidermophyton floccosum*.

Tinea versicolor (treatment)—Tolnaftate is indicated in the topical treatment of tinea versicolor (pityriasis versicolor, or "sun fungus") caused by *Malassezia furfur*.

Tinea barbae (treatment)—Tolnaftate is used in the topical treatment of tinea barbae.

Aerosol powder/Aerosol solution/Cream/Gel/Powder/Solution

Adults/Pediatrics ≥2 years of age: Apply to affected area 2 times a day.

For more information, refer to the complete monograph for tolnaftate in "Athlete's Foot and Jock Itch" under Dermatological Conditions.

TERBINAFINE PRODUCTS	
Brand Name	**Dosage Form**
Lamisil AT Athlete's Foot (Novartis)	**Cream:** 1%**Spray:** 1%
Lamisil AT Jock Itch (Novartis)	**Cream:** 1% **Spray:** 1%
Lamisil AT for Women (Novartis)	**Cream:** 1%
TOLNAFTATE PRODUCTS	
Brand Name	**Dosage Form**
Tinactin (Schering)	**Cream:** 1% **Powder:** 1% **Solution:** 1% **Spray:** 1%
Tinactin Jock Itch (Schering)	**Cream:** 1% **Powder:** 1%
Absorbine JR. Antifungal (W.F. Young)	**Cream:** 1%

UNDECYLENIC ACID

Compound undecylenic acid has a fungistatic action. The zinc present in the zinc undecylenate component provides a beneficial astringent action, which aids in reducing rawness and irritation.

Compound undecylenic acid has been used for the topical treatment of tinea cruris, tinea pedis, and other tinea infections. However, in the opinion of USP medical experts, it has been superseded by newer and more effective topical antifungal agents.

Aerosol foam/Aerosol powder/Cream/Ointment/Powder/ Solution

Adults/Pediatrics ≥2 years of age: Apple to affected area 2 times a day.

For more information, refer to the complete monograph for undecylenic acid in "Athlete's Foot and Jock Itch" under Dermatological Conditions.

CALCIUM UNDECYLENATE AND UNDECYLENIC ACID PRODUCTS	
Brand Name	**Dosage Form**
Caldesene (Heritage)	**Powder:** 10%
Cruex (Novartis)	**Powder:** 10%
Elon Dual Defense (Dartmouth)	**Tincture:** 25%
Sanafitil (Tarmac)	**Spray:** 10%

DOSING INFORMATION FOR ANTIFUNGAL PRODUCTS

The following table provides a quick comparison of the ingredients and dosages of common brand-name OTC drugs. Products are listed alphabetically by generic ingredient and brand name.

Brand Name	Generic Ingredient/Strength	Dose
BUTENAFINE		
Lotrimin Ultra Antifungal cream (*Schering-Plough*)	Butenafine Hydrochloride 1%	**Adults & Peds ≥12 yo:** Use bid.
CLOTRIMAZOLE		
Clearly Confident Triple Action Toenail & Foot Treatment (*Gandeden Biotech*)	Clotrimazole 1%	**Adult:** Apply to affected area qd.
Cruex spray powder (*Novartis Consumer Health*)	Miconazole Nitrate 2%	**Adults:** Apply to affected area bid.
FungiCure Anti-Fungal Liquid Spray (*Alva-Amco Pharmacal*)	Clotrimazole 1%	**Adults & Peds:** Use bid.
Lotrimin AF Antifungal Athlete's Foot cream (*Schering-Plough*)	Clotrimazole 1%	**Adults & Peds ≥2 yo:** Use bid.
Lotrimin AF Antifungal Athlete's Foot topical solution (*Schering-Plough*)	Clotrimazole 1%	**Adults & Peds ≥2 yo:** Use bid.
Swabplus Foot Care Athlete's Foot Relief Swabs (*Swabplus*)	Clotrimazole 1%	**Adults & Peds:** Use bid.
MICONAZOLE		
Baza Antifungal cream	Miconazole Nitrate 2%	**Adults & Peds:** Apply to affected area bid.
Desenex Antifungal liquid spray (*Novartis Consumer Health*)	Miconazole Nitrate 2%	**Adults:** Apply to affected area bid.
Desenex Antifungal powder (*Novartis Consumer Health*)	Miconazole Nitrate 2%	**Adults:** Apply to affected area bid.
Desenex Antifungal spray powder (*Novartis Consumer Health*)	Miconazole Nitrate 2%	**Adults:** Apply to affected area bid.
DiabetAid Antifungal Foot Bath tablets (*Del Pharmaceuticals*)	Miconazole Nitrate 2%	**Adults & Peds ≥2 yo:** Use prn.
Diabet-X Antifungal Skin Treatment cream (*Del Pharmaceuticals*)	Miconazole Nitrate 2%	**Adults & Peds ≥2 yo:** Use prn.
Lotrimin AF Antifungal Aerosol liquid spray (*Schering-Plough*)	Miconazole Nitrate 2%	**Adults & Peds ≥2 yo:** Use bid.
Lotrimin AF Antifungal Jock Itch aerosol powder spray (*Schering-Plough*)	Miconazole Nitrate 2%	**Adults & Peds ≥2 yo:** Use bid.
Lotrimin AF Antifungal powder (*Schering-Plough*)	Miconazole Nitrate 2%	**Adults & Peds ≥2 yo:** Use bid.
Micatin Antifungal liquid spray (*Pfizer Consumer Healthcare*)	Miconazole Nitrate 2%	**Adults & Peds ≥12 yo:** Use bid.

DOSING INFORMATION FOR ANTIFUNGAL PRODUCTS (cont.)

BRAND NAME	GENERIC INGREDIENT/STRENGTH	DOSE
Micatin Antifungal Spray Powder *(Pfizer Consumer Healthcare)*	Miconazole Nitrate 2%	**Adults & Peds ≥12 yo:** Use bid.
Micatin Athlete's Foot cream *(Pfizer Consumer Healthcare)*	Miconazole Nitrate 2%	**Adults:** Apply to affected area bid. **Max:** 2 weeks.
Micatin Athlete's Foot spray liquid *(Pfizer Consumer Healthcare)*	Miconazole Nitrate 2%	**Adults:** Apply to affected area bid. **Max:** 2 weeks.
Micatin Athlete's Foot spray powder *(Pfizer Consumer Healthcare)*	Miconazole Nitrate 2%	**Adults:** Apply to affected area bid. **Max:** 2 weeks.
Micatin Jock Itch Spray powder *(Pfizer Consumer Healthcare)*	Miconazole Nitrate 2%	**Adults:** Apply to affected area bid. **Max:** 2 weeks.
Neosporin AF Antifungal cream *(Pfizer Consumer Healthcare)*	Miconazole Nitrate 2%	**Adults & Peds ≥12 yo:** Use bid.
Neosporin AF Athlete's Foot Spray liquid *(Pfizer Consumer Healthcare)*	Miconazole Nitrate 2%	**Adults & Peds ≥12 yo:** Use bid.
Neosporin AF Athlete's Foot, Spray powder *(Pfizer Consumer Healthcare)*	Miconazole Nitrate 2%	**Adults & Peds ≥12 yo:** Use bid.
Zeasorb Super Absorbent Antifungal powder *(Steifel Laboratories)*	Miconazole Nitrate 2%	**Adults & Peds:** Use bid.
TERBINAFINE		
Lamisil AT Athlete's Foot cream *(Novartis Consumer Health)*	Terbinafine Hydrochloride 1%	**Adults & Peds ≥12 yo:** Use bid.
Lamisil AT Athlete's Foot Spray Pump *(Novartis Consumer Health)*	Terbinafine Hydrochloride 1%	**Adults & Peds ≥12 yo:** Use bid.
Lamisil AT for Women cream *(Novartis Consumer Health)*	Terbinafine Hydrochloride 1%	**Adults & Peds ≥12 yo:** Use bid.
Lamisil AT Jock Itch cream *(Novartis Consumer Health)*	Terbinafine Hydrochloride 1%	**Adults & Peds ≥12 yo:** Use bid.
Lamisil AT Jock Itch Spray Pump *(Novartis Consumer Health)*	Terbinafine Hydrochloride 1%	**Adults & Peds ≥12 yo:** Use bid.
TOLNAFTATE		
Aftate Antifungal Liquid Spray for Athlete's Foot *(Schering-Plough)*	Tolnaftate 1%	**Adults:** Apply to affected area qd-bid.
FungiCure Anti-Fungal Gel *(Alva-Amco Pharmacal)*	Tolnaflate 1%	**Adults & Peds:** Use bid.
Gold Bond Antifungal Foot Swabs *(Chattem)*	Tolnaftate 1%	**Adults & Peds:** Use bid.
Miracle of Aloe Miracle Anti-Fungal *(Ontel Products)*	Tolnaftate 1%	**Adults & Peds ≥12 yo:** Use bid.
Swabplus Foot Care Fungus Relief Swabs *(Swabplus)*	Tolnaftate 1%	**Adults & Peds:** Use bid.
Tinactin Antifungal Aerosol Deodorant Powder Spray *(Schering-Plough)*	Tolnaftate 1%	**Adults & Peds:** Use bid.
Tinactin Antifungal Aerosol liquid spray *(Schering-Plough)*	Tolnaftate 1%	**Adults & Peds:** Use bid.
Tinactin Antifungal Aerosol powder spray *(Schering-Plough)*	Tolnaftate 1%	**Adults & Peds:** Use bid.
Tinactin Antifungal cream *(Schering-Plough)*	Tolnaftate 1%	**Adults & Peds:** Use bid.
Tinactin Antifungal Foot powder *(Schering-Plough)*	Tolnaftate 1%	**Adults & Peds:** Use bid.
Tinactin Antifungal Jock Itch powder spray *(Schering-Plough)*	Tolnaftate 1%	**Adults & Peds:** Use bid.
UNDECYLENIC ACID		
Fungi Nail Anti-fungal Solution *(Kramer Laboratories)*	Undecylenic Acid 25%	**Adults & Peds:** Use bid.
FungiCure Anti-fungal Liquid *(Alva-Amco Pharmacal Cos)*	Undecylenic Acid 10%	**Adults & Peds:** Use bid.
Tineacide Antifungal cream *(Blaine Labs)*	Undecylenic Acid 10%	**Adults & Peds ≥12 yo:** Use bid.

Insect Bites and Stings

Bites and stings inflicted by different species of insects, arachnids (spiders), and acarids (mites)—all members of the phylum Arthropoda—cause two kinds of reactions in humans: (1) physical trauma resulting from the puncture of the skin and feeding, and (2) a toxic or allergic reaction to the irritating toxic substances and/or antigenic substances introduced into the host. Anaphylaxis, potentially the most life-threatening reaction to an insect sting or arthropod bite, is IgE mediated and is caused by sensitization of the host to antigenic substances in either the arthropod's saliva or its venom. Sensitization of the host can also lead to large local reactions, which may be caused by one or more allergic mechanisms. The first allergic mechanism is IgE-mediated hypersensitivity, as in the cutaneous late-phase reaction; the second is cell-mediated hypersensitivity. The rare neurologic sequelae also seem to be mediated by IgE or by an immune complex reaction.

Bites—The salivary proteins of various arthropods are implicated in the pathogenesis of local and systemic reactions. For example, the high-molecular-weight protein F-1 is the major skin-reactive substance of the mosquito *Aedes aegypti*. When injected into the skin of sensitized individuals, F-1 produces a dose-response reaction proportionate to the amount injected. Papular urticaria to flea bites is associated with two components, components A and B, of the oral secretions of the cat flea, *Ctenocephalides felis*.

Bites, local reactions—People without a history of flea bites usually follow a predictable sequence of skin reactions when they are repeatedly bitten over a 1-year period. In *stage I*, the induction period, there is no observable skin reaction or abnormality on skin biopsy. *Stage II* is characterized by a delayed skin reaction that occurs 18 to 24 hours after a bite and is accompanied by infiltration of lymphocytes and other mononuclear cells into the dermis and extending into the epidermis. These pruritic, erythematous, and indurated lesions may persist for 10 to 14 days. *Stage III* manifests as an immediate skin reaction (within 15 to 60 minutes) that clears in 4 hours and is followed by a delayed skin reaction. At the immediate phase of this stage, the primary infiltrating cells are eosinophils, whereas mononuclear cells characterize the delayed skin reaction. *Stage IV* is characterized by an immediate skin reaction (within 20 minutes) and eosinophilic response and a mild or absent delayed reaction (within 24 hours) with a mononuclear response. With continued challenge, both responses diminish. *Stage V* is the stage of nonreactivity, in which the biopsy site at 20 minutes and at 24 hours reveals little or no cellular response.

Studies performed over the past 40 years have demonstrated a similar sequence of events in subjects exposed to mosquito bites over a period of time. This suggests that during natural exposure, desensitization to bites occurs. Papular urticaria in humans is characterized by pruritic erythematous papules, vesicles, or bullae grouped in clusters. They are associated with multiple flea, mosquito, and bedbug bites. Papular urticaria develops only in subjects with delayed reactions to such bites. It commonly occurs in children 2 to 7 years of age and usually involves the extremities. Chigger (Trombiculidae) bites can result in similar lesions, but the lesions typically occur under areas covered by tight clothing.

Bites, systemic allergic reactions—Anaphylactic reactions from bites are rare; they occur most commonly with insects of the orders Hemiptera and Diptera. Insects of the order Hemiptera, genus *Triatoma*—known as kissing, conenose, or assassin bugs—are endemic from Texas to California. Typically, these bugs bite at night, when the victim is asleep. Although the bite is painless, the victim may subsequently awaken with itching, respiratory distress, and other allergic symptoms. Several anaphylactic deaths have been reported in subjects with evidence of IgE sensitization to the insect's saliva. The most common insect bites are from mosquitoes, which rarely appear to cause systemic reactions. Black flies are a plague in areas of the Northern Hemisphere, and their bites have been associated with anaphylactic reactions. The large horseflies and deerflies administer painful bites that have been associated with verified systemic reactions. Evidently, systemic reactions caused by some of the insects in the order Diptera are IgE mediated.

Insect stings—More than 16,000 species of Hymenoptera are found in the United States. Many of the workers and adult females of this order have a modified ovipositor and venom sac for stinging. Humans stung by hymenopteran insects suffer local cutaneous reactions at the sting site, ranging from transient erythema to edema with or (rarely) without pain, extensive erythema, or edema and induration lasting more than 48 hours. Members of three families of Hymenoptera are responsible for most insect sting reactions: Apidae (honeybees and bumblebees), Vespidae (wasps, yellow jackets, and hornets), and Formicidae (native and imported fire ants and harvester ants). The apids and vespids are found in most regions of the United States. *Solenopsis invicta* and the less prevalent and aggressive *Solenopsis richteri*, collectively referred to as the imported fire ant, have largely replaced the native fire ants (*Solenopsis geminata, Solenopsis aurea,* and *Solenopsis xyloni*) in the United States. Harvester ants (genus *Pogonomyrmex*), which can also cause systemic reactions, are found primarily in the southwestern and western parts of the country. *Pogonomyrmex badius* is found east of the Mississippi. Stingers of the various families of Hymenoptera are different in size but similar in design: they are ensheathed, barbed instruments with an attached venom sac located at the tip of the insect's abdomen. The larger barbs of the honeybee stinger anchor firmly in the human skin, so the honeybee cannot withdraw the stinger. The stinger then becomes detached when the animal flies away, resulting in the bee's evisceration and death. Muscles associated with the remaining venom sac can continue to expel venom into the sting site for several minutes, delivering approximately 50 to 100mcg of venom protein. Most other hymenopterans are able to withdraw their stinger from the skin and are thus able to sting again. The venoms are collected from hymenopteran insects using several techniques.

Insect stings, local, nonallergic (toxic)—A nonallergic local reaction begins immediately following the sting and is a toxic response to venom constituents that induce mast cell degranulation. Characteristic local manifestations include erythema, edema, pain, and pruritus. The reaction may persist for several hours and then resolve.

Insect stings, local, allergic—Allergic local reactions to Hymenoptera stings are larger and last longer than nonallergic reactions. These large local reactions are arbitrarily defined as local cutaneous reactions. They are pruritic and sometimes painful, with erythema and edema of greater than 10cm (>4 inches) in diameter that persist for at least 48 hours to 5 days.

Insect stings, systemic allergic reactions—Most systemic allergic reactions begin within 30 minutes, and almost all begin within 100 minutes after a sting; rarely, reactions begin hours afterward. Urticaria and generalized pruritus are the most common clinical manifestations, especially in children; however, generalized erythema, angioedema and upper airway edema, asthma, abdominal cramps, diarrhea, seizures, and hypotension secondary to vascular collapse can occur and even result in death.

Preventing bites and stings can often be accomplished by avoidance, physical barriers, and insect repellents. Most OTC insect repellents contain DEET. There are also a number of OTC products available to treat the symptoms of bites and stings, including topical and oral antihistamines, topical anesthetics, topical corticosteroids, and counterirritants.

ANTIHISTAMINES

Antihistaminic (H_1-receptor)—Antihistamines used in the treatment of allergy act by competing with histamine for H_1-receptor sites on effector cells. They thereby prevent, but do not reverse, responses mediated by histamine alone. Antihistamines antagonize, in varying degrees, most of the pharmacological effects of histamine, including urticaria and pruritus. Also, the anticholinergic actions of most antihistamines provide a drying effect on the nasal mucosa.

Pruritus (treatment); *urticaria* (treatment); *angioedema* (treatment); *dermatographism* (treatment); *transfusion reactions, urticarial* (treatment)—Antihistamines are indicated for the symptomatic treatment of pruritus associated with allergic reactions and of mild, uncomplicated allergic skin manifestations of urticaria and angioedema, in dermatographism, and in urticaria associated with transfusions.

Brompheniramine

Capsules/Elixir/Tablets

Adults/Pediatrics ≥*12 years of age*: 4mg every 4 to 6 hours as needed.

Pediatrics 2 to 6 years of age: 1mg every 4 to 6 hours as needed.

Pediatrics 6 to 12 years of age: 2mg every 4 to 6 hours as needed.

Chlorpheniramine

Capsules, extended-release/Tablets, extended-release

Adults/Pediatrics ≥*12 years of age*: 8 to 12mg every 8 to 12 hours as needed.

Syrup/Tablets

Adults/Pediatrics ≥*12 years of age*: 4mg every 4 to 6 hours as needed.

Pediatrics 6 to 12 years of age: 2mg 3 or 4 times a day as needed. Max: 12mg per day.

Clemastine

Syrup/Tablets

Adults/Pediatrics ≥*12 years of age*: 1.34mg 2 times a day; or 2.68mg 1 to 3 times a day as needed.

Pediatrics 6 to 12 years of age: 0.67mg to 1.34mg 2 times a day; not to exceed 4.02mg/day.

Diphenhydramine

Capsules

Adults/Pediatrics ≥*12 years of age*: 25 to 50mg every 4 to 6 hours as needed.

Pediatrics up to 6 years of age: 6.25 to 12.5mg every 4 to 6 hours.

Pediatrics 6 to 12 years of age: 12.5 to 25mg every 4 to 6 hours; not to exceed 150mg/day.

Elixir/Tablets

Adults/Pediatrics ≥*12 years of age*: 25 to 50mg every 4 to 6 hours as needed.

Pediatrics: 1.25mg/kg of body weight or 37.5mg/m^2 of body surface, every 4 to 6 hours; not to exceed 300mg/day.

Pediatrics weighing up to 9.1kg: 6.25 to 12.5mg every 4 to 6 hours.

Pediatrics weighing 9.1kg and over: 12.5 to 25mg every 4 to 6 hours.

BROMPHENIRAMINE PRODUCTS	
Brand Name	**Dosage Form**
Dimetapp Allergy (Wyeth)	**Capsule:** 4mg **Tablet:** 4mg
Dimetapp Allergy Children's (Wyeth)	**Elixir:** 2mg/5ml
Dimetane Extentabs (Wyeth)	**Tablet:** 12 mg
CHLORPHENIRAMINE PRODUCTS	
Brand Name	**Dosage Form**
Chlor-Trimeton (Schering)	**Syrup:** 2mg/5mL **Tablet:** 4mg,8mg,12mg
Efidac 24 (Novartis)	**Tablet:** 16mg
CLEMASTINE PRODUCTS	
Brand Name	**Dosage Form**
Tavist-1 (Novartis)	**Tablet:** 1.34mg

Loratadine

Syrup

Adults/Pediatrics ≥6 years of age: 10mg once a day.

Pediatrics 2 to 6 years of age: 5mg once a day.

For more information, refer to the complete monograph for antihistamines in "Allergic Rhinitis" under Respiratory System.

TOPICAL ANTIHISTAMINES

Antihistaminic (H_1-receptor)—Antihistamines used in the treatment of allergy act by competing with histamine for H_1-receptor sites on effector cells. They thereby prevent, but do not reverse, responses mediated by histamine alone. Antihistamines antagonize, in varying degrees, most of the pharmacological effects of histamine, including urticaria and pruritus.

Pruritus (treatment)—Antihistamines are indicated for the symptomatic treatment of pruritus and pain associated with insect bites, minor burns, sunburn, minor skin irritations, minor cuts, scrapes, and rashes due to poison ivy, poison oak, and poison sumac.

Diphenhydramine

Cream/Gel

Adults/Pediatrics ≥2 years of age: Apply to affected area not more than 3 to 4 times daily.

For more information, refer to the complete monograph for antihistamines in "Contact Dermatitis" under Dermatological conditions

TOPICAL CORTICOSTEROIDS

Corticosteroids diffuse across cell membranes and complex with specific cytoplasmic receptors. These complexes then enter the cell nucleus, bind to DNA (chromatin), and stimulate transcription of messenger RNA (mRNA) and subsequent protein synthesis of various inhibitory enzymes responsible for the anti-inflammatory effects of topical corticosteroids. These anti-inflammatory effects include inhibition of early processes such as edema, fibrin deposition, capillary dilatation, movement of phagocytes into the area, and phagocytic activities. Later processes, such as capillary production, collagen deposition, and keloid formation, are also inhibited by corticosteroids. The overall actions of topical corticosteroids are catabolic.

Relief of inflammation and/or pruritus (treatment)—Topical corticosteroids are indicated to provide symptomatic relief of inflammation and/or pruritus associated with acute and chronic corticosteroid-responsive disorders.

Hydrocortisone (only available OTC topical corticosteroid)

Cream/Lotion/Ointment *(See next page for products)*

Adults: Apply to affected area 1 to 4 times a day.

Pediatrics ≥2 years of age: 0.25%-0.05%: Apply to affected area 1 to 4 times a day. 1%: Apply to affected area 1 to 2 times a day.

Topical solution *(See next page for products)*

Adults: Apply to affected area 1 to 4 times a day.

Pediatrics ≥2 years of age: Apply to affected area 1 to 2 times a day.

For more information, refer to the complete monograph for antihistamines in "Contact Dermatitis" under Dermatological conditions.

DIPHENHYDRAMINE PRODUCTS (ORAL)	
Brand Name	**Dosage Form**
Benadryl (Pfizer)	**Capsule:** 25mg **Tablet:** 25mg
Benadryl Allergy (Pfizer)	**Solution:** 12.5mg/5mL **Tablet:** 12.5mg
Benadryl Allergy Fastmelt (Pfizer)	**Tablet:** 19mg
LORATADINE PRODUCTS	
Brand Name	**Dosage Form**
Alavert (Wyeth)	**Tablet:** 10mg
Claritin (Schering)	**Solution:** 5mg/5mL **Tablet:** 10mg
Claritin Hives Releif (Schering)	**Tablet:** 10mg
Claritin Reditabs (Schering)	**Tablet:** 10mg

DIPHENHYDRAMINE PRODUCTS (TOPICAL)	
Brand Name	**Dosage Form**
Benadryl Itch Relief Stick Extra Strength (Pfizer)	**Stick:** 2%
Benadryl Itch stopping cream Original (Pfizer)	**Cream:** 1%
Benadryl Itch Stopping cream Extra Strength (Pfizer)	**Cream:** 2%
Benadryl Itch Stopping Gel Extra Strength (Pfizer)	**Gel:** 2%
Benadryl Itch Stopping Spray Extra Strength (Pfizer)	**Spray:** 2%

HYDROCORTISONE PRODUCTS (DERMATITIS)

Brand Name	Dosage Form
Aveeno Anti-itch (J & J)	Cream: 1%
Caldecort (Novartis)	Cream: 1% Spray: 0.5%
Caldecort Light (Novartis)	Cream: 1%
Cortaid Intensive Therapy (Pharmacia)	Cream: 1%
Cortaid Maximum Strength (Pharmacia)	Cream: 1% Ointment: 1% Spray: 1%
Cortaid Sensitive Skin w/aloe (Pharmacia)	Cream: 0.05%
Cortixaine (UCB)	Cream: 0.05%
Cortizone-5 (Pfizer)	Ointment: 0.50%
Cortizone-10 (Pfizer)	Cream: 1% Ointment: 1%
Cortizone-10 Plus (Pfizer)	Cream: 1%
Cortizone 10 Quick Shot (Pfizer)	Spray: 1%
Dermarest Dricort (Del)	Cream: 1%
Dermarest Eczema Medicated (Del)	Lotion: 1%
Gynecort Anti-itch (Combe)	Cream: 1%
Hytone (Dermik)	Lotion: 1%
Ivy Soothe (Enviroderm)	Cream: 1%
Ivy State Dual Action Poison Ivy Exfoliant and Treatment (Tec)	Gel: 1%
Lanacort (Combe)	Cream: 1%
Massengill Medicated Towelettes (GSK)	Pads: 0.50%
Neutrogena T/Scalp (Neutrogena)	Liquid: 1%
Nupercainal HC 1% (Novartis)	Cream: 1%
Scalpicin (Combe)	Liquid: 1%

DOSING INFORMATION FOR ANTI-ITCH PRODUCTS

The following table provides a quick comparison of the ingredients and dosages of common brand-name OTC drugs. Products are listed alphabetically by drug category and brand name.

BRAND NAME	GENERIC INGREDIENT/STRENGTH	DOSE
ANTIHISTAMINE		
Benadryl Extra Strength Gel Pump (Pfizer Consumer Healthcare)	Diphenhydramine HCl 2%	**Adults & Peds ≥12 yo:** Apply to affected area tid-qid.
ANTIHISTAMINE COMBINATION		
Benadryl Extra Strength Cream (Pfizer Consumer Healthcare)	Diphenhydramine HCl/Zinc Acetate 2%-0.1%	**Adults & Peds ≥12 yo:** Apply to affected area tid-qid.
Benadryl Extra Strength Spray (Pfizer Consumer Healthcare)	Diphenhydramine HCl/Zinc Acetate 2%-0.1%	**Adults & Peds ≥12 yo:** Apply to affected area tid-qid.
Benadryl Itch Relief Stick (Pfizer Consumer Healthcare)	Diphenhydramine HCl/Zinc Acetate 2%-0.1%	**Adults & Peds ≥2 yo:** Apply to affected area tid-qid.
Benadryl Original Cream (Pfizer Consumer Healthcare)	Diphenhydramine HCl/Zinc Acetate 1%-0.1%	**Adults & Peds ≥2 yo:** Apply to affected area tid-qid.
CalaGel Anti-Itch Gel (Tec Laboratories)	Diphenhydramine HCl/Zinc Acetate/ Benzenthonium Chloride 1.8%-0.21%-15%	**Adults & Peds ≥2 yo:** Apply to affected area tid-qid.
CORTICOSTEROIDS		
Aveeno Anti-Itch Cream 1% (Johnson & Johnson/Merck Consumer)	Hydrocortisone 1%	**Adults & Peds ≥2 yo:** Apply to affected area tid-qid.
Cortaid Intensive Therapy Cooling Spray (Pharmacia Consumer Healthcare)	Hydrocortisone 1%	**Adults & Peds ≥2 yo:** Apply to affected area tid-qid.
Cortaid Intensive Therapy Moisturizing cream (Pharmacia Consumer Healthcare)	Hydrocortisone 1%	**Adults & Peds ≥2 yo:** Apply to affected area tid-qid.
Cortaid Maximum Strength cream (Pharmacia Consumer Healthcare)	Hydrocortisone 1%	**Adults & Peds ≥2 yo:** Apply to affected area tid-qid.

DOSING INFORMATION FOR ANTI-ITCH PRODUCTS (cont.)

Brand Name	Generic Ingredient/Strength	Dose
Cortizone-10 Cream *(Pfizer Consumer Healthcare)*	Hydrocortisone 1%	**Adults & Peds ≥2 yo:** Apply to affected area tid-qid.
Cortizone-10 Maximum Strength Anti-itch oinment *(Pfizer Consumer Healthcare)*	Hydrocortisone 1%	**Adults & Peds ≥2 yo:** Apply to affected area tid-qid.
Cortizone-10 Ointment *(Pfizer Consumer Healthcare)*	Hydrocortisone 1%	**Adults & Peds ≥2 yo:** Apply to affected area tid-qid.
Cortizone-10 plus Maximum Strength cream *(Pfizer Consumer Healthcare)*	Hydrocortisone 1%	**Adults & Peds ≥2 yo:** Apply to affected area tid-qid.
Cortizone-10 Quick Shot Spray *(Pfizer Consumer Healthcare)*	Hydrocortisone 1%	**Adults & Peds ≥2 yo:** Apply to affected area tid-qid.
COUNTERIRRITANT		
After Bite Fast Relief Itch Eraser, Gentle Kids Cream *(Tender Corp.)*	Eucalyptus Oil/Tea Tree Oil 1.3%-1.0%	**Adults & Peds ≥2 yo:** Apply to affected area tid-qid.
After Bite Fast Relief Itch Eraser, Xtra Soothing Gel *(Tender Corp.)*	Ammonia 2.0%	**Adults & Peds ≥2 yo:** Apply to affected area tid-qid.
After Bite The Itch Eraser for Insect Bites *(Tender Corp.)*	Ammonia 3.5%	**Adults & Peds ≥2 yo:** Apply to affected area tid-qid.
Eucerin Itch Relief Moisturizing Spray *(Beiersdorf)*	Menthol 0.15%	**Adults:** Apply to affected area prn.
Gold Bond First Aid Quick Spray *(Chattem)*	Menthol/Benzethonium Chloride 1%-0.13%	**Adults & Peds ≥2 yo:** Apply to affected area tid-qid.
Gold Bond Medicated Maximum Strength Anti-Itch Cream *(Chattem)*	Menthol/Pramoxine HCl 1%-1%	**Adults & Peds ≥2 yo:** Apply to affected area tid-qid.

Pediculosis (Lice)

The phylum Arthropoda includes more species than all the other phyla combined, comprising billions of organisms. Some of their distinguishing characteristics are a hard external skeleton, jointed legs, and other appendages. The arthropods that cause human skin disease include four classes: Arachnida, Chilopoda, Diplopoda, and Insecta. The class Insecta includes various orders such as Anoplura and Hymenoptera. Various arthropods, some of which serve as vectors of disease, parasitize humans whether for a meal or as part of their life cycle. For example, bedbugs and lice tend to bite and then return to their nearby living areas, whereas scabies mites prefer to remain on their host upon infestation. These arthropod assaults on humans may have many manifestations clinically, histologically, and immunologically.

Lice belong to Anoplura, the order of sucking lice. Infestation by head or body lice is referred to as pediculiasis and the associated "disease" as pediculosis. Louse infestation remains a major health and economic problem throughout the world. Over the past several decades, the incidence of pediculosis has risen steadily. Head-lice infestation among schoolchildren has reached near epidemic proportions in some parts of the United States. Body lice are important vectors of some serious human diseases. Three main types of lice parasitize humans: *Pediculus humanus capitis* (head louse), *Pediculus humanus corporis* (body louse), and *Phthirus pubis* (pubic louse).

Lice are wingless and have three pairs of legs, each ending in a talus designed for grasping. Body lice infest clothing, while head and pubic lice infest hairs. Head and pubic lice feed approximately 5 times a day, about 30 to 45 minutes per feeding. Unlike head and public lice, which can live only 1 day away from the host, the body louse can survive as long as 10 days away from the host without a blood meal.

Head lice are 1 to 2mm in length and whitish gray in color with a long, segmented abdomen. The female louse usually lays her eggs at night, at the base of a hair shaft, often in the posterior hairline or postauricular region. Body lice are larger, ranging from 2 to 4mm in length and are also whitish gray with a long, segmented abdomen. They tend to live in human clothing, crawling on the body to feed, usually at night. The female body louse lays her eggs in cooler temperatures than the female head louse, preferring the fibers of clothing, close to the seams. Pubic lice are approximately 1mm in length and whitish gray, with a shorter, broader body and larger front claws, for which they have earned the nickname "crabs." They infest and lay eggs most frequently on pubic hair shafts but may also infest axillary, eyelash, eyebrow, facial, and even scalp hair.

The nits, or eggs, of the louse attach to the hair shaft or clothing fibers with a highly insoluble cement. Nits usually hatch in 8 to 10 days. The hollow egg casing remains attached to the hair or fiber. In the case of head-lice infestation, the duration of the disease can be measured by assuming that the egg was laid at or near the base of the hair shaft and that hair grows approximately 1cm a month. There are several OTC products available to treat lice, most containing permethrin or pyrethrins.

PERMETHRIN

PHARMACOLOGY

Permethrin acts on the nerve cell membrane of the louse or mite to disrupt the sodium channel current that regulates the polarization of the membrane. This leads to delayed repolarization and subsequent paralysis of the louse or mite.

INDICATIONS

Pediculosis capitis (treatment)—Permethrin 1% is indicated for the treatment of infestation caused by *Pediculus humanus* var *capitis* (head louse) and its ova.

Scabies (treatment)—Permethrin 5% is indicated for the treatment of scabies infestation caused by *Sarcoptes scabiei* (human mites).

CONTRAINDICATIONS

Risk-benefit should be considered when the following medical problems exist:

- Inflammation of the scalp, acute (condition may be exacerbated).
- Sensitivity to permethrin.

WARNINGS/PRECAUTIONS

Patients sensitive to veterinary insecticides containing permethrin will be sensitive to permethrin cream or lotion. In addition, patients sensitive to other synthetic pyrethroids, such as those found in household insecticides, or to pyrethrins or chrysanthemums may be sensitive to this medication also.

Pregnancy: FDA Category B.

Breastfeeding: Problems in humans have not been documented. Although it is not known whether permethrin is distributed into human milk, permethrin has been shown to have tumorigenic potential in some animal studies.

ADVERSE REACTIONS

Those indicating need for medical attention only if they continue or are bothersome:

Incidence less frequent or rare

Burning, itching, numbness, rash, redness, stinging, swelling, or tingling of the scalp.

PERMETHRIN PRODUCTS	
Brand Name	**Dosage Form**
Nix (Heritage)	**Shampoo:** 1%
Rid Bedding & Furniture (Bayer Healthcare)	**Spray:** 0.50%

ADMINISTRATION AND DOSAGE

General Dosing Information

Pediculosis: Permethrin is used as a single-application treatment. Less than 1% of patients will require an additional treatment. If live lice are observed after 7 or more days following initial treatment, a second treatment may be administered.

Shampoo, rinse, and dry hair and scalp before application of permethrin. The lotion should be worked into dry hair until the hair and scalp are thoroughly wet. The lotion should be allowed to remain in place for 10 minutes. Then the hair and scalp should be rinsed thoroughly and dried with a clean towel. Although not necessary for the success of the treatment, when the hair is dry after the treatment, the patient may use a fine-toothed comb to remove any remaining nits or nit shells. After treatment, a residual amount of permethrin remains on the hair providing protection against reinfestation for approximately 2 weeks. This protection is unaffected by regular shampooing.

Scabies (available as prescription only): Scabies rarely infests the scalp of adults, although the hairline, neck, temple, and forehead may be infested in geriatric patients and in infants. Infants should be treated on the scalp, temple, and forehead. The cream should be massaged into the skin from the head to the soles of the feet. Usually 30g are sufficient for an average adult. The medication should be left on for 8 to 14 hours, then removed by thorough washing (shower or bath). Persistent pruritus may be experienced after treatment. This is rarely a sign of treatment failure and is not an indication for retreatment. Demonstrable living mites after 14 days indicate that retreatment is necessary.

For pediculosis capitis:

Lotion/Shampoo

Adults/Pediatrics ≥2 years of age: Apply to the hair and scalp or skin, for one application.

PYRETHRINS/PIPERONYL BUTOXIDE

PHARMACOLOGY

Pyrethrins—Are absorbed through the chitinous exoskeleton of arthropods and stimulate the nervous system, probably by competitively interfering with cationic conductances in the lipid layer of nerve cells, thereby blocking nerve impulse transmissions, which results in paralysis and death.

Piperonyl butoxide—Has little or no insecticidal activity but potentiates that of pyrethrins by inhibiting the hydrolytic enzymes responsible for metabolism of pyrethrins in arthropods, thereby increasing the insecticidal activity of pyrethrins by 2 to 12 times.

INDICATIONS

Pediculosis corporis (treatment); *pediculosis capitis* (treatment); *pediculosis pubis* (treatment)—Pyrethrins and piperonyl butoxide combination is indicated for the treatment of pediculosis (lice) infestations caused by *Pediculus humanus* var *corporis* (body louse), *Pediculus humanus* var *capitis* (head louse), and *Phthirus pubis* (pubic or crab louse).

CONTRAINDICATIONS

Risk-benefit should be considered when the following medical problems exist:

- Inflammation of skin, acute (condition may be exacerbated).
- Sensitivity to pyrethrins or piperonyl butoxide.

WARNINGS/PRECAUTIONS

Patients allergic to the ragweed or chrysanthemum plant may be allergic to the pyrethrins in this medication also. Patients sensitive to kerosene may also be sensitive to the pyrethrins and piperonyl butoxide combination preparations that contain kerosene.

Pregnancy: Problems in humans have not been documented; however, pyrethrins and piperonyl butoxide may be absorbed systemically in small amounts through intact skin.

Breastfeeding: Problems in humans have not been documented; however, pyrethrins and piperonyl butoxide may be absorbed systemically in small amounts through intact skin.

ADVERSE REACTIONS

Those indicating need for medical attention: Incidence less frequent or rare

Allergic reaction (skin rash, sudden attacks of sneezing, stuffy or runny nose, wheezing or difficulty in breathing); skin infection; skin irritation not present before therapy.

ADMINISTRATION AND DOSAGE

General Dosing Information

Following the initial treatment, a second treatment should be made in 7 to 10 days to kill any newly hatched lice. When used in the treatment of pediculosis pubis, the sexual partner should receive concurrent therapy, since the infestation may spread to persons in close contact.

Gel/Shampoo/Topical solution

Adults: Apply to the hair and scalp or skin for one application, repeated once in 7 to 10 days.

PYRETHRINS/PIPERONYL BUTOXIDE PRODUCTS	
Brand Name	**Dosage Form**
Licide (Reese)	**Kit:** 0.3%-3% **Shampoo:** 0.3%-3% **Spray:** 0.2%-1%
Rid (Bayer)	**Shampoo:** 0.33%-4%
Rid Lice Killing Mousse Maximum Strength (Bayer)	**Foam:** 0.33%-4%
Rid Lice Elimination Kit (Bayer)	**Kit:** 0.33%-4%

DOSING INFORMATION FOR LICE PRODUCTS

The following table provides a quick comparison of the ingredients and dosages of common brand-name OTC drugs. Products are listed alphabetically by generic ingredient and brand name.

BRAND NAME	GENERIC INGREDIENT/STRENGTH	DOSE
PERMETHRIN		
Nix Lice Control spray *(Heritage)*	Permethrin 0.25%	**Adults & Peds:** Spray to objects (furniture/ bedding etc.) prn.
Nix Lice Treatment *(Heritage)*	Permethrin 1%	**Adults & Peds:** Wash hair with shampoo without conditioner. Appply to damp but not wet hair and leave on hair for 10 minutes. Rinse with warm water. Repeat in seven days if needed.
Rid Lice Control spray *(Bayer Healthcare)*	Permethrin 0.50%	**Adults & Peds:** Spray to objects (furniture/ bedding etc.) prn.
PIPERONYL BUTOXIDE/PYRETHRUM EXTRACT		
Rid Maximum Strength shampoo *(Bayer Healthcare)*	Piperonyl butoxide/pyrethrum extract 4%-0.33%	**Adults & Peds:** Appply to dry hair and leave on hair for 10 minutes. Rinse with warm water. Repeat in 10 days.
Rid Maximum Strength mousse *(Bayer Healthcare)*	Piperonyl butoxide/pyrethrum extract 4%-0.33%	**Adults & Peds:** Appply to dry hair and leave on hair for 10 minutes. Rinse with warm water. Repeat in 7 to 10 days.
Rid Lice Elimination Kit *(Bayer Healthcare)*	Piperonyl butoxide/pyrethrum extract 4%-0.33%	**Adults & Peds:** Appply to dry hair and leave on hair for 10 minutes. Rinse with warm water. Repeat in 7 to 10 days.
ALTERNATIVE AGENTS & ADJUNCTS		
Rid Pure Alternative Lice & Egg Removal System *(Bayer Healthcare)*	Dimethicone	**Adults:** Apply q10d prn.
Rid Egg & Nit Comb-Out Gel *(Bayer Healthcare)*	Water, Glycerin, Hydroxyethylcellulose, Behenamidopropyl Dimethylamine Behenate, Cabbage Extract, Cysteine, Disodium EDTA, Disodium Phosphate, DMDM Hydantoin, Fragrance, Iodopropynyl Butylcarbamate, PG-Hydroxyethylcellulose Cocodimonium Chloride, Pineapple Extract, Polysorbate 20, Sodium Chloride, Sodium Phosphate, Tocopheryl Acetate	**Adults & Peds:** Apply to damp hair prn.

Psoriasis

Psoriasis is an idiopathic disease that manifests as erythematous, scaling plaques over the skin. Its name is derived from the Greek word *psōra*, meaning "itch." Psoriasis ranges from a mild disease to one that is severely debilitating. Psoriasis is a genetic disease with several known environmental triggers. It appears that more than one gene is involved. As evidence of its genetic basis, there is a 70% concordance rate of psoriasis among identical twins versus a 23% concordance rate among fraternal twins. Known environmental triggers include stress, streptococcal infections, and several drugs. One third of psoriasis patients report flare-ups of their disease after stressful life events. Streptococcal infections appear to activate T cells nonspecifically through a superantigen, thereby exacerbating psoriasis, particularly a small-plaque form called *guttate psoriasis*. Several drugs can also exacerbate psoriasis (e.g., ß-blockers, antimalarials, and lithium). Psoriasis afflicts 1% to 2% of the population, with men and women equally affected. The age of onset is bimodal, with one peak between the ages of 20 and 30 years and a second peak between the ages of 50 and 60 years. Separate histocompatibility antigens are seen with the different ages of onset. There are several OTC topical products available to treat psoriasis, including coal tar, topical corticosteroids, and urea.

COAL TAR

PHARMACOLOGY

Coal tar suppresses the hyperplastic skin in some proliferative disorders. Although there is no confirmed evidence as to its pharmacologic effects, its actions in humans have been reported as antiseptic, antipruritic, antiparasitic, antifungal, antibacterial, keratoplastic, and antiacantholic. Vasoconstrictive activity has also been reported.

INDICATIONS

Dandruff (treatment); *dermatitis, seborrheic* (treatment); *dermatitis, atopic* (treatment); *eczema* (treatment); *psoriasis* (treatment)—Indicated for the relief of itching, burning, and other symptoms associated with generalized persistent dermatoses, such as psoriasis, eczema, atopic dermatitis, and seborrheic dermatitis, and for the control of dandruff.

Coal tar preparations are also used in conjunction with ultraviolet (UV) light or sunlight, under the supervision of a physician, in the treatment of psoriasis or other conditions responding to this combined therapy.

CONTRAINDICATIONS

Risk-benefit should be considered when the following medical problems exist:

- *Major clinical significance*—Acute inflammation, open wounds, or infection of skin
- Sensitivity to coal tar

WARNINGS/PRECAUTIONS

Patients sensitive to any of the tars may be sensitive to coal tar also.

Pregnancy: FDA Category C. Studies have not been done in humans.

Breastfeeding: It is not known whether coal tar is distributed into breast milk. Problems in humans have not been documented.

Pediatrics: Infants—Coal tar products should not be used on infants unless under close supervision of a physician.

DRUG INTERACTIONS

Photosensitizing medications (concurrent use of coal tar with these medications may cause additive photosensitizing effects; concurrent use of coal tar with systemic or topical methoxsalen or trioxsalen is not recommended).

ADVERSE REACTIONS

Those indicating need for medical attention: Incidence rare

Allergic or irritant contact dermatitis, folliculitis, or pustular or keratocystic response (skin rash); skin irritation not present before therapy.

COAL TAR PRODUCTS	
Brand Name	**Dosage Form**
Denorex Therapeutic Protection (Wyeth)	**Shampoo:** 2.5%
Denorex Therapeutic Protection 2-in-1 (Wyeth)	**Shampoo:** 2.5%
Doak Tar (Doak)	**Shampoo:** 0.5%
Ionil-T (Healthpoint)	**Shampoo:** 1%
Ionil-T Plus (Healthpoint)	**Shampoo:** 2%
MG 217 (Triton)	**Ointment:** 2% **Shampoo:** 3%
Neutrogena T/Gel Extra Strength (Neutrogena)	**Shampoo:** 1%
Neutrogena T/Gel Original Formula (Neutrogena)	**Shampoo:** 0.5%
Neutrogena T/Gel Stubborn Itch (Neutrogena)	**Shampoo:** 0.5%
Pentrax (Medicis)	**Shampoo:** 0.5%
Polytar (Stiefel)	**Shampoo:** 0.5% **Soap:** 0.5%
Psoriasin (Alva-Amco)	**Gel:** 1.25% **Liquid:** 0.66%
Tegrin (GSK)	**Cream:** 0.8% **Shampoo:** 1.1%

Those indicating need for medical attention only if they continue or are bothersome:

Incidence more frequent

Stinging, mild—especially for gel and solution dosage forms.

ADMINISTRATION AND DOSAGE

General Dosing Information

After using this medication, patient should avoid exposure of treated areas to sunlamps or direct sunlight for 72 hours unless otherwise directed by a physician, since a photosensitivity reaction may occur. Before subsequent exposure to direct sunlight or sunlamps, all coal tar should be removed from patient's skin. If coal tar is used in conjunction with UV light or sunlight, exposure to light may be undertaken 2 to 72 hours after coal tar is applied. A determination of the minimal erythemal dosage (MED) should be made for each patient, and the initial irradiation should not exceed the MED.

For cleansing bar dosage form:

- For best results on hard scales, patient should soak in a warm bath first, then lather with the cleansing bar.

For gel dosage form:

- If dryness occurs, an emollient may be applied 1 hour after the gel is applied and between applications as needed.

For lotion dosage form:

- This medication may be applied directly to dry or wet skin or added to lukewarm bath water, depending on the product.

For shampoo dosage form:

- The scalp should be moistened with lukewarm water, and a liberal amount of shampoo massaged into the scalp, then rinsed. Application is to be repeated and the shampoo allowed to remain on the scalp for 5 minutes, then rinsed thoroughly. The shampoo may be reapplied as necessary or as directed by the physician.

For solution dosage form:

- The solution may be used full strength or diluted with 3 parts of water and applied to a cotton or gauze pad and then massaged gently on the affected area.
- A coal tar solution bath may be prepared by adding 4 to 6 tablespoonfuls of the solution to a tubful of lukewarm water.

Cleansing bar

Adults: Apply to affected area 1 to 2 times a day.

Cream

Adults: Apply to affected area up to 4 times a day.

Gel

Adults: Apply to affected area 1 to 2 times a day.

Lotion

Adults: Apply to the affected area as a direct application, as a bath, as a hand or foot soak, or as a hair rinse, depending on the product.

Ointment

Adults: Apply to affected area 2 to 3 times a day

Shampoo

Adults: Apply to scalp once a week to once a day.

Topical solution

Adults: Apply to affected area as a direct application to wet skin or scalp or as a bath, depending on the product.

Topical suspension

Adults: Apply to affected area as a bath.

SALICYLIC ACID

Salicylic acid facilitates desquamation by solubilizing the intercellular cement that binds scales in the stratum corneum, thereby loosening the keratin. This keratolytic effect may provide an antifungal action because removal of the stratum corneum suppresses fungal growth; it also aids in the penetration of other antifungal agents. Salicylic acid also has a mild antiseptic action.

Psoriasis (treatment)—Salicylic acid gel and ointment are indicated as adjuncts in the treatment of psoriasis.

For more information, refer to the complete monograph for salicylic acid in "Calluses, Corns, and Warts" under Dermatological Conditions.

TOPICAL CORTICOSTEROIDS

Corticosteroids diffuse across cell membranes and complex with specific cytoplasmic receptors. These complexes then enter the cell nucleus, bind to DNA (chromatin), and stimulate transcription of messenger RNA (mRNA) and subsequent protein synthesis of various inhibitory enzymes responsible for the anti-inflammatory effects of topical corticosteroids. These anti-inflammatory effects include inhibition of early processes such as edema, fibrin deposition, capillary dilatation, movement of phagocytes into the area, and phagocytic activities. Later processes, such as capillary production, collagen deposition, and keloid formation, are also inhibited by corticosteroids. The overall actions of topical corticosteroids are catabolic.

Relief of inflammation and/or pruritus (treatment)—Topical corticosteroids are indicated to provide symptomatic relief of inflammation and/or pruritus associated with acute and chronic corticosteroid-responsive disorders. The location of the skin lesion to be treated should be considered in selecting a formulation. In areas with thinner skin, such as facial, eye, and intertriginous areas, low-potency corticosteroid preparations are preferred for long-term therapy. Low- to medium-potency products may be used on the ears, trunk, arms, legs, and scalp. Medium- to very high-potency formulations may be required for treatment of dermatologic disorders in areas with thicker skin, such as the palms and soles. Lotion, aerosol, and gel formulations are cosmetically better suited for hairy areas.

The type of lesion to be treated should also be considered in product selection. For dry, scaly, cracked, thickened, or hardened

SALICYLIC ACID PRODUCTS (PSORIASIS/SEBORRHEIC DERMATITIS)	
Brand Name	**Dosage Form**
Dermarest Psoriasis (Del)	**Shampoo**: 3%
Dermarest Psoriasis Medicated Moisturizer (Del)	**Lotion**: 2%
Dermarest Psoriasis Skin Treatment (Del)	**Gel**: 3%
Dermarest Psoriasis Scalp Treatment (Del)	**Gel**: 3%
Neutrogena Healthy Scalp (Neutrogena)	**Shampoo**: 1.80%
Neutrogena T/Sal Maximum Strength (Neutrogena)	**Liquid**: 3%

skin, ointments of medium potency are often used. Medium-potency lotions, aerosols, or creams are preferred in treating moister, weeping lesions or areas or in treating conditions with intense inflammation. High- to very high-potency ointments may be required to treat hyperkeratotic or thick skin lesions.

Hydrocortisone (only available OTC topical corticosteroid)

Cream/Lotion/Ointment

Adults: Apply to affected area 1 to 4 times a day.

Pediatrics >2 years of age—0.25%-0.05%: Apply to affected area 1 to 4 times a day. *1%*: Apply to affected area 1 to 2 times a day.

Topical solution

Adults: Apply to affected area 1 to 4 times a day.

Pediatrics ≥2 years of age: Apply to affected area 1 to 2 times a day.

For more information, refer to the complete monograph for topical corticosteroids in "Contact Dermatitis" under Dermatological Conditions.

HYDROCORTISONE PRODUCTS (DERMATITIS)	
Brand Name	**Dosage Form**
Aveeno Anti-itch (J&J)	**Cream:** 1%
Caldecort (Novartis)	**Cream:** 1% **Spray:** 0.50%
Caldecort Light (Novartis)	**Cream:** 1%
Cortaid Intensive Therapy (Pharmacia)	**Cream:** 1%
Cortaid Maximum Strength (Pharmacia)	**Cream:** 1% **Ointment:** 1% **Stick:** 1%
Cortaid Sensitive Skin w/aloe (Pharmacia)	**Cream:** 0.05%
Cortixaine (UCB)	**Cream:** 0.05%
Cortizone-5 (Pfizer)	**Ointment:** 0.50%
Cortizone-10 (Pfizer)	**Cream:** 1% **Ointment:** 1%
Cortizone-10 Plus (Pfizer)	**Cream:** 1%
Cortizone 10 Quick Shot (Pfizer)	**Spray:** 1%
Dermarest Dricort (Del)	**Cream:** 1%
Dermarest Eczema Medicated (Del)	**Lotion:** 1%
Gynecort Anti-itch (Combe)	**Cream:** 1%
Hytone (Dermik)	**Lotion:** 1%
Ivy Soothe (Enviroderm)	**Cream:** 1%
Ivy State Dual Action Poison Ivy Exfoliant and Treatment (Tec)	**Gel:** 1%
Lanacort (Combe)	**Cream:** 1%
Massengill Medicated Towelettes (GSK)	**Pads:** 0.50%
Neutrogena T/Scalp (Neutrogena)	**Liquid:** 1%
Nupercainal HC 1% (Novartis)	**Cream:** 1%
Scalpicin (Combe)	**Liquid:** 1%

DOSING INFORMATION FOR PSORIASIS PRODUCTS

The following table provides a quick comparison of the ingredients and dosages of common brand-name OTC drugs. Products are listed alphabetically by generic ingredient and brand name.

BRAND NAME	GENERIC INGREDIENT/STRENGTH	DOSE
COAL TAR		
Denorex Psoriasis Overnight Treatment cream *(Wyeth Consumer Healthcare)*	Coal Tar	**Adults & Peds:** Apply to affected area qhs prn.
Denorex Therapeutic Protection 2-in-1 shampoo *(Wyeth Consumer Healthcare)*	Coal Tar 2.5%	**Adults & Peds:** Use at least biw.
Denorex Therapeutic Protection shampoo *(Wyeth Consumer Healthcare)*	Coal Tar 2.5%	**Adults & Peds:** Use at least biw.
DHS Tar Shampoo *(Person & Covey)*	Coal Tar 0.5%	**Adults & Peds:** Use at least biw.
Ionil-T Plus Shampoo *(Healthpoint)*	Coal Tar 2%	**Adults & Peds:** Use at least biw.

DOSING INFORMATION FOR PSORIASIS PRODUCTS (cont.)

Brand Name	Generic Ingredient/Strength	Dose
Ionil-T Shampoo *(Healthpoint)*	Coal Tar 1%	**Adults & Peds:** Use at least biw.
MG217 Ointment *(Trenton)*	Coal Tar 2%	**Adults & Peds:** Apply to affected area qd-qid.
MG217 Tar Shampoo *(Trenton)*	Coal Tar 3%	**Adults & Peds:** Use at least biw.
Neutrogena T/Gel Shampoo Extra Strength *(Neutrogena)*	Coal Tar 1%	**Adults & Peds:** Use at least biw.
Neutrogena T/Gel Shampoo Orignial Formula *(Neutrogena)*	Coal Tar 0.5%	**Adults & Peds:** Use at least biw.
Neutrogena T/Gel Stubborn Itch Shampoo *(Neutrogena)*	Coal Tar 0.5%	**Adults & Peds:** Use at least biw.
Pentrax Shampoo *(Medicis)*	Coal Tar 5.0%	**Adults & Peds:** Use at least biw.
Polytar shampoo *(Stiefel)*	Coal Tar 0.5%	**Adults & Peds:** Use at least biw.
Polytar soap *(Stiefel)*	Coal Tar 0.5%	**Adults & Peds:** Apply to affected area prn.
Psoriasin Multi-Symptom Psoriasis Relief Gel *(Alva-Amco Pharmacal)*	Coal Tar 1.25%	**Adults & Peds:** Apply to affected area qd-qid.
Psoriasin Multi-Symptom Psoriasis Relief Ointment *(Alva-Amco Pharmacal)*	Coal Tar 2%	**Adults & Peds:** Apply to affected area qd-qid.
CORTICOSTEROIDS		
Aveeno Anti-Itch Cream 1% *(Johnson & Johnson/Merck Consumer)*	Hydrocortisone 1%	**Adults & Peds ≥2 yo:** Apply to affected area tid-qid.
Cortaid Intensive Therapy Cooling Spray *(Pharmacia Consumer Healthcare)*	Hydrocortisone 1%	**Adults & Peds ≥2 yo:** Apply to affected area tid-qid.
Cortaid Intensive Therapy Moisturizing Cream *(Pharmacia Consumer Healthcare)*	Hydrocortisone 1%	**Adults & Peds ≥2 yo:** Apply to affected area tid-qid.
Cortaid Maximum Strength Cream *(Pharmacia Consumer Healthcare)*	Hydrocortisone 1%	**Adults & Peds ≥2 yo:** Apply to affected area tid-qid.
Cortizone-10 Cream *(Pfizer Consumer Healthcare)*	Hydrocortisone 1%	**Adults & Peds ≥2 yo:** Apply to affected area tid-qid.
Cortizone-10 Maximum Strength Anti-Itch Ointment *(Pfizer Consumer Healthcare)*	Hydrocortisone 1%	**Adults & Peds ≥2 yo:** Apply to affected area tid-qid.
Cortizone-10 Ointment *(Pfizer Consumer Healthcare)*	Hydrocortisone 1%	**Adults & Peds ≥2 yo:** Apply to affected area tid-qid.
Cortizone-10 Plus Maximum Strength Cream *(Pfizer Consumer Healthcare)*	Hydrocortisone 1%	**Adults & Peds ≥2 yo:** Apply to affected area tid-qid.
Cortizone-10 Quick Shot Spray *(Pfizer Consumer Healthcare)*	Hydrocortisone 1%	**Adults & Peds ≥2 yo:** Apply to affected area tid-qid.
SALICYLIC ACID		
Denorex Psoriasis Daytime Treatment cream *(Wyeth Consumer Healthcare)*	Salicylic Acid 3%	**Adults & Peds:** Apply to affected area qd-qid.
Dermarest Psoriasis Medicated Foam Shampoo *(Del Laboratories)*	Salicylic Acid 3%	**Adults & Peds:** Apply to affected at least biw.
Dermarest Psoriasis Medicated Moisturizer *(Del Laboratories)*	Salicylic Acid 2%	**Adults & Peds:** Apply to affected area qd-qid.
Dermarest Psoriasis Medicated Scalp Treatment *(Del Laboratories)*	Salicylic Acid 3%	**Adults & Peds:** Apply to affected area qd-qid.
Dermarest Psoriasis Medicated Scalp Treatment mousse *(Del Laboratories)*	Salicylic Acid 3%	**Adults & Peds:** Apply to affected area qd-qid.
Dermarest Psoriasis Medicated Shampoo/Conditioner *(Del Laboratories)*	Salicylic Acid 3%	**Adults & Peds:** Apply to affected at least biw.
Dermarest Psoriasis Skin Treatment *(Del Laboratories)*	Salicylic Acid 3%	**Adults & Peds:** Apply to affected area qd-qid.
Neutrogena T/Gel Conditioner *(Neutrogena)*	Salicylic Acid 2%	**Adults & Peds:** Use at least biw.
Psoriasin Therapeutic Body Wash With Aloe *(Alva-Amco Pharmacal)*	Salicylic Acid 3%	**Adults & Peds:** Use biw.
Psoriasin Therapeutic Shampoo With Panthenol *(Alva-Amco Pharmacal)*	Salicylic Acid 3%	**Adults & Peds:** Use biw.

Seborrheic Dermatitis

Seborrheic dermatitis is a chronic inflammatory, erythematous skin condition characterized by loose, greasy or dry, white to yellowish scales. Seborrheic dermatitis is most commonly seen on the scalp, sides of the nose, eyebrows, eyelids, behind the ears, and middle of the chest. Other areas, such as the navel, buttocks, skin folds under the arms, axillary regions, breasts, and groin, may also be involved. Seborrheic dermatitis is called cradle cap (crusta lactea) when it affects infants. Cradle cap appears as thick, crusty, yellow or brown scales over the child's scalp and also sometimes affects the eyelids, ears, area around the nose, and groin. Seborrheic dermatitis appears to run in families and is often linked to stress, fatigue, weather extremes, oily skin, infrequent shampoos or skin cleansing, use of lotions that contain alcohol, skin disorders, and obesity. Nonprescription shampoos containing tar, pyrithione zinc, selenium sulfide, ketoconazole, and/or salicylic acid are available.

COAL TAR

Coal tar suppresses hyperplastic skin associated with some proliferative disorders. Although there is no confirmed evidence explaining its pharmacologic effects, its actions in humans have been reported as antiseptic, antipruritic, antiparasitic, antifungal, antibacterial, keratoplastic, and antiacantholic. Vasoconstrictive activity has also been reported.

Dermatitis, seborrheic (treatment)—Indicated for the relief of itching, burning, and other symptoms associated with generalized persistent dermatoses, such as psoriasis, eczema, atopic dermatitis, and seborrheic dermatitis, and for the control of dandruff.

Coal tar preparations are also used in conjunction with ultraviolet (UV) light or sunlight, under the supervision of a physician, in the treatment of psoriasis or other conditions responding to this combined therapy.

Cleansing bar

Adults: Apply to affected area 1 to 2 times a day.

Cream

Adults: Apply to affected area up to 4 times a day.

Gel

Adults: Apply to affected area 1 to 2 times a day.

Lotion

Adults: Apply to the affected area, as a direct application, as a bath, as hand or foot soak, or as a hair rinse, depending on the product.

Ointment

Adults: Apply to affected area 2 to 3 times a day

Shampoo

Adults: Apply to scalp once a week to once a day.

Topical solution

Adults: Apply to affected area, as a direct application to wet skin or scalp or as a bath, depending on the product.

Topical suspension:

Adults: Apply to affected area as a bath.

For more information, refer to the complete monograph for coal tar in "Psoriasis" under Dermatological Conditions.

COAL TAR PRODUCTS	
Brand Name	**Dosage Form**
Denorex Therapeutic Protection (Wyeth)	**Shampoo:** 2.5%
Denorex Therapeutic Protection 2-in-1 (Wyeth)	**Shampoo:** 2.5%
Doak Tar (Doak)	**Shampoo:** 0.5%
Ionil-T (Healthpoint)	**Shampoo:** 1%
Ionil-T Plus (Healthpoint)	**Shampoo:** 2%
MG 217 (Triton)	**Ointment:** 2% **Shampoo:** 3%
Neutrogena T/Gel Extra Strength (Neutrogena)	**Shampoo:** 1%
Neutrogena T/Gel Original Formula (Neutrogena)	**Shampoo:** 0.5%
Neutrogena T/Gel Stubborn Itch (Neutrogena)	**Shampoo:** 0.5%
Pentrax (Medicis)	**Shampoo:** 0.5%
Polytar (Stiefel)	**Shampoo:** 0.5% **Soap:** 0.5%
Psoriasin (Alva-Amco)	**Gel:** 1.25% **Liquid:** 0.66%
Tegrin (GSK)	**Cream:** 0.8% **Shampoo:** 1.1%

PYRITHIONE ZINC

Pyrithione zinc may act by an antimitotic action, resulting in a reduction in the turnover of epidermal cells. It also has bacteriostatic and fungistatic activity, but it is not known if this action contributes to the antiseborrheic effects of the drug.

Dermatitis, seborrheic (treatment)—Depending on the formulation, pyrithione zinc is indicated to help control dandruff and seborrheic dermatitis of the scalp and/or seborrheic dermatitis of the body, face, and scalp.

Bar

Adults/Pediatrics: Apply to affected areas of the body, face, or scalp once a day for at least 2 times a week. Lather, massage into affected skin or scalp, rinse, and repeat.

Cream/Lotion

Adults/Pediatrics: Apply to affected areas of the body, face, or scalp 1 to 3 times a day.

Shampoo

Adults/Pediatrics: Apply to scalp once a day for at least 2 times a week. Apply after wetting hair, leave on scalp for several minutes or massage vigorously, then rinse. May be used once a day if needed.

For more information, refer to the complete monograph for pyrithione zinc in "Dandruff" under Dermatological Conditions.

SALICYLIC ACID

Salicylic acid facilitates desquamation by solubilizing the intercellular cement that binds scales in the stratum corneum, thereby loosening the keratin. This keratolytic effect may provide an antifungal action because removal of the stratum corneum suppresses fungal growth; it also aids in the penetration of other antifungal agents. Salicylic acid also has a mild antiseptic action.

Dermatitis, seborrheic (treatment); *dermatitis, seborrheic, of scalp* (treatment)—Salicylic acid lotion and shampoo are indicated to help control scaling of the scalp associated with dandruff and seborrheic dermatitis. Salicylic acid ointment is indicated in the treatment of seborrheic dermatitis.

Cream/Lotion 2%-3%

Adults/Pediatrics: Apply to affected area 1 to 4 times a day.

Shampoo 2%-3%

Adults/Pediatrics: Apply to the scalp 1 to 2 times a week.

For more information, refer to the complete monograph for salicylic acid in "Calluses, Corns, and Warts" under Dermatological Conditions.

SALICYLIC ACID/SULFUR

Salicylic acid facilitates desquamation by solubilizing the intercellular cement that binds scales in the stratum corneum, thereby loosening the keratin. This keratolytic effect may provide an antifungal action because removal of the stratum corneum suppresses fungal growth; it also aids in the penetration of other antifungal agents. Salicylic acid also has a mild antiseptic action.

Sulfur has germicidal, fungicidal, parasiticidal, and keratolytic actions. Its germicidal activity may be the result of its conversion to pentathionic acid by epidermal cells or by certain microorganisms.

Dermatitis, seborrheic, of scalp (treatment)—Salicylic acid and sulfur (bar or shampoo) is indicated for the temporary control of scaling and itching associated with dandruff and seborrheic dermatitis of the scalp.

Liquid/Shampoo

Adults/Pediatrics: Apply to affected area of the scalp once a day at least 2 times a week to maintain control, or as directed by a physician. Apply after wetting hair, lather, massage into affected scalp, leave on scalp for five minutes, rinse, and repeat. May be used once a day if needed.

For more information, refer to the complete monograph for salicylic acid/sulfur in "Calluses, Corns, and Warts" under Dermatological Conditions.

PYRITHIONE ZINC PRODUCTS	
Brand Name	**Dosage Form**
Dermazinc (Dermalogix)	**Cream:** 0.25% **Shampoo:** 2% **Spray:** 0.25%
Denorex (Wyeth)	**Shampoo:** 2%
DHS Zinc Shampoo (Person & Covey)	**Shampoo:** 2%
Head & Shoulders Dandruff Conditioner (Procter & Gamble)	**Shampoo:** 0.5%
Head & Shoulders Dandruff Shampoo (Procter & Gamble)	**Shampoo:** 1%
Head & Shoulders Soothing Lotion (Procter & Gamble)	**Lotion:** 0.1%
Neutrogena Triple Moisture Active Soothing Shampoo (Neutrogena)	**Shampoo:** 0.5%
Pert Plus Dandruff Control (Procter & Gamble)	**Shampoo:** 1%
Selsun Blue Dandruff Conditioner (Chattem)	**Shampoo:** 0.75%
Zincon (Medtech)	**Shampoo:** 1%
ZNP (Stiefel)	**Soap** 2%

SALICYLIC ACID PRODUCTS (PSORIASIS/SEBORRHEIC DERMATITIS)	
Brand Name	**Dosage Form**
Dermarest Psoriasis (Del)	**Shampoo:** 3%
Dermarest Psoriasis Medicated Moisturizer (Del)	**Lotion:** 2%
Dermarest Psoriasis Skin Treatment (Del)	**Gel:** 3%
Dermarest Psoriasis Scalp Treatment (Del)	**Gel:** 3%
Neutrogena Healthy Scalp (Neutrogena)	**Shampoo:** 1.80%
Neutrogena T/Sal Maximum Strength (Neutrogena)	**Liquid:** 3%

SALICYLIC ACID/SULFUR/COAL TAR

PHARMACOLOGY

Salicylic acid facilitates desquamation by solubilizing the intercellular cement that binds scales in the stratum corneum, thereby loosening the keratin. This keratolytic effect may provide an antifungal action because removal of the stratum corneum suppresses fungal growth; it also aids in the penetration of other antifungal agents. Salicylic acid also has a mild antiseptic action.

Sulfur has germicidal, fungicidal, parasiticidal, and keratolytic actions. Its germicidal activity may be the result of its conversion to pentathionic acid by epidermal cells or by certain microorganisms.

Coal tar suppresses the hyperplastic skin in some proliferative disorders. Although there is no confirmed evidence as to its pharmacologic effects, its actions in humans have been reported as antiseptic, antipruritic, antiparasitic, antifungal, antibacterial, keratoplastic, and antiacantholic. Vasoconstrictive activity has also been reported.

INDICATIONS

Dandruff (treatment); *dermatitis, seborrheic, of scalp* (treatment)—Salicylic acid, sulfur, and coal tar shampoo is indicated as adjunctive treatment for dandruff and seborrheic dermatitis to relieve itching and scaling of the scalp.

Psoriasis, of scalp (treatment)—Salicylic acid, sulfur, and coal tar shampoo is indicated in the treatment of psoriasis to relieve itching and scaling of the scalp.

WARNINGS/PRECAUTIONS

Salicylic Acid—*See the complete monograph in "Calluses, Corns, and Warts" under Dermatological Conditions.*

Sulfur—*See the complete monograph in "Acne" under Dermatological Conditions.*

Coal Tar—*See the complete monograph in "Psoriasis" under Dermatological Conditions.*

ADVERSE REACTIONS

Salicylic Acid—*See the complete monograph in "Calluses, Corns, and Warts" under Dermatological Conditions.*

Sulfur—*See the complete monograph in "Acne" under Dermatological Conditions.*

Coal Tar—*See the complete monograph in "Psoriasis" under Dermatological Conditions.*

ADMINISTRATION AND DOSAGE

Shampoo

Adults/Pediatrics: Apply to scalp 1 or 2 times a week.

SELENIUM SULFIDE

Selenium sulfide may act by an antimitotic action, resulting in a reduction in the turnover of epidermal cells. It also has local irritant, antibacterial, and mild antifungal activity, which may contribute to its effectiveness.

Dermatitis, seborrheic, of scalp(treatment)—Selenium sulfide is indicated for the treatment of dandruff or seborrheic dermatitis of the scalp.

Shampoo

Adults/Pediatrics: Apply to scalp 2 times a week for 2 weeks and then at less frequent intervals of once a week or once every 2 or more weeks.

TOPICAL CORTICOSTEROIDS

Corticosteroids diffuse across cell membranes and complex with specific cytoplasmic receptors. These complexes then enter the cell nucleus, bind to DNA (chromatin), and stimulate transcription of messenger RNA (mRNA) and subsequent protein synthesis of various inhibitory enzymes responsible for the anti-inflammatory effects of topical corticosteroids. These anti-inflammatory effects include inhibition of early processes such as edema, fibrin deposition, capillary dilatation, movement of phagocytes into the area, and phagocytic activities. Later processes, such as capillary production, collagen deposition, and keloid formation, are also inhibited by corticosteroids. The overall actions of topical corticosteroids are catabolic.

Relief of inflammation and/or pruritus (treatment)—Topical corticosteroids are indicated to provide symptomatic relief of inflammation and/or pruritus associated with acute and chronic corticosteroid-responsive disorders. The location of the skin lesion to be treated should be considered in selecting a formulation. In areas with thinner skin, such as facial, eye, and intertriginous areas, low-potency corticosteroid preparations are preferred for long-term therapy. Low- to medium-potency products may be used on the ears, trunk, arms, legs, and scalp. Medium- to very high-potency formulations may be required for treatment of dermatologic disorders in areas with thicker skin, such as the palms and soles. Lotion, aerosol, and gel formulations are cosmetically better suited for hairy areas.

The type of lesion to be treated should also be considered in product selection. For dry, scaly, cracked, thickened, or hardened skin, ointments of medium potency are often used. Medium-potency lotions, aerosols, or creams are preferred in treating moister, weeping lesions or areas or in treating conditions with intense inflammation. High- to very high-potency ointments may be required to treat hyperkeratotic or thick skin lesions.

SALICYLIC ACID/SULFUR PRODUCTS	
Brand Name	**Dosage Form**
Meted (Sirius)	**Shampoo:** 3%-5%
Sebex (Rugby)	**Liquid:** 2%-2%
Sebulex (Westwood-Squibb)	**Liquid:** 2%-2%
SALICYLIC ACID/SULFUR/COAL TAR PRODUCTS	
Brand Name	**Dosage Form**
Sebex-T (Clay-Park)	**Liquid:** 2%-2%-5%
Sebutone (Westwood-Squibb)	**Liquid:** 2%-2%-1.5%
SELENIUM SULFIDE PRODUCTS	
Brand Name	**Dosage Form**
Head & Shoulders Intensive Treatment (Proctor&Gamble)	**Shampoo:** 1%
Selsun Blue Dandruff (Chattem)	**Shampoo:** 1%

114/SEBORRHEIC DERMATITIS

Hydrocortisone (only available OTC topical corticosteroid)

Cream/Lotion/Ointment

Adults: Apply to affected area 1 to 4 times a day.

Pediatrics >2 years of age—0.25%-0.05%: Apply to affected area 1 to 4 times a day. *1%*: Apply to affected area 1 to 2 times a day.

Topical solution

Adults: Apply to affected area 1 to 4 times a day.

Pediatrics >2 years of age: Apply to affected area 1 to 2 times a day.

HYDROCORTISONE PRODUCTS (DERMATITIS)

Brand Name	Dosage Form
Aveeno Anti-itch (J & J)	Cream: 1%
Caldecort (Novartis)	Cream: 1% Spray: 0.50%
Caldecort Light (Novartis)	Cream: 1%
Cortaid Intensive Therapy (Pharmacia)	Cream: 1%
Cortaid Maximum Strength (Pharmacia)	Cream: 1% Ointment: 1% Stick: 1%
Cortaid Sensitive Skin w/aloe (Pharmacia)	Cream: 0.05%
Cortixaine (UCB)	Cream: 0.05%
Cortizone-5 (Pfizer)	Ointment: 0.50%
Cortizone-10 (Pfizer)	Cream: 1% Ointment: 1%
Cortizone-10 Plus (Pfizer)	Cream: 1%
Cortizone 10 Quick Shot (Pfizer)	Spray: 1%
Dermarest Dricort (Del)	Cream: 1%
Dermarest Eczema Medicated (Del)	Lotion: 1%
Gynecort Anti-itch (Combe)	Cream: 1%
Hytone (Dermik)	Lotion: 1%
Ivy Soothe (Enviroderm)	Cream: 1%
Ivy State Dual Action Poison Ivy Exfoliant and Treatment (Tec)	Gel: 1%
Lanacort (Combe)	Cream: 1%
Massengill Medicated Towelettes (GSK)	Pads: 0.50%
Neutrogena T/Scalp (Neutrogena)	Liquid: 1%
Nupercainal HC 1% (Novartis)	Cream: 1%
Scalpicin (Combe)	Liquid: 1%

DOSING INFORMATION FOR ANTISEBORRHEAL PRODUCTS

The following table provides a quick comparison of the ingredients and dosages of common brand-name OTC drugs. Products are listed alphabetically by generic ingredient and brand name.

BRAND NAME	GENERIC INGREDIENT/STRENGTH	DOSE
COAL TAR		
DHS Tar Dermatological Hair & Scalp Shampoo *(Person & Covey)*	Coal Tar 0.5%	**Adults & Peds:** Use biw.
DHS Tar Shampoo *(Person & Covey)*	Coal Tar 0.5%	**Adults & Peds:** Use at least biw.
Neutrogena T/Gel Shampoo Orignial Formula *(Neutrogena)*	Coal Tar 0.5%	**Adults & Peds:** Use at least biw.
Neutrogena T/Gel Stubborn Itch Shampoo *(Neutrogena)*	Coal Tar 0.5%	**Adults & Peds:** Use at least biw.
Polytar shampoo *(Stiefel)*	Coal Tar 0.5%	**Adults & Peds:** Use at least biw.
Polytar soap *(Stiefel)*	Coal Tar 0.5%	**Adults & Peds:** Apply to affected area prn.
Psoriasin Liquid dab-on *(Alva-Amco Pharmacal)*	Coal Tar 0.66%	**Adults:** Apply to affected area qd-qid.
Ionil-T Shampoo *(Healthpoint)*	Coal Tar 1%	**Adults & Peds:** Use at least biw.
Neutrogena T/Gel Shampoo Extra Strength *(Neutrogena)*	Coal Tar 1%	**Adults & Peds:** Use at least biw.
Psoriasin gel *(Alva-Amco Pharmacal)*	Coal Tar 1.25%	**Adults:** Apply to affected area qd-qid.
Ionil-T Plus Shampoo *(Healthpoint)*	Coal Tar 2%	**Adults & Peds:** Use at least biw.

DOSING INFORMATION FOR ANTISEBORRHEAL PRODUCTS (cont.)

BRAND NAME	GENERIC INGREDIENT/STRENGTH	DOSE
MG217 Ointment (Trenton)	Coal Tar 2%	**Adults & Peds:** Apply to affected area qd-qid.
Denorex Therapeutic Protection 2-in-1 shampoo (Wyeth Consumer Healthcare)	Coal Tar 2.5%	**Adults & Peds:** Use at least biw.
Denorex Therapeutic Protection shampoo (Wyeth Consumer Healthcare)	Coal Tar 2.5%	**Adults & Peds:** Use at least biw.
MG217 Tar Shampoo (Trenton)	Coal Tar 3%	**Adults & Peds:** Use at least biw.
Ionil T Therapeutic Coal Tar Shampoo (Healthpoint)	Coal Tar 5%	**Adults & Peds:** Use biw.
Pentrax Shampoo (Medicis)	Coal Tar 5.0%	**Adults & Peds:** Use at least biw.
CORTICOSTEROIDS		
Aveeno Anti-Itch Cream 1% (Johnson & Johnson/Merck Consumer)	Hydrocortisone 1%	**Adults & Peds ≥2 yo:** Apply to affected area tid-qid.
Cortaid Intensive Therapy Cooling Spray (Pharmacia Consumer Healthcare)	Hydrocortisone 1%	**Adults & Peds ≥2 yo:** Apply to affected area tid-qid.
Cortaid Intensive Therapy Moisturizing Cream (Pharmacia Consumer Healthcare)	Hydrocortisone 1%	**Adults & Peds ≥2 yo:** Apply to affected area tid-qid.
Cortaid Maximum Strength Cream (Pharmacia Consumer Healthcare)	Hydrocortisone 1%	**Adults & Peds ≥2 yo:** Apply to affected area tid-qid.
Cortizone-10 Cream (Pfizer Consumer Healthcare)	Hydrocortisone 1%	**Adults & Peds ≥2 yo:** Apply to affected area tid-qid.
Cortizone-10 Maximum Strength Anti-Itch Ointment (Pfizer Consumer Healthcare)	Hydrocortisone 1%	**Adults & Peds ≥2 yo:** Apply to affected area tid-qid.
Cortizone-10 Ointment (Pfizer Consumer Healthcare)	Hydrocortisone 1%	**Adults & Peds ≥2 yo:** Apply to affected area tid-qid.
Cortizone-10 Plus Maximum Strength Cream (Pfizer Consumer Healthcare)	Hydrocortisone 1%	**Adults & Peds ≥2 yo:** Apply to affected area tid-qid.
Cortizone-10 Quick Shot Spray (Pfizer Consumer Healthcare)	Hydrocortisone 1%	**Adults & Peds ≥2 yo:** Apply to affected area tid-qid.
PYRITHIONE ZINC		
Denorex Dandruff Shampoo, Daily Protection (Medtech Products)	Pyrithione zinc 2%	**Adults & Peds:** Use biw.
Garnier Fructis Fortifying Shampoo, Anti-Dandruff (Garnier)	Pyrithione zinc 1%	**Adults & Peds:** Use biw.
Head & Shoulders Dandruff Conditioner, Dry Scalp Care (Procter & Gamble)	Pyrithione zinc 0.5%	**Adults & Peds:** Use biw.
Head & Shoulders Dandruff Conditioner, Extra Fullness (Procter & Gamble)	Pyrithione zinc 0.5%	**Adults & Peds:** Use biw.
Head & Shoulders Dandruff Shampoo Plus Conditioner, Smooth & Silky (Procter & Gamble)	Pyrithione zinc 1%	**Adults & Peds:** Use biw.
Head & Shoulders Dandruff Shampoo, Citrus Breeze (Procter & Gamble)	Pyrithione zinc 1%	**Adults & Peds:** Use biw.
Head & Shoulders Dandruff Shampoo, Classic Clean (Procter & Gamble)	Pyrithione zinc 1%	**Adults & Peds:** Use biw.
Head & Shoulders Dandruff Shampoo, Dry Scalp Care (Procter & Gamble)	Pyrithione zinc 1%	**Adults & Peds:** Use biw.
Head & Shoulders Dandruff Shampoo, Extra Volume (Procter & Gamble)	Pyrithione zinc 1%	**Adults & Peds:** Use biw.
Head & Shoulders Dandruff Shampoo, Refresh (Procter & Gamble)	Pyrithione zinc 1%	**Adults & Peds:** Use biw.
Head & Shoulders Dandruff Shampoo, Sensitive Care (Procter & Gamble)	Pyrithione zinc 1%	**Adults & Peds:** Use biw.
L'Oreal VIVE for Men Shampoo, Thickening Anti-Dandruff (L'Oreal)	Pyrithione zinc 1%	**Adults & Peds:** Use biw.
Neutrogena T-Gel Daily Control Dandruff Shampoo (Neutrogena)	Pyrithione zinc 1%	**Adults & Peds:** Use biw.

DOSING INFORMATION FOR ANTISEBORRHEAL PRODUCTS (cont.)

BRAND NAME	GENERIC INGREDIENT/STRENGTH	DOSE
Nexxus Dandarrest Dandruff Control Shampoo (Nexxus Products)	Pyrithione zinc 1.1%	**Adults & Peds:** Use biw.
Pantene Pro-V Shampoo + Conditioner, Anti-Dandruff (Procter & Gamble)	Pyrithione zinc 1%	**Adults & Peds:** Use biw.
Pert Plus Shampoo Plus Conditioner, Dandruff Control (Procter & Gamble)	Pyrithione zinc 1%	**Adults & Peds:** Use biw.
Selsun Blue Dandruff Conditioner (Ross Products)	Pyrithione zinc 0.75%	**Adults & Peds:** Use biw.
Suave for Men 2 in 1 Shampoo/Conditioner, Dandruff (Suave)	Pyrithione zinc 0.5%	**Adults & Peds:** Use biw.
SALICYLIC ACID		
Neutrogena T/Gel Conditioner (Neutrogena)	Salicylic Acid 2%	**Adults & Peds:** Use at least biw.
Psoriasin Therapeutic Body Wash With Aloe (Alva-Amco Pharmacal Cos)	Salicylic Acid 3%	**Adults & Peds:** Use biw.
Psoriasin Therapeutic Shampoo With Panthenol (Alva-Amco Pharmacal)	Salicylic Acid 3%	**Adults & Peds:** Use biw.
Neutrogena T/Sal Shampoo, Scalp Build-up Control (Neutrogena)	Salicylic Acid 3.0%	**Adults & Peds:** Use biw.
Scalpicin Anti-Itch Liquid Scalp Treatment (Combe)	Salicylic Acid 3.0%	**Adults:** Apply to affected area qd-qid.
SALICYLIC ACID/SULFUR/COAL TAR		
Sebex-T Tar Shampoo (Clay-Park)	Salicylic acid/sulfur/coal tar 2%-2%-5%	**Adults & Peds:** Use qw to biw.
Sebutone (Westwood-Squibb)	Salicylic acid/sulfur/coal tar 2%-2%-1.5%	**Adults & Peds:** Use qw to biw.
SELENIUM SULFIDE		
Head & Shoulders Dandruff Shampoo, Intensive Treatment (Procter & Gamble)	Selenium Sulfide 1%	**Adults & Peds:** Use biw.
Selsun Blue Dandruff Shampoo, Medicated Treatment (Ross Products)	Selenium Sulfide 1%	**Adults & Peds:** Use biw.
Selsun Blue Dandruff Shampoo Plus Conditioner (Ross Products)	Selenium Sulfide 1%	**Adults & Peds:** Use biw.
Selsun Blue Dandruff Shampoo, Balanced Treatment (Ross Products)	Selenium Sulfide 1%	**Adults & Peds:** Use biw.
Selsun Blue Dandruff Shampoo, Moisturizing Treatment (Chattem)	Selenium Sulfide 1%	**Adults & Peds:** Use biw.
SULFUR/SALICYLIC ACID		
Sebulex Medicated Dandruff Shampoo (Westwood-Squibb)	Sulfur/Salicylic Acid 2%-2%	**Adults & Peds:** Use qd.

Sunburn

Sunburn correlates inversely with the degree of melanin pigmentation in the skin. Sunburn occurs primarily in fair-complexioned persons with little epidermal melanin. Immediate pigmentation due to the oxidation of preformed melanin develops soon after exposure, lasts only a few hours, and does not protect against further radiation damage. Delayed pigmentation develops a few days after exposure, does protect against subsequent ultraviolet (UV) injury and produces suntan. An increase in the thickness of the epidermis develops a few days following exposure and provides some protection against subsequent UV penetration.

The mechanism of sunburn is not well understood but is believed to be due to a series of biochemical events leading to inflammation most likely initiated by DNA absorption of UVB. When unprotected skin is exposed to a thrice minimal erythema dose of UV rays, the first sign of its effect is redness. Reaction typically begins 3 to 6 hours after exposure, peaks at 12 to 48 hours, and subsides in 3 to 5 days if there is no subsequent sun exposure. Greater exposure to sunlight produces more rapid and progressively severe reactions extending to marked blistering and shock. Pruritus and skin peeling occur as the initial burn heals and blisters. Severe sunburn consists of topical symptoms similar to a superficial partial-thickness burn accompanied by systemic symptoms including chills, fever, nausea and vomiting, fatigue, weakness, headache, and prostration. Sunburn is a significant risk factor for subsequent development of skin cancer. UV keratitis, also known as snow blindness, is characterized by the onset of severe pain, photophobia, blurred vision, lacrimation, and scleral erythema 6 to 12 hours after prolonged exposure to UV light.

Sunburn should be prevented with the use of a sunscreen. There are many sunscreens available; most include agents such as avobenzone, oxybenzone, octocrylene, titanium dioxide, and zinc oxide. If sunburn does occur, there are many OTC products used to relieve the symptoms, including topical anesthetics, NSAIDs, and moisturizing agents such as aloe vera.

SUNSCREEN AGENTS

PHARMACOLOGY

Chemical sunscreen agents—These products diminish the penetration of ultraviolet (UV) light through the epidermis by absorbing UV radiation within a specific wavelength range. The amount and wavelength of UV radiation absorbed are affected by the molecular structure of the sunscreen agent.

Physical sunscreen agents—These products minimize UV penetration through the epidermis by creating a physical barrier that reflects, scatters, absorbs, and blocks UV and visible radiations.

INDICATIONS

Sunburn (prophylaxis)—Sunscreen agents are indicated for the prevention of sunburn. In addition to limiting the skin's exposure to the sun, using sunscreen agents regularly when in the sun may help reduce long-term sun damage such as premature wrinkling and skin cancer.

General considerations:

The degree of protection provided by a sunscreen product may be determined by the following: the sunscreen protection factor (SPF), which evaluates ultraviolet B (UVB) light-blocking capacity; phototoxic protection factor (or other protection factors), which evaluates ultraviolet A (UVA) light-blocking activity; and substantivity.

UVB light is known as the "sunburn ray" because of its tendency to cause erythema of the skin. A sunscreen agent should be effective in reducing erythema due to sun exposure. The SPF displayed on sunscreen agent containers is a measure of the amount of UVB light needed to produce a minimal erythema reaction in sunscreen-protected skin compared with unprotected skin. Sunscreen agents with SPF of 15 or greater are considered sunblocks because they may absorb more than 92% of UVB radiation.

UVA light may also induce erythema but at considerably higher doses than UVB light. Currently, there is no standard method to assess sunscreen agents for UVA protection. Difficulty in determining UVA protection may be due to the extremely long exposure time to UVA needed to produce erythema. One method utilizes the phototoxic protection factor (this is not usually required in the labeling of sunscreen products), which represents the amount of UVA light needed to produce a minimal phototoxic response in sunscreen-protected photosensitized skin compared with unprotected photosensitized skin.

Substantivity is defined as the sunscreen's resistance to removal by physical means, such as being washed off by water or sweating. The substantivity of sunscreen agents is determined by the design of the vehicle and the active ingredients. Sweat resistance is determined by measuring the SPF after 30 minutes on a person who is sweating profusely. Water-resistant and waterproof sunscreens are determined by measuring the SPFs after water exposures of 40 and 80 minutes, respectively.

CONTRAINDICATIONS

Risk-benefit should be considered when the following medical problems exist:

- Sensitivity to the sunscreen or other ingredients of the preparation
- Using sunscreens may aggravate the following conditions due to increased sensitivity of the skin to the chemicals; patch testing before use may be advisable.
- Photodermatoses, such as dermatitis (atopic, chronic actinic, or seborrheic)
- Herpes labialis
- Lichen rubeo planus
- Lupus erythematosus
- Persistent light reaction
- Photosensitivity, idiopathic
- Phytophotodermatitis
- Polymorphous light eruption
- Xeroderma pigmentosum

Pharmacology of Sunscreen Agents

Sunscreen Agent Category	Drug	Concentration (%)	Absorbance Wavelength (nanometer)
UVA Absorbers*			
	Avobenzone	3	320-400
	Dioxybenzone	3	250-390
	Menthyl anthranilate	3.5-5	260-380
	Oxybenzone	2-6	270-350
	Sulisobenzone	5-10	260-375
UVB Absorbers†			
	Aminobenzoic acid	5-15	260-313
	Homosalate	4-15	295-315
	Lisadimate	2-3	264-315
	Octocrylene	7-10	250-360
	Octyl methoxycinnamate	2-7.5	290-320
	Octyl salicylate	3-5	280-320
	Padimate O	1.4-8	290-315
	2-Phenylbenzimidazole-5-sulfonic acid	1-4	290-340
	Roxadimate	1-5	280-330
	Trolamine salicylate	5-12	260-320
Physical Blockers			
	Titanium dioxide	2-25	290-700
	Zinc oxide		290-700

* FDA-proposed UVA protection defined as absorption spectrum ≥360 nanometers.

† FDA-approved UVB protection defined as absorption spectrum 290-320 nanometers.

WARNINGS/PRECAUTIONS

Patients sensitive to artificial sweeteners (e.g., saccharin, sodium cyclamate); ester-type anesthetics (e.g., benzocaine, procaine, tetracaine); para-amino type azo dyes (e.g., aniline, paraphenylenediamine); sulfonamide antibiotics; sulfonamide-based oral hypoglycemics; or thiazide diuretics may be sensitive to sunscreen agents containing para-aminobenzoic acid (PABA) or its derivatives.

Patients sensitive to cinnamon derivatives (balsam of Peru, balsam of Tolu, Cassia, cinnamic acid, cinnamic alcohol, cinnamic aldehyde, cinnamon oil, coca leaves), which are used in cosmetics and perfumes and as flavoring agents in medications and toothpastes, may be sensitive to cinnamate-containing sunscreen agents. Cross-sensitivity may occur among sunscreens containing benzophenone, dibenzoylmethane, and aminobenzoic acid or its derivatives.

Pregnancy: Problems in humans have not been documented.

Breastfeeding: Problems in humans have not been documented.

Pediatrics: Sun protection for children is very important. Studies show the risk of developing skin cancer is increased by excessive exposure to the sun during childhood. It is reported also that in cutaneous melanoma a large proportion of skin damage caused by the sun has been acquired during the first 10 to 20 years of life. Furthermore, the regular use of a sunscreen with an SPF of 15 during the first 18 years of life may help reduce the lifetime incidence of nonmelanoma skin cancer by about 75%, provided children using sunscreens do not stay out in the sun longer than they would have if sunscreens had not been used.

Infants under 6 months of age should be kept out of the sun and be physically protected from direct sun exposure. Sunscreen agents should not be used on infants less than 6 months old because of possible irritation and accidental ingestion.

Children 6 months of age and older should not be exposed or should receive only moderate exposure to the sun and should be protected by sunscreen agents with an SPF of 15 or higher when in the sun. Lotion sunscreen products are preferred for use in children. Alcohol-based sunscreen products should be avoided because they can cause irritation.

Geriatrics: Studies have suggested a possibility that frequent use of sunscreen agents may put the US population—especially the elderly, who spend little time in the sun—at risk of vitamin D deficiency, which could lead to osteomalacia, osteoporosis, or bone fractures. However, a recent study failed to confirm this finding. Oral vitamin D supplementation in addition to adequate food intake rich in vitamin D may be advisable for elderly patients who use sunscreens.

ADVERSE REACTIONS

Those indicating need for medical attention: Incidence rare

Acne; allergic contact dermatitis (burning, itching, or stinging of skin); folliculitis (burning, itching, and pain in hairy areas; pus in hair follicles); photoallergic contact dermatitis (early appearance of redness or swelling of the skin; late appearance of rash with or without weeping blisters that become crusted, especially in sun-exposed areas of skin, and that may extend to unexposed areas); skin irritation (burning, itching, redness, or stinging of skin); skin rash.

Factors to Consider When Selecting a Sunscreen Agent

Basic Factors	Determining Factors	Appropriate Sunscreen Agent
Type of activity	High-altitude activities such as mountain climbing and snow skiing	Use SPF 15 or higher with UVA and UVB coverage.
	Prolonged sunbathing Sweat-generating activities such as outdoor jobs (e.g., gardening, construction work), outdoor sports or exercise, or water sports such as swimming, waterskiing, or windsurfing	Use SPF 15 or higher; water-resistant* or waterproof.†
	Reflective surfaces (e.g., concrete, sand, snow, water)	It's best to avoid such surfaces. Use SPF 15 or higher with UVA and UVB coverage.
Age	Less than 6 months of age	Do not use sunscreen agents; keep out of sun.
	6 months of age and older	Use SPF 15 or higher. For children, use lotion sunscreen products; avoid alcohol-based products.
Site of application	Ear, nose	Use physical sunscreen agent.
	Lips	Use gel-based agent.
Skin condition	Dry	Use cream or lotion.
	Oily	Use alcohol- or gel-based agent.
	Eczematous or inflamed	Avoid alcohol-based agent.
Skin type (complexion)‡		**Recommended Sunscreen Agent§**
Very fair—Always burns easily; rarely tans		SPF 20 to 30
Fair—Always burns easily; tans minimally		SPF 12 to 20
Light—Burns moderately; tans gradually (light brown)		SPF 8 to 12
Medium—Burns minimally; always tans well (moderate brown)		SPF 4 to 8
Dark—Rarely burns; tans profusely (dark brown)		SPF 2 to 4

* Water-resistant sunscreen's photoprotective effect remains for up to 40 minutes of active immersion.

† Waterproof (FDA has proposed name change to "very water-resistant") sunscreen's photoprotective effect remains after 80 minutes of active immersion.

‡ Skin types are based on response to initial summer sun exposure for 30 minutes or longer.

§ Proposed FDA recommendations.

Those indicating need for medical attention only if they continue or are bothersome:

Incidence more frequent

Drying, stinging, or tightening of skin—may occur with alcohol-based sunscreen agents.

ADMINISTRATION AND DOSAGE

General Dosing Information

When choosing a sunscreen agent, some of the factors that should be taken into consideration are: type of activity, age, site of application, skin condition, and skin type.

Before every exposure to the sun, an appropriate sunscreen agent that protects against UV radiation should be used. Sunscreens should be applied uniformly and generously to all exposed skin surfaces (including lips, using lip sunscreen or a balm) prior to sun exposure. Sunscreen agents containing aminobenzoic acid and derivatives should be applied 1 to 2 hours before sun exposure, while all other sunscreen products should be applied 30 minutes beforehand. Lip sunscreens should be applied 45 to 60 minutes before exposure.

Sunscreen agents should be reapplied liberally after swimming or profuse sweating. Because most sunscreens agents are easily removed from the skin, reapplication every 1 to 2 hours usually is required for adequate protection. Lip sunscreens should be reapplied liberally at least once every hour and also before and after swimming, after eating and drinking, and during other activities that remove it from the lips.

In addition to using sunscreen agents, sun exposure should be minimized during the hours of 10 a.m. to 2 p.m. (11 a.m. to 3 p.m. daylight savings time) when the sun is strongest. Extra precautions should be utilized on cloudy or overcast days and around reflective surfaces such as concrete, sand, snow, or water, since these surfaces can reflect up to 85% of the sun's damaging rays. Sunlamps and tanning parlors should be avoided. Because UV radiation can cause cataract formation, UV-rated, opaque sunglasses should be worn.

For specific product information, see the dosing table at the end of this section.

TOPICAL ANESTHETICS

Local anesthetics block both the initiation and conduction of nerve impulses by decreasing the neuronal membrane's permeability to sodium ions. This reversibly stabilizes the membrane and inhibits depolarization, resulting in the failure of a propagated action potential and subsequent conduction blockade.

Skin disorders, minor (treatment)—Topical anesthetics are indicated to relieve pain, pruritus, and inflammation associated with minor skin disorders, including:

● Burns, minor (including sunburn).

● Bites or stings (insect).

● Dermatitis, contact (including poison ivy, poison oak, and poison sumac).

● Wounds, minor (including cuts and scratches).

ADMINISTRATION AND DOSAGE

Benzocaine/Dibucaine/Pramoxine/Tetracaine

Adults/Pediatrics ≥2 years of age: Apply to the affected area 3 or 4 times a day as needed.

Butamben

Adults: Apply to the affected area 3 or 4 times a day as needed.

Lidocaine

Adults: Apply to the affected area 3 or 4 times a day as needed.

Pediatrics: Dosage must be individualized, depending on the child's age, weight, and physical condition, up to a maximum of 4.5 mg per kg of body weight.

For more information, refer to the complete monograph for topical anesthetics in "Burns" under Dermatological Conditions.

BENZOCAINE PRODUCTS	
Brand Name	Dosage Form
Solarcaine (Schering)	Spray: 20%

BENZOCAINE/BENZETHONIUM CHLORIDE PRODUCTS	
Brand Name	Dosage Form
Lanacane Original Formula (Combe)	Cream: 6%-0.2%
Lanacane First-Aid (Combe)	Cream: 20%-0.2%
Lanacane Maximum Strength (Combe)	Cream: 20%-0.2% Spray: 20%-0.2%

BENZOCAINE/CHLOROXYLENOL PRODUCTS	
Brand Name	Dosage Form
Foille Medicated First Aid (Blistex)	Ointment: 5%-0.1% Spray: 5%-01%

DIBUCAINE PRODUCTS	
Brand Name	Dosage Form
Nupercainal (Novartis)	Cream: 0.50% Ointment: 1%

LIDOCAINE PRODUCTS	
Brand Name	Dosage Form
Solarcaine Aloe Extract (Schering)	Gel: 0.5% Spray: 0.50%

PRAMOXINE PRODUCTS	
Brand Name	Dosage Form
Sarna Sensitive (Stiefel)	Lotion: 1%

PRAMOXINE/MENTHOL PRODUCTS	
Brand Name	Dosage Form
Gold Bond Medicated Anti-itch Maximum Strength (Chattem)	Cream: 1%-1%

DOSING INFORMATION FOR SUNSCREEN PRODUCTS

The following table provides a quick comparison of the ingredients and dosages of common brand-name OTC drugs. Products are listed alphabetically by brand name.

BRAND NAME	INGREDIENT/STRENGTH	DOSE
Aveeno Radiant Skin Daily Moisturizer with SPF 15 *(Johnson & Johnson Consumer)*	Octinoxate/Avobenzone/Octisalate 7.5%-3%-2%	**Adults & Peds ≥2 yo:** Apply 15 minutes prior to sun exposure.
Baby Blanket Sunblock Stick for Babies, SPF 45+ *(Children's Healthcare Research Group)*	Octocrylene/Octyl/Methoxycinnamate/Oxybenzone/Zinc Oxide 6%-7.5%-3%-15.0%	**Adults & Peds:** Apply 15 minutes prior to sun exposure.
Banana Boat Baby Magic Sunblock Spray, SPF 48 *(Playtex Family Products)*	Homosalate/Octinoxate/Oxybenzone/Octisalate/Titanium Dioxide 10%-7.5%-6.0%-5.0%-2.14%	**Adults & Peds:** Apply 15 minutes prior to sun exposure.
Banana Boat Faces Plus Sunblock Stick, SPF 30 *(Playtex Family Products)*	Homosalate/Octocrylene/Octyl Methoxycinnamate/Octyl Salicylate/Oxybenzone 7%-8%-7.5%-5%-6%	**Adults & Peds ≥2 yo:** Apply 15 minutes prior to sun exposure.
Banana Boat Kids Quickblock UVA & UVB Sunblock Spray Lotion, SPF 35 *(Playtex Family Products)*	Avobenzone/Octinoxate/Octisalate/Octocrylene/Oxybenzone 3%-7.5%-5%-2.5%-5%	**Adults & Peds ≥2 yo:** Apply 15 minutes prior to sun exposure.
Banana Boat Kids Sunblock Lotion SPF 30 *(Playtex Family Products)*	Octinoxate/Oxybenzone/Octisalate/Titanium Dioxide 7.5%-5.25%-4.75%-1.2%	**Adults & Peds ≥2 yo:** Apply 15 minutes prior to sun exposure.
Banana Boat Sport Quick Dry Sunblock spray *(Playtex Family Products)*	Avobenzone/Homosalate/Octinoxate/Octisalate/Oxybenzone 1%-8.78%-7.5%-5%-5%	**Adults & Peds ≥2 yo:** Apply 15 minutes prior to sun exposure.
Banana Boat Sport Sunblock Lotion SPF 15 *(Playtex Family Products)*	Octyl Methoxycinnamate, Oxybenzone, Octyl Salicylate	**Adults & Peds ≥2 yo:** Apply 15 minutes prior to sun exposure.
Banana Boat Sport Sunblock Lotion SPF 30+ *(Playtex Family Products)*	Octyl Methoxycinnamate, Oxybenzone, Octyl Salicylate	**Adults & Peds ≥2 yo:** Apply 15 minutes prior to sun exposure.
Banana Boat Sunblock Lotion Maximum SPF 50 *(Playtex Family Products)*	Octocrylene/Oxybenzone/Octisalate 10%-7.5%-5%	**Adults & Peds ≥2 yo:** Apply 15 minutes prior to sun exposure.
Banana Boat Sunblock Lotion SPF 15 *(Playtex Family Products)*	Padimate O/Oxybenzone/Octinoxate 5%-3%-2%	**Adults & Peds ≥2 yo:** Apply 15 minutes prior to sun exposure.
Banana Boat Sunblock Lotion, Surf Waterproof SPF 15 *(Playtex Family Products)*	Octinoxate/Octisalate/Oxybenzone/Titanium Dioxide 5%-5%-3%-1.6%	**Adults & Peds ≥2 yo:** Apply 15 minutes prior to sun exposure.
Banana Boat Sunscreen Lotion SPF8 *(Playtex Family Products)*	Padimate O, Oxybenzone	**Adults & Peds ≥2 yo:** Apply 15 minutes prior to sun exposure.
Banana Boat Suntanicals Sunscreen Lotion, SPF 15 *(Playtex Family Products)*	Octinoxate/Octocrylene 7.5%-2.75%	**Adults & Peds ≥2 yo:** Apply 15 minutes prior to sun exposure.
Banana Boat Suntanicals Sunscreen Lotion, SPF 30 *(Playtex Family Products)*	Avobenzone/Octinoxate/Octisalate/Oxybenzone 1.5%-7.5%-5%-4.1%	**Adults & Peds ≥2 yo:** Apply 15 minutes prior to sun exposure.
Banana Boat Suntanicals Sunscreen Lotion, SPF 8 *(Playtex Family Products)*	Octinoxate/Octisalate 5.5%-1.5%	**Adults & Peds ≥2 yo:** Apply 15 minutes prior to sun exposure.
Banana Boat Ultra Sunblock Lotion SPF 30+ *(Playtex Family Products)*	Octyl Methoxycinnamate; Oxybenzone; Octyl Salicylate	**Adults & Peds ≥2 yo:** Apply 15 minutes prior to sun exposure.
Bodyglide SPF 25 *(Sternoff)*	Tribehenin, Octyl Methoxy Cinnamate, Benzophenone-3, Octyl Salicylate	**Adults & Peds ≥6 mos:** Apply 20 mins prior to sun exposure.
Coppertone Bug and Sun Sunscreen SPF 30 *(Schering-Plough)*	DEET 10.0%, Octocrylene, Octinoxate, Oxybenzone	**Adults & Peds ≥2 yo:** Apply 15 minutes prior to sun exposure.
Coppertone Endless Summer Ultrasheer Sunscreen Stick, SPF 30 *(Schering-Plough)*	Octinoxate, Octocrylene, Zinc Oxide	**Adults & Peds ≥6 mos:** Apply exposed areas before sun or water exposure.
Coppertone Endless Summer Ultrasheer Sunscreen, SPF 15 *(Schering-Plough)*	Avobenzone, Homosalate, Octisalate, Octocrylene, Oxybenzone	**Adults & Peds ≥6 mos:** Apply exposed areas before sun or water exposure.
Coppertone Endless Summer Ultrasheer Sunscreen, SPF 30 *(Schering-Plough)*	Avobenzone, Homosalate, Octisalate, Octocrylene, Oxybenzone	**Adults & Peds ≥6 mos:** Apply exposed areas before sun or water exposure.
Coppertone Kids Sunblock Lotion SPF 30 Trigger Spray *(Schering-Plough)*	Homosalate, Octinoxate, Octisalate, Oxybenzone	**Adults & Peds ≥2 yo:** Apply exposed areas prior to sun exposure.
Coppertone Kids Sunblock Lotion SPF 40 *(Schering-Plough)*	Homosalate, Octinoxate, Octisalate, Oxybenzone	**Adults & Peds ≥2 yo:** Apply exposed areas prior to sun exposure.
Coppertone Kids Sunblock Stick SPF 30 *(Schering-Plough)*	Octinoxate, Oxybenzone, Octisalate, Homosalate	**Adults & Peds ≥2 yo:** Apply exposed areas prior to sun exposure.

DOSING INFORMATION FOR SUNSCREEN PRODUCTS (cont.)

BRAND NAME	INGREDIENT/STRENGTH	DOSE
Coppertone Oil Free Sunblock Lotion for Faces, SPF 30 *(Schering-Plough)*	Avobenzone, Homosalate, Octocrylene, Octyl Salicylate, Oxybenzone	**Adults & Peds ≥6 mos:** Apply exposed areas before sun or water exposure.
Coppertone Oil Free Sunblock Lotion SPF 15 *(Schering-Plough)*	Octinoxate, Oxybenzone	**Adults & Peds ≥2 yo:** Apply 15 minutes prior to sun exposure.
Coppertone Oil Free Sunblock Lotion SPF 30 *(Schering-Plough)*	Octinoxate, Homosalate, Oxybenzone, Octisalate, Avobenzone	**Adults & Peds ≥6 mos:** Apply exposed areas before sun or water exposure.
Coppertone Oil Free Sunblock Lotion, SPF 45 *(Schering-Plough)*	Ethylhexyl P-Methoxycinnamate, Oxybenzone, 2-Ethylhexyl Salicylate, Homosalate	**Adults & Peds ≥2 yo:** Apply 15 minutes prior to sun exposure.
Coppertone Shade Sunblock Lotion, SPF 45 *(Schering-Plough)*	Avobenzone, Homosalate, Octocrylene, Octisalate, Oxybenzone	**Adults & Peds ≥6 mos:** Apply exposed areas before sun or water exposure.
Coppertone Shade Sunblock Stick, SPF 30 *(Schering-Plough)*	Ethylhexyl P-Methoxycinnamate, Oxybenzone, 2-ethylexyl Salicylate, Homosalate	**Adults & Peds ≥6 mos:** Apply exposed areas before sun or water exposure.
Coppertone Spectra3 Kids Sunblock Lotion SPF 50 *(Schering-Plough)*	Homosalate, Octinoxate, Octisalate, Octocrylene, Oxybenzone, Zinc Oxide	**Adults & Peds ≥6 mos:** Apply exposed areas before sun or water exposure.
Coppertone Spectra3 Sunblock Lotion SPF 30 *(Schering-Plough)*	Homosalate, Octocrylene, Octinoxate, Octisalate, Zinc Oxide	**Adults & Peds ≥6 mos:** Apply exposed areas before sun or water exposure.
Coppertone Spectra3 Sunblock Lotion SPF 50 *(Schering-Plough)*	Homosalate, Octinoxate, Octocrylene, Oxybenzone, Zinc Oxide	**Adults & Peds ≥6 mos:** Apply exposed areas before sun or water exposure.
Coppertone Spectra3 Waterbabies Sunblock Lotion SPF 50 *(Schering-Plough)*	Homosalate, Octinoxate, Octisalate, Octocrylene, Oxybenzone, Zinc Oxide	**Adults & Peds ≥6 mos:** Apply exposed areas before sun or water exposure.
Coppertone Sport Sunblock Gel, SPF 30 *(Schering-Plough)*	Avobenzone, Octocrylene, Octyl Salicylate, Oxybenzone	**Adults & Peds ≥6 mos:** Apply exposed areas before sun or water exposure.
Coppertone Sport Sunblock Lotion SPF 15 *(Schering-Plough)*	Octyl Methoxycinnamate, Octyl Salicylate, Oxybenzone	**Adults & Peds ≥6 mos:** Apply exposed areas before sun or water exposure.
Coppertone Sport Sunblock Lotion SPF 30 Trigger Spray *(Schering-Plough)*	Homosalate, Octinoxate, Octisalate, Oxybenzone	**Adults & Peds ≥6 mos:** Apply exposed areas before sun or water exposure.
Coppertone Sport Sunblock Lotion SPF 30 with Caribiner *(Schering-Plough)*	Homosalate, Octinoxate, Octisalate, Oxybenzone	**Adults & Peds ≥6 mos:** Apply exposed areas before sun or water exposure.
Coppertone Sport Sunblock Lotion SPF 45 *(Schering-Plough)*	Homosalate, Octinoxate, Octisalate, Oxybenzone	**Adults & Peds ≥6 mos:** Apply exposed areas before sun or water exposure.
Coppertone Sport Sunblock Spray SPF 30 *(Schering-Plough)*	Homosalate, Octyl Methoxycinnamate, Octyl Salicylate, Oxybenzone	**Adults & Peds ≥6 mos:** Apply exposed areas before sun or water exposure.
Coppertone Sport Sunblock Spray, Continuous SPF 30 *(Schering-Plough)*	Homosalate, Octinoxate, Octisalate, Oxybenzone	**Adults & Peds ≥6 mos:** Apply exposed areas before sun or water exposure.
Coppertone Sport Sunblock Stick, SPF 30 *(Schering-Plough)*	Octyl Methoxycinnamate, Oxybenzone, Octyl Salicylate, Homosalate	**Adults & Peds ≥6 mos:** Apply exposed areas before sun or water exposure.
Coppertone Sport Ultra Sweatproof/ Waterproof Sunblock Lotion, SPF 30 *(Schering-Plough)*	Octyl Methoxycinnamate, Oxybenzone, Octyl Salicylate, Homosalate	**Adults & Peds ≥2 yo:** Apply exposed areas prior to sun exposure.
Coppertone Sunblock Lotion SPF 15, UVA/ UVB Protection, Waterproof *(Schering-Plough)*	Octyl Methoxycinnamate, Oxybenzone	**Adults & Peds ≥2 yo:** Apply 15 minutes prior to sun exposure.
Coppertone Sunblock Lotion, SPF 45 *(Schering-Plough)*	Avobenzone, Homosalate, Octyl Salicylate, Oxybenzone	**Adults & Peds ≥6 mos:** Apply exposed areas before sun or water exposure.
Coppertone Sunblock Spray SPF 30 *(Schering-Plough)*	Homosalate, Octinoxate, Octisalate, Oxybenzone	**Adults & Peds ≥2 yo:** Apply exposed areas prior to sun exposure.
Coppertone Sunscreen Lotion SPF 8, UVA/ UVB Protection, Waterproof *(Schering-Plough)*	Octyl Methoxycinnamate, Oxybenzone	**Adults & Peds ≥2 yo:** Apply exposed areas prior to sun exposure.
Coppertone Ultra Sheer, Faces SPF 30 *(Schering-Plough)*	Avobenzone, Homosalate, Octisalate, Octocrylene, Oxybenzone	**Adults & Peds ≥6 mos:** Apply exposed areas before sun or water exposure.
Coppertone Ultrasheer Sunscreen, SPF 45 *(Schering-Plough)*	Avobenzone, Homosalate, Octisalate, Octocrylene, Oxybenzone	**Adults & Peds ≥6 mos:** Apply exposed areas before sun or water exposure.
Coppertone Water Babies Sunblock Lotion SPF 45 *(Schering-Plough)*	Octinoxate, Oxybenzone, Octisalate, Homosalate	**Adults & Peds ≥2 yo:** Apply exposed areas prior to sun exposure.

DOSING INFORMATION FOR SUNSCREEN PRODUCTS (cont.)

Brand Name	Ingredient/Strength	Dose
Coppertone Water Babies Sunblock Spray, SPF 45 *(Schering-Plough)*	Octyl Methoxycinnamate, Oxybenzone, Octyl Salicylate, Homosalate	**Adults & Peds ≥2 yo:** Apply exposed areas prior to sun exposure.
Cotz Sunscreen SPF 58 *(Fallene)*	Titanium Dioxide; Zinc Oxide	**Adults & Peds ≥2 yo:** Apply 15 minutes prior to sun exposure.
DML Daily Facial Moisturizer, SPF 25 *(Person & Covey)*	Avobenzone 3.0%/Octyl Methoxycinnamate/ Homosalate/Octocrylene 3.0%-7.5%-6%- 1.5%	**Adults:** Apply qd.
Eucerin Extra Protective Moisture Lotion, SPF 30 *(Beiersdorf)*	Octocrylene, Octinoxate, Zinc Oxide, Titanium Dioxide, Ensulizole	**Adults:** Apply to affected area qd.
Eucerin Skin Renewal Day Lotion, SPF 15 *(Beiersdorf)*	Octinoxate, Octisalate, Oxybenzone	**Adults:** Apply to affected area prn.
Hawaiian Tropic 15 Plus Sunblock *(HT Marketing)*	Octinoxate, Octisalate, Titanium Dioxide	**Adults & Peds ≥2 yo:** Apply 15 minutes prior to sun exposure.
Hawaiian Tropic Ozone Sport Sunblock SPF 60+ *(HT Marketing)*	Octocrylene, Oxybenzone, Avobenzone	**Adults & Peds ≥2 yo:** Apply 15 minutes prior to sun exposure.
Mustela Bebe Moderate Sun Protection Lotion, SPF 25 *(Laboratoirs Expanscience)*	Titanium Dioxide/Zinc Oxide 9.8%-5%	**Adults & Peds ≥6 mos:** Apply 20 mins prior to sun exposure.
Neutrogena Intensified Day Moisture SPF 15 *(Neutrogena)*	Titanium Dioxide, Triethanolamine	**Adults:** Apply every morning after cleansing.
Neutrogena Active Breathable Sunblock SPF 30 *(Neutrogena)*	Avobenzone/Homosalate/Octinoxate/ Octisalate/Oxybenzone 2%-7%-7.5%-5%-3%	**Adults:** Apply 15-30 minutes before sun exposure.
Neutrogena Active Breathable Sunblock SPF 45 *(Neutrogena)*	Avobenzone/Homosalate/Octinoxate/ Octisalate/Oxybenzone 2%-7%-7.5%-5%-3%	**Adults:** Apply 15-30 minutes before sun exposure.
Neutrogena Healthy Defense Daily Moisturizer SPF 30 *(Neutrogena)*	Isohexadecane, Cyclopentasiloxane, Dimethicone, Triethanolamine, Codium Tomentosum, B Trimethylolpropane Triethylhexanoate	**Adults:** Apply 15-30 minutes before sun exposure.
Neutrogena Healthy Defense Oil-Free Sunblock SPF 30 *(Neutrogena)*	Isohexadecane, Butyloctyl Salicylate, Cyclopentasiloxane, Dimethicone, Triethanolamine, Codium Tomentosum, Trimethylolpropane Triethylhexanoate	**Adults:** Apply 15-30 minutes before sun exposure.
Neutrogena Healthy Defense Oil-Free Sunblock SPF 45 *(Neutrogena)*	Methylpropanediol, PVP/Eicosene Copolymer, Triethanolamine	**Adults:** Apply 15 minutes before sun exposure.
Neutrogena Healthy Defense Oil-Free Sunblock Spray SPF 30 *(Neutrogena)*	SD Alcohol 40 (54%), Dibutyl Adipate, PPG- 12/SMDI Copolymer, Acrylates/ Octylacrylamide Copolymer, Ascorbyl Palmitate, Retinyl Palmitate	**Adults:** Apply 15 minutes before sun exposure.
Neutrogena Healthy Defense Oil-Free Sunblock Stick SPF 30 *(Neutrogena)*	Ozokerite, Cyclopentasiloxane, Neopentyl Glycol Dioctanoate, Polyethylene, Dimethicone	**Adults:** Apply 15-30 minutes before sun exposure
Neutrogena Moisture SPF 15 - Sheer *(Neutrogena)*	Octinoxate/Octisalate/Oxybenzone 7.5%-5%- 3%	**Adults:** Use qd.
Neutrogena Sensitive Skin Sunblock Lotion SPF 30 *(Neutrogena)*	Titanium Dioxide 9.1%	**Adults:** Apply 15 minutes before sun exposure.
Neutrogena Triple Protect Face Lotion SPF 20 *(Neutrogena)*	Ensulizole/Octinoxate/Oxybenzone	**Adults:** Use qd.
Neutrogena Ultra Sheer Sunblock SPF 30 *(Neutrogena)*	VP-Hexadecene Copolymer, Dimethicone, Hydroxyethyl Acrylate/Sodium Acryloyldimethyltaurate Copolymer, Dimethicone, Cetyl Dimethicone, Dipotassium Glycyrrhizate, Trimethylsiloxysilicate	**Adults:** Apply 15 mins prior to sun exposure.
Neutrogena Ultra Sheer Sunblock SPF 45 *(Neutrogena)*	VP-Hexadecene Copolymer, Dimethicone, Hydroxyethyl Acrylate/Sodium Acryloyldimethyltaurate Copolymer, Dimethicone, Cetyl Dimethicone, Trimethylsiloxysilicate	**Adults:** Apply 15 mins prior to sun exposure.
NO-AD Sun Block Lotion SPF 15 *(Solar Cosmetics Lab)*	Octyl Methoxycinnamate/Octyl Salicylate/ Benzophenone-3 5%-3%-2%	**Adults & Peds ≥2 yo:** Apply 30 minutes before sun exposure.

DOSING INFORMATION FOR SUNSCREEN PRODUCTS (cont.)

BRAND NAME	INGREDIENT/STRENGTH	DOSE
NO-AD Sunblock, Babies, Waterproof, SPF 45 *(Solar Cosmetics Lab)*	Octyl Methoxycinnamate/Octyl Salicylate/ Benzophenone 3, Zinc Oxide 4%-5%-0.28%	**Adults & Peds ≥2 yo:** Apply 30 minutes before sun exposure.
NO-AD Sunblock, Kids, Waterproof, SPF 30 *(Solar Cosmetics Lab)*	Octyl Methoxycinnamate, Octyl Salicyclate, Benzophenone-3 7.5%-4%-3%	**Adults & Peds ≥2 yo:** Apply 30 minutes before sun exposure.
NO-AD Sunblock, Lotion, Waterproof, SPF 15 *(Solar Cosmetics Lab)*	Octyl Methoxycinnamate (Octinoxate)(5%), Octyl Salicyclate (Octisalate)(3%), Benzophenone-3 (Oxybenzone)(2%	**Adults & Peds ≥2 yo:** Apply 30 minutes before sun exposure.
NO-AD Sunblock, Maximum Lotion, Waterproof SPF 45 *(Solar Cosmetics Lab)*	Octyl Methoxy Cinnamate, Octyl Salicylate, Benzophenone	**Adults & Peds ≥2 yo:** Apply 30 minutes before sun exposure.
NO-AD Sunblock, Sport Lotion, Waterproof, SPF 50 *(Solar Cosmetics Lab)*	Homosalate/Octinoxate/Oxybenzone/ Octisalate 15%-6%-6%-5%	**Adults & Peds ≥2 yo:** Apply 30 minutes before sun exposure.
NO-AD Sunblock, Sport Ultra, Waterproof, SPF 30 *(Solar Cosmetics Lab)*	Octyl Methoxycinnamate, Octyl Salicylate, Benzophenone 7.5%-4%-3 3%	**Adults & Peds ≥2 yo:** Apply 30 minutes before sun exposure.

DOSING INFORMATION FOR TOPICAL ANESTHETIC PRODUCTS

The following table provides a quick comparison of the ingredients and dosages of common brand-name OTC drugs. Products are listed alphabetically by brand name.

BRAND NAME	INGREDIENT/STRENGTH	DOSE
Lanacane Maximum Strength cream *(Combe)*	Benzocaine/Benzethonium Chloride 20%-0.2%	**Adults & Peds ≥2 yo:** Apply to clean dry affected area qd-tid.
Lanacane Maximum Strength spray *(Combe)*	Benzocaine/Benzethonium Chloride 20%-0.2%	**Adults & Peds ≥2 yo:** Apply to clean dry affected area qd-tid.
Lanacane Original Formula cream *(Combe)*	Benzocaine/Benzethonium Chloride 6%-0.2%	**Adults & Peds ≥2 yo:** Apply to clean dry affected area qd-tid.
Solarcaine Aloe Extra Burn Relief gel *(Schering-Plough)*	Lidocaine HCl 0.5%	**Adults & Peds ≥2 yo:** Apply to clean dry affected area tid-qid.
Solarcaine Aloe Extra Burn Relief spray *(Schering-Plough)*	Lidocaine 0.5%	**Adults & Peds ≥2 yo:** Apply to clean dry affected area tid-qid.
Tender's Afterburn Aloe gel *(Tender Corporation)*	Lidocaine 0.5%	**Adults & Peds ≥2 yo:** Apply to clean dry affected area tid-qid.
Water Jel Burn Jel, For Fast Relief of Minor Burns *(Water-Jel Technologies)*	Lidocaine HCl 2.0%	**Adults & Peds ≥2 yo:** Apply to clean dry affected area tid-qid.

Wound Care

Minor cuts and scrapes usually do not require medical attention and can often be cared for at home. The best way to clean an abrasion, laceration, or puncture wound is with cool water. Soap and a washcloth should be used to clean the skin around the wound. Most small cuts and scrapes will stop bleeding on their own in a short time. Applying firm but gentle pressure with a clean cloth, tissue, or gauze continuously for 20 to 30 minutes can help stop bleeding. Bandages can be used to cover the wound and keep it from becoming irritated and infected. Bandages should be changed daily. There are a number of OTC products available to cleanse wounds (chlorhexidine gluconate, hydrogen peroxide, iodine, etc.) and to aid in healing and prevent infection (topical antibiotics such as neomycin, polymyxin B, and bacitracin).

BENZALKONIUM CHLORIDE

PHARMACOLOGY

The mechanism of action of benzalkonium chloride is not known but is thought to be related to bacterial enzyme inactivation. Benzalkonium chloride is said to be rapidly microbicidal against a wide variety of bacteria, fungi, and protozoa. However, bacterial endospores, viruses, and certain genera of gram-negative bacteria (i.e., *Pseudomonas, Mycobacteria*, and enteric gram-negative rods) are generally considered resistant.

INDICATIONS

Skin infection (prophylaxis and treatment)—A 1:750 concentration of benzalkonium chloride is used for preoperative skin preparation, treatment of minor wounds, and lacerations, as a surgical scrub, and for sterilizing metallic instruments.

CONTRAINDICATIONS

Risk-benefit should be considered when the following medical problems exist:

- Hypersensitivity to benzalkonium chloride

WARNINGS/PRECAUTIONS

Pregnancy: Unknown.

Breastfeeding: Unknown.

ADVERSE REACTIONS

Those indicating need for medical attention: Incidence rare

Anaphylaxis.

Those indicating need for medical attention: Only if bothersome

Skin irritation.

ADMINISTRATION AND DOSAGE

Solution:

Adults/Pediatrics: Apply to the affected area as needed in 1:750 concentration.

CHLORHEXIDINE GLUCONATE

PHARMACOLOGY

Chlorhexidine is an antiseptic antimicrobial that is used as a topical skin cleanser or as a dental mouth rinse to reduce plaque. Chlorhexidine, a polybiguanide is an antiseptic and antimicrobial drug with bactericidal activity. The drug is a base and is stable as a salt, the most commonly studied being chlorhexidine gluconate. At physiologic pH, chlorhexidine salts dissociate releasing a positively charged component. The bactericidal effect of chlorhexidine is a result of the binding of this cationic molecule to negatively charged bacterial cell walls and extramicrobial complexes. At low concentrations, this causes an alteration of bacterial cell osmotic equilibrium and leakage of potassium and phosphorous resulting in a bacteriostatic effect. At high concentrations of chlorhexidine, the cytoplasmic contents of the bacterial cell precipitate and result in cell death.

Chlorhexidine is indicated for topical use in preoperative skin preparation, skin wound and general skin cleansing, and as a surgical hand scrub for health care professionals.

INDICATIONS

Skin infection (prophylaxis and treatment)—Chlorhexidine is indicated for topical use in preoperative skin preparation, skin wound and general skin cleansing, and as a surgical hand scrub for health care professionals.

CONTRAINDICATIONS

Risk-benefit should be considered when the following medical problems exist:

- Hypersensitivity to chlorhexidine

WARNINGS/PRECAUTIONS

Pregnancy: FDA Category C.

Breastfeeding: Potential risk; change in therapy or care plan may be advisable.

CHLORHEXIDINE GLUCONATE PRODUCTS	
Brand Name	**Dosage Form**
Betasept (Purdue)	**Liquid:** 4%
Hibiclens (Regent)	**Liquid:** 4%
Hibistat (Regent)	**Pad:** 0.50%

ADVERSE REACTIONS

Those indicating need for medical attention: Incidence rare
Anaphylaxis; corneal injury due to eye contact.

Those indicating need for medical attention only if bothersome:
Skin irritation.

ADMINISTRATION AND DOSAGE

Solution 4%

Adults/Pediatrics: Apply to the affected area for at least 2 minutes. The area should then be dried with a sterile towel and the washing procedure repeated for an additional 2 minutes.

NEOMYCIN/POLYMYXIN B/BACITRACIN

Neomycin is actively transported across the bacterial cell membrane, binds to a specific receptor protein on the 30 S subunit of bacterial ribosomes, and interferes with an initiation complex between mRNA (messenger RNA) and the 30 S subunit, inhibiting protein synthesis. DNA may be misread, thus producing nonfunctional proteins; polyribosomes are split and are unable to synthesize protein.

Polymyxin B is bactericidal and active against *Pseudomonas aeruginosa* and other gram-negative bacteria. It is a surface-active basic polypeptide that binds to anionic phospholipid sites in bacterial cytoplasmic membranes, disrupts membrane structure, and alters membrane permeability to allow leakage of intracellular contents. Its action is antagonized by calcium and magnesium.

Bacitracin, a polypeptide antibiotic, is usually bactericidal against gram-positive organisms. It acts within the bacterial cell membrane and interferes with bacterial cell wall synthesis by binding to and inhibiting the dephosphorylation of a membrane-bound lipid pyrophosphate. Pyrophosphate is the precursor of a carrier molecule, undecaprenyl phosphate, which is involved in peptidoglycan polymerization.

Skin infections, bacterial, minor (prophylaxis)—Topical neomycin, polymyxin B, and bacitracin combination is indicated in the prophylaxis of superficial skin infections caused by susceptible organisms in minor abrasions, burns, and cuts.

Skin infections, bacterial, minor (treatment); *ulcer, dermal* (treatment)—Topical neomycin, polymyxin B, and bacitracin combination is used in the treatment of minor bacterial skin infections and dermal ulcer.

Cream

Adults/Pediatrics >2 year of age: Apply to affected area 1 to 3 times a day.

Ointment

Adults/Pediatrics: Apply to affected area 2 to 5 times a day.

For more information, refer to the complete monographs for bacitracin; neomycin; neomycin/polymyxin B; and neomycin/polymyxin B/bacitracin in "Bacterial Infections" under Dermatological Conditions.

NEOMYCIN/POLYMYXIN B/PRAMOXINE PRODUCTS	
Brand Name	**Dosage Form**
Neosporin Plus Pain Relief (Pfizer)	**Cream:** 3.5mg-10,000 U-10mg
BACITRACIN PRODUCTS	
Brand Name	**Dosage Form**
Bacitracin (Various)	**Ointment:** 500 U/g
NEOMYCIN/POLYMYXIN B/BACITRACIN PRODUCTS	
Brand Name	**Dosage Form**
Neosporin (Pfizer)	**Ointment:** 3.5g-5,000 U-400 U
Neosporin Neo to Go (Pfizer)	**Ointment:** 3.5g-5,000 U-400 U
NEOMYCIN/POLYMYXIN B/BACITRACIN/PRAMOXINE PRODUCTS	
Brand Name	**Dosage Form**
Neosporin Plus Pain Relief (Pfizer)	**Ointment:** 3.5g-10,000 U-500 U-10mg

DOSING INFORMATION FOR WOUND CARE PRODUCTS

The following table provides a quick comparison of the ingredients and dosages of common brand-name OTC drugs. Products are listed alphabetically by drug category and brand name.

BRAND NAME	INGREDIENT/STRENGTH	DOSE
NEOMYCIN/POLYMYXIN B/BACITRACIN COMBINATIONS		
Bacitracin ointment (*Various*)	Bacitracin 500 U	**Adults & Peds:** Apply to affected area qd-tid.
Neosporin ointment (*Pfizer Consumer Healthcare*)	Neomycin/polymyxin B/bacitracin 3.5mg-5,000 U-400 U	**Adults & Peds:** Apply to affected area qd-tid.
Neosporin Plus Pain Relief cream (*Pfizer Consumer Healthcare*)	Neomycin/polymyxin B/pramoxine 3.5mg-10,000 U-10mg	**Adults & Peds:** Apply to affected area qd-tid.
Neosporin Plus Pain Relief ointment (*Pfizer Consumer Healthcare*)	Neomycin/polymyxin B/bacitracin/pramoxine 3.5mg-10,000 U-500 U-10mg	**Adults & Peds:** Apply to affected area qd-tid.
Neosporin To Go ointment (*Pfizer Consumer Healthcare*)	Neomycin/polymyxin B/bacitracin 3.5mg-5,000 U-400 U	**Adults & Peds:** Apply to affected area qd-tid.
Polysporin ointment (*Pfizer Consumer Healthcare*)	Polymyxin B/Bacitracin 10,000 U-500 U	**Adults & Peds:** Apply to affected area qd-tid.
BENZALKONIUM CHLORIDE COMBINATIONS		
Bactine First Aid Liquid (*Bayer Healthcare*)	Lidocaine HCl/Benzalkonium Cl 2.5%-0.13%	**Adults & Peds ≥2 yo:** Apply to affected area qd-tid.
Bactine Pain Relieving Cleansing Wipes (*Bayer Healthcare*)	Benzalkonium Chloride/Pramoxine Hydrochloride 0.13%-1.0%	**Adults & Peds ≥2 yo:** Use 1 wipe qd-tid.
Band-Aid Antiseptic Foam, One-Step Cleansing and Infection Protection (*Johnson & Johnson/Merck Consumer*)	Benzalkonium Chloride 0.13%	**Adults & Peds ≥3 yo:** Use tid.
BENZETHONIUM CHLORIDE COMBINATIONS		
Bactine Pain Relieving Cleansing Spray (*Bayer Healthcare*)	Lidocaine HCl/Benzalkonium Cl 2.5%-0.13%	**Adults & Peds ≥2 yo:** Apply to affected area qd-tid.
Gold Bond First Aid Quick Spray (*Chattem*)	Menthol/Benzethonium Chloride 1%-0.13%	**Adults & Peds ≥2 yo:** Apply to affected area tid-qid.
Gold Bond First Aid, Medicated Wipes (*Chattem*)	Benzethonium Chloride/Menthol 0.13%-1%	**Adults & Peds ≥2 yo:** Apply to affected area tid-qid.
Gold Bond First Aid, Medicated Wipes (*Chattem*)	Benzethonium Chloride/Menthol 0.13%-1%	**Adults & Peds ≥2 yo:** Apply to affected area tid-qid.
Lanacane Maximum Strength Cream (*Combe*)	Benzocaine/Benzethonium Chloride 20%-0.2%	**Adults & Peds ≥2 yo:** Apply to affected area qd-tid.
CHLORHEXIDINE GLUCONATE		
Hibiclens (*Regent*)	Chlorhexidine gluconate 4%	**Adults & Peds:** Apply the sparingly to affected area prn.
IODINE		
Betadine ointment (*Purdue*)	Povidone-Iodine 10%	**Adults & Peds:** Apply to affected area qd-tid.
Betadine Skin Cleanser (*Purdue*)	Povidone-Iodine 7.5%	**Adults & Peds:** Apply to affected area for 3 minutes and rinse. Repeat bid-tid.
Betadine solution (*Purdue*)	Povidone-Iodine 10%	**Adults & Peds:** Apply to affected area qd-tid.
Betadine spray (*Purdue*)	Povidone-Iodine 10%	**Adults & Peds:** Apply to affected area qd-tid.
Betadine Surgical Scrub (*Purdue*)	Povidone-Iodine 7.5%	**Adults & Peds:** Apply to affected area for 5 minutes.
Betadine swab (*Purdue*)	Povidone-Iodine 10%	**Adults & Peds:** Apply to affected area qd-tid.
MISCELLANEOUS		
Aquaphor Healing Ointment (*Beiersdorf*)	Petrolatum, Mineral Oil, Ceresin, Lanolin Alcohol, Panthenol, Glycerin, Bisabolol	**Adults & Peds:** Apply to affected area prn.
Curad Spray Bandage (*Beiersdorf*)	Ethyl Acetate, Pentane, Methylacrylate, Menthol, Carbon Dioxide	**Adults & Peds:** Apply to affected area prn.
Proxacol Hydrogen Peroxide (*Pfizer Consumer Healthcare*)	Hydrogen peroxide 3%	**Adults:** Apply to affected area qd to tid.
Wound Wash Sterile Saline spray (*Blairex Laboratories*)	Sterile Sodium Chloride Solution 0.9%	**Adults & Peds:** Apply to affected area prn.

Diabetes Mellitus

Diabetes mellitus (DM) is a disorder of carbohydrate, fat, and protein metabolism that is associated with an absolute or relative deficiency of insulin and/or varying degrees of insulin resistance. DM is a syndrome that includes a heterogeneous group of disorders characterized by fasting hyperglycemia and/or elevated plasma glucose levels following a standard oral glucose tolerance test (OGTT). The Expert Committee on the Diagnosis and Classification of Diabetes Mellitus of the American Diabetes Association defines the following major groups of DM and impaired glucose tolerance:

I. *Type 1 DM*: patients with autoimmune pancreatic islet B-cell destruction who are prone to ketoacidosis

II. *Type 2 DM*: patients with both insulin resistance and an insulin secretory defect

III. *Other forms*: uncommon forms of DM, usually from conditions that predispose to insulin resistance or are associated with nonimmune-mediated pancreatic islet B-cell destruction

IV. *Gestational DM*: glucose intolerance discovered or developed during pregnancy.

Impaired glucose tolerance (IGT) and impaired fasting glucose (IFG) refer to patients with plasma glucose levels above the normal range but not high enough to be labeled DM. IGT and IFG represent metabolic states intermediate between normal glucose homeostasis and DM and are referred to as prediabetes. Within 5 years, 10% to 25% of people with IGT or IFG will develop DM, some will revert to normal glucose tolerance, and others will continue to have IGT or IFG.

Type 1 DM is an autoimmune disorder characterized by autoantibodies to B-cell antigens or insulin; by cellular infiltration (insulitis) and B-cell destruction; and, ultimately, by insulinopenia and ketoacidosis. Incompletely understood genetic factors are important in the pathogenesis of type 1 DM. For example, certain human leukocyte antigens (HLA) are closely associated with type 1 DM. Compared with 40% to 50% of the Caucasian population, approximately 95% of type 1 DM patients have either HLA-DR3 or HLA-DR4. Apparently, HLA immune response genes predispose patients to an autoimmune response to the pancreatic B cells that is primarily mediated by cytotoxic T cells. The large geographic variation in incidence suggests that environmental factors are also important in the pathogenesis.

Type 2 DM represents a heterogeneous group of disorders with different pathophysiologic mechanisms contributing to hyperglycemia. These mechanisms range from uncommon but well-defined genetic abnormalities (such as mutations in insulin or its receptors) to unexplained insulin resistance and impaired insulin secretion (associated with obesity). The strongest evidence of a genetic predisposition to type 2 DM comes from studies of twins—monozygotic twins have concordance rates between 55% and 100%.

Although the inheritance pattern for most forms of type 2 DM is unclear, maturity-onset diabetes of the young (MODY) has autosomal dominant transmission. The prevalence of type 2 DM in populations migrating to the United States differs from that in their countries of origin, suggesting that environmental factors are involved in the expression of type 2 DM. In a genetically predisposed person, the development of obesity and changes in lifestyle (decreased exercise) and eating patterns significantly increase the risk of developing type 2 DM. Type 2 DM is characterized by two major pathophysiologic abnormalities: peripheral insulin resistance and impaired insulin secretion, both of which lead to excessive hepatic glucose production. In type 2 DM, insulin resistance associated with abdominal obesity augments genetically determined insulin resistance. In early-stage disease, pancreatic B cells compensate for increased insulin resistance by increasing insulin output. With time, the B cells cannot sustain sufficient hyperinsulinemia to compensate for the progressively increasing insulin resistance. Early B-cell decline is characterized by impaired glucose tolerance and by postprandial hyperglycemia; further B-cell decline is characterized by fasting hyperglycemia and overt DM. Others believe that B-cell failure contributes to hepatic glucose overproduction from the beginning and that the insulin response in diabetics to a glucose clamp is always deficient, even before glucose intolerance develops.

According to the "two-hit" hypothesis, the clinical expression of type 2 DM depends on the inheritance of two sets of genetic variants: one set determines the early development of insulin resistance, and the other set predisposes to B-cell dysfunction following chronic metabolic stress (hyperglycemia). Insulin resistance is associated with a variety of cardiovascular risk factors such as abdominal obesity, high blood pressure, and dyslipidemia. Insulin-resistant nondiabetic or prediabetic patients with several of these risk factors are sometimes considered to have *metabolic syndrome* (also known as insulin-resistance syndrome or syndrome X). Although some researchers doubt its existence, the metabolic syndrome concept may have important implications for prevention, identification, and management of cardiovascular risk. Unfortunately, diagnostic criteria are not yet completely standardized, but recent recommendations of the National Cholesterol Education Program Adult Treatment Panel III (ATP III) are likely to set a precedent.

Other types of DM are associated with genetic defects of B-cell function, genetic defects in insulin action, pancreatic diseases, endocrinopathies, drugs, chemicals, infections, uncommon forms of immune-mediated DM, and other genetic syndromes.

Gestational DM occurs in about 7% of pregnancies and is associated with increased perinatal mortality and morbidity. Although most women with gestational DM have normal glucose tolerance postpartum, up to 60% will develop type 2 DM within 15 years. Thus, after completion of pregnancy, it is important to reclassify these patients as having IGT/IFG, DM, or "previous abnormality of glucose tolerance."

There are many products available to treat and manage diabetes. Regular insulin, NPH insulin, and Lente insulin are available OTC, and there are numerous blood-glucose monitors available to monitor therapy.

INSULIN

PHARMACOLOGY

Insulin is a polypeptide hormone that controls the storage and metabolism of carbohydrates, proteins, and fats. This activity occurs primarily in the liver, in muscle, and in adipose tissues after binding of the insulin molecules to receptor sites on cellular plasma membranes. Although the mechanisms of insulin's molecular actions in the cellular area are still being explored, it is known that cell membrane transport characteristics, cellular growth, enzyme activation and inhibition, and alterations in protein and fat metabolism are all influenced by insulin. More specifically, insulin promotes uptake of carbohydrates, proteins, and fats in most tissues. Also, insulin influences carbohydrate, protein, and fat metabolism by stimulating protein and free fatty acid synthesis, and by inhibiting release of free fatty acid from adipose cells. Insulin increases active glucose transport through muscle and adipose cellular membranes, and promotes conversion of intracellular glucose and free fatty acid to the appropriate storage forms (glycogen and triglyceride, respectively). Although the liver does not require active glucose transport, insulin increases hepatic glucose conversion to glycogen and suppresses hepatic glucose output. Even though the actions of exogenous insulin are identical to those of endogenous insulin, the ability to negatively affect hepatic glucose output differs because a smaller quantity of exogenous insulin reaches the portal vein.

Antidiabetic agent: Administered insulin substitutes for the lack of endogenous insulin secretion and partially corrects the disordered metabolism and inappropriate hyperglycemia of diabetes mellitus, which are caused by either an absolute deficiency or a reduction in the biological effectiveness of insulin, or possibly both. Maintenance of good blood glucose control by insulin, which is facilitated by increasing glucose uptake and use, may slow the progression of the serious long-term complications of diabetes.

Diagnostic aid, pituitary growth hormone reserve: Regular insulin administered intravenously (IV) stimulates growth hormone secretion by producing hypoglycemia, which is used to evaluate pituitary growth hormone reserve.

INDICATIONS

Diabetes, type 1—Insulin is indicated in the treatment of type 1 diabetes (previously called Type I, ketosis-prone, brittle, or juvenile-onset diabetes), which occurs in individuals who produce little or no endogenous insulin. One of two regimens (conventional or intensive therapy) is commonly used to treat this condition. The intensive regimen provides more rigid control of blood glucose than the conventional regimen does, but requires more frequent monitoring and more frequent dosage adjustment and, unless insulin is administered via an insulin pump, a larger number of injections.

Diabetes, type 2—Insulin is indicated in the treatment of certain patients with type 2 diabetes (previously known as Type II, adult-onset, maturity-onset, ketosis-resistant, or stable diabetes), which occurs in individuals who produce or secrete insufficient quantities of endogenous insulin or who have developed resistance to endogenous insulin. Insulin therapy in type 2 diabetes is reserved for patients whose disease is not controlled by other measures, such as diet, exercise, or oral antidiabetic agents, or for patients who cannot tolerate oral antidiabetic agents.

Diabetes mellitus, gestational (GDM); *diabetes mellitus, malnutrition-related*; *diabetes mellitus, other, associated with certain conditions or syndromes, such as pancreatic disease (congenital*

Pharmacology/Pharmacokinetics of Insulin

USP Insulin Type	Onset of Action (hrs)*	Time to Peak (hrs)*	Duration of Action (hrs)*
Intravenous Insulin injection U-100 (regular insulin) pork, purified pork, biosynthetic human, semisynthetic human	1/6-1/2	1/4-1/2	1/2-1
Subcutaneous Insulin injection U-100 (regular insulin) pork, purified pork, biosynthetic human, semisynthetic human	1/2-1	2-4	5-7
Insulin injection U-500 (regular insulin) purified pork, biosynthetic human			24†
Isophane insulin suspension U-100 (NPH insulin) mixed, ‡ pork, purified pork, biosynthetic human	3-4	6-12	18-28
Isophane insulin suspension (70%) and insulin injection (30%) U-100 biosynthetic human	1/2	4-8	24
Insulin zinc suspension U-100 (lente insulin) mixed, ‡ pork, purified pork, biosynthetic human	1-3	8-12	18-28
Extended insulin zinc suspension U-100 (ultralente) biosynthetic human	4-6	18-24	36
Prompt insulin zinc suspension U-100 (semilente)	1-3	2-8	12-16

* Mean values; individual responses vary widely.

† U-500 strength is absorbed slowly, resulting in a long duration of action.

‡ Mixture of beef and pork insulins.

absence of the pancreatic islets, transient diabetes of the new-born, functional immaturity of insulin secretion in the neonate, or cystic fibrosis), endocrine disease (endocrine overactivity due to Cushing's syndrome, hyperthyroidism, pheochromocytoma, somatostatinoma, or aldosteronoma; endocrine underactivity due to hypoparathyroidism-hypocalcemia, type I isolated growth hormone deficiency, or multitropic pituitary deficiency), and genetic syndromes, including inborn errors of metabolism (glycogen-storage disease type I or insulin-resistant syndromes, such as muscular dystrophies, late onset proximal myopathy, and Huntington's chorea)—Insulin is indicated for the treatment of GDM and for the treatment of diabetes mellitus associated with certain conditions and syndromes uncontrolled by other treatment measures (diet, exercise, and oral antidiabetic agents). Insulin requirements eventually increase during pregnancy for all patients with diabetes. Need for additional exogenous insulin usually stops postpartum for GDM patients due to hormonal and metabolic changes; however, in some patients, GDM progresses to type 1 or type 2 diabetes within 5 to 10 years. Insulin is also used to treat diabetes induced by hormones, medications, or chemicals. Insulin has been added to total parenteral nutrition and glucose solutions in order to facilitate glucose utilization in patients with poor glucose tolerance.

—Insulin is also used to treat acute complications associated with diabetes, such as ketoacidosis, significant acidosis, ketosis, hyperglycemic hyperosmolar nonketotic coma, and diabetic coma. Also, temporary insulin dosing for patients with diabetes who do not usually require insulin or an increased insulin dosage for patients with type 1 diabetes or patients with type 2 diabetes who require insulin may be warranted when these patients are subjected to physical stress (e.g., pregnancy, fever, severe infection, severe burns, major surgery, or other severe trauma).

—Combination use of insulin and oral antidiabetic agents in patients with type 1 diabetes is controversial because many studies have indicated that oral antidiabetic agents are not effective in the treatment of these patients. Some patients with type 2 diabetes who are resistant to sulfonylureas alone may benefit from the combination of low-dose insulin and oral sulfonylurea agents for diabetes; however, resultant weight gain and effects of hyperinsulinemia should be considered. In addition, the combination of metformin and sulfonylurea agents has been used successfully before discontinuation of oral agents and initiation of insulin therapy.

—Concentrated insulin (500 USP Insulin Units per mL) is used to treat only insulin-resistant patients needing a high dosage (>200 USP Units) of insulin.

Nephropathy, diabetic (prophylaxis); *retinopathy, diabetic* (prophylaxis)—Insulin, used in an intensified regimen, is indicated to prevent the development or slow the progression of microvascular complications, including diabetic nephropathy, neuropathy, and retinopathy, in patients with type 1 and type 2 diabetes.

—In 2 large, long-term clinical trials (the Diabetes Control and Complications Trial [DCCT] and the Stockholm Diabetes Intervention Study [SDIS]), patients with type 1 diabetes who followed an intensified regimen that included at least 3 insulin injections each day realized improved microvascular outcomes compared to patients who followed a conventional regimen that included only 1 or 2 insulin injections each day. In addition to the 3 daily insulin injections, intensive therapy involved self-monitoring of blood glucose concentrations at least 4 times a day with adjustments in insulin dosage made as necessary, monthly clinic visits, individualized diabetes education, and continuous tutoring. The goal of intensive therapy was to achieve and maintain blood glucose concentrations and glycosylated hemoglobin (HbA1c) values as close to normal as possible. In the DCCT, in which patients were followed for an average of 6.5 years, this goal was met by 44% of patients who achieved HbA1c values of 6.05% or less at least one time during the study; however, less than 5% of patients were able to maintain values within the normal range. In the SDIS, in which patients were followed for 7.5 years, patients in the intensive therapy group achieved a mean HbA1c value of slightly more than 7%. This value was higher than normal, but it was statistically significant compared to the baseline values obtained in the same group ($9.5\% \pm 1.3\%$) and to the outcome values obtained in patients who received conventional therapy ($8.5\% \pm 0.7\%$; $P = 0.001$). As a result of the lowered blood glucose concentrations achieved with intensive insulin therapy, the risk of development of nephropathy, neuropathy, and retinopathy was reduced by 35% to 76% in patients with no existing disease, and the progression of disease was slowed by approximately 55% in patients with mild forms of disease.

—Intensive insulin therapy also has been shown to significantly reduce the risk of development of microvascular complications in patients with type 2 diabetes. Several long-term, randomized, controlled clinical trials, including the 10-year United Kingdom Prospective Diabetes Study (UKPDS), have demonstrated that patients who received intensive insulin therapy consisting of at least 3 insulin injections each day were able to maintain HbA1c values of approximately 7%. This value was significantly lower than the HbA1c values achieved by patients who received conventional therapy consisting of 1 or 2 insulin injections each day and, in the UKPDS, represented an 11% reduction over baseline values. Consequently, the onset and the progression of diabetic nephropathy, neuropathy, and retinopathy were effectively delayed in type 2 patients who followed an intensified regimen compared with type 2 patients who followed a conventional regimen.

Growth hormone deficiency (diagnosis)—Regular insulin administered IV is used to assess the capacity of the pituitary gland to release growth hormone. Reliable results may require that more than one test be performed, using either regular insulin or arginine. This test may also be used to obtain information regarding release of corticotropin from the pituitary. A physician experienced in the use of the insulin tolerance test should be present because of the risk of hypoglycemia.

Hyperglycemia during IV nutrition in low birth weight infants (treatment)—Insulin is indicated for the treatment of hyperglycemia caused by IV nutrition in low birth weight infants.

Drug Interactions for Insulin

Precipitant Drug	Object Drug	Effect On Object Drug	Description
◆ Alcohol	Insulin	↑	Consumption of moderate or large amounts of alcohol enhances insulin's hypoglycemic effect, increasing the risk of prolonged, severe hypoglycemia, especially under fasting conditions or when liver glycogen stores are low; small amounts of alcohol consumed with meals do not usually present problems.
Anabolic steroids (stanozolol, oxandrolone, methandrostenolone)	Insulin	↑	Increased tissue sensitivity to insulin and increased tissue resistance to glucagon may occur, resulting in hypoglycemia, especially when insulin resistance is present; a decrease in insulin dosage may be required.
Antidiabetic agents Carbonic anhydrase inhibitors (acetazolamide) Sulfonylurea	Insulin	↑	These medications chronically stimulate the pancreatic ß cell to release insulin and increase receptor and tissue sensitivity to insulin; although concurrent use of these medications with insulin may increase the hypoglycemic response, the effect may be unpredictable.
◆ Beta-adrenergic blocking agents	Insulin	↔	May inhibit insulin secretion, modify carbohydrate metabolism, and increase peripheral insulin resistance, leading to hyperglycemia; however, they may also cause hypoglycemia and block the normal catecholamine-mediated response to hypoglycemia (glycogenolysis and mobilization of glucose), thereby prolonging the time it takes to achieve euglycemia and increasing the risk of a severe hypoglycemic reaction. Selective ß$_1$-adrenergic blocking agents (such as acebutolol, atenolol, betaxolol, bisoprolol, and metoprolol) exhibit the above actions to a lesser extent; however, any of these agents can blunt some of the symptoms of developing hypoglycemia, such as increased heart rate or blood pressure (increased sweating may not be altered), making detection of this complication more difficult.
Chloroquine Quinidine Quinine	Insulin	↑	Concurrent use with insulin may increase the risk of hypoglycemia and increased blood insulin concentrations because of decreased insulin degradation.
◆ Corticosteroids	Insulin	↓	These agents antagonize insulin's effects by stimulating release of catecholamines, causing hyperglycemia; corticosteroid-induced diabetes can occur in up to 14% of the patients taking systemic corticosteroids for several weeks or with prolonged use of topical corticosteroids, but this condition rarely produces acidosis or ketonuria even with high glucose concentrations; reversal of effects may take several weeks or months; changes in insulin dosage may be necessary for patients with diabetes during and following concurrent use.
Diuretics, loop or thiazide	Insulin	↓	Concurrent use with insulin may increase the risk of hyperglycemia because the potassium-depleting effect of these diuretics may inhibit insulin secretion and decrease tissue sensitivity to insulin.
Guanethidine MAOIs (furazolidone, procarbazine, selegiline)	Insulin	↔	Epinephrine release by these agents may cause hyperglycemia; however, chronic use results in hypoglycemia; the mechanism of the latter is unknown but may include stored catecholamine depletion and interference with the compensatory adrenergic response to a fall in blood glucose; a change in dosage of insulin before, during, and after treatment with these agents may be necessary.

Drug Interactions for Insulin (cont.)

Precipitant Drug	Object Drug	Effect On Object Drug	Description
Hyperglycemia-causing agents (eg, calcium channel blockers; clonidine; danazol; dextrothyroxine; diazoxide, parenteral; epinephrine; estrogen; estrogen-progestin-containing oral contraceptives; glucagons; growth hormone; heparin; histamine H_2-receptor antagonists; marijuana; morphine; nicotine; phenytoin; sulfinpyrazone; thyroid hormones)	Insulin	↓	These medications may change metabolic control of glucose concentrations and, unless the changes can be controlled with diet, may necessitate an increase in the amount or a change in the timing of the insulin dosage.
Hypoglycemia-causing agents (eg, ACE inhibitors; bromocriptine; clofibrate; ketoconazole; lithium; mebendazole; pyridoxine; sulfonamides; theophylline)	Insulin	↑	These medications may change metabolic control of glucose concentrations and, unless the changes can be controlled with diet, may necessitate a decrease in the amount or a change in the timing of the insulin dosage.
NSAIDs	Insulin	↑	These medications inhibit synthesis of prostaglandin E (which inhibits endogenous insulin secretion), thereby increasing basal insulin secretion, the response to a glucose load, and the hypoglycemic effect of concurrently administered insulin; dosage adjustment of the NSAID or salicylate and/or insulin may be necessary, especially during and following chronic concurrent use.
Octreotide	Insulin	↔	Octreotide can cause changes in the counterregulatory hormones' secretion (insulin, glucagon, and growth hormone) and slow gastric emptying and gastrointestinal contractility, resulting in delayed meal absorption and mild transient hypoglycemia or hyperglycemia in individuals with or without diabetes; in patients with diabetes, insulin therapy may need to be reduced following the initiation of octreotide and monitored for adjustments during and after octreotide treatment.
♦ Pentamidine	Insulin	↔	Pentamidine has a toxic effect on pancreatic beta cells, resulting in a biphasic effect on glucose concentration (i.e., initial insulin release and hypoglycemia followed by hypoinsulinemia and hyperglycemia) with continued use of pentamidine; initially, insulin dosage should be reduced, then the dosage should be increased with continued use of pentamidine.
Tetracycline	Insulin	↔	A delayed onset of increased tissue sensitivity to insulin may occur in patients with diabetes; this reaction has not occurred in individuals with normal glucose tolerance.
Tobacco, smoking	Insulin	↓	May antagonize insulin effects by stimulating release of catecholamines, causing hyperglycemia; also, smoking reduces subcutaneous insulin absorption; dosage reduction of insulin may be necessary when an insulin-dependent patient suddenly stops smoking.

♦ = Major clinical significance. ACE = angiotensin-converting enzyme; MAOI = monoamine oxidase inhibitor; NSAID = nonsteroidal anti-inflammatory drug.

CONTRAINDICATIONS

Risk-benefit should be considered when the following medical problems exist:

- Allergy or local skin sensitivity to insulins.

- Diarrhea, gastroparesis, intestinal obstruction, vomiting, or other conditions causing delayed food absorption or malabsorption—*major clinical significance* (vomiting or delayed stomach emptying may require a change in timing of the insulin dose to realign peak action to peak blood glucose concentrations).

- Hepatic disease (insulin requirements are complex, and an increase or decrease of dosage may be needed partly because of modifications in hepatic metabolism of insulin and alterations in hepatic and plasma glucose concentrations).

- Hyperglycemia-causing conditions, such as female hormonal changes; fever, high; hyperadrenalism, not optimally controlled; infection, severe; psychological stress—*major clinical significance* (these conditions may increase blood glucose, increase or change the insulin requirement, and necessitate more frequent blood glucose monitoring; insulin requirements may be increased near or during a menstrual cycle and may return to normal after menstruation; also, a change to IV insulin administration may be needed during labor when close glucose control is necessary).

- Hyperthyroidism, not optimally controlled (hyperthyroidism increases both the activity and the clearance of insulin, making glycemic control difficult until the patient is euthyroid).

- Hypoglycemia-causing conditions, such as adrenal insufficiency, not optimally controlled; pituitary insufficiency, not optimally controlled—*major clinical significance* (these conditions, by reducing blood glucose concentrations, may decrease the insulin requirement and necessitate more frequent blood glucose monitoring; also, untreated or not optimally controlled adrenal or pituitary insufficiency may increase tissue sensitivity to insulin and reduce the patient's insulin requirement).

- Renal disease (insulin requirements are complex, and an increase or decrease of dosage may be needed due to modifications in renal clearance of insulin).

- Surgery or trauma (hypoglycemia or hyperglycemia may occur, depending on the surgery or trauma; a change to IV insulin administration may be needed when close glucose control is necessary).

WARNINGS/PRECAUTIONS

Patients intolerant of beef or pork insulins may use the alternative single-source insulin under the direction of their physician. Intolerance of beef insulin is more common than intolerance of pork insulin. Intolerance is often reduced by the use of purified pork insulin, biosynthetic human insulin, or semisynthetic human insulin. Patients hypersensitive to protamine sulfate may also be hypersensitive to protamine-containing insulins. Patients who have become sensitized to protamine through administration of a protamine-containing insulin are at risk for severe anaphylactoid reactions if protamine sulfate is subsequently administered for reversal of heparin effect.

Pregnancy: Insulin does not cross the placenta. However, maternal glucose and maternal insulin antibodies do cross the placenta and can cause fetal hyperinsulinemia and related problems, such as large-for-gestational-age infants and macrosomnia, possibly resulting in a need for early induced or cesarean delivery. Furthermore, high blood glucose concentrations occurring during early pregnancy (5-8 weeks' gestation) have been associated with a higher incidence of major congenital abnormalities and, later in pregnancy, increased perinatal morbidity and mortality.

Women with diabetes must be educated about the necessity of maintaining strict metabolic control before conception and throughout pregnancy, especially during early pregnancy, to significantly decrease the risk of maternal mortality, congenital anomalies, and perinatal morbidity and mortality. Use of insulin rather than oral antidiabetic agents for the treatment of type 2 diabetes and GDM permits maintenance of blood glucose at concentrations as close to normal as possible. Insulin requirements in pregnant patients with diabetes often are decreased during the first trimester. Requirements usually are increased in the last 2 trimesters of pregnancy in response to the anti-insulin hormone activity associated with increased concentrations of human placental estrogen, progesterone, chorionic gonadotropin, and prolactin; peripheral insulin resistance due to increasing levels of fatty acids and triglycerides; and increased degradation of insulin by the placenta.

Postpartum: Insulin requirements drop quickly after childbirth, and GDM patients usually no longer need insulin. Inadequately controlled maternal blood glucose late in pregnancy may cause increased insulin production in the fetus, resulting in neonatal hypoglycemia. Treatment may be necessary until euglycemic control is established by the neonate.

Breastfeeding: Insulin is not distributed into breast milk. Problems in humans have not been documented. The insulin requirement in lactating women is reduced because of hormonal changes; in patients with type 1 diabetes, insulin requirements during lactation may be up to 27% lower than the patient's pre-pregnancy requirements. Daily monitoring for several months is important until insulin needs stabilize or until insulin is no longer needed.

ADVERSE REACTIONS

Those indicating need for medical attention: Incidence more frequent

Hypoglycemia—mild, including nocturnal hypoglycemia (anxiety; behavior change similar to drunkenness; blurred vision; cold sweats; confusion; cool, pale skin; difficulty in concentrating; drowsiness; excessive hunger; fast heartbeat; headache; nausea; nervousness; nightmares; restless sleep; shakiness; slurred speech; unusual tiredness or weakness); hypoglycemia—severe (coma; seizures); weight gain.

Incidence rare:

Edema (swelling of face, fingers, feet, or ankles); lipoatrophy at injection site (depression of the skin at the injection site); lipohypertrophy at injection site (thickening of the skin at the injection site).

ADMINISTRATION AND DOSAGE

General Dosing Information

In the United States, the potency of insulin is expressed in terms of USP Insulin Units or USP Insulin Human Units. Bovine or porcine insulin contains not less than 26 USP Insulin Units per mg of insulin on the dried basis. Human insulin contains not less than 27.5 USP Insulin Human Units per mg of insulin on the dried basis. International Units cannot be compared directly to USP Units because the reference standards and the methodologies for manufacturing are different. It is generally not recommended that patients whose diabetes is well controlled with animal insulins automatically be switched to human insulins. Human insulins may not offer any significant advantage over the highly purified pork insulins, with the exception of reduced antibody concentrations, which may be a consideration for some patients, especially children, young adults, patients who are pregnant or considering pregnancy, patients with allergies, or patients using insulin intermittently. Patients should be informed of the possible need for dosage adjustment during the first 1 to 2 weeks following a change in the source of their insulin products (bovine and porcine, porcine, or human) and advised not to make such a change without first consulting their physician. Transferring patients from oral hypoglycemic agents to insulin can be immediate, although blood glucose concentrations should be evaluated for several days following the change, and the prolonged effects of chlorpropamide should be considered when determining the insulin dosage.

The vial of insulin must not be shaken hard before being used. Frothing or bubble formation can cause an incorrect dose. Contents are mixed well by rolling the bottle slowly between the palms of the hands or by gently tipping the bottle over a few times. Insulin should not be used if it looks lumpy or grainy or sticks to the bottle. Also, regular insulin should not be used if it becomes viscous or cloudy; only clear, colorless solutions should be used. Dilution of insulin preparations generally should be avoided. However, some pediatric doses may be too small to measure accurately. If needed, diluting from U-100 to U-10 has been suggested to aid in accurate dosing for very small doses in pediatric patients. Such dilutions are stable for 2 months when stored at 4°C (39°F) or until the date of expiration of the insulin, whichever occurs first. Occasionally, insulin must be diluted to avoid crystallization in the catheters when it is administered as a low-dose infusion via an insulin pump. In these rare cases, dilution should be performed aseptically in a laminar flow hood using diluents and mixing vials provided or recommended by the manufacturer. The differences in strength, dosage volume, and expiration date should be clearly labeled by the pharmacist and emphasized to the patient. If insulin needs to be diluted during an emergency and the diluents are not readily available, 0.9% sodium chloride injection without preservative may be used for dilution of small insulin doses. However, these solutions are not stable and should be used promptly. Stinging or burning at the site of injection also may occur due to the lower pH of these solutions.

Different types of insulin are sometimes mixed in the syringe in proportions ordered by the physician in order to achieve a more accurate matching of insulin availability to the patient's requirements in a single dose. If insulins are to be mixed, several factors should be considered:

- Each patient should always follow the same sequence of mixing the separate insulin preparations. As a rule, regular insulin should be drawn first to avoid contamination and clouding of the vial of regular insulin by the other insulin. A mixture of regular insulin and another insulin will have a longer duration of action than does regular insulin alone.

- Insulin zinc, prompt insulin zinc, and extended insulin zinc may be mixed in any proportion without loss of the characteristics of the individual insulins. Such mixtures are stable for up to 18 months.

- Unbuffered regular insulin and isophane insulin may be mixed in any proportion in a syringe and stored upright if possible. The prefilled syringe can be used immediately, stored at room temperature and used within 14 days, or stored in a refrigerator for use within 3 weeks. Mixtures containing buffered regular insulin should be used immediately.

- Mixing unbuffered regular insulin and insulin zinc insulins (lente, semilente, and ultralente) is not recommended because the excess zinc in the insulin zinc insulin can form an extra zinc insulin complex with the regular insulin. This can lengthen the insulin's duration of action and give unpredict-

able clinical results. However, if these insulins are combined, it is recommended that the mixture be used immediately.

- Phosphate buffered regular insulin or isophane insulins should not be mixed with insulin zinc insulins. Zinc phosphate may precipitate from the mixture, which can shorten the expected duration of action and provide unpredictable clinical results.

- Phosphate buffered regular insulin should not be mixed with any other insulin when used in an external insulin infusion pump because of the potential problem of precipitation.

After receiving insulin at first diagnosis of type 1 diabetes, 20% to 30% of patients appear to normalize for a few weeks or months (called the honeymoon phase). Some clinicians continue insulin treatment in small doses of 0.2 to 0.5 USP Units per kg of body weight during this time. Conventional and intensive insulin therapies are individualized insulin regimens that provide different levels of blood glucose control. Conventional therapy consists of 1or 2 insulin injections a day and daily self-monitoring of urine or blood glucose, but not daily adjustments of insulin dosage. Intensive insulin therapy provides tighter blood glucose control via administration of 3 or more injections a day or by use of an insulin pump. Also, adjustments of insulin dose according to the results of self-monitoring of blood glucose determinations are performed at least 4 times a day and before anticipated dietary intake and exercise. The dosage and timing of administration of insulin can vary greatly and must therefore be determined for each individual patient by the attending physician. Matching the patient's specific insulin needs over a 24-hour period through the use of short-acting and longer-acting preparations may decrease long-term complications of diabetes mellitus.

If a pattern of metabolic noncontrol ensues (blood glucose concentrations changing for 3 days), the total daily insulin dosage usually is adjusted by changing only one type of insulin and only one segment of the daily dosage; the first preprandial dose is the one most commonly changed because it more prominently affects the other doses of the day. Insulin requirements may change with diet or physical activity. Algorithms can be developed to aid a patient with supplemental or anticipatory insulin dosing needs based on the patient's sensitivity to insulin. Supplemental doses of regular insulin can be used to correct excessive preprandial blood glucose concentrations after the basic dosage of insulin is established. Anticipatory insulin doses are based on anticipated dietary or physical activity changes. Because of the increased risk of secondary hyperglycemia due to exercise, patients should be cautioned against exercising if the blood glucose concentration exceeds 240mg/dL (13.3mmol/L) or when a condition exists that causes low glucagon stores. Additional low doses of regular insulin (1-2 USP Units for each 30-40mg/dL [1.7-2.2mmol/L] incremental rise above the target blood glucose concentration) every 3 to 4 hours may be needed on sick days. Patients should be warned to inform the physician if the concentration remains above 240mg/dL (13.3mmol/L) after 3 supplementary insulin doses or if symptoms of ketoacidosis develop. The patient should always use only one brand or type of syringe and should consult the physician before changing brands or syringe types. Among different brands or syringe types, the unmeasured volume between the needle point and the bottom calibration on the syringe barrel (called dead space) may differ enough to cause improper dosage.

The use of a disposable syringe and needle to administer more than one injection is controversial. Although USP medical advisory panels do not recommend this practice, it must be recognized that some patients reuse disposable syringes and needles because of economic constraints. Where this is occurring, it must be emphasized that the syringe and needle be used for only one particular patient; that the needle be wiped with alcohol; and that the cap of the needle be replaced after each use. Also, the syringe and needle should be reused only for a limited number of injections. Disposable syringes and needles should not be reused on a continuing basis.

For intravenous infusion:

Regular insulin (Insulin Injection USP and Insulin Human Injection USP) in the 100-USP-Unit concentration is the only insulin type suitable for IV administration. Insulin can be adsorbed to the surfaces of glass and plastic IV infusion containers (including polyvinyl chloride [PVC], ethylene vinyl acetate, and polyethylene). Adsorption is unpredictable, and the clinical significance is uncertain. Recommendations for minimizing adsorption include adding 0.35% serum albumin human or approximately 5mL of the patient's blood or using a syringe pump with a short cannula. For admixtures of insulin greater than 100 USP Units per 500mL of IV solution, decant 50mL of IV solution containing insulin through the administration apparatus and store for 30 minutes before using for optimal results. Afterward, insulin dosage should be adjusted to meet the patient's targeted blood glucose concentration. Regular insulin is compatible with dextrose injection, 0.9% sodium chloride injection, and combinations of these.

For continuous subcutaneous insulin infusion pump:

Generally, buffered regular insulin is used in insulin pumps, although unbuffered regular insulin has been used. Phosphate buffered regular insulin is less likely to crystallize and block insulin pump catheters and is preferred over unbuffered regular insulin. Following the recommendations and suggested maintenance procedures of insulin pump manufacturers is important to ensure optimal performance and to avoid problems, such as insulin adhesion or clogging. Consult the individual manufacturer's package inserts. When initiating a continuous subcutaneous insulin infusion with an insulin pump, a priming dose may be needed. Without an initial priming dose, the depot forms at a very slow rate. Pumps with a short pulse-rate interval have little superiority over pumps with a longer interval in relation to the depot formation. An additional priming dose is not necessary when the infusion site is changed. Absorption of insulin from the depot at the first site continues after discontinuation of the infusion, preventing insulin concentrations from decreasing to subtherapeutic values while another depot is forming at the new site.

INSULIN PORK REGULAR PRODUCTS	
Brand Name	**Dosage Form**
Iletin II Regular Pork (Lilly)	**Solution:** 100 U/mL
INSULIN PORK ISOPHANE (LENTE) PRODUCTS	
Brand Name	**Dosage Form**
Iletin II Lente Pork (Lilly)	**Suspension:** 100 U/mL
INSULIN PORK ISOPHANE (NPH) PRODUCTS	
Brand Name	**Dosage Form**
Iletin II NPH Pork (Lilly)	**Suspension:** 100 U/mL
INSULIN HUMAN REGULAR PRODUCTS	
Brand Name	**Dosage Form**
Humulin R (Lilly)	**Solution:** 100 U/mL
Novolin R (Novo Nordisk)	**Solution:** 100 U/mL
Novolin R Innolet (Novo Nordisk)	**Solution:** 100 U/mL
Novolin R Penfill (Novo Nordisk)	**Solution:** 100 U/mL
INSULIN HUMAN ZINC (LENTE) PRODUCTS	
Brand Name	**Dosage Form**
Humulin L (Lilly)	**Suspension:** 100 U/mL
INSULIN HUMAN ZINC, EXTENDED (ULTRALENTE) PRODUCTS	
Brand Name	**Dosage Form**
Humulin U (Lilly)	**Suspension:** 100 U/mL
INSULIN HUMAN NPH/REGULAR PRODUCTS	
Brand Name	**Dosage Form**
Humulin 50/50 (Lilly)	**Suspension:** 50 U/mL-50 U/mL
Humulin 70/30 (Lilly)	**Suspension:** 70 U/mL-50 U/mL
Novolin 70/30 (Novo Nordisk)	**Suspension:** 70 U/mL-50 U/mL
Novolin 70/30 Innolet (Novo Nordisk)	**Suspension:** 70 U/mL-50 U/mL
Novolin 70/30 Penfill (Novo Nordisk)	**Suspension:** 70 U/mL-50 U/mL

PRODUCT INFORMATION FOR BLOOD GLUCOSE METERS

The following table provides a quick comparison of the ingredients and dosages of common brand-name OTC drugs. Products are listed alphabetically by category and brand name.

GLUCOMETER	TEST STRIPS
Accu-Chek Active System (Roche)	Accu-Chek Active
Accu-Chek Advantage (Roche)	Accu-Chek Comfort Curve
Accu-Chek Aviva System (Roche)	Accu-Chek Aviva
Accu-Chek Compact System (Roche)	Accu-Chek Compact
Accu-Chek Compact Plus System (Roche)	Accu-Chek Compact
Accu-Chek Complete System (Roche)	Accu-Chek Comfort Curve
Accu-Chek Go System (Roche)	Accu-Chek Go
Accu-Chek Inform System (Roche)	Accu-Chek Comfort
Ascensia Breeze (Bayer)	Ascensia Autodisc
Ascensia Contour (Bayer)	Ascensia Microfill
Ascensia Dex (Bayer)	Ascensia Autodisc
Ascensia Elite (Bayer)	Ascensia Elite
Ascenia Elite XL (Bayer)	Acensia Elite
CoZmonitor (Abbott)	FreeStyle
FreeStyle (Abbott)	FreeStyle
FreeStyle Flash (Abbott)	FreeStyle
InDuo System (LifeScan)	OneTouch Ultra
OneTouch Ultra (LifeScan)	OneTouch Ultra
OneTouch UltraSmart (LifeScan)	OneTouch Ultra
OneTouch Basic (LifeScan)	OneTouch
OneTouch FastTake (LifeScan)	OneTouch FastTake
OneTouch Profile (LifeScan)	OneTouch
OneTouch SureStep (LifeScan)	OneTouch SureStep
Precision Xtra (Abbott)	Precision Xtra

Constipation

Constipation can be defined as infrequent or difficult evacuation of stool. Normal stool frequency ranges from three times a week to twice a day; infrequency is passage of two or fewer evacuations per week. Difficult evacuation is variously described as the inability to initiate defecation, straining, or incomplete evacuation. It is essential to know exactly what the patient means by "constipation" before planning management.

Persistent constipation that is caused by some definable disease is called *secondary constipation*. Causes of secondary constipation include endocrine and metabolic conditions, neurologic diseases, organic anorectal and colonic diseases, and drugs. When no primary (underlying) cause for constipation is identified, it is classified as *idiopathic constipation*. The two major syndromes of idiopathic constipation are slow transit and functional outlet obstruction. These are also the pathophysiologic mechanisms for secondary constipation.

Slow transit constipation is a failure of propulsion through the colon, thought to result from dysfunction of the enteric nerves or of the smooth muscle of the colon. Clinically, patients with slow transit constipation have infrequent stools as their primary symptom. Once stool gets into position for evacuation, it can be expelled relatively easily. Slow transit is the most common mechanism of idiopathic constipation. *Functional outlet obstruction constipation* is caused by ineffective opening or blockage of the anal canal during defecation or by failure of expulsion by the rectum. The normal process of defecation involves removal of a series of barriers to the evacuation of stool. Errors in the execution of any of these steps can lead to constipation. Patients may have a normal stool frequency but typically complain about difficulty with evacuation. Functional outlet obstruction may coexist with slow transit constipation and may limit the effectiveness of treatment for slow transit constipation if not dealt with first.

An otherwise healthy patient less than 45 years of age with mild symptoms and no evidence of structural, medical, or neurologic disease can usually be treated initially with fiber supplements and, if needed, osmotic laxatives. Patients aged 45 years and older, patients who fail conservative treatment, or patients with anemia or occult blood in the stool should undergo colonoscopy or sigmoidoscopy and barium enema to identify structural colonic diseases. Consultation with a gastroenterologist is recommended for patients with constipation that does not respond to standard medical management. Such patients may require further investigations, such as colonic transit and/or pelvic floor function studies.

Constipation affects all age groups and both sexes. Children may have problems with congenital disorders, such as Hirschsprung's disease, or functional problems such as encopresis (constipation associated with overflow incontinence). Young adults most often have functional problems related to abnormal colonic motility or pelvic floor dysfunction. Older individuals develop constipation due to other disorders, drug therapy, dementia, or structural problems. Constipation and associated problems account for more than 2.5 million patient visits to physicians each year. An even larger number of people with constipation manage it themselves with OTC or herbal laxatives such as bisacodyl, docusate, senna, polycarbophil, psyllium, castor oil, mineral oil, and glycerin.

LAXATIVES

PHARMACOLOGY

Bulk-forming: Absorbs water and expands to provide increased bulk and moisture content to the stool. The increased bulk encourages normal peristalsis and bowel motility.

Carbon dioxide-releasing: Carbon dioxide released from combined potassium bitartrate and sodium bicarbonate induces gentle pressure in the rectum, thus promoting bowel movement.

Hyperosmotic: Glycerin: Attracts water into the stool, thereby stimulating rectal contraction; also, lubricates and softens inspissated fecal mass.

Lactulose: Produces osmotic effect in the colon resulting from biodegradation by colonic bacterial flora into lactic, formic, and acetic acids. Fluid accumulation produces distention, which in turn promotes increased peristalsis and bowel evacuation.

Polyethylene glycol: Prevents absorption by the intestinal tract of the portion of water ingested, serving to hydrate and soften the stool and promote peristalsis.

Saline: Produces osmotic effect primarily in the small intestine by drawing water into the intestinal lumen. Fluid accumulation produces distention, which in turn promotes increased peristalsis and bowel evacuation. During the use of saline laxatives, the release of cholecystokinin from the intestinal mucosa may enhance the laxative effect.

Lubricant: Increases water retention in the stool by coating surfaces of the stool and intestines with a water-immiscible film. Lubricant effect eases passage of the contents through intestines. Emulsification of the lubricant tends to enhance its ability to soften the stool mass.

Stool softener: Reduces surface film tension of the interfacing liquid contents of the bowel, promoting permeation of additional liquid into the stool to form a softer mass.

Stimulant: Precise mechanism of action is unknown. Thought to increase peristalsis by a direct effect on the smooth intestinal musculature by stimulation of intramural nerve plexi. Also has been shown to promote fluid and ion accumulation in the colon (castor oil acts on the small intestine) to increase the laxative effect.

Antihyperammonemic: Lactulose decreases blood ammonia concentrations probably as a result of its bacterial degradation, in the colon, into low molecular weight organic acids that decrease the pH of the colonic contents. Acidification of colonic contents results in the retention of ammonia in the colon as the ammonium ion. The osmotic laxative action of the metabolites of lactulose expels the trapped ammonium from the colon.

Hydrocholeretic: Dehydrocholic acid has no effect on the production of bile salts; however, it increases bile volume and flow by increasing water output, thus producing bile of relatively low specific gravity, viscosity, and total solid content.

Antidiarrheal: Psyllium hydrophilic mucilloid and polycarbophil's water and bile salt-binding capacity may result in fewer and bulkier stools.

Antihyperlipidemic: Psyllium hydrophilic mucilloid has an antihyperlipidemic effect. It decreases serum total cholesterol, low-density lipoprotein (LDL) cholesterol, and the ratio of LDL cholesterol to high-density lipoprotein (HDL) cholesterol. Although the exact mechanism of psyllium's antihyperlipidemic effect is not known, it is believed that psyllium increases bile acid secretion, thus draining cholesterol products from the body.

INDICATIONS

Constipation (prophylaxis)—Oral bulk-forming, lubricant, and stool softener laxatives are indicated prophylactically in patients who should not strain during defecation, such as those with an episiotomy wound, painful thrombosed hemorrhoids, fissures or perianal abscesses, body wall and diaphragmatic hernias, anorectal stenosis, or postmyocardial infarction. An oral hyperosmotic laxative (polyethylene glycol 3350) is indicated for the prevention of constipation.

Constipation (treatment)—Oral laxatives are indicated for the short-term relief of constipation. Oral bulk-forming laxatives, stimulant laxatives, and carbon dioxide-releasing suppositories are indicated to facilitate defecation in geriatric patients with diminished colonic motor response. Oral bulk-forming laxatives and stool softener laxatives are preferred to treat constipation that may occur during pregnancy and postpartum to help reestablish normal bowel function or to avoid straining if hemorrhoids are present. An oral hyperosmotic laxative (polyethylene glycol 3350) is indicated for the treatment of occasional constipation. In severe cases of constipation, such as with fecal impaction, mineral oil and stool softener laxatives administered orally or rectally are indicated to soften the impacted feces. To help complete the evacuation of the impacted colon, a rectal stimulant or saline laxative may follow.

Bowel evacuation—Pre- and postpartum: Carbon dioxide-releasing suppositories are indicated to evacuate the colon in preparation for delivery and for a few days after to help reestablish normal bowel function.

—Preoperative and Preradiography: Oral or rectal stimulant and oral saline laxatives, rectal preparations of glycerin, and carbon dioxide-releasing suppositories are also indicated to evacuate the colon in preparation for rectal and bowel examinations and for elective colon surgery.

—Parasites, intestinal (treatment adjunct): Oral saline laxatives are indicated to accelerate excretion of various parasites including nematodes, after anthelmintic therapy.

—Toxicity, nonspecific (treatment adjunct): Oral saline laxatives are also indicated to hasten excretion of poisonous substances (except acids or alkalies) from the gastrointestinal tract.

Laxative dependency (treatment)—Glycerin suppositories are indicated temporarily to reestablish normal bowel function in laxative-dependent patients.

Pharmacology/Pharmacokinetics of Laxatives

Type of Laxative	Absorption		Onset of action		Type of stool formed	Elimination (of absorbed doses)
	Oral	Rectal	Oral	Rectal		
Bulk-forming	Not absorbed		12-24 hrs (up to 3 days)		Soft formed stool	
Carbon dioxide-releasing				5-30 min		
Stool softener or emollient	Unknown amount	Unknown amount	24-48 hrs (up to 3-5 days)	2-15 min	Soft formed stool	Fecal
Hyperosmotic						
Glycerin		Poor		1/4-1 hr		
Lactulose	Minimal (<3% dose)		24-48 hrs		Soft formed stool	Renal
Polyethylene Glycol 3350	None		48-96 hrs			
Saline	Up to 20%dose		1/2-3 hrs	2-5 min	Watery stool (with high doses)	Renal
Lubricant	Minimal*	Minimal	6-8 hrs	2-15 min		
Stimulant			6-8 hrs †			
Anthraquinone derivatives	Minimal			1/2-2 hrs	Soft or formed stool	Fecal and/or renal
Bisacodyl	Minimal	Minimal		1/4-1 hr		Renal
Castor oil	Unknown amount ‡		2-6 hrs		Watery stool	
Danthron	Significant amount				Soft or formed stool	Fecal and/or renal
Dehydrocholic acid	Significant amount					Fecal

* Emulsified mineral oil may be absorbed 30% to 60%.

† Action may be prolonged up to 3 to 4 days.

‡ Ricinoleic acid, the active principle of castor oil produced by hydrolysis, is absorbed to a small extent and metabolized like other fatty acids.

Hyperammonemia (prophylaxis and treatment)—Lactulose is indicated for the prevention and treatment of portal-systemic encephalopathy, including the stages of hepatic precoma and coma.

Biliary tract disorders (treatment)—Dehydrocholic acid is indicated as an adjunct in conditions involving the biliary tract.

Diarrhea (treatment)—Polycarbophil is indicated in the treatment of diarrhea associated with irritable bowel syndrome and diverticulosis and of acute nonspecific diarrhea. Psyllium hydrophilic mucilloid is used in the treatment of choleretic diarrhea and diarrhea caused by vagotomy, small bowel resection, or disease of the terminal ileum.

Bowel syndrome, irritable (treatment adjunct)— Polycarbophil is indicated (and other bulk-forming laxatives are used) to relieve constipation associated with irritable or spastic bowel.

Hyperlipidemia (treatment)—Psyllium hydrophilic mucilloid is used as an adjunct to diet in the treatment of mild to moderate hypercholesterolemia.

CONTRAINDICATIONS

Except under special circumstances, this medication should not be used when the following medical problems exist:

For all classes:

- Appendicitis, or symptoms of—*major clinical significance.*
- Bleeding, rectal, undiagnosed—*major clinical significance.*
- Congestive heart failure—*major clinical significance.*
- Hypertension—*major clinical significance.*
- Diabetes mellitus—*major clinical significance.*
- Intestinal obstruction—*major clinical significance.*
- Sensitivity to the class of laxative being used—*major clinical significance.*

For bulk-forming:

- Dysphagia—*major clinical significance* (esophageal obstruction may occur).

For hyperosmotic—saline:

- Dehydration—*major clinical significance* (may be aggravated by repeated use of saline laxatives).
- Renal function impairment—*major clinical significance* (hyperkalemia and hypermagnesemia may result, especially with preparations containing magnesium and potassium salts; tetany with hypocalcemia and hyperphosphatemia may occur with the use of phosphate salts).

For hyperosmotic—saline and lubricant:

- Colostomy—*major clinical significance.*
- Ileostomy—*major clinical significance* (increased risk of electrolyte or fluid imbalance).

For lubricant:

- Dysphagia—*major clinical significance* (oral mineral oil may be aspirated and cause lipid pneumonitis).

WARNINGS/PRECAUTIONS

Pregnancy:

Hyperosmotic: Saline: Sodium-containing preparations may promote sodium retention with resultant edema. *Polyethylene glycol 3350*: FDA Category C. Studies have not been done in animals or humans.

Lubricant: Repeated oral use of mineral oil may decrease absorption of foods, fat-soluble vitamins, and some oral medications. Hypoprothrombinemia and hemorrhagic disease of the neonate have occurred following chronic use during pregnancy.

Stimulant: Castor oil is contraindicated since its use often results in pelvic area engorgement, which may initiate reflex stimulation of the gravid uterus.

Breastfeeding:

Stimulant: Cascara sagrada and danthron preparations may be distributed into breast milk. The amounts are reportedly large enough to produce loose stools in the infant, although this still remains controversial.

Pediatrics:

For all laxatives: Laxatives should not be given to young children (up to 6 years of age) unless prescribed by a physician. Since children are not usually able to describe their symptoms precisely, proper diagnosis should precede the use of a laxative. This will avoid the complication of an existing condition (eg, appendicitis) or the appearance of more severe side effects.

For lubricant: Oral mineral oil is not recommended for children up to 6 years of age since patients in this age group are more prone to aspiration of oil droplets, which may produce lipid pneumonia.

For stimulant: Bisacodyl enteric-coated tablets are not recommended for children up to 6 years of age since patients in this age group may have difficulty swallowing the tablet without chewing it. Gastric irritation may occur if the enteric coating is destroyed by chewing.

For rectal solutions: Weakness, excessive perspiration, shock, seizures, and/or coma may occur in children with the use of rectal solutions due to water intoxication or dilutional hyponatremia. Seizures with hypocalcemia may occur as a result of absorption of large amounts of phosphate in children receiving sodium phosphates rectal solution.

Geriatrics:

For lubricant: Oral mineral oil is not recommended for bedridden elderly patients since they are more prone to aspiration of oil droplets, which may produce lipid pneumonia.

For osmotic: Polyethylene glycol 3350: There is no evidence for special considerations when polyethylene glycol 3350 is administered to elderly patients. However, a higher incidence of diarrhea occurred in elderly nursing home patients when given the recommended dose of 17g. Polyethylene glycol 3350 should be discontinued if diarrhea occurs.

For stimulant: Weakness, incoordination, and orthostatic hypotension may be exacerbated in elderly patients as a result of significant electrolyte loss when stimulant laxatives are used repeatedly to evacuate the colon.

For rectal solutions: Weakness, excessive perspiration, shock, seizures, and/or coma may occur in elderly patients with the use of rectal solutions due to water intoxication or dilutional hyponatremia.

Drug Interactions for Laxatives

Precipitant Drug	Object Drug	Effect On Object Drug	Description
Antacids Histamine H2-receptor antagonists (cimetidine, famotidine, nizatidine, ranitidine) Milk	Bisacodyl	↔	Administration within 1 hour of bisacodyl tablets may cause the enteric coating to dissolve too rapidly, resulting in gastric or duodenal irritation.
Bulk-forming laxatives	Anticoagulants, oral Digitalis glycosides Salicylates	↓	Concurrent use with cellulose bulk-forming laxatives may reduce the desired effect because of physical binding or other absorptive hindrance; a 2-hour interval between dosage with such medication and laxative dosage is recommended.
♦ Calcium polycarbophil	Tetracyclines, oral	↓	Concurrent use with calcium polycarbophil may decrease absorption because of possible formation of nonabsorbable complexes with free calcium released after ingestion; patients should be advised not to take calcium polycarbophil laxative within 1-2 hours of tetracyclines.
♦ Hyperosmotic-saline, magnesium-containing laxatives	Anticoagulants, coumarin- or indandione-derivatives, oral Digitalis glycosides Phenothiazines (chlorpromazine)	↓	These medications have been shown to have reduced effectiveness in the presence of aluminum- and magnesium-containing antacids; pending further studies, their concurrent administration with magnesium-containing, hyperosmotic-saline laxatives is best avoided.
♦ Hyperosmotic-saline, magnesium containing laxatives	Ciprofloxacin	↓	Magnesium-containing laxatives may reduce absorption by chelation of ciprofloxacin, resulting in lower serum and urine concentrations of the antibiotic; therefore, concurrent use is not recommended.
♦ Hyperosmotic-saline, magnesium containing laxatives	Etidronate	↓	Concurrent use may prevent absorption of oral etidronate; patients should be advised to avoid using magnesium-containing laxatives within 2 hours of etidronate.
Hyperosmotic-saline, magnesium containing laxatives	Sodium polystyrene sulfonate	↔	Sodium polystyrene sulfonate may bind with magnesium, preventing neutralization of bicarbonate ions and leading to systemic alkalosis, which may be severe; concurrent use is not recommended, although the risk may be less with rectal administration of the resin.
♦ Hyperosmotic-saline, magnesium containing laxatives	Tetracyclines, oral	↓	Concurrent use with magnesium-containing laxatives may result in formation of nonabsorbable complexes; patients should be advised not to take these laxatives within 1-2 hours of tetracyclines.
Laxatives, all classes	Potassium-sparing diuretics Potassium supplements	↓	Chronic use or overuse of laxatives may reduce serum potassium concentrations by promoting excessive potassium loss from the intestinal tract; may interfere with potassium-retaining effects of potassium-sparing diuretics.

Drug Interactions for Laxatives (cont.)

Precipitant Drug	Object Drug	Effect On Object Drug	Description
Lubricant laxatives	Anticoagulants, coumarin- or indandione-derivatives, oral Contraceptives, oral Digitalis glycosides Vitamins, fat soluble (A, D, E, K)	↓	Concurrent use with mineral oil may interfere with the proper absorption of these or other medications and reduce their effectiveness. In addition to interfering with absorption of oral anticoagulants, mineral oil also decreases absorption of vitamin K, which may lead to increased anticoagulant effects.
Stool softeners	Danthron Mineral oil	↑	Concurrent use with a stool softener laxative may enhance the systemic absorption of these agents. Although such combinations are intentionally used in some "fixed-dose" laxative preparations, the propensity for toxic effects is greatly increased. Liver injury has been reported with the danthron combination following repeated dosage.

♦ = Major clinical significance.

ADVERSE REACTIONS

Those indicating need for medical attention: Incidence less frequent

For rectal solutions (more frequent with sodium phosphates):

Rectal irritation (rectal bleeding, blistering, burning, itching, or pain).

Incidence rare:

For bulk-forming:

Allergies to some vegetable components (difficulty breathing; skin rash or itching).

Esophageal blockage or intestinal impaction.

For hyperosmotic-saline:

Electrolyte imbalance (confusion; irregular heartbeat; muscle cramps; unusual tiredness or weakness)—due to acute overdosage or chronic misuse.

Magnesium accumulation in presence of renal function impairment (dizziness or light-headedness).

For stimulant:

Allergic reaction to dehydrocholic acid (skin rash).

Electrolyte imbalance (confusion; irregular heartbeat; muscle cramps; unusual tiredness or weakness)—due to acute overdosage or chronic misuse.

Pink to red, red to violet, or red to brown discoloration of alkaline urine—with cascara, danthron, and/or senna only.

Yellow to brown discoloration of acid urine—with cascara and/or senna only.

For stool softeners:

Allergies, undetermined (skin rash).

Those indicating need for medical attention only if they continue or are bothersome: Incidence less frequent

For hyperosmotic—glycerin:

Skin irritation surrounding rectal area.

For hyperosmotic—polyethylene glycol 3350:

While taking other medications that contain polyethylene glycol: urticaria suggestive of allergic reaction (hives or welts; itching; redness of skin; skin rash).

For hyperosmotic—lactulose, polyethylene glycol 3350, or saline:

Bloating.

Cramping.

Diarrhea.

Nausea.

Gas formation.

Increased thirst.

For lubricant:

Skin irritation surrounding rectal area.

For stimulant:

Belching

Cramping—more frequent with aloe and certain senna preparations.

Diarrhea.

Nausea.

Rectal irritation (skin irritation surrounding rectal area)—with suppository dosage form.

For stool softeners:

Stomach and/or intestinal cramping.

Throat irritation —with liquid forms.

ADMINISTRATION AND DOSAGE

General Dosing Information

For bulk-forming:

Bulk-forming laxatives are suitable for long-term therapy, if necessary.

For polycarbophil when used as an antidiarrheal:

Polycarbophil is available as chewable tablets that absorb up to 60 times their weight in water. They are sometimes utilized to control diarrheal conditions by administering less fluid with each dose. The usual oral adult dosage of calcium polycarbophil when used as an antidiarrheal is 1g, 1 to 4 times a day. The usual oral pediatric dosage for children 3 to 6 years of age is 500mg, 2 times a day; for children 6 to 12 years of age the dosage may be given 3 times a day, but not to exceed 3g/d.

For psyllium hydrophilic mucilloid when used as an antihyperlipidemic:

Reduced values for serum total cholesterol, LDL, and the ratio of LDL cholesterol to HDL cholesterol have been achieved with three 3.4g doses of psyllium per day.

For lactulose:

Has no effect on small intestine; lowers pH of colon. Use with caution in diabetics—Contains up to 1.2g of lactose and up to 2.2g of galactose per 15 mL. Dose may be mixed with milk or fruit juice to improve flavor.

For lactulose when used as an antihyperammonemic:

The usual oral adult dosage of lactulose when used as antihyperammonemic is 20 to 30g (30-45mL) 3 or 4 times a day. This dose may be adjusted every day or two to produce 2 to 3 soft stools daily. In the initial phase of therapy, 20 to 30g (30-45mL) may be given every hour to induce rapid laxation. Concurrent use of other laxatives during the initial phase of therapy for portal-systemic encephalopathy may result in loose stools and falsely suggest that adequate lactulose dosage has been obtained.

For polyethylene glycol 3350:

Has no effect on active absorption or secretion of glucose or electrolytes. Should be used for 2 weeks or less. No evidence of tachyphylaxis.

For saline:

Solid forms must be completely dissolved before swallowing. Because of relatively short response time, saline laxatives are not usually given at bedtime or late in the day unless the dose is relatively small and given with food. This type of laxative may contain large amounts of sodium (up to 1g or more per dose in some preparations).

For lubricant:

Commonly administered at bedtime, when slower peristalsis allows longer transit time to improve laxative effect. If administered at bedtime, patient should not be reclining to avoid aspiration of oil droplets. Because mineral oil may interfere with absorption of oil-soluble nutrients and/or medications, this type of laxative is not administered within 2 hours of meals or other medications. To avoid oil leakage through the anal sphincter, the dose of mineral oil may be reduced or divided, or a stable emulsion may be used instead.

For stimulant:

Many preparations of this group are administered at bedtime with a snack to produce results in the morning— except castor oil. Because of its shorter response time, castor oil is not usually taken at bedtime or late in the day. Bisacodyl tannex (bisacodyl and tannic acid complex) should not be used if multiple enemas are required. If absorbed in sufficient amounts, tannic acid is hepatotoxic. Cascara, danthron, and/or senna preparations may discolor alkaline urine pink to red, red to violet, or red to brown. Acid urine may be discolored yellow to brown with cascara and/ or senna preparations.

For dehydrocholic acid when used as a hydrocholeretic:

The usual oral adult dosage of dehydrocholic acid when used as hydrocholeretic is 244 to 500mg 3 times a day after meals.

For stool softeners:

Because stool softener laxatives may increase absorption of other laxatives, including mineral oil, they are not given within 2 hours of such preparations. Patients should be informed. The bitter taste of some liquid preparations of this type of laxative may be improved by diluting each dose in milk or fruit juice.

For oral dosage forms:

With the possible exception of bulk-forming laxatives, more rapid results are obtained when laxatives are taken on an empty stomach. When taken with food and/or at bedtime, results tend to be delayed. Intake of at least 6 to 8 full glasses (240mL each) of fluid per day is necessary to aid in producing a soft stool and to protect the patient against dehydration when large volumes of water are lost with passage of the stool.

For rectal dosage forms:

Lubrication of the anus with petroleum jelly is recommended to prevent rectal abrasion and/or laceration produced by the insertion of a hard enema tip. Lubrication of suppositories with mineral oil or petrolatum is not recommended since it may interfere with the action of the suppository. Instead, the suppository should be moistened with water by placing it under a water tap for 30 seconds or in a cup of water for at least 10 seconds before rectal insertion.

For specific OTC dosing information, please refer to the comprehensive product table at the end of this chapter.

BISACODYL PRODUCTS	
Brand Name	**Dosage Form**
Correctol (Schering)	**Tablet:** 5mg
Doxidan (Pharmacia)	**Tablet:** 5mg
Dulcolax (Boehringer Ingelheim)	**Suppository:** 10mg
	Tablet: 5mg
Ex-Lax Ultra (Novartis)	**Tablet:** 5mg
Fleet Bisacodyl (CB Fleet)	**Suppository:** 10mg
	Suspension: 10mg/37.5mL
	Tablet: 5mg

CALCIUM POLYCARBOPHIL PRODUCTS	
Brand Name	**Dosage Form**
Fiberall (Novartis)	**Tablet:** 1250mg
Equalactin (Numark)	**Tablet:** 625mg
Fibercon (Lederle)	**Tablet:** 625mg
Fiber-Lax (Rugby)	**Tablet:** 625mg
Konsyl Fiber (Konsyl)	**Tablet:** 625mg
Perdiem (Novartis)	**Tablet:** 625mg
Phillips' Fibercaps (Bayer)	**Tablet:** 625mg

OCUSATE PRODUCTS	
Brand Name	**Dosage Form**
Colace (Purdue)	**Capsule:** 50mg, 100mg
	Liquid: 100mg/10mL
	Solution: 20mg/5mL
Dulcolax (Boehringer Ingelheim)	**Capsule:** 100mg
Ex-Lax Stool Softener (Novartis)	**Tablet:** 100mg
Fleet Sof-Lax (CB Fleet)	**Tablet:** 100mg
Phillips' Stool Softener (Bayer)	**Capsule:** 100mg
Surfax Stool Softener (Pharmacia)	**Capsule:** 240mg

GLYCERIN PRODUCTS	
Brand Name	**Dosage Form**
Fleet Children's Babylax (CB Fleet)	**Suppository:** 2.3g
Fleet Liquid Glycerin (CB Fleet)	**Suppository:** 5.6g

MAGNESIUM HYDROXIDE PRODUCTS	
Brand Name	**Dosage Form**
Dulcolax Milk of Magnesia (Boehringer Ingelheim)	**Suppository:** 400mg/5mL
Freelax (Wyeth)	**Tablet:** 1200mg
Phillips' Milk of Magnesia (Bayer)	**Liquid:** 400mg/5mL
	Tablet: 311mg
Phillips' Milk of Magnesia Concentrated (Bayer)	**Liquid:** 800mg/5mL

METHYLCELLULOSE PRODUCTS	
Brand Name	**Dosage Form**
Citrucel (GSK)	**Powder:** 2g/tblsp **Tablet:** 500mg

MINERAL OIL PRODUCTS	
Brand Name	**Dosage Form**
Fleet Mineral Oil Enema (CB Fleet)	**Enema:** 133mL

MONOBASIC/DIBASIC SODIUM PHOSPATE PRODUCTS	
Brand Name	**Dosage Form**
Fleet Children's Enema (CB Fleet)	**Enema:** 19g-7g/133mL
Fleet Enema (CB Fleet)	**Enema:** 19g-7g/133mL
Fleet Phospho-Soda (CB Fleet)	**Liquid:** 2.4g-0.9g/5mL

SENNA/SENNOSIDES PRODUCTS	
Brand Name	**Dosage Form**
Ex-Lax (Novartis)	**Tablet:** 15mg
Ex-Lax Maximum Strength (Novartis)	**Tablet:** 25mg
Perdiem (Novartis)	**Tablet:** 15mg
Senokot (Purdue)	**Syrup:** 8.8mg/5mL **Tablet:** 8.6mg
SenokotXTRA (Purdue)	**Tablet:** 17mg
X-prep (Purdue)	**Syrup:** 8.8mg/5mL

DOSING INFORMATION FOR LAXATIVE PRODUCTS

The following table provides a quick comparison of the ingredients and dosages of common brand-name OTC drugs. Products are listed alphabetically by drug category and brand name.

BRAND NAME	INGREDIENT/STRENGTH	DOSE
BULK-FORMING		
Citrucel caplets *(GlaxoSmithKline Consumer Healthcare)*	Methylcellulose 500mg	**Adults** ≥**12 yo:** 2-4 tabs qd. **Max:** 12 tabs q24h. **Peds 6-12 yo:** 1 tabs qd. **Max:** 6 tabs q24h.
Citrucel powder *(GlaxoSmithKline Consumer Healthcare)*	Methylcellulose 2g/tbl	**Adults** ≥**12 yo:** 1 tbl (11.5g) qd-tid. **Peds 6-12 yo:** 1/2 tbl (5.75g) qd.
Equalactin chewable tablet *(Numark Laboratories)*	Calcium Polycarbophil 625mg	**Adults & Peds** ≥**12 yo:** 2 tabs qd. **Max:** 8 tabs qd.
Fiberall powder *(Novartis Consumer Health)*	Psyllium 3.4g/tsp	**Adults** ≥**12 yo:** 1 tsp qd-tid. **Peds 6-12 yo:** 1/2 tbl (5.75g) qd.
Equalactin chewable tablet *(Numark Laboratories)*	Calcium Polycarbophil 625mg	**Adults & Peds** ≥**12 yo:** 2 tabs qd. **Max:** 8 tabs qd.
Fiberall powder *(Novartis Consumer Health)*	Psyllium 3.4g/tsp	**Adults** ≥**12 yo:** 1 tsp qd-tid. **Peds 6-12 yo:** 1/2 tbl (5.75g) qd.
Equalactin chewable tablet *(Numark Laboratories)*	Calcium Polycarbophil 625mg	**Adults & Peds** ≥**12 yo:** 2 tabs qd. **Max:** 8 tabs qd.
Fiberall powder *(Novartis Consumer Health)*	Psyllium 3.4g/tsp	**Adults** ≥**12 yo:** 1 tsp qd-tid. **Peds 6-12 yo:** 1/2 tsp qd-tid.
Fiberall tablets *(Novartis Consumer Health)*	Calcium Polycarbophil 1250mg	**Adults & Peds** ≥**12 yo:** 1 tabs qd. **Max:** 4 tabs qd.
Fibercon caplets *(Lederle Consumer Health)*	Calcium Polycarbophil 625mg	**Adults & Peds** ≥**12 yo:** 2 tabs qd. **Max:** 8 tabs qd.
Fiber-Lax tablets *(Rugby Laboratories)*	Calcium Polycarbophil 625mg	**Adults & Peds** ≥**12 yo:** 2 tabs qd. **Max:** 8 tabs qd.
Konsyl Easy Mix powder *(Konsyl Pharmaceuticals)*	Psyllium 6g/tsp	**Adults** ≥**12 yo:** 1 tsp qd-tid. **Peds 6-12 yo:** 1/2 tsp qd-tid.
Konsyl Fiber tablets *(Konsyl Pharmaceuticals)*	Calcium Polycarbophil 625mg	**Adults & Peds** ≥**12 yo:** 2 tabs qd. **Max:** 8 tabs qd.
Konsyl Orange powder *(Konsyl Pharmaceuticals)*	Psyllium 3.4g	**Adults** ≥**12 yo:** 1 tsp qd-tid. **Peds 6-12 yo:** 1/2 tsp qd-tid.
Konsyl Original powder *(Konsyl Pharmaceuticals)*	Psyllium 6g/tsp	**Adults** ≥**12 yo:** 1 tsp qd-tid. **Peds 6-12 yo:** 1/2 tsp qd-tid.
Konsyl-D powder *(Konsyl Pharmaceuticals)*	Psyllium 3.4g/tsp	**Adults** ≥**12 yo:** 1 tsp qd-tid. **Peds 6-12 yo:** 1/2 tsp qd-tid.
Metamucil capsules *(Procter & Gamble)*	Psyllium 0.52g	**Adults & Peds** ≥**12 yo:** 4 caps qd-tid.
Metamucil Original Texture powder *(Procter & Gamble)*	Psyllium 3.4g/tsp	**Adults** ≥**12 yo:** 1 tsp qd-tid. **Peds 6-12 yo:** 1/2 tsp qd-tid.
Metamucil Smooth Texture powder *(Procter & Gamble)*	Psyllium 3.4g/tsp	**Adults** ≥**12 yo:** 1 tsp qd-tid. **Peds 6-12 yo:** 1/2 tsp qd-tid.
Metamucil wafers *(Procter & Gamble)*	Psyllium 1.7g/tsp	**Adults** ≥**12 yo:** 2 wafers qd-tid. **Peds 6-12 yo:** 1 wafer qd-tid.
Phillips Fibercaps *(Bayer Healthcare)*	Calcium Polycarbophil 625mg	**Adults** ≥**12 yo:** 2 tabs qd. **Max:** 8 tabs qd. **Peds 6-12 yo:** 1 tab qd. **Max:** 4 tabs qd.
HYPEROSMOTIC		
Fleet Children's Babylax suppositories *(CB Fleet)*	Glycerin 2.3g	**Peds 2-5 yo:** 1 supp. qd.
Fleet Glycerin Suppositories *(CB Fleet)*	Glycerin 2g	**Adults & Peds** ≥**6 yo:** 1 supp. qd.
Fleet Liquid Glycerin Suppositories *(CB Fleet)*	Glycerin 5.6g	**Adults & Peds** ≥**6 yo:** 1 supp. qd.
Fleet Mineral Oil Enema *(CB Fleet)*	Mineral Oil 133mL	**Adults** ≥**12 yo:** 1 bottle (133mL). **Peds 2-12 yo:** 1/2 bottle (66.5mL)
HYPEROSMOTIC COMBINATION		
Fleet Pain Relief Pre-Moistened Anorectal Pads *(CB Fleet)*	Glycerin/Pramoxine Hydrochloride 12%-1%	**Adults & Peds** ≥**12 yo:** Apply to affected area five times daily.

DOSING INFORMATION FOR LAXATIVE PRODUCTS (cont.)

BRAND NAME	INGREDIENT/STRENGTH	DOSE
SALINE		
Dulcolax Milk of Magnesia liquid *(Boehringer Ingelheim Consumer Healthcare)*	Magnesium Hydroxide 400mg/5mL	**Adults ≥12 yo:** 30-60mL qd. **Peds 6-11 yo:** 15-30mL qd. **2-5 yo:** 5-15mL qd.
Ex-Lax Milk of Magnesia liquid *(Novartis Consumer Health)*	Magnesium Hydroxide 400 mg/5 ml	**Adults & Peds ≥12 yo:** Take 1-3 tsp qid **Max:** 12 tsp q24h
Fleet Children's Enema *(CB Fleet)*	Monobasic Sodium Phosphate/Dibasic Sodium Phosphate 9.5g-3.5g/66mL	**Peds 5-11 yo:** 1 bottle (66mL). **2-5 yo:** 1/2 bottle (33mL).
Fleet Enema *(CB Fleet)*	Monobasic Sodium Phosphate/Dibasic Sodium Phosphate 19g-7g/133mL	**Adults & Peds ≥12 yo:** 1 bottle (133mL).
Fleet Phospho-Soda *(CB Fleet)*	Monobasic Sodium Phosphate/Dibasic Sodium Phosphate 2.4g-0.9g/5mL	**Adults ≥12 yo:** 4-9 tsp qd. **Peds 10-11 yo:** 2-4 tsp qd. **5-9 yo:** 1-2 tsp qd.
Freelax caplets *(Wyeth Consumer Healthcare)*	Magnesium Hydroxide 1200mg	**Adults & Peds ≥12 yo:** 2 tabs qd. **Max:** 4 tabs q24h.
Magnesium Citrate solution *(Various)*	Magnesium Citrate 1.75gm/30mL	**Adults ≥12 yo:** 300ml. **Peds 6-12 yo:** 90-210mL. **2-6 yo:** 60-90mL.
Phillips Antacid/Laxative chewable tablets *(Bayer Healthcare)*	Magnesium Hydroxide 311mg	**Adults ≥ 12 yo:** 6-8 tabs qd. **Peds 6-11 yo:** 3-4 tabs qd. **2-5 yo:** 1-2 tabs qd.
Phillips Soft Chews, Laxative *(Bayer Healthcare)*	Magnesium/Sodium 500mg-10 mg	**Adults & Peds ≥12 yo:** Take 2-4 tab qd. **Max:** 4 tab q24h
Phillips Cramp-free Laxative caplets *(Bayer Healthcare)*	Magnesium 500 mg	**Adults & Peds ≥12 yo:** Take 2-4 tab qd. **Max:** 4 tab q24h
Phillips Milk of Magnesia Concentrated liquid *(Bayer Healthcare)*	Magnesium Hydroxide 800mg/5mL	**Adults ≥12 yo:** 15-30mL qd. **Peds 6-11 yo:** 7.5-15mL qd. **2-5 yo:** 2.5-7.5mL qd.
Phillips Milk of Magnesia liquid *(Bayer Healthcare)*	Magnesium Hydroxide 400mg/5mL	**Adults ≥12 yo:** 30-60mL qd. **Peds 6-11 yo:** 15-30mL qd. **2-5 yo:** 5-15mL qd.
SALINE COMBINATION		
Phillips M-O liquid *(Bayer Healthcare)*	Magnesium Hydroxide/Mineral Oil 300mg-1.25mL/5mL	**Adults ≥12 yo:** 30-60mL qd. **Peds 6-11 yo:** 5-15mL qd.
STIMULANT		
Alophen Enteric Coated Stimulant Laxative pills *(Newmark Laboratories)*	Bisacodyl 5mg	**Adults ≥12 yo:** Take 1-3 tab qd. **Peds 6-12 yo:** Take 1 tab qd
Carter's Laxative, Sodium Free pills *(Carter-Wallace)*	Bisacodyl 5 mg	**Adults ≥12 yo:** Take 1-3 tab (usually 2 tab) qd. **Peds 6-12 yo:** Take 1 tab qd
Castor Oil *(Various)*	Castor Oil	**Adults ≥12 yo:** 15-60mL. **Peds 2-12 yo:** 5-15mL.
Correctol Stimulant Laxative tablets For Women *(Schering-Plough)*	Bisacodyl 5mg	**Adults ≥12 yo:** Take 1-3 tab qd. **Peds 6-12 yo:** Take 1 tab qd
Doxidan capsules *(Pharmacia Consumer Healthcare)*	Bisacodyl 5mg	**Adults ≥12 yo:** 1-3 caps (usually 2) qd. **Peds 6-12 yo:** 1 cap qd.
Dulcolax Overnight Relief Laxative tablets *(Boehringer Ingelheim Consumer Healthcare)*	Bisacodyl 5mg	**Adults ≥12 yo:** 1-3 tabs (usually 2) qd. **Peds 6-12 yo:** 1 tab qd.
Dulcolax suppository *(Boehringer Ingelheim Consumer Healthcare)*	Bisacodyl 10mg	**Adults ≥12 yo:** 1 supp. qd. **Peds 6-12 yo:** 1/2 supp. qd.
Dulcolax tablets *(Boehringer Ingelheim Consumer Healthcare)*	Bisacodyl 5mg	**Adults ≥12 yo:** 1-3 tabs (usually 2) qd. **Peds 6-12 yo:** 1 tab qd.
Ex-Lax Maximum Strength tablets *(Novartis Consumer Health)*	Sennosides 25mg	**Adults ≥12 yo:** 2 tabs qd-bid. **Peds 6-12 yo:** 1 tab qd-bid.
Ex-Lax tablets *(Novartis Consumer Health)*	Sennosides 15mg	**Adults ≥12 yo:** 2 tabs qd-bid. **Peds 6-12 yo:** 1 tab qd-bid.
Ex-Lax Ultra Stimulant Laxative tablets *(Novartis Consumer Health)*	Bisacodyl 5mg	**Adults ≥12 yo:** 1-3 tabs qd. **Peds 6-12 yo:** 1 tab qd.
Fleet Bisacodyl Suppositories *(CB Fleet)*	Bisacodyl 10mg	**Adults ≥12 yo:** 1 supp. qd. **Peds 6-12 yo:** 1/2 supp. qd.
Fleet Stimulant Laxative tablets *(CB Fleet)*	Bisacodyl 5mg	**Adults ≥12 yo:** 1-3 tabs (usually 2) qd. **Peds 6-12 yo:** 1 tab qd.

DOSING INFORMATION FOR LAXATIVE PRODUCTS (cont.)

BRAND NAME	INGREDIENT/STRENGTH	DOSE
Nature's Remedy caplets (GlaxoSmithKline Consumer Healthcare)	Aloe/Cascara Sagrada 100mg-150mg	Adults ≥12 yo: 2 tabs qd-bid. Max: 4 tabs bid. Peds 6-12 yo: 1 tab qd-bid. Max: 2 tab bid. 2-6 yo: 1/2 tab qd-bid. Max: 1 tab bid.
Perdiem Overnight Relief tablets (Novartis Consumer Health)	Sennosides 15mg	Adults ≥12 yo: 2 tabs qd-bid. Peds 6-12 yo: 1 tab qd-bid.
Senokot tablets (Purdue Products)	Sennosides 8.6mg	Adults ≥12 yo: 2 tabs qd. Max: 4 tabs bid. Peds 6-12 yo: 1 tab qd. Max: 2 tabs bid. 2-6 yo: 1/2 tab qd. Max: 1 tab bid.
SenoSol Laxative, Tablets (Western Research Laboratories)	Sennosides 8.6mg	Adults ≥12 yo: Take 2 tab qd. Max: 8 tab q24h Peds 6-12 yo: Take 1 tab qd. Max: 4 tab q24h. Peds 2-6 yo: Take 1/2 tab qd. Max: 2 tab q24h.
SenoSolXtra Laxative, Tablets (Western Research Laboratories)	Sennosides 17mg	Adults ≥12 yo: Take 2 tab qd. Max: 8 tab q24h Peds 6-12 yo: Take 1 tab qd. Max: 4 tab q24h. Peds 2-6 yo: Take 1/2 tab qd. Max: 2 tab q24h.
STIMULANT COMBINATION		
Perdiem powder (Novartis Consumer Health)	Senna/Psyllium 0.74g-3.25g/6g	Adults ≥12 yo: 1-2 tsp qd-bid. Peds 6-12 yo: 1 tsp qd-bid.
Peri-Colace tablets (Purdue Products)	Sennosides/Docusate 8.6mg-50mg	Adults ≥12 yo: 2-4 tabs qd. Peds 6-12 yo: 1-2 tabs qd. 2-6 yo: 1 tab qd.
SennaPrompt capsules (Konsyl Pharmaceuticals)	Sennosides/Psyllium 500mg/9mg	Adults & Peds ≥12 yo: 5 caps qd-bid.
Senokot S tablets (Purdue Products)	Sennosides/Docusate 8.6mg-50mg	Adults ≥12 yo: 2 tabs qd. Max: 4 tabs bid. Peds 6-12 yo: 1 tab qd. Max: 2 tabs bid. 2-6 yo: 1/2 tab qd. Max: 1 tab bid.
SenoSol-S Laxative, Tablets (Western Research Laboratories)	Sennosides/Docusate Sodium 8.6 mg-50mg	Adults ≥12 yo: Take 2 tab qd. Max: 8 tab q24h Peds 6-12 yo: Take 1 tab qd. Max: 4 tab q24h. Peds 2-6 yo: Take 1/2 tab qd. Max: 2 tab q24h
SURFACTANT (STOOL SOFTENER)		
Colace capsules (Purdue Products)	Docusate Sodium 100mg	Adults ≥12 yo: 1-3 caps qd. Peds 2-12 yo: 1 cap qd.
Colace capsules (Purdue Products)	Docusate Sodium 50mg	Adults ≥12 yo: 1-6 caps qd. Peds 2-12 yo: 1-3 caps qd.
Colace Glycerin Suppositories (Purdue Products)	Glycerin 2.1g; 1.2g	Adults ≥6 yo: 2.1g supp. qd. Peds 2-6 yo: 1.2g supp. qd.
Colace liquid (Purdue Products)	Docusate Sodium 10mg/mL	Adults ≥12 yo: 5-15mL qd-bid. Peds 2-12 yo: 5-15mL qd.
Colace syrup (Purdue Products)	Docusate Sodium 60mg/15mL	Adults ≥12 yo: 15-90mL qd. Peds 2-12 yo: 5-37.5mL qd.
Correctol Stool Softener Laxative soft-gels (Schering-Plough)	Docusate Sodium 100mg	Adults ≥12 yo: Take 1-3 cap qd. Peds 6-12 yo: Take 1 cap qd
Doculase Constipation Relief softgels (Western Research Laboratories)	Docusate Sodium 100mg	Adults ≥12 yo: Take 1-3 cap qd. Peds 6-12 yo: Take 1 cap qd
Doculase Constipation Relief softgels (Western Research Laboratories)	Docusate Sodium 50mg	Adults ≥12 yo: Take 1-3 cap qd. Peds 6-12 yo: Take 1 cap qd
Docusol Constipation Relief, Mini Enemas (Western Research Laboratories)	Docusate Sodium 283mg	Adults ≥12 yo: Take 1-3 units qd. Peds 6-12 yo: Take 1 unit qd
Dulcolax Stool Softener capsules (Boehringer Ingelheim Consumer Healthcare)	Docusate Sodium 100mg	Adults ≥12 yo: 1-3 caps qd. Peds 2-12 yo: 1 cap qd.
Ex-Lax Stool Softener tablets (Novartis Consumer Health)	Docusate Sodium 100mg	Adults ≥12 yo: 1-3 caps qd. Peds 2-12 yo: 1 cap qd.
Fleet Sof-Lax tablets (CB Fleet)	Docusate Sodium 100mg	Adults ≥12 yo: 1-3 caps qd. Peds 2-12 yo: 1 cap qd.
Kaopectate Liqui-Gels (Pharmacia Consumer Healthcare)	Docusate Sodium 240mg	Adults & Peds ≥12 yo: 1 cap qd until normal bowel movement.
Phillips Stool Softener capsules (Bayer Healthcare)	Docusate Sodium 100mg	Adults ≥12 yo: 1-3 caps qd. Peds 2-12 yo: 1 cap qd.

Contraception

Artificial contraception methods work in different ways to decrease the likelihood that sexual intercourse will result in pregnancy. Barrier methods such as condoms (male or female), diaphragms (with or without spermicide), and sponges (with spermicide) have as their first line of defense the physical blocking of the sperm's entry into the uterus. If sperm cannot enter the uterus, it cannot fertilize an egg and pregnancy cannot occur. An IUD works in a different way, by making the uterus toxic to sperm and disturbing the lining of the uterus so that it won't allow egg implantation. The hormones in oral contraceptives and hormone implants fool the ovaries into refraining from ovulation, and without a fertile egg, pregnancy will not occur. IUDs, certain oral contraceptives, and other hormonal medication (e.g., Plan B and Preven) may be used as emergency contraception in the case of unprotected sex, but none of them will protect against sexually transmitted diseases.

There are two main types of contraceptives available over-the-counter: condoms and nonoxynol-9. The male condom is a barrier contraceptive made of latex or polyurethane that must be fitted over the erect penis. The female condom, which is also a barrier contraceptive, is a thin, loose-fitting, flexible plastic tube that is worn inside the vagina. Condoms are sold over-the-counter and when used properly are an inexpensive, effective barrier to pregnancy and sexually transmitted diseases. Nonoxynol-9 is a spermicidal agent often used in combination with a diaphragm, condom, or sponge. Nonoxynol-9 is available over-the-counter in a jelly, foam, suppository, and film.

NONOXYNOL-9

PHARMACOLOGY

Chemically, nonoxynol-9 is a nonionic surfactant. The spermicidal action of nonoxynol-9 is related to its ability to alter the permeability of the lipid membrane of spermatozoa. When applied prior to coitus, nonoxynol-9 causes immediate disruption of the cell and acrosomal membranes and midpiece of the sperm, resulting in rapid loss of motility and inability to penetrate the ovum.

The antibacterial/antiviral mechanism of action of nonoxynol-9 has been attributed to its surfactant properties; specifically, immobilization of viral and bacterial pathogens via disruption of cell membranes and viral envelopes. Against chlamydia, however, the mechanism may depend on antimicrobial activity against chlamydia receptors on the target cells as opposed to disruption of the cell membrane.

INDICATIONS

Contraception—Nonoxynol-9 is a nonprescription vaginal spermicide which may also possess antimicrobial/antiviral properties.

CONTRAINDICATIONS

This medication should not be used when the following medical problems exist:

- History of toxic shock syndrome

- Hypersensitivity to nonoxynol-9 or any component of the preparation

WARNINGS/PRECAUTIONS

Pregnancy: FDA Category C.

Breastfeeding: Potential risk; change in therapy or care may be advisable.

ADVERSE REACTIONS

Those indicating need for medical attention: Incidence less frequent or rare

Allergic-type reactions; genital ulcerations; toxic shock syndrome.

Those indicating need for medical attention only if they continue:

Incidence more frequent:

Contact dermatitis; vaginal or penile irritation.

Incidence less frequent or rare:

Vaginal discharge; vaginal dryness; vaginal burning; and dysuria.

ADMINISTRATION AND DOSAGE

General Dosing Information

Foams, gels, creams, and suppositories containing nonoxynol-9 are inserted vaginally between 30 to 60 minutes before intercourse, with applications being repeated prior to each subsequent act of intercourse; a 10- to 15-minute delay prior to intercourse is required for suppositories. The vaginal film is inserted at least 15 minutes prior to every act of intercourse.

Vaginal Film: insert vaginally 5 to 15 minutes prior to intercourse; effective for 2 hours.

Vaginal Foam/Gel: 1 applicatorful inserted vaginally immediately or up to 1 hour prior to intercourse.

Vaginal Jelly (used with diaphragm): 1 applicatorful applied to dome cup and around rim of diaphragm prior to insertion up to 6 hours prior to intercourse; leave diaphragm in place for 6 hours after intercourse, then remove.

Vaginal Jelly (used with condom): 1 applicatorful inserted vaginally within 1 hour of intercourse.

Vaginal Suppository: 1 suppository inserted vaginally; wait 10 to 15 minutes but no more than 1 hour before intercourse.

MALE CONDOM PRODUCTS	
Brand Name	**Description**
Durex Avanti	Non-latex
Durex Extra-Sensitive	
Durex Her Sensation	
Durex High Sensation	
Durex Intense Sensation	
Durex Love	
Durex Mutual Pleasure	
Durex Natural Feeling	
Durex Performax	5% Benzocaine
Durex Tingling Pleasure	
Durex Tropical	
Durex Ultimate Feeling	
Durex Warming Pleasure	
Durex XXL	Extra-large
LifeStyles Lasting Pleasure	4.5% Benzociane
LifeStyles Sheer Pleasure	
LifeStyles Ultra Sensitive	
LifeStyles Ultra Sensitive w/Spermicide	25mg Nonoxynol-9
LifeStyles Ultra Thin	
LifeStyles Warming Pleasure	
Trojan-Enz	
Trojan-Enz Large Spermicidal	7% Nonoxynol-9/Large
Trojan-Enz Non-Lubricated	
Trojan-Enz Spermicidal	7% Nonoxynol-9
Trojan Extended Pleasure	4% Benzocaine
Trojan Extra Strength	
Trojan Her Pleasure	
Trojan Her Pleasure Spermicidal	7% Nonoxynol-9
Trojan Mint Tingle	
Trojan Magnum Warm Sensations	Large
Trojan Magnum	
Trojan Magnum XL	Extra-large
Trojan Non-Lubricated	
Trojan Shared Sensation	
Trojan Shared Sensation Spermicidal	7% Nonoxynol-9
Trojan Supra	8% Nonoxynol-9/Non-latex
Trojan Twisted Pleasure	
Trojan Ultra Pleasure	
Trojan Ultra Pleasure Spermicidal	7% Nonoxynol-9
Trojan Ultra Ribbed	
Trojan Ultra-Ribbed Spermicidal	7% Nonoxynol-9
Trojan Warm Sensations	

NONOXYNOL-9 PRODUCTS	
Brand Name	**Dosage Form**
Conceptrol (Personal Products)	**Gel:** 4%
Delfen Foam (Personal Products)	**Foam:** 12.5%
Emko (Schering-Plough)	**Foam:** 8%
Encare (Blairex Labs)	**Suppository:** 100mg
Gynol II (Personal Products)	**Gel:** 2%
Semicid (Wyeth)	**Suppository:** 100mg
VCF (Apothecus)	**Film:** 28%

DOSING INFORMATION FOR SPERMICIDAL AGENTS

The following table provides a quick comparison of the ingredients and dosages of common brand-name OTC drugs. Products are listed alphabetically by brand name.

BRAND NAME	INGREDIENT/STRENGTH	DOSE
Encare suppositories *(Blairex Laboratories)*	Nonoxynol-9 100mg	**Adults:** 1 suppository inserted vaginally, wait 10 to 15 minutes but no more than 1 hr before intercourse.
Gynol II Extra Strength Contraceptive Jelly *(Advanced Care Product)*	Nonoxynol-9 3%	**Adults:** Apply 1 applicatorful to dome cup of diaphragm and round rim prior to insertion, up to 6 hr prior to intercourse. Or 1 applicatorful inserted vaginally 1 hour before intercourse when used with a condom.
Gynol II Vaginal Contraceptive Jelly *(Advanced Care Product)*	Nonoxynol-9 2%	**Adults:** Apply 1 applicatorful to dome cup of diaphragm and round rim prior to insertion, up to 6 hr prior to intercourse.
Ortho Options Delfen Vaginal Contraceptive Foam *(Ortho Pharmaceuticals)*	Nonoxynol-9 12.5%	**Adults:** 1 applicatorful inserted vaginally immediately or up to 1 hr prior to intercourse.
Ortho Options Vaginal Contraceptive Gel *(Ortho Pharmaceuticals)*	Nonoxynol-9 4%	**Adults:** 1 applicatorful inserted vaginally immediately or up to 1 hr prior to intercourse.
VCF films *(Apothecus)*	Nonoxynol-9 28%	**Adults:** Insert 1 film and place against the cervix. Insert film not less than 15 minutes and not more than 3 hours before intercourse. Use one film before each act of intercourse.

Diarrhea

As an objective diagnosis, diarrhea has been defined as more than 200g or 200mL of stool per 24 hours while consuming a typical Western diet. In recent years, as many people's dietary fiber intake has increased, 250g or 250mL has become the more appropriate normal value. Essentially, diarrhea consists of a change in bowel habits that has become annoying or distressing in terms of the symptoms or physiologic consequences. Diarrhea can involve changes in the number of stools per day, increased volume of stool with a single bowel movement, increased fluid content of stool resulting in loss of stool form, or the onset of urgency. *Fecal incontinence* is often perceived as diarrhea, even when the stool volume and consistency of the stool would be considered normal. In this instance, the patient defines diarrhea as the inability to maintain continence from the time of sensing an impending bowel movement to the actual passage of stool. Allowing the patient to define diarrhea is useful; this leads to the selection of appropriate diagnostic tests and ultimately the most effective therapy.

Osmotic diarrhea occurs when the osmotic gradient from the vascular space to the intestinal lumen either prevents the absorption of tissue water or draws tissue water from the bloodstream into the colonic lumen. The high level of luminal osmoles required to cause this diarrhea most often arises from carbohydrate malabsorption. The three main subtypes of osmotic diarrhea include: (1) ingestion of poorly absorbable solutes (e.g., saline purgatives), (2) maldigestion of nutrients (e.g., disaccharidase deficiency), and (3) failure of mucosal transport mechanisms (e.g., glucose-galactose malabsorption). Osmotically active solutes cause water and salts to be retained within the intestinal lumen, resulting in diarrhea. Carbohydrate malabsorption also stimulates intestinal motility through the short chain fatty acids, which arise as a result of bacterial metabolism of the small carbohydrates. The characteristic clinical feature of osmotic diarrhea is that it stops when the patient fasts or stops ingesting the offending substance.

Secretory diarrhea results when normal absorptive mechanisms are inhibited or when there is net luminal secretion of water and electrolytes. In many patients with secretory diarrhea, both mechanisms can be active. Unlike those with osmotic diarrhea, patients with secretory diarrhea may have an increase in stool volume even when fasting, because severe secretory diarrhea often has an osmotic component that further worsens the condition. Common causes of secretory diarrhea include enterotoxin-induced secretions (*Escherichia coli, Vibrio cholerae*), pancreatic cholera syndrome (vasoactive intestinal polypeptide syndrome), carcinoid syndrome, medullary carcinoma of the thyroid, Zollinger-Ellison syndrome, and bile acid-induced secretion.

Motility dysfunction can occur at any level of the GI tract. Accelerated gastric emptying or small bowel transit may decrease the time for absorption of nutrients and fluid. Disturbed colonic motility may accelerate the transit from the cecum to the rectum. Abnormal motility of the sigmoid colon, rectosigmoid junction, or rectum may result in a feeling of urgency and fecal incontinence. Suspected motility disturbances are often quite difficult to confirm. Although altered intestinal motility as a cause of diarrhea is most commonly associated with rapid intestinal transit, poor motility with intestinal stasis may cause diarrhea as a consequence of bacterial overgrowth.

Absorption defect: Pancreatic insufficiency can lead to diarrhea related to maldigestion of fat and other nutrients, which prevents absorption. Thus, food passes undigested through the GI tract to the colon. Voluminous nutrient loss may predispose to the production of toxic bacterial products from degradation of the nutrient-rich colonic contents, resulting in osmotic diarrhea. If the small bowel surface area is reduced, malabsorption may also occur.

There are many OTC products available to treat diarrhea, including bulk-forming agents (eg, polycarbophil), adsorbents, bismuth subsalicylate, and antiperistaltic agents (eg, loperamide).

ATTAPULGITE

PHARMACOLOGY

Adsorbent and protectant. Attapulgite is a hydrated magnesium aluminum silicate that supposedly adsorbs large numbers of bacteria and toxins and reduces water loss. Activated attapulgite (contained in most of the products commercially available) is attapulgite that has been carefully heated to increase its adsorptive capacity. Results of animal studies with adsorbent antidiarrheals suggest that the fluidity of the stool is decreased but total water loss appears to be unchanged and sodium and potassium loss may be exacerbated.

INDICATIONS

Diarrhea (treatment)—Attapulgite may be indicated as an adjunct to rest, fluids, and an appropriate diet in the symptomatic treatment of mild to moderately acute diarrhea. Use is recommended in chronic diarrhea only as temporary symptomatic treatment until the etiology is determined. Attapulgite should not be used if diarrhea is accompanied by fever, or if there is blood or mucus in the stool.

CONTRAINDICATIONS

Risk-benefit should be considered when the following medical problems exist:

- Dehydration—*major clinical significance* (although adsorbent antidiarrheals may increase the consistency of feces and decrease the frequency of evacuation, they do not reduce the amount of fluid loss, but only mask its extent; rehydration therapy is essential if symptoms of dehydration, such as dryness of mouth, excessive thirst, wrinkled skin, decreased urination, and dizziness or lightheadedness, are present; fluid loss may have serious consequences, such as circulatory collapse and renal failure, especially in young children and the elderly)

- Diarrhea, parasite-associated, suspected (use of adsorbent antidiarrheals may make recognition of parasitic causes of diarrhea more difficult; if parasitic agents are suspected pathogens, appropriate stool analyses should be performed prior to therapy with adsorbents)

- Dysentery, acute, characterized by bloody stools and elevated temperature—*major clinical significance* (sole treatment with adsorbent antidiarrheals may be inadequate; antibiotic therapy may be required)

- Obstruction of the bowel, suspected (condition may be aggravated)

Drug Interactions for Attapulgite

Precipitant Drug	Object Drug	Effect On Object Drug	Description
Attapulgite	Anticholinergics; antidyskinetics; digitalis glycosides; lincomycins; phenothiazines; thioxanthenes; xanthines (aminophylline, caffeine, dyphylline, oxtriphylline, theophylline)	↓	Attapulgite may impair absorption.

ATTAPULGITE PRODUCTS	
Brand Name	**Dosage Form**
Diarrest (Dover)	**Tablet:** 300mg
Diatrol (Otis Clapp)	**Tablet:** 300mg
K-Pec (Hi-Tech)	**Suspension:** 750mg/15mL

WARNINGS/PRECAUTIONS

Pregnancy: Problems in humans have not been documented. Attapulgite is not absorbed after oral administration.

Breastfeeding: Problems in humans have not been documented. Attapulgite is not absorbed after oral administration.

Pediatrics: In infants and children up to 3 years of age with diarrhea, use is not recommended unless directed by a physician because of the risk of fluid and electrolyte loss. Oral rehydration therapy is recommended in children with diarrhea to prevent loss of fluids and electrolytes.

Geriatrics: In geriatric patients with diarrhea, caution is recommended because of the risk of fluid and electrolyte loss; these patients should be referred to a physician.

ADVERSE REACTIONS

Constipation.

ADMINISTRATION AND DOSAGE

Adults/Pediatrics ≥12 years of age: 1.2g to 1.5g after each loose bowel movement, not to exceed 9g/d.

Pediatrics 6 to 12 years of age: 600mg after each loose bowel movement, not to exceed 4.2g/d.

Pediatrics 3 to 6 years of age: 300mg after each loose bowel movement, not to exceed 2.1g/d.

BISMUTH SUBSALICYLATE

PHARMACOLOGY

Antidiarrheal—Exact mechanism has not been determined. Bismuth subsalicylate may exert its antidiarrheal action not only by stimulating absorption of fluid and electrolytes across the intestinal wall (antisecretory action) but also, when hydrolyzed to salicylic acid, by inhibiting synthesis of a prostaglandin responsible for intestinal inflammation and hypermotility. In addition, bismuth subsalicylate binds toxins produced by *Escherichia coli.* Both bismuth subsalicylate and the intestinal reaction products, bismuth oxychloride and bismuth hydroxide, are believed to have bactericidal action.

Antacid—Bismuth has weak antacid properties.

INDICATIONS

Diarrhea (treatment)—Bismuth subsalicylate is indicated for the symptomatic treatment of nonspecific diarrhea in adults and children 12 years of age and older.

Gastric distress (treatment)—Bismuth subsalicylate is indicated for the symptomatic relief of upset stomach, including heartburn, acid indigestion, and nausea in adults and children 12 years of age and older.

Traveler's diarrhea (prophylaxis)—Bismuth subsalicylate is used for the prevention of secretory diarrhea produced by enterotoxigenic *Escherichia coli* (traveler's diarrhea) and viral infections.

Ulcer, duodenal, Helicobacter pylori-*associated* (treatment adjunct) or

Gastritis, Helicobacter pylori-*associated* (treatment adjunct)— Bismuth subsalicylate is used, in combination with oral antibiotic therapy, in the treatment of *Helicobacter pylori*-associated gastritis and duodenal ulcer.

CONTRAINDICATIONS

Except under special circumstances, this medication should not be used when the following medical problem exists:

- Hypersensitivity to bismuth subsalicylate or any component of this product or to salicylates including aspirin

Risk-benefit should be considered when the following medical problems exist:

- Bleeding ulcers or other active hemorrhagic states—*major clinical significance* (may be exacerbated by the salicylate)

- Dehydration—major clinical significance (rehydration therapy is essential if signs of dehydration, such as dry mouth, excessive thirst, wrinkled skin, decreased urination, and dizziness or lightheadedness, are present with the diarrhea; fluid loss may have serious consequences, such as circulatory collapse and renal failure, especially in young children)

- Dysentery, acute, characterized by bloody stools and elevated temperature—*major clinical significance* (sole treatment with bismuth subsalicylate may be inadequate; antibiotic therapy may be required)

- Gout (salicylates may have variable dose-dependent effects on serum uric acid concentrations; also, salicylates may interfere with efficacy of uricosuric antigout agents)

- Hemophilia—*major clinical significance* (salicylate may increase risk of hemorrhage)

- Renal function impairment (increased risk of bismuth and salicylate toxicity because of decreased excretion)

WARNINGS/PRECAUTIONS

Patients sensitive to salicylates including methyl salicylate (oil of wintergreen), or to other nonsteroidal anti-inflammatory drugs (NSAIDs), may be sensitive to bismuth subsalicylate also.

Pregnancy—First trimester: Salicylates readily cross the placenta. Studies in animals have shown that salicylates cause birth defects including fissure of the spine and skull; facial clefts; eye defects; and malformations of the central nervous system (CNS), viscera, and skeleton (especially the vertebrae and ribs). It has been reported that salicylate use during pregnancy may increase the risk of birth defects in humans.

Pregnancy—Third trimester: Chronic, high-dose salicylate therapy may result in prolonged gestation, increased risk of postmaturity syndrome (fetal damage or death due to decreased placental function if pregnancy is greatly prolonged), and increased risk of maternal antenatal hemorrhage. Also, ingestion of salicylates during the last 2 weeks of pregnancy may increase the risk of fetal or neonatal hemorrhage. The possibility that regular use late in pregnancy may result in constriction or premature closure of the fetal ductus arteriosus, possibly leading to persistent pulmonary hypertension and heart failure in the neonate, must also be considered. Chronic, high-dose salicylate therapy late in pregnancy may result in prolonged labor, complicated delivery, and increased risk of maternal or fetal hemorrhage. Salicylate is distributed into breast milk; with chronic, high-dose use, intake by the infant may be high enough to cause adverse effects.

Geriatrics: In geriatric patients with diarrhea, caution is recommended because of the risk of fluid and electrolyte loss; these patients should be referred to a physician. Also, elderly patients are more likely to have age-related renal function impairment, which may increase the risk of salicylate toxicity. Dosage reduction may be required to prevent accumulation of the medication. Bismuth is more likely to cause impaction in elderly patients.

ADVERSE REACTIONS

Those indicating need for medical attention: Incidence rare

Bismuth encephalopathy, severe constipation; salicylism

Those not indicating need for medical attention: Incidence more frequent

Discoloration produced by bismuth (darkening of tongue or grayish black stools)

ADMINISTRATION AND DOSAGE

Adults/Pediatrics ≥12 years of age: 524mg every 30 minutes to 1 hour as needed, up to 8 doses in 24 hours.

Pediatrics 9 to 12 years of age: 262mg every 30 minutes to 1 hour as needed, up to 8 doses in 24 hours.

Pediatrics 6 to 9 years of age: 174mg every 30 minutes to 1 hour as needed, up to 8 doses in 24 hours.

Pediatrics 3 to 6 years of age: 87mg every 30 minutes to 1 hour as needed, up to 8 doses in 24 hours.

Drug Interactions for Bismuth Subsalicylate

Precipitant Drug	Object Drug	Effect On Object Drug	Description
Bismuth Subsalicylate	♦ Salicylates (aspirin)	↑	Ingestion of large repeated doses of bismuth subsalicylate, as for traveler's diarrhea, may produce substantial plasma salicylate concentrations, thus increasing the risk of salicylate toxicity during concurrent use.
Bismuth Subsalicylate	♦ Tetracyclines, oral	↓	Calcium carbonate contained in the tablet dosage form may decrease gastrointestinal absorption and bioavailability of tetracyclines; patients should be advised not to take bismuth subsalicylate tablets within 1 to 3 hours of oral tetracyclines.
Bismuth Subsalicylate	♦ Probenacid; Sulfinpyrazone	♦	Concurrent use is not recommended when used to treat hyperuricemia or gout because uricosuric effects may be decreased by doses of salicylates that produce serum salicylate concentrations above 50 mcg/mL.
Bismuth Subsalicylate	♦ Antidiabetic agents; Insulin	↑	Large doses of salicylate may enhance the hypoglycemic effect.
Bismuth Subsalicylate	♦ Anticoagulants (coumarin or indandione derivative or heparin); Thrombolytic agents (alteplase, anistreplase, streptokinase, urokinase)	↑	Increased risk of bleeding may occur when these medications are used concurrently with salicylates.

♦ = Major clinical significance.

BISMUTH SUBSALICYLATE PRODUCTS	
Brand Name	**Dosage Form**
Kaopectate (Pharmacia)	**Caplet:** 262mg **Liquid:** 262mg/15mL
Kaopectate Extra Strength (Pharmacia)	**Liquid:** 525mg/15mL
Pepto Bismol (Procter & Gamble)	**Caplet/Chewable Tablet:** 262mg **Liquid:** 262mg/15mL
Pepto Bismol Maximum Strength (Procter & Gamble)	**Liquid:** 525mg/15mL

Drug Interactions for Calcium Polycarbophil

Precipitant Drug	Object Drug	Effect On Object Drug	Description
Calcium polycarbophil	Anticoagulants, oral; digitalis glycosides; salicylates	↓	Bulk-forming laxatives may reduce desired effect because of physical binding or other absorptive hindrance.
Calcium polycarbophil	◆ Tetracylines, oral	↓	Concurrent use with calcium polycarbophil may decrease absorption because of possible formation of nonabsorbable complexes with free calcium released after ingestion. Patients should not take calcium polycarbophil within 1-2 hours of tetracyclines.

◆ = Major clinical significance.

CALCIUM POLYCARBOPHIL PRODUCTS	
Brand Name	**Dosage Form**
Fiberall (Novartis)	**Tablet:** 1250mg
Equalactin (Numark)	**Tablet:** 625mg
Fibercon (Lederle)	**Tablet:** 625mg
Fiber-Lax (Rugby)	**Tablet:** 625mg
Konsyl Fiber (Konsyl)	**Tablet:** 625mg
Perdiem (Novartis)	**Tablet:** 625mg
Phillip's Fibercaps (Bayer)	**Tablet:** 625mg

CALCIUM POLYCARBOPHIL

PHARMACOLOGY
Calcium polycarbophil absorbs water and expands to provide increased bulk and moisture content to the stool. The increased bulk encourages normal peristalsis and bowel motility.

INDICATIONS
Polycarbophil is indicated in the treatment of diarrhea associated with irritable bowel syndrome and diverticulosis, and acute non-specific diarrhea.

CONTRAINDICATIONS
Dysphagia—*major clinical significance* (esophageal obstruction may occur)

WARNINGS/PRECAUTIONS
Impaction or obstruction may be caused by bulk-forming agents. Caution in patients with diabetes and patients on sodium-restricted diet—some products are high in sugar and/or sodium content.

ADVERSE REACTIONS
Allergic reaction (difficulty breathing, skin rash, itching), esophageal blockage, intestinal impaction.

ADMINISTRATION AND DOSAGE
Adults/Pediatrics ≥12 years of age: 1g qd-qid as needed, not to exceed 6g/d.

Pediatrics 6 to 12 years of age: 500mg qd-qid as needed, not to exceed 3g/d.

Pediatrics 3 to 5 years of age: 500mg qd-bid as needed, not to exceed 1.5g/d.

KAOLIN/PECTIN

PHARMACOLOGY
Adsorbent and protectant. Kaolin is a natural hydrated aluminum silicate that is believed to adsorb large numbers of bacteria and toxins and reduce water loss. Pectin is a polyuronic polymer for which the mechanism of action is unknown. Pectin consists of purified carbohydrate extracted from citrus fruit or apple pomace. Studies have shown no decrease in stool frequency or fecal weight and water content with this combination even though stools appeared more formed.

INDICATIONS
Diarrhea (treatment)—Kaolin and pectin may be indicated as an adjunct to rest, fluids, and an appropriate diet in the symptomatic treatment of mild to moderately acute diarrhea. Use is recommended in chronic diarrhea only as temporary symptomatic treatment until the etiology is determined. Kaolin and pectin combination should not be used if diarrhea is accompanied by fever or if there is blood or mucus in the stool.

CONTRAINDICATIONS
Risk-benefit should be considered when the following medical problems exist:
- Dehydration—*major clinical significance* (although adsorbent antidiarrheals may increase the consistency of feces and decrease the frequency of evacuation, they do not reduce the amount of fluid loss, but only mask its extent; rehydration therapy is essential if signs or symptoms of dehydration, such as dryness of mouth, excessive thirst, wrinkled skin, decreased urination, and dizziness or lightheadedness are present; fluid loss may have serious consequences, such as circulatory collapse and renal failure, especially in young children).

Drug Interactions for Kaolin/Pectin

Precipitant Drug	Object Drug	Effect On Object Drug	Description
Kaolin/pectin	Anticholinergics; antidyskinetics; digitalis glycosides; lincomycins; loxapine; phenothiazines; thioxanthenes	↓	Kaolin/pectin may impair the absorption.

KAOLIN/PECTIN PRODUCTS	
Brand Name	**Dosage Form**
Kaodene NN (Pfeiffer)	**Suspension:** 3.9g-194.4mg/30mL
Kaolinpec (Truxton)	**Suspension:** 5.2g-260mg/30mL
Kapectolin (Consolidated Midland)	**Suspension:** 15g-330mg/5mL

LOPERAMIDE PRODUCTS	
Brand Name	**Dosage Form**
Immodium A-D (McNeil)	**Caplet:** 2mg **Liquid:** 1mg/5mL
Immodium Advanced (McNeil)	**Caplet/Tablet:** 2-125mg (simethicone)

- Diarrhea, parasite-associated, suspected (use of adsorbent antidiarrheals may make recognition of parasitic causes of diarrhea more difficult; if parasitic agents are suspected pathogens, appropriate stool analyses should be performed prior to therapy with adsorbents).

- Dysentery, acute, characterized by bloody stools and elevated temperature—*major clinical significance* (sole treatment with adsorbent antidiarrheals may be inadequate; antibiotic therapy may be required).

WARNINGS/PRECAUTIONS

In infants and children up to 3 years of age with diarrhea, use is not recommended unless directed by a physician because of the risk of fluid and electrolyte loss. Oral rehydration therapy is recommended in children with diarrhea to prevent loss of fluids and electrolytes. In geriatric patients with diarrhea, caution is recommended because of the risk of fluid and electrolyte loss; these patients should be referred to a physician.

ADVERSE REACTIONS

Constipation.

ADMINISTRATION AND DOSAGE

Adults: 60 to 120mL after each loose bowel movement.

Pediatrics ≥12 years of age: 45 to 60mL after each loose bowel movement.

Pediatrics 6 to 12 years of age: 30 to 60mL after each loose bowel movement.

Pediatrics 3 to 6 years of age: 15 to 30mL after each loose bowel movement.

LOPERAMIDE

PHARMACOLOGY

Loperamide acts on receptors along the small intestine to decrease circular and longitudinal muscle activity. Loperamide exerts its antidiarrheal action by slowing intestinal transit and increasing contact time, and perhaps also by directly inhibiting fluid and electrolyte secretion and/or stimulating salt and water absorption.

INDICATIONS

Diarrhea (treatment)—Loperamide is indicated in adults for the control and symptomatic relief of acute nonspecific diarrhea and of chronic diarrhea associated with inflammatory bowel disease. Loperamide is also indicated to reduce the volume of discharge from ileostomies, colostomies, and other intestinal resections.

Traveler's diarrhea (treatment)—Loperamide is indicated for symptomatic relief of secretory diarrhea produced by bacteria, viruses, and parasites.

CONTRAINDICATIONS

Except under special circumstances, this medication should not be used when the following medical problems exist:

- Colitis, severe—*major clinical significance* (patient may develop toxic megacolon)

- Diarrhea associated with *Clostridium difficile* resulting from treatment with broad-spectrum antibiotics—*major clinical significance* (loperamide may prolong transit time, causing a delay in the removal of toxins from the colon, thereby prolonging and/or worsening the diarrhea).

- Dysentery, acute, characterized by bloody stools and elevated temperature—*major clinical significance* (sole treatment with loperamide may be inadequate; antibiotic therapy may be required).

- Previous allergic reaction to loperamide—*major clinical significance.*

Risk-benefit should be considered when the following medical problems exist:

- Dehydration—*major clinical significance* (rehydration therapy is essential if signs or symptoms of dehydration, such as dryness of mouth, excessive thirst, wrinkled skin, decreased urination, and dizziness or lightheadedness, are present; fluid loss may have serious consequences, such as circulatory collapse and renal failure, especially in young children).

- Diarrhea caused by infectious organisms (bacterial diarrhea may, on rare occasions, worsen due to the increased contact time between the mucosa and the penetrating microorganism; however, there is no evidence of this occurring in actual practice).

- Hepatic function impairment (loperamide undergoes extensive first pass metabolism in the liver; therefore, patients with hepatic function impairment may have an increased risk of developing CNS toxicity).

WARNINGS/PRECAUTIONS

Pregnancy: FDA Category B. Adequate and well-controlled studies have not been done in humans.

Breastfeeding: Use with caution. It is not known whether loperamide is distributed into breast milk. However, in pre- and post-natal studies, loperamide administered to female nursing rats at a dose of 40 mg per kg of body weight caused a decrease in pup survival.

Geriatrics: In geriatric patients with diarrhea, caution is recommended because loperamide may mask dehydration and depletion of electrolytes. Dehydration may further increase the variability in the response to loperamide.

Fluid/Electrolyte Depletion: Fluid/electrolyte depletion may occur in patients who have diarrhea. The use of loperamide does not preclude administration of appropriate fluid and electrolyte therapy.

DRUG INTERACTIONS

Opioid analgesics—major clinical significance (concurrent use of loperamide with an opioid analgesic may increase the risk of severe constipation).

ADVERSE REACTIONS

Those indicating need for medical attention: Incidence rare

Allergic reaction; toxic megacolon

Those indicating need for medical attention only if they continue or are bothersome: Incidence rare

Dizziness or drowsiness; dryness of mouth

ADMINISTRATION AND DOSAGE

Adults/Pediatrics ≥12 years of age: 4mg after first loose bowel movement, then 2mg after each subsequent loose bowel movement, not to exceed 8mg/d for no more than 2 days.

Pediatrics 9 to 11 years of age (60-95lb): 2mg after first loose bowel movement, then 1mg after each subsequent loose bowel movement, not to exceed 6mg/d for no more than 2 days.

Pediatrics 6 to 8 years of age (48-59lb): 1mg after first loose bowel movement, then 1mg after each subsequent loose bowel movement, not to exceed 4mg/d for no more than 2 days.

DOSING INFORMATION FOR ANTIDIARRHEAL PRODUCTS

The following table provides a quick comparison of the ingredients and dosages of common brand-name OTC drugs. Products are listed alphabetically by drug category and brand name.

BRAND NAME	INGREDIENT/STRENGTH	DOSE
ABSORBENT AGENT		
Equalactin chewable tablets *(Numark Laboratories)*	Calcium Polycarbophil 625mg	**Adults ≥12 yo:** 2 tabs q30min. prn. **Max:** 6 doses q24h. **Peds 6-12 yo:** 1 tab q30min. **Max:** 6 doses q24h. **3-6 yo:** 1 tab q30min. **Max:** 3 doses q24h.
Fiberall tablets *(Novartis Consumer Health)*	Calcium Polycarbophil 1250mg	**Adults ≥12 yo:** 1 tab q30min. prn. **Max:** 6 tabs q24h. **Peds 6-12 yo:** 1/2 tab q30min. **Max:** 3 doses q24h. **3-6 yo:** 1/2 tab q30min. **Max:** 1.5 tabs q24h.
Fibercon caplets *(Lederle Consumer Health)*	Calcium Polycarbophil 625mg	**Adults ≥12 yo:** 2 tabs q30min. prn. **Max:** 6 doses q24h. **Peds 6-12 yo:** 1 tab q30min. **Max:** 6 doses q24h. **3-6 yo:** 1 tab q30min. **Max:** 3 doses q24h.
Fiber-Lax tablets *(Rugby Laboratories)*	Calcium Polycarbophil 625mg	**Adults ≥12 yo:** 2 tabs q30min. prn. **Max:** 6 doses q24h. **Peds 6-12 yo:** 1 tab q30min. **Max:** 6 doses q24h. **3-6 yo:** 1 tab q30min. **Max:** 3 doses q24h.
Kapectolin *(Consolidated Midland Corp)*	Kaolin/Pectin 90g-2g/30mL	**Adults:** 60-120mL after each loose bowel movement. **Peds ≤12 yo:** 45-60mL after each loose bowel movement. **6-12 yo:** 30-60mL after each loose bowel movement. **3-6 yo:** 15-30mL after each loose bowel movement.
Konsyl Fiber tablets *(Konsyl Pharmaceuticals)*	Calcium Polycarbophil 625mg	**Adults ≥12 yo:** 2 tabs q30min. prn. **Max:** 6 doses q24h. **Peds 6-12 yo:** 1 tab q30min. **Max:** 6 doses q24h. **3-6 yo:** 1 tab q30min. **Max:** 3 doses q24h.
K-pec *(Hi-tech Pharmacal)*	Attapulgite 750mg/15mL	**Adults ≥12 yo:** 30mL (1500mg) after each loose bowel movement. **Max:** of 9000mg q24h. **Peds 6-12 yo:** 12mL (600mg) after each loose bowel movement. **Max:** 4200mg q24h. **3-6 yo:** 6mL (300mg) after each loose bowel movement. **Max:** 2100mg q24h.
Perdiem tablets *(Novartis Consumer Health)*	Calcium Polycarbophil 625mg	**Adults ≥12 yo:** 2 tabs q30min. prn. **Max:** 6 doses q24h. **Peds 6-12 yo:** 1 tab q30min. **Max:** 6 doses q24h. **3-6 yo:** 1 tab q30min. **Max:** 3 doses q24h.

DOSING INFORMATION FOR ANTIDIARRHEAL PRODUCTS (cont.)

BRAND NAME	GENERIC INGREDIENT/STRENGTH	DOSE
Phillip's Fibercaps *(Bayer Healthcare)*	Calcium Polycarbophil 625mg	**Adults ≥12 yo:** 2 tabs q30min. prn. **Max:** 6 doses q24h. **Peds 6-12 yo:** 1 tab q30min. **Max:** 6 doses q24h. **3-6 yo:** 1 tab q30min. **Max:** 3 doses q24h.
ANTIPERISTALTIC AGENT		
Imodium A-D caplet *(McNeil Consumer)*	Loperamide HCl 2mg	**Adults ≥12 yo:** 2 caplets after first loose stool; 1 caplet after each subsequent loose stool. **Max:** 4 caplets q24h. **Peds 9-11 yo (60-95lbs):** 1 caplet after first loose stool; 1/2 caplet after each subsequent loose stool. **Max:** 3 caplets q24h. **6-8 yo (48-59lbs):** 1 caplet after first loose stool; 1/2 caplet after each subsequent loose stool. **Max:** 2 caplets q24h.
Imodium A-D liquid *(McNeil Consumer)*	Loperamide HCl 1mg/7.5mL	**Adults ≥12 yo:** 30mL (6 tsp) after first loose stool; 15mL (3 tsp) after each subsequent loose stool. **Max:** 60mL (12 tsp) q24h. **Peds 9-11 yo (60-95lbs):** 15mL (3 tsp) after first loose stool; 7.5mL (1-1/2 tsp) after each subsequent loose stool. Max: 45mL (9 tsp) q24h. **6-8 yo (48-59lbs):** 15 mL (3 tsp) after first loose stool; 7.5mL (1-1/2 tsp) after each subsequent loose stool. **Max:** 30mL (6 tsp) q24h.
ANTIPERISTALTIC AGENT/ANTIFLATULENT		
Imodium Advanced caplet *(McNeil Consumer)*	Loperamide HCl/Simethicone 2mg-125mg	**Adults ≥12 yo:** 2 caplets after first loose stool; 1 caplet after each subsequent loose stool. **Max:** 4 caplets q24h. **Peds 9-11 yo (60-95lbs):** 1 caplet after first loose stool; 1/2 caplet after each subsequent loose stool. **Max:** 3 caplets q24h. **6-8 yo (48-59lbs):** 1 caplet after first loose stool; 1/2 caplet after each subsequent loose stool. **Max:** 2 caplets q24h.
Imodium Advanced chewable tablet *(McNeil Consumer)*	Loperamide HCl/Simethicone 2mg-125mg	**Adults ≥12 yo:** 2 tabs after first loose stool; 1 tab after each subsequent loose stool. **Max:** 4 tabs q24h. **Peds 9-11 yo (60-95lbs):** 1 tab after first loose stool; 1/2 tab after each subsequent loose stool. **Max:** 3 tabs q24h. **6-8 yo (48-59lbs):** 1 tab after first loose stool; 1/2 tab after each subsequent loose stool. **Max:** 2 q24h.
BISMUTH SUBSALICYLATE		
Kaopectate caplet *(Pharmacia Consumer Healthcare)*	Bismuth Subsalicylate 262mg caplets	**Adults & Peds ≥12 yo:** 2 tabs q1/2-1h. **Max:** 8 doses q24h.
Kaopectate Extra Strength liquid *(Pharmacia Consumer Healthcare)*	Bismuth Subsalicylate 525mg/15mL	**Adults ≥12 yo:** 2 tbl (30mL). **Peds 9-12 yo:** 1 tbl (15mL) q1h prn. **6-9 yo:** 2 tsp (10mL) q1h prn. **3-6 yo:** 1 tsp (5mL) q1h prn. **Max:** 8 doses q24h.
Kaopectate liquid *(Pharmacia Consumer Healthcare)*	Bismuth Subsalicylate 262mg/15mL	**Adults ≥12 yo:** 2 tbl (30mL). **Peds 9-12 yo:** 1 tbl (15mL) q1h prn. **6-9 yo:** 2 tsp (10mL) q1h prn. **3-6 yo:** 1 tsp (5mL) q1h prn. **Max:** 8 doses q24h.
Pepto Bismol chewable tablets *(Procter & Gamble)*	Bismuth Subsalicylate 262mg	**Adults & Peds ≥12 yo:** 2 tabs q1/2-1h. **Max:** 8 doses q24h.
Pepto Bismol caplets *(Procter & Gamble)*	Bismuth Subsalicylate 262mg	**Adults & Peds ≥12 yo:** 2 tabs q1/2-1h. **Max:** 8 doses q24h.
Pepto Bismol liquid *(Procter & Gamble)*	Bismuth Subsalicylate 262mg/15mL	**Adults & Peds ≥12 yo:** 2 tbl (30mL) q1/2-1h. **Max:** 8 doses q24h.
Pepto Bismol Maximum Strength *(Procter & Gamble)*	Bismuth Subsalicylate 525mg/15mL	**Adults ≥12 yo:** 2 tbl (30mL). **Peds 9-12 yo:** 1 tbl (15mL) q1h prn. **6-9 yo:** 2 tsp (10mL) q1h prn. **3-6 yo:** 1 tsp (5mL) q1h prn. **Max:** 8 doses q24h.

Dyspepsia

Dyspepsia (from Greek *dys*, bad, and *pepsia*, digestion) refers to symptoms of upper abdominal pain or discomfort that are thought to arise in the upper gastrointestinal tract. They may have some relationship to food, but often do not. Because patients do not use the term "dyspepsia" and because the pain may be associated with other symptoms such as nausea, bloating, heartburn, and early satiety, the physician must determine from the patient's description of the symptoms whether the patient has "true" dyspepsia or the complaints are more suggestive of gastroesophageal reflux disease (GERD), irritable bowel syndrome, aerophagia, dysphagia, or myocardial infarction.

There are four major causes of dyspepsia: nonulcer dyspepsia, GERD/esophagitis, peptic ulcer disease (gastric or duodenal), and gastric cancer. In studies of dyspeptic patients who undergo endoscopy, no abnormality is detected in approximately 60% of patients. By definition, the diagnosis of dyspeptic patients without a structural abnormality (usually documented by upper endoscopy) is nonulcer dyspepsia (also referred to as functional dyspepsia). The three main structural abnormalities typical of dyspepsia are esophagitis (15%), peptic ulcer disease (20%), and gastric cancer (<1%). A small proportion of patients will have gastric or duodenal erosions of uncertain relationship to their symptoms. Also, some patients with normal endoscopy undoubtedly have GERD. Nonetheless, clearly the majority of patients who present with dyspepsia without alarm features will have no detectable organic disease. Hiatal hernia may be uncovered during the evaluation. Hiatal hernia is considered a contributing factor, but not a causative one. The presence of a hiatal hernia does not mean that GERD is present, but it should raise one's suspicions, especially in those patients who report heartburn or acid regurgitation.

Organic disease is more common in patients older than 45 years. In particular, gastric cancer is uncommon in patients younger than 45 years. For example, in a study of 1386 patients with dyspepsia referred for endoscopy or upper gastrointestinal barium imaging, no cancer was diagnosed in those less than 45 years of age.

A prior history of peptic ulcer disease, a family history of peptic ulcer disease, a history of smoking, and the use of NSAIDs are also associated with finding a structural abnormality. Another study showed that a history of pain on an empty stomach and smoking are associated with peptic ulcer disease. Biliary disease, pancreatitis, irritable bowel disease, ischemic bowel disease, gastroparesis, drugs, and ischemic heart disease are other less common causes of dyspepsia.

Dyspepsia is very common. Approximately 2% to 5% of all patient visits to primary care physicians are related to dyspepsia. There are several OTC products available to treat dyspepsia, including antacids (calcium carbonate, magnesium hydroxide, aluminum hydroxide, etc), H_2-receptor antagonists (cimetidine, famotidine, ranitidine, nizatidine), and proton-pump inhibitors (omeprazole).

ANTACIDS

These medications react chemically to neutralize or buffer existing quantities of stomach acid, but have no direct effect on its output. This action results in increased pH value of stomach contents, thus providing relief of hyperacidity symptoms. Also, these medications reduce acid concentration within the lumen of the esophagus. This causes an increase in intra-esophageal pH and a decrease in pepsin activity.

Antacids are indicated for relief of symptoms associated with hyperacidity (heartburn, acid indigestion, and sour stomach). In addition, antacids are used in hyperacidity associated with gastric and duodenal ulcers.

For specific dosing information, refer to the complete monograph for antacids in "Heartburn/Gastroesophageal Reflux Disease" under Gastrointestinal/Genitourinary System.

BISMUTH SUBSALICYLATE

Bismuth has weak antacid properties and is indicated for the symptomatic relief of upset stomach, including heartburn, acid ingestion, and nausea.

Adults/Pediatrics ≥12 year of age: 524mg every 30 minutes to 1 hour as needed, up to 8 doses in 24 hours.

Pediatrics 9 to 12 years of age: 262mg every 30 minutes to 1 hour as needed, up to 8 doses in 24 hours.

Pediatrics 6 to 9 years of age: 174mg every 30 minutes to 1 hour as needed, up to 8 doses in 24 hours.

Pediatrics 3 to 6 years of age: 87mg every 30 minutes to 1 hour as needed, up to 8 doses in 24 hours.

For more information, refer to the complete monograph for bismuth subsalicylate in "Diarrhea" under Gastrointestinal/Genitourinary System.

ALUMINUM HYDROXIDE/MAGNESIUM CARBONATE PRODUCTS	
Brand Name	**Dosage Form**
Gaviscon Extra Strength (GSK)	**Liquid:** 254mg-237.5mg/5mL
	Tablet: 160mg-105mg
Gaviscon Original (GSK)	**Tablet:** 80mg-20mg
ALUMINUM HYDROXIDE/MAGNESIUM CARBONATE SIMETHICONE PRODUCTS	
Brand Name	**Dosage Form**
Gelusil (Pfizer)	**Tablet:** 200mg-200mg-25mg
Maalox Maximum Strength (Novartis)	**Liquid:** 400mg-400mg-40mg/5mL
Maalox Regular Strength (Novartis)	**Tablet:** 200mg-200mg-20mg/5mL
Mylanta Maximum Strength (J&J/Merck)	**Liquid:** 400mg-400mg-40mg/5mL
Mylanta Regular Strength (J&J/Merck)	**Liquid:** 200mg-200mg-20mg/5mL

CALCIUM CARBONATE PRODUCTS	
Brand Name	**Dosage Form**
Alka-Mints (Bayer)	**Tablet:** 850mg
Maalox Quick Dissolve (Novartis)	**Tablet:** 600mg
Rolaids Extra Strength (Pfizer)	**Tablet:** 1177mg
Titralac (3M)	**Tablet:** 420mg
Titralac Extra Strength (3M)	**Tablet:** 750mg
Tums (GSK)	**Tablet:** 500mg
Tums E-X (GSK)	**Tablet:** 750mg
Tums Lasting Effects (GSK)	**Tablet:** 500mg
Tums Smooth Dissolve (GSK)	**Tablet:** 750mg
Tums Ultra Maximum Strength (GSK)	**Tablet:** 1000mg

CALCIUM CARBONATE/MAGNESIUM HYDROXIDE PRODUCTS	
Brand Name	**Dosage Form**
Mylanta (J&J/Merck)	**Capsule:** 550mg-125mg
Mylanta Supreme (J&J/Merck)	**Liquid:** 400mg-135mg/5mL
Mylanta Ultra (J&J/Merck)	**Tablet:** 700mg-300mg
Rolaids Extra Strength (Pfizer)	**Tablet:** 675mg-135mg
Rolaids (Pfizer)	**Tablet:** 550mg-110mg

CALCIUM CARBONATE/MAGNESIUM HYDROXIDE/SIMETHICONE PRODUCTS	
Brand Name	**Dosage Form**
Rolaids Multi-Symptom (Pfizer)	**Tablet:** 675mg-135mg-60mg

MAGNESIUM HYDROXIDE PRODUCTS	
Brand Name	**Dosage Form**
Riopan (Wyeth)	**Liquid:** 540ml/5ml

MAGNESIUM HYDROXIDE/SIMETHICONE PRODUCTS	
Brand Name	**Dosage Form**
Riopan Plus (Wyeth)	**Suspension:** 540mg-20mg/5mL
	Tablet: 540mg-20mg
Riopan Plus Double Strength (Wyeth)	**Suspension:** 1080mg-40mg/5mL

BISMUTH SUBSALICYLATE PRODUCTS	
Brand Name	**Dosage Form**
Kaopectate (Pharmacia)	**Caplet:** 262mg
	Liquid: 262mg/15mL
Kaopectate Extra Strength (Pharmacia)	**Liquid:** 525mg/15mL
Pepto Bismol (Procter & Gamble)	**Caplet/Chewable Tablet:** 262mg
	Liquid: 262mg/15mL
Pepto Bismol Maximum Strength (Procter & Gamble)	**Liquid:** 525mg/15mL

H$_2$-RECEPTOR ANTAGONISTS

H$_2$-receptor antagonists inhibit basal and nocturnal gastric acid secretion by competitive inhibition of the action of histamine at the histamine H$_2$-receptors of the parietal cells. They also inhibit gastric acid secretion stimulated by food, betazole, pentagastrin, caffeine, insulin, and physiological vagal reflex.

Heartburn, acid indigestion, and sour stomach associated with hyperacidity (prophylaxis and treatment)—Nonprescription strengths of the histamine H$_2$-receptor antagonists cimetidine, famotidine, and ranitidine are indicated for relief of symptoms associated with hyperacidity, including heartburn, acid indigestion, and sour stomach. Nonprescription strengths of cimetidine, famotidine, nizatidine, and ranitidine are also indicated in prevention of hyperacidity symptoms brought on by the consumption of food or beverages.

Cimetidine

Adults/Pediatrics ≥*12 years of age*: 200mg qd, max of 400mg qd.

Famotidine

Adults/Pediatrics ≥*12 years of age*: 10-20mg qd, max of 40mg qd.

Nizatidine

Adults/Pediatrics ≥*12 years of age*: 75mg qd, max of 150mg qd.

Ranitidine

Adults/Pediatrics ≥*12 years of age*: 75-150mg qd, max of 300mg qd.

For more information, refer to the complete monograph for H$_2$-receptor antagonists in "Heartburn/Gastroesophageal Reflux Disease" under Gastrointestinal/Genitourinary System.

FAMOTIDINE PRODUCTS	
Brand Name	**Dosage Form**
Pepcid AC (J&J/Merck)	**Tablet:** 10mg
	Capsule: 10mg
Pepcid AC Maximum Strength (J&J/Merck)	**Tablet:** 20mg
RANITIDINE PRODUCTS	
Brand Name	**Dosage Form**
Zantac 150 (Pfizer)	**Tablet:** 150mg
Zantac 75 (Pfizer)	**Tablet:** 75mg

DOSING INFORMATION FOR DYSPEPSIA PRODUCTS

The following table provides a quick comparison of the ingredients and dosages of common brand-name OTC drugs. Products are listed alphabetically by drug category and brand name.

BRAND NAME	INGREDIENT/STRENGTH	DOSE
ANTACID		
Alka-Mints chewable tablets *(Bayer Healthcare)*	Calcium Carbonate 850mg	**Adults & Peds** ≥**12 yo:** 1-2 tabs q2h. **Max:** 9 tabs q24h.
Alka-Seltzer Gold tablets *(Bayer Healthcare)*	Citric Acid/Potassium Bicarbonate/Sodium Bicarbonate 1000mg-344mg-1050mg	**Adults** ≥**60 yo:** 2 tabs q4h prn. **Max:** 7 tabs q24h. **Adults & Peds** ≥**12 yo:** 2 tabs q4h prn. **Max:** 8 tabs q24h. **Peds** ≤**12 yo:** 1 tab q4h prn. **Max:** 4 tabs q24h.
Alka-Seltzer Heartburn Relief tablets *(Bayer Healthcare)*	Citric Acid/Sodium Bicarbonate 1000mg-1940mg	**Adults** ≥**60 yo:** 2 tabs q4h prn. **Max:** 4 tabs q24h. **Adults & Peds** ≥**12 yo:** 2 tabs q4h prn. **Max:** 8 tabs q24h.
Alka-Seltzer Tablets, Antacid & Pain Relief *(Bayer Healthcare)*	Aspirin/Sodium Bicarbonate/Citric Acid 325 mg-1916 mg-1000 mg	**Adults** ≥**60 yo:** 2 tabs q4h prn. **Max:** 4 tabs q24h. **Adults & Peds** ≥**12 yo:** 2 tabs q4h prn. **Max:** 8 tabs q24h.
Brioschi powder *(Brioschi)*	Sodium Bicarbonate/Tartaric Acid 2.69g-2.43g/dose	**Adults & Peds** ≥**12 yo:** 1 capful (6g) dissolved in 4-6 oz water q1h. **Max:** 6 doses q24h.
Dulcolax Milk of Magnesia liquid *(Boehringer Ingelheim Consumer Healthcare)*	Magnesium Hydroxide 400mg/5mL	**Adults & Peds** ≥**12 yo:** 1-3 tsp (5-15mL) qd-qid.
Gaviscon Extra Strength liquid *(GlaxoSmithKline Consumer Healthcare)*	Aluminum Hydroxide/Magnesium Carbonate 254mg-237.5mg/5mL	**Adults:** 2-4 tsp (10-20mL) qid.
Gaviscon Extra Strength tablets *(GlaxoSmithKline Consumer Healthcare)*	Aluminum Hydroxide/Magnesium Carbonate 160mg-105mg	**Adults:** 2-4 tabs qid.
Gaviscon Original chewable tablets *(GlaxoSmithKline Consumer Healthcare)*	Aluminum Hydroxide/Magnesium Trisilicate 80mg-20mg	**Adults:** 2-4 tabs qid.
Gaviscon Regular Strength Liquid *(GlaxoSmithKline Consumer Healthcare)*	Aluminum Hydroxide/Magnesium Carbonate 95mg-358mg/5ml	**Adults:** 2-4 tsp (10-20mL) qid.
Maalox Quick Dissolve Regular Strength chewable tablets *(Novartis Consumer Health)*	Calcium Carbonate 600mg	**Adults:** 1-2 tabs prn. **Max:** 12 tabs q24h.

DOSING INFORMATION FOR DYSPEPSIA PRODUCTS (cont.)

BRAND NAME	INGREDIENT/STRENGTH	DOSE
Mylanta - Children's chewable tablets, bubble gum (Johnson & Johnson/Merck Consumer)	Calcium Carbonate 400 mg	**Peds 6-11 yo (48-95 lbs):** Take 2 tab prn. **Peds 2-5 yo (24-47 lbs):** Take 1 tab prn
Mylanta gelcaps (Johnson & Johnson/Merck Consumer)	Calcium Carbonate/Magnesium Hydroxide 550mg-125mg	**Adults:** 2-4 caps prn. **Max:** 12 caps q24h.
Mylanta Supreme Antacid liquid (Johnson & Johnson/Merck Consumer)	Calcium Carbonate/Magnesium Hydroxide 400mg-135mg/5mL	**Adults:** 2-4 tsp (10-20mL) qid. **Max:** 18 tsp (90mL) q24h.
Mylanta Ultra chewable tablets (Johnson & Johnson/Merck Consumer)	Calcium Carbonate/Magnesium Hydroxide 700mg-300mg	**Adults:** 2-4 tabs qid. **Max:** 10 tabs q24h.
Phillips Milk of Magnesia liquid (Bayer Healthcare)	Magnesium Hydroxide 400mg/5mL	**Adults & Peds ≥12 yo:** 30-60mL qd. **Peds 6-11 yo:** 15-30mL qd. **2-5 yo:** 5-15mL qd.
Riopan suspension (Wyeth Consumer Healthcare)	Magaldrate 540mg/5mL	**Adults:** 1-4 tsp (5-20mL) qid.
Rolaids Extra Strength Softchews (Pfizer Consumer Healthcare)	Calcium Carbonate 1177mg	**Adults:** 2-3 chews q1h prn. **Max:** 6 chews q24h.
Rolaids Extra Strength tablets (Pfizer Consumer Healthcare)	Calcium Carbonate/Magnesium Hydroxide 675mg-135mg	**Adults:** 2-4 tabs q1h prn. **Max:** 10 tabs q24h.
Rolaids tablets (Pfizer Consumer Healthcare)	Calcium Carbonate/Magnesium Hydroxide 550mg-110mg	**Adults:** 2-4 tabs q1h prn. **Max:** 12 tabs q24h.
Titralac chewable tablets (3M Consumer Healthcare)	Calcium Carbonate 420mg	**Adults:** 2 tabs q2-3h prn. **Max:** 19 tabs q24h.
Titralac Extra Strength chewable tablets (3M Consumer Healthcare)	Calcium Carbonate 750mg	**Adults:** 1-2 tabs q2-3h prn. **Max:** 10 tabs q24h.
Tums chewable tablets (GlaxoSmithKline Consumer Healthcare)	Calcium Carbonate 500mg	**Adults:** 2-4 tabs q1h prn. **Max:** 15 tabs q24h.
Tums E-X chewable tablets (GlaxoSmithKline Consumer Healthcare)	Calcium Carbonate 750mg	**Adults:** 2-4 tabs prn. **Max:** 10 tabs q24h.
Tums Lasting Effects chewable tablets (GlaxoSmithKline Consumer Healthcare)	Calcium Carbonate 500mg	**Adults:** 2 tabs prn. **Max:** 15 tabs q24h.
Tums Smooth Dissolve tablets (GlaxoSmithKline Consumer Healthcare)	Calcium Carbonate 750mg	**Adults:** 2-4 tabs prn. **Max:** 10 tabs q24h.
Tums Ultra Maximum Strength chewable tablets (GlaxoSmithKline Consumer Healthcare)	Calcium Carbonate 1000mg	**Adults:** 2-3 tabs prn. **Max:** 7 tabs q24h.

ANTACID/ANTIFLATULENT

Gas-X with Maalox capsules (Novartis Consumer Health)	Calcium Carbonate/Simethicone 250mg-62.5mg	**Adults:** 2-4 caps prn. **Max:** 8 caps q24h.
Gelusil chewable tablets (Pfizer Consumer Healthcare)	Aluminum Hydroxide/Magnesium Hydroxide/Simethicone 200mg-200mg-20mg	**Adults:** 2-4 tabs qid.
Maalox Max liquid (Novartis Consumer Health)	Aluminum Hydroxide/Magnesium Hydroxide/Simethicone 400mg-400mg-40mg/5mL	**Adults & Peds ≥12 yo:** 2-4 tsp (10-20mL) qid. **Max:** 12 tsp (60mL) q24h.
Maalox Max Quick Dissolve Maximum Strength tablets (Novartis Consumer Health)	Calcium Carbonate/Simethicone 1000mg-60mg	**Adults:** 1-2 tabs prn. **Max:** 8 tabs q24h.
Maalox Regular Strength liquid (Novartis Consumer Health)	Aluminum Hydroxide/Magnesium Hydroxide/Simethicone 200mg-200mg-20mg/5mL	**Adults & Peds ≥12 yo:** 2-4 tsp (10-20mL) qid. **Max:** 16 tsp (80mL) q24h.
Mylanta Maximum Strength liquid (Johnson & Johnson/Merck Consumer)	Aluminum Hydroxide/Magnesium Hydroxide/Simethicone 400mg-400mg-40mg/5mL	**Adults & Peds ≥12 yo:** 2-4 tsp (10-20mL) qid. **Max:** 12 tsp (60mL) q24h.
Mylanta Regular Strength liquid (Johnson & Johnson/Merck Consumer)	Aluminum Hydroxide/Magnesium Hydroxide/Simethicone 200mg-200mg-20mg/5mL	**Adults & Peds ≥12 yo:** 2-4 tsp (10-20mL) qid. **Max:** 24 tsp (120mL) q24h.
Riopan Plus Double Strength suspension (Wyeth Consumer Healthcare)	Magaldrate/Simethicone 1080mg-40mg/5mL	**Adults:** 2-4 tsp (5-20mL) qid.
Riopan Plus suspension (Wyeth Consumer Healthcare)	Magaldrate/Simethicone 540mg-20mg/5mL	**Adults:** 2-4 tsp (5-20mL) qid.
Riopan Plus tablets (Wyeth Consumer Healthcare)	Magaldrate/Simethicone 540mg-20mg	**Adults:** 2-4 tabs qid.
Rolaids Multi-Sympton chewable tablets (Pfizer Consumer Healthcare)	Calcium Carbonate/Magnesium Hydroxide/Simethicone 675mg-135mg-60mg	**Adults:** 2 tabs qid prn. **Max:** 8 tabs q24h.

DOSING INFORMATION FOR DYSPEPSIA PRODUCTS (cont.)

Brand Name	Ingredient/Strength	Dose
Titralac Plus chewable tablets (*3M Consumer Healthcare*)	Calcium Carbonate/Simethicone 420mg-21mg	**Adults:** 2 tabs q2-3h prn. **Max:** 19 tabs q24h.
BISMUTH SUBSALICYLATE		
Maalox Total Stomach Relief Maximum Strength liquid (*Novartis Consumer Health*)	Bismuth Subsalicylate 525mg/15mL	**Adults & Peds ≥12 yo:** 2 tbl (30mL) q1/2-1h. **Max:** 8 tbl (120mL) q24h.
Pepto Bismol chewable tablets (*Procter & Gamble*)	Bismuth Subsalicylate 262mg	**Adults & Peds ≥12 yo:** 2 tabs q1/2-1h. **Max:** 8 doses q24h.
Pepto Bismol caplets (*Procter & Gamble*)	Bismuth Subsalicylate 262mg	**Adults & Peds ≥12 yo:** 2 tabs q1/2-1h. **Max:** 8 doses q24h.
Pepto Bismol liquid (*Procter & Gamble*)	Bismuth Subsalicylate 262mg/15mL	**Adults & Peds ≥12 yo:** 2 tbl (30mL) q1/2-1h. **Max:** 8 doses (240mL) q24h.
Pepto Bismol Maximum Strength liquid (*Procter & Gamble*)	Bismuth Subsalicylate 525mg/15mL	**Adults ≥12 yo:** 2 tbl (30mL) q1h. **Peds 9-12 yo:** 1 tbl (15mL) q1h. **6-9 yo:** 2 tsp (10mL) q1h. **3-6 yo:** 1 tsp (5mL). **Max:** of 8 doses (240mL) q24h.
H₂-RECEPTOR ANTAGONIST		
Tagamet HB tablets (*GlaxoSmithKline Consumer Healthcare*)	Cimetidine 200mg	**Adults & Peds ≥12 yo:** 1 tab qd. **Max:** 2 tabs q24h.
Axid AR tablets (*Wyeth Consumer Healthcare*)	Nizatidine 75mg	**Adults:** 1 tab qd. **Max:** 2 tabs q24h.
Pepcid AC chewable tablets (*Johnson & Johnson/Merck Consumer*)	Famotidine 10mg	**Adults & Peds ≥12 yo:** 1 tab qd. **Max:** 2 tabs q24h.
Pepcid AC gelcaps (*Johnson & Johnson/ Merck Consumer*)	Famotidine 10mg	**Adults & Peds ≥12 yo:** 1 cap qd. **Max:** 2 caps q24h.
Pepcid AC Maximum Strength tablets (*Johnson & Johnson/Merck Consumer*)	Famotidine 20mg	**Adults & Peds ≥12 yo:** 1 tab qd. **Max:** 2 tabs q24h.
Pepcid AC tablets (*Johnson & Johnson/ Merck Consumer*)	Famotidine 10mg	**Adults & Peds ≥12 yo:** 1 tab qd. **Max:** 2 tabs q24h.
Zantac 150 tablets (*Pfizer Consumer Healthcare*)	Ranitidine 150mg	**Adults & Peds ≥12 yo:** 1 tab qd. **Max:** 2 tabs q24h.
Zantac 75 tablets (*Pfizer Consumer Healthcare*)	Ranitidine 75mg	**Adults & Peds ≥12 yo:** 1 tab qd. **Max:** 2 tabs q24h.
H₂-RECEPTOR ANTAGONIST/ANTACID		
Pepcid Complete chewable tablets (*Johnson & Johnson/Merck Consumer*)	Famotidine/Calcium Carbonate/Magnesium Hydroxide 10mg-800mg-165mg	**Adults & Peds ≥12 yo:** 1 tab qd. **Max:** 2 tabs q24h.

Flatulence

Flatulence (gas) is defined as the expulsion of air in the intestine through the rectum. Gas comes from two main sources: swallowed air and the normal breakdown of certain foods by the flora naturally present in the large intestine. The body does not digest some forms of carbohydrates in the small intestine because of the shortage or absence of certain enzymes. As a result, these undigested carbohydrates are broken down in the large intestine by bacteria, producing hydrogen, carbon dioxide, and methane that eventually exit through the rectum. There are a number of OTC products available to treat flatulence, most of which contain simethicone.

ACTIVATED CHARCOAL

PHARMACOLOGY

Antidote (adsorbent): *Single-dose therapy*—Activated charcoal adsorbs the toxic substance ingested, thus inhibiting gastrointestinal absorption and reducing or preventing toxicity. *Multiple-dose therapy*—When administered in multiple doses, activated charcoal creates and maintains a concentration gradient across the wall of the gastrointestinal tract that facilitates passive diffusion of the toxic substance from the bloodstream into the gastrointestinal tract lumen where it is adsorbed and thereby prevented from being reabsorbed. In this manner, activated charcoal interrupts the enterohepatic or enteroenteric cycle and enhances the rate of elimination of the toxic substance from the body. This process has been termed "gastrointestinal dialysis."

INDICATIONS

Toxicity, nonspecific (treatment)—A single dose of activated charcoal, in the form of activated charcoal powder (prepared as an aqueous slurry) or oral suspension, or activated charcoal and sorbitol oral suspension, is indicated for use as an emergency antidote in the treatment of poisoning by most drugs and chemicals. Activated charcoal is most effective when it is administered within 1 hour following ingestion of the toxic substance. However, use may be considered more than 1 hour after the toxic ingestion. Activated charcoal may be beneficial when administered several hours after ingestion of long-acting or extended-release drugs, or drugs that slow gastrointestinal motility. But the efficacy of activated charcoal when administered more than 1 hour after most other toxic ingestions has been neither proven nor disproven.

Activated charcoal administered in multiple doses (MDAC) is indicated in the treatment of severe intoxications with drugs that are secreted into the stomach or that undergo clinically significant enterohepatic or enteroenteric cycling; or with drugs that have low intrinsic clearances, long half-lives, nonrestrictive protein binding, and small volumes of distribution. Some drugs for which MDAC therapy may be effective include carbamazepine, dapsone, phenobarbital, quinine, and theophylline. MDAC may also be used to accelerate the elimination of some industrial and environmental toxicants and heavy metals and their radioactive isotopes.

The Food and Drug Administration (FDA) has classified activated charcoal as lacking substantial evidence of efficacy as an antiflatulent or digestive aid.

CONTRAINDICATIONS

Except under special circumstances, this medication should not be used when the following medical problems exist:

- Bowel sounds, absence of—*major clinical significance.*
- Hemorrhage, gastrointestinal, risk of—*major clinical significance*
- Obstruction, gastrointestinal—*major clinical significance*
- Perforation, gastrointestinal—*major clinical significance*
- Surgery, recent—*major clinical significance* (increased risk of gastrointestinal complications)
- Electrolyte imbalance—*major clinical significance*
- Volume depletion—*major clinical significance* (use of cathartics, such as sorbitol, is not recommended)

Risk-benefit should be considered when the following medical problems exist:

- Decreased patient alertness—*major clinical significance* (endotracheal intubation is required prior to administration of activated charcoal to assist in prevention of pulmonary aspiration).
- Gastrointestinal motility, impaired (efficacy of activated charcoal in increasing elimination of toxic substances may be decreased).

WARNINGS/PRECAUTIONS

Pregnancy: Problems in humans have not been documented.

Breastfeeding: Problems in humans have not been documented.

Pediatrics: Preparations of activated charcoal with sorbitol usually are not recommended for use in children younger than 1 year of age because of the risk of fluid and electrolyte imbalance. In older children, the weight of the child must be taken into account to determine a safe dosage of sorbitol, which should not exceed 3g/kg of body weight. Children should not receive preparations of activated charcoal with sorbitol unless they are under the direct supervision of a physician, so proper attention may be given to the patients' fluid and electrolyte needs.

Geriatrics: Although adequate and well-controlled studies have not been done in the geriatric population, caution is recommended when using preparations of activated charcoal with sorbitol because of the increased risk of catharsis, which may result in fluid and electrolyte loss in geriatric patients. Caution also is recommended when using multiple doses of activated charcoal in geriatric patients with poor gastrointestinal motility because of the increased risk of constipation in this population.

ADVERSE REACTIONS

Those indicating need for medical attention: Incidence less frequent or rare

Electrolyte disturbances; hypotension; pain or swelling in abdomen.

Those indicating need for medical attention only if they continue: Incidence more frequent

Diarrhea.

Incidence less frequent or rare:

Constipation; vomiting—incidence increased with administration of sorbitol.

Those not indicating need for medical attention: Incidence more frequent

Black stools.

ADMINISTRATION AND DOSING

General Dosing Information

Activated charcoal is most effective when it is administered early in acute poisoning, preferably within 1 hour following ingestion of the poison. However, use still may be considered more than 1 hour after the toxic ingestion. Activated charcoal may be beneficial when administered several hours after ingestion of long-acting or extended-release drugs, or drugs that slow gastrointestinal motility. But the efficacy of activated charcoal when administered more than 1 hour after most other toxic ingestions has been neither proven nor disproven.

To ensure that a full dose of activated charcoal is received, the container should be shaken vigorously just before administration and, after administration, rinsed with water, shaken, and the mixture drunk. The administration of activated charcoal as an aqueous slurry is generally preferred. However, to improve the palatability of activated charcoal, it has been administered in combination with suspending agents such as bentonite or carboxymethylcellulose. Also, a flavoring agent such as chocolate syrup has been added to the combination at the time of administration. However, some studies have shown that these agents, especially the flavoring agents, decrease the adsorptive capacity of activated charcoal and should not be used.

Following administration of activated charcoal, cathartics have been administered to enhance removal of the drug/charcoal complex. However, based on available data, the use of cathartics in combination with activated charcoal cannot be recommended. If an activated charcoal product containing sorbitol is used, additional cathartic should not be administered. When multiple doses of activated charcoal are required, preparations that contain sorbitol should not be used in each dose of the multiple-dose regimen since they may produce excessive catharsis, which may result in dehydration and hypotension. Instead, 1 to 2 doses of cathartic may be administered every 24 hours, with the first dose administered with the first dose of activated charcoal.

The presence of normal bowel sounds is necessary to determine whether to continue multiple-dose activated charcoal therapy. If bowel sounds are absent or hypoactive, continuing multiple dosing of activated charcoal with or without sorbitol is not recommended because of the possibility of (or aggravation of) constipation and the possibility of pooling of fluids in the colon if sorbitol continues to be administered with the activated charcoal. Multiple-dose activated charcoal therapy should continue until the patient recovers or the major symptoms of toxicity resolve.

Adults/Pediatrics ≥13 years of age: Single-dose therapy: 25 to 100g as a slurry in water. *Multiple-dose therapy: Initial*: 50 to 100g as a slurry in water. Then 12.5g every hour, 25g every 2 hours, 50g every 4 hours.

Pediatrics ≤1 year of age: Single-dose therapy: 10 to 25g or 1g/kg of body weight as a slurry in water. *Multiple-dose therapy: Initial*: 10 to 25g as a slurry in water. Then 1 to 2g/kg every 2 to 4 hours.

Pediatrics 1 to 12 years of age: Single-dose therapy: 25 to 50g or 0.5 to1g/kg of body weight as a slurry in water. *Multiple-dose therapy: Initial*: 10 to 25g as a slurry in water. Then 1 to 2g/kg every 2 to 4 hours.

Drug Interactions for Activated Charcoal

Precipitant Drug	Object Drug	Effect On Object Drug	Description
Activated charcoal	Acetylcysteine	↔	Adsorbed by activated charcoal in in vitro studies; however, studies in humans have demonstrated that the efficacy of acetylcysteine is not significantly affected by administration of activated charcoal.
Activated charcoal	Ipecac	↔	If both ipecac and activated charcoal are to be used in the treatment of oral poisoning, it is generally recommended that the charcoal be administered only after vomiting has been completed; however, in some clinical trials in which activated charcoal was administered preemesis 10 minutes after high doses of ipecac, the emetic properties of ipecac were not inhibited.
Activated charcoal	Oral medications, other	↓	The efficacy of other concurrently used medications may be decreased because of decreased adsorption caused by the activated charcoal; patients should be advised not to take any other medication within at least 2 hours of the activated charcoal.
Polyethylene glycol and electrolytes	Activated charcoal	↓	Concurrent use may decrease the binding capacity of activated charcoal.

ACTIVATED CHARCOAL PRODUCTS

Brand Name	Dosage Form
Actidose-Aqua (Paddock)	**Suspension:** 15g/72mL
Char-Caps (The Key Company)	**Capsule:** 260mg
Charcoal (Nature's Bounty)	**Capsule:** 260mg
Ez-Char (Paddock)	**Powder:** 25g/29.4g

SIMETHICONE

PHARMACOLOGY

Simethicone acts in vitro to lower the surface tension of gas bubbles. Its relevance to action in vivo is not clearly established.

INDICATIONS

Gas, gastrointestinal (treatment)—Simethicone's clinical use is based on its antifoam properties demonstrated in vitro. It is indicated in the treatment of functional conditions in which the retention of gas may be a problem.

Gastroscopy (adjunct); *radiography, bowel* (adjunct)—Simethicone is used as an antifoaming agent during gastroscopy to enhance visualization and prior to radiography of the bowel to reduce gas shadows.

CONTRAINDICATIONS

Risk-benefit should be considered when the following medical problem exists:

- Sensitivity to simethicone.

WARNINGS/PRECAUTIONS

Pregnancy: Problems in humans have not been documented.

Breastfeeding: Problems in humans have not been documented.

ADMINISTRATION AND DOSAGE

General Dosing Information

Dosage or frequency of administration may be doubled with the advice of a physician.

Pediatric dosage should be based on the severity of the condition and the surface area of the patient rather than on body weight.

Capsules

Adults: 95 to 125mg 4 times a day, after meals and at bedtime, or as needed.

Tablets

Adults: 40 to 125mg 4 times a day, after meals and at bedtime, or as needed.

Or 150mg 3 times a day after meals, or as needed.

Suspension

Adults: 40 to 95mg 4 times a day, after meals and at bedtime, or as needed.

ACTIVATED CHARCOAL/SIMETHICONE PRODUCTS	
Brand Name	Dosage Form
Bicarsim (Kramer-Novis)	Tablet: 250mg-80mg
Bicarsim Forte (Kramer-Novis)	Tablet: 250mg-125mg
Flatulex (Dayton)	Tablet: 250mg-80mg
Flatulex Maximum Strength (Dayton)	Tablet: 250mg-125mg
SIMETHICONE PRODUCTS	
Brand Name	Dosage Form
Gas-X (Novartis)	Tablet: 80mg
Gas-X Extra Strength (Novartis)	Tablet: 125mg
Maalox Anti-Gas (Novartis)	Tablet: 80mg
Maalox Anti-Gas Extra Strength (Novartis)	Tablet: 150mg
Mylanta Gas (J & J/Merck)	Tablet: 80mg
Mylanta Gas Maximum Strength (J & J/Merck)	Tablet: 125mg
2Mylicon Infants' (J & J/Merck)	Suspension: 40mg/0.6mL
Phazyme (GSK)	Tablet: 125mg
Phazyme Ultra Strength (GSK)	Tablet: 180mg

DOSING INFORMATION FOR ANTIFLATULANT PRODUCTS

The following table provides a quick comparison of the ingredients and dosages of common brand-name OTC drugs. Products are listed alphabetically by drug category and brand name.

BRAND NAME	INGREDIENT/STRENGTH	DOSE
ALPHA-GALACTOSIDASE		
Beano Food Enzyme Dietary Supplement drops (AkPharma)	Alpha-Galactosidase Enzyme 150 GalU	**Adults:** Add 5 drops before meals.
Beano Food Enzyme Dietary Supplement tablets (AkPharma)	Alpha-Galactosidase Enzyme 150 GalU	**Adults:** Take 3 tabs before meals.
ANTACID/ANTIFLATULANT		
Gas-X with Maalox capsules (Novartis Consumer Health)	Calcium Carbonate/Simethicone 250mg-62.5mg	**Adults:** 2-4 caps prn. **Max:** 8 caps q24h.
Gelusil chewable tablets (Pfizer Consumer Healthcare)	Aluminum Hydroxide/Magnesium Hydroxide/Simethicone 200mg-200mg-20mg	**Adults:** 2-4 tabs qid.
Maalox Max liquid (Novartis Consumer Health)	Aluminum Hydroxide/Magnesium Hydroxide/Simethicone 400mg-400mg-40mg/5mL	**Adults & Peds ≥12 yo:** 2-4 tsp (10-20mL) qid. **Max:** 12 tsp (60mL) q24h.
Maalox Max Quick Dissolve Maximum Strength tablets (Novartis Consumer Health)	Calcium Carbonate/Simethicone 1000mg-60mg	**Adults:** 1-2 tabs prn. **Max:** 8 tabs q24h.
Maalox Regular Strength liquid (Novartis Consumer Health)	Aluminum Hydroxide/Magnesium Hydroxide/Simethicone 200mg-200mg-20mg/5mL	**Adults & Peds ≥12 yo:** 2-4 tsp (10-20mL) qid. **Max:** 16 tsp (80mL) q24h.
Mylanta Maximum Strength liquid (Johnson & Johnson/Merck Consumer)	Aluminum Hydroxide/Magnesium Hydroxide/Simethicone 400mg-400mg-40mg/5mL	**Adults & Peds ≥12 yo:** 2-4 tsp (10-20mL) qid. **Max:** 12 tsp (60mL) q24h.
Mylanta Regular Strength liquid (Johnson & Johnson/Merck Consumer)	Aluminum Hydroxide/Magnesium Hydroxide/Simethicone 200mg-200mg-20mg/5mL	**Adults & Peds ≥12 yo:** 2-4 tsp (10-20mL) qid. **Max:** 24 tsp (120mL) q24h.
Riopan Plus Double Strength suspension (Wyeth Consumer Healthcare)	Magaldrate/Simethicone 1080mg-40mg/5mL	**Adults:** 2-4 tsp (5-20mL) qid.
Riopan Plus suspension (Wyeth Consumer Healthcare)	Magaldrate/Simethicone 540mg-20mg/5mL	**Adults:** 2-4 tsp (5-20mL) qid.
Riopan Plus tablets (Wyeth Consumer Healthcare)	Magaldrate/Simethicone 540mg-20mg	**Adults:** 2-4 tabs qid.
Rolaids Multi-Sympton chewable tablets (Pfizer Consumer Healthcare)	Calcium Carbonate/Magnesium Hydroxide/Simethicone 675mg-135mg-60mg	**Adults:** 2 tabs qid prn. **Max:** 8 tabs q24h.
Titralac Plus chewable tablets (3M Consumer Healthcare)	Calcium Carbonate/Simethicone 420mg-21mg	**Adults:** 2 tabs q2-3h prn. **Max:** 19 tabs q24h.
SIMETHICONE		
GasAid Maximum Strength Anti-Gas softgels (McNeil Consumer)	Simethicone 125mg	**Adults:** Take 1-2 cap prn and qhs. **Max:** 4 cap q24h.
Gas-X Antigas tablets (Novartis Consumer Health)	Simethicone 80mg	**Adults:** Take 1-2 cap prn and qhs. **Max:** 6 cap q24h.
Gas-X Extra Strength Antigas softgels (Novartis Consumer Health)	Simethicone 125mg	**Adults:** Take 1-2 cap prn and qhs. **Max:** 4 cap q24h.
Gas-X Maximum Strength Antigas softgels (Novartis Consumer Health)	Simethicone 166mg	**Adults:** Take 1-2 cap prn and qhs. **Max:** 3 cap q24h.
Little Tummys Gas Relief drops (Vetco)	Simethicone 20 mg/0.3ml	**Peds ≥2 yo (≥24 lbs):** 0.6ml prn. **Peds <2 yo (<24 lbs):** 0.3ml prn. **Max:** 12 doses q24h.
Mylanta Gas Maximum Strength Chewable tablets (Johnson & Johnson/Merck Consumer)	Simethicone 125 mg	**Adults:** Chew 1-2 tab prn and qhs.
Mylanta Gas Regular Strength Chewable tablets (Johnson & Johnson/Merck Consumer)	Simethicone 80 mg	**Adults:** Chew 1-2 tab prn and qhs.
Mylicon Infant's Gas Relief drops (Johnson & Johnson/Merck Consumer)	Simethicone 20mg	**Peds ≥2 yo (≥24lbs):** 0.6ml prn. **Peds <2 yo (<24lbs):** 0.3ml prn. **Max:** 12 doses q24h

Heartburn/Gastroesophageal Reflux Disease (GERD)

GERD results from a failure of the antireflux barrier, which allows the contents of the stomach (and occasionally the duodenum) back into the esophagus. Normal peristalsis rapidly returns most refluxed material to the stomach. The small amount of acid remaining on the esophageal mucosa is neutralized by swallowed saliva. Although not as resistant to acid as the columnar-lined stomach and duodenum, the squamous lining of the esophageal mucosa has some inherent resistance. Patients with GERD have defects in one or more of these processes. Delayed gastric emptying may contribute to increased symptoms. The antireflux barrier comprises the lower esophageal sphincter (LES), the crura of the diaphragm, and the phrenoesophageal ligament, which anchors the gastroesophageal junction in the abdomen. Until recently, the LES received most of the blame for reflux, but it is now recognized that active contraction of the diaphragmatic crura plays an important role in the antireflux barrier.

Additionally, hiatal hernias are closely associated with GERD. In the presence of a hiatal hernia, two of the three components of the antireflux barrier are lost, with only the LES intact. Although the LES can still work well, esophageal clearance of acid is impaired. This increases the time during which acid is in contact with the esophageal mucosa, leading to symptoms, esophageal mucosal disease, or extraesophageal manifestations of GERD. Up to half of the people over age 50 have hiatal hernias; most are asymptomatic, but patients with severe GERD inevitably have a hiatal hernia.

Although acid is the most easily measured (and treated) component of GERD, bile and pancreatic enzymes refluxing from the duodenum via the stomach may play a role in mucosal damage and symptoms. Even after the acid component of reflux is therapeutically eliminated, the patient may still complain of regurgitation-type symptoms. In addition, the presence of reflux into the oropharynx and trachea can produce pulmonary and oropharyngeal manifestations of GERD.

GERD is diagnosed when patients have symptoms 2 to 3 times a week, have symptoms that cause them to self-medicate regularly or seek medical attention, or have documented esophageal or extraesophageal changes due to reflux. The foremost symptom is heartburn (i.e., epigastric or substernal burning that typically moves upward) that is usually worse after meals, in the supine position, when bending over, or with any movement (e.g., lifting or straining) that increases intra-abdominal pressure. Many patients are bothered by nocturnal symptoms that awaken them from sleep. Fatty, greasy foods, which slow gastric emptying and relax the lower esophageal sphincter, are common offenders, as are chocolate, citrus products, tomato sauces, mints, and alcoholic beverages.

Other typical but less specific symptoms include regurgitation (the reflux of detectable volumes of material, often into the oropharynx), water brash (the appearance of salivary secretions in the mouth, as occurs prior to vomiting), and belching. Atypical chest pain may also be due to GERD, which can mimic symptoms of angina or myocardial infarction. However, GERD should only be considered the cause of atypical chest pain after a cardiac etiology has been ruled out. Although esophageal motil-ity disorders are classically suspected, GERD is the most common esophageal cause of atypical chest pain. Oropharyngeal problems such as hoarseness, sore throat, globus sensation, and even damage to the teeth are sometimes reported as atypical symptoms of GERD.

Most patients suffering from gastroesophageal reflux do not see physicians and instead self-medicate from the wide variety of acid-reducing medications available over the counter, such as H_2-receptor antagonists (cimetidine, ranitidine, famotidine, nizatidine), proton pump inhibitors (omeprazole), antacids (aluminum carbonate, calcium carbonate, magnesium carbonate, etc) and bismuth subsalicylate.

ANTACIDS

PHARMACOLOGY

Antacid—These medications react chemically to neutralize or buffer existing quantities of stomach acid but have no direct effect on its output. This action results in increased pH value of stomach contents, thus providing relief of hyperacidity symptoms. Also, these medications reduce acid concentration within the lumen of the esophagus. This causes an increase in intra-esophageal pH and a decrease in pepsin activity.

Antiurolithic—Aluminum carbonate and aluminum hydroxide bind phosphate ions in the intestine to form insoluble aluminum phosphate, which is excreted in the feces. They thereby reduce phosphates in the urine and prevent formation of phosphatic (struvite) urinary stones. Magnesium hydroxide inhibits the precipitation of calcium oxalate and calcium phosphate, thus preventing the formation of calcium stones.

Antihyperphosphatemic—Aluminum carbonate and aluminum hydroxide reduce serum phosphate levels by binding with phosphate ions in the intestine to form insoluble aluminum phosphate, which passes through the intestinal tract unabsorbed.

Antihypocalcemic—Aluminum hydroxide may increase the release of calcium from bone as a result of the decreased serum phosphate levels.

Antidiarrheal—Aluminum hydroxide's constipating properties help decrease the fluidity of stools.

INDICATIONS

Hyperacidity; duodenal ulcers; gastric ulcers (treatment)—Antacids are indicated for relief of symptoms associated with hyperacidity (heartburn, acid indigestion, and sour stomach). In addition, antacids are used in hyperacidity associated with gastric and duodenal ulcers.

GERD (treatment)—Antacids are indicated in the symptomatic treatment of gastroesophageal reflux disease.

Stress-related mucosal damage (prophylaxis and treatment)—Antacids are indicated to prevent and treat upper gastrointestinal, stress-induced ulceration and bleeding, especially in intensive care patients.

Gastric hypersecretory conditions; Zollinger-Ellison syndrome; systemic mastocytosis; nultiple endocrine adenoma (adjunct treatment)—Antacids are indicated in conjunction with histamine H_2-receptor antagonists or omeprazole for transient symptomatic relief in the treatment of pathological gastric hypersecretion associated with Zollinger-Ellison syndrome (alone or as part of multiple endocrine neoplasia Type I), systemic mastocytosis, and multiple endocrine adenoma.

Hyperphosphatemia (treatment)—Aluminum carbonate and aluminum hydroxide may be used in conjunction with a low-phosphate diet to reduce elevated phosphate levels and demineralization of bones in patients with renal insufficiency. However, use of aluminum-containing antacids as phosphate binders may lead to aluminum toxicity in patients with renal insufficiency. Other agents may be preferable for treating hyperphosphatemia in patients with renal insufficiency.

Hypocalcemia (treatment)—Calcium carbonate is indicated for treating low levels of calcium in the blood. Aluminum hydroxide has been used in the treatment of neonatal hypocalcemia and diarrhea; however, it generally has been replaced by other agents. Aluminum carbonate and aluminum hydroxide have been used along with a low-phosphate diet to prevent formation of phosphatic (struvite) urinary stones; however, their use has been replaced by other agents. Magnesium hydroxide has been used to prevent recurrence of calcium stones; however, it has been replaced by other agents. Use of aluminum-containing antacids in young children and premature infants may lead to aluminum toxicity, especially in those patients with renal failure.

Some of the antacid combinations contain other ingredients that have no antacid properties. Simethicone, an antiflatulent, has been added as an aid in those conditions in which the retention of gas may be a problem.

Antacid	Onset of action	Duration of action
Aluminum Carbonate	Slow	Short
Aluminum Hydroxide	Slow	Prolonged *
Aluminum Phosphate	Slow	Short
Calcium Carbonate	Fast	Prolonged
Magaldrate	Intermediate	Prolonged
Magnesium Carbonate	Intermediate	Short
Magnesium Hydroxide	Fast	Short
Magnesium Oxide	Fast	Short
Magnesium Trisilicate	Slow	Prolonged †
Sodium Bicarbonate	Fast	Short

* Absorptive properties of the gel prolong its duration of action.

† If gastric emptying is rapid, stomach may empty before much of the acid is neutralized.

WARNINGS/PRECAUTIONS

Antacids should not be given to young children (up to 6 years of age) unless prescribed by a physician. Since children are not usually able to describe their symptoms precisely, proper diagnosis should precede the use of an antacid. This will avoid the complication of an existing condition (eg, appendicitis) or the appearance of severe adverse effects.

Use of magnesium-containing antacids is contraindicated in very young children because there is a risk of hypermagnesemia, especially in dehydrated children or children with renal failure.

Use of aluminum-containing antacids is contraindicated in very young children because there is a risk of aluminum toxicity, especially in dehydrated infants and children or infants and children with renal failure.

Metabolic bone disease commonly seen in the elderly may be aggravated by the phosphorus depletion, hypercalciuria, and inhibition of absorption of intestinal fluoride caused by the chronic use of aluminum-containing antacids. Also, elderly patients are more likely to have age-related renal function impairment, which may lead to aluminum retention.

Although it is not known whether high intake of aluminum leads to Alzheimer's disease, the use of aluminum-containing antacids in Alzheimer's patients is not generally recommended. Research suggests that aluminum may contribute to the disease's development since it has been found to concentrate in neurofibrillary tangles in brain tissue.

ADMINISTRATION AND DOSAGE

General Dosing Information

For antacid use:

The dose of antacid needed to neutralize gastric acid varies among patients, depending on the amount of acid secreted and the buffering capacity of the particular preparation. It is estimated that 99% of the gastric acid will be neutralized when a gastric pH of 3.3 is achieved. The amount (in mEq) of 1 N hydrochloric acid that can be titrated to pH 3.5 in 15 minutes by a certain dose of antacid is referred to as the neutralizing capacity of the antacid. Approximately 15 to 20mEq of an aluminum- and magnesium-containing antacid are required to neutralize 1mEq of gastric hydrochloric acid.

Patients with hypersecretory disorders (eg, duodenal ulcer, Zollinger-Ellison syndrome, multiple endocrine adenomas, and systemic mastocytosis) may require 80 to 160mEq of buffer at each dose for symptomatic relief; this is approximately 30 to 60mL of most antacids. Only half of this dose is needed for patients with normal acid secretion.

The liquid dosage form of antacids is considered to be more effective than the solid or powder dosage form. In most cases, tablets must be thoroughly chewed before being swallowed; otherwise, they may not dissolve completely in the stomach before entering the small intestine. The maximum recommended dosage should not be taken for more than 2 weeks, except under the advice or supervision of a physician. Combinations of antacids containing aluminum and/or calcium compounds with magnesium salts may offer the advantage of balancing the constipating qualities of aluminum and/or calcium and the laxative qualities of magnesium.

(Continued on page 174)

Contraindications for Antacids

♦ = Major clinical significance
Al = Aluminum-containing
Ca = Calcium-containing
MGL = Magaldrate
Mg = Magnesium-containing
NaHCO₃ = Sodium-bicarbonate-containing

	Al	Ca	MGL	Mg	NaHCO₃
Except under special circumstances, these medications should not be used when the following medical problems exist:					
♦ **Hypercalcemia** (increased risk of exacerbation)		✓			
♦ **Intestinal obstruction**	✓	✓	✓	✓	✓
♦ **Renal function impairment, severe** (increased risk of hypermagnesemia)			✓	✓	
Risk-benefit should be considered when the following medical problems exist:					
♦ **Alzheimer's disease** (may be exacerbated)	✓		✓		
♦ **Appendicitis, or symptoms of** (may complicate existing condition; laxative or constipating effects may increase danger of perforation or rupture)	✓	✓	✓	✓	✓
Bleeding, gastrointestinal or rectal, undiagnosed (condition may be exacerbated)	✓	✓	✓	✓	✓
Bone fractures	*		*		
♦ **Cirrhosis of liver, congestive heart failure, edema, toxemia of pregnancy** (fluid retention may be increased; low-sodium antacids should be used)	†	†			✓
Colitis, ulcerative (may be aggravated by laxative effect of magnesium-containing antacids)			✓	✓	
Colostomy, diverticulitis ♦ **Ileostomy** (increased risk of fluid or electrolyte imbalance)			✓	✓	
♦ **Constipation, fecal impaction** (may be exacerbated)	✓	✓			
Diarrhea, chronic (possible increased danger of phosphate depletion with aluminum-containing antacids; and possible increased laxative effect with magnesium-containing antacids)	✓		✓	✓	
♦ **Gastric outlet obstruction**	✓		✓		
♦ **Hemorrhoids** (may be aggravated)	✓	✓			
♦ **Hypoparathyroidism** (calcium excretion may be decreased)		✓			
♦ **Hypophosphatemia**	*		*		
♦ **Renal function impairment** (possible increased risk of aluminum toxicity to brain tissue, bone, and parathyroid glands; possible onset of the neurological syndrome "dialysis dementia" in dialysis patients with long-term use of aluminum-containing antacids)	✓		✓		
(possible increased danger of milk-alkali syndrome and hypercalcemia with calcium-containing antacids)		✓			
(possible increased danger of hypermagnesemia)			‡	‡	
(may cause metabolic alkalosis)					✓
♦ **Sarcoidosis** (increased risk of hypercalcemia or renal disease with calcium-containing antacids)		✓			
Sensitivity to aluminum-, calcium-, magnesium-, simethicone-, or sodium bicarbonate-containing medications	✓	✓	✓	✓	✓

* Aluminum hydroxide has the ability to form the insoluble complex of aluminum phosphate, which is excreted in the feces. This may lead to lowered serum phosphate concentrations and phosphorus mobilization from the bone. If phosphate depletion (e.g., malabsorption syndrome) is already present, osteomalacia, osteoporosis, and fracture may result, especially in patients with other bone disease. In such patients predisposed to phosphate depletion, other aluminum-containing antacids (except aluminum phosphate) will be of concern only in relation to their ability to form an aluminum phosphate complex.

† Antacids containing more than 5mEq (115mg) of sodium per total daily dose should not be used without first checking with physician. The usual amount of sodium allowed in restricted diets is 3g or less per day.

‡ In patients with renal function impairment, use of antacids containing more than 50mEq (608mg) of magnesium per total daily dose should be carefully considered

Drug Interactions for Antacids

Note: Combinations containing any of the following medications, depending on the amount present, may also interact with antacids. Only specific interactions between antacids and other oral medications have been identified in this monograph. However, because of the ability of antacids to change gastric or urinary pH and to adsorb or form complexes with other drugs, the rate and/or extent of absorption of other medications may be increased or reduced when the medication is used concurrently with antacids. In general, patients should be advised not to take any other oral medications within 1 to 2 hours of antacids.

♦ = **Major clinical significance**
Al = **Aluminum-containing**
Ca = **Calcium-containing**
MGL = **Magaldrate**
Mg = **Magnesium-containing**
NaHCO₃ = **Sodium-bicarbonate-containing**

	Al	Ca	MGL	Mg	NaHCO₃
Acidifiers, urinary, such as: **Ammonium chloride, ascorbic acid, potassium or sodium phosphates, racemethionine** (antacids may alkalinize the urine and counteract the effect of urinary acidifiers; frequent use of antacids, especially in high doses, is best avoided by patients receiving therapy to acidify the urine)	✓	✓	✓	✓	✓
Amphetamines (urinary excretion may be inhibited when amphetamines are used concurrently with antacids in doses that cause the urine to become alkaline, possibly resulting in toxicity; dosage adjustment may be needed when therapy with these antacids is initiated or discontinued or if dosage is changed)	✓	✓	✓	✓	✓
Anticholinergics or other medications with anticholinergic activity (concurrent use with antacids may decrease absorption, reducing the effectiveness of anticholinergics; doses of these medications should be spaced 1 hour apart from doses of antacids; also, urinary excretion may be delayed by alkalinization of the urine, thus potentiating anticholinergic side effects)	✓	✓	✓	✓	✓
Calcitonin, etidronate, gallium nitrate, pamidronate, plicamycin (concurrent use with calcium carbonate may antagonize the effect of these medications in the treatment of hypercalcemia)		✓			
Calcium-containing preparations (concurrent and prolonged use with sodium bicarbonate may result in the milk-alkali syndrome)					✓
♦ **Cellulose sodium phosphate** (concurrent use with calcium-containing antacids may decrease effectiveness of cellulose sodium phosphate in preventing hypercalciuria)		✓			
(concurrent use with magnesium-containing antacids may result in binding of magnesium; patients should be advised not to take these medications within 1 hour of cellulose sodium phosphate)			✓	✓	
Chenodiol (concurrent use with aluminum-containing antacids may result in binding of chenodiol, thus decreasing its absorption)	✓	✓			
Citrates (concurrent use with antacids containing aluminum, calcium carbonates, magaldrate, or sodium bicarbonate may result in systemic alkalosis)	✓	✓	✓		✓
(concurrent use of sodium citrate with sodium bicarbonate may promote the development of calcium stones in patients with uric acid stones, due to sodium ion opposition to the hypocalciuric effect of the alkaline load; may also cause hypernatremia)					✓
(concurrent use of aluminum-containing antacids and magaldrate with citrate salts can increase aluminum absorption, possibly resulting in acute aluminum toxicity, especially in patients with renal insufficiency)	✓		✓		
Digitalis glycosides (concurrent use with aluminum- and magnesium-containing antacids may inhibit absorption, possibly decreasing plasma concentrations of digitalis glycosides; although actual clinical importance of this interaction has not been established, it is recommended that doses of antacids and digitalis glycosides be separated by several hours)	✓		✓	✓	
Diuretics, potassium-depleting, such as bumetanide, ethacrynic acid, furosemide, indapamide, thiazide diuretics (concurrent use of thiazide diuretics with large doses of calcium carbonate may result in hypercalcemia)		✓			
Enteric-coated medications, such as bisacodyl (concurrent administration of antacids with enteric-coated medications may cause the enteric coating to dissolve too rapidly, resulting in gastric or duodenal irritation)	✓	✓	✓	✓	✓

Drug Interactions for Antacids (cont.)

	Al	Ca	MGL	Mg	NaHCO₃
Ephedrine (urine alkalinization induced by sodium bicarbonate may increase the half-life of ephedrine and prolong its duration of action, especially if the urine remains alkaline for several days or longer; dosage adjustment of ephedrine may be necessary)					✓
◆ **Fluoroquinolones** (alkalinization of the urine may reduce the solubility of ciprofloxacin and norfloxacin in the urine, especially when the urinary pH exceeds 7.0; if antacids and one of these medications are used concurrently, patients should be observed for signs of crystalluria and nephrotoxicity)	✓	✓	✓	✓	✓
(aluminum- and magnesium-containing antacids may reduce absorption of fluoroquinolones, resulting in lower serum and urine concentrations of these medications; therefore, concurrent use is not recommended; however, if aluminum- and magnesium-containing antacids must be used concurrently with these medications, it is recommended that enoxacin be taken at least 2 hours before or 8 hours after the antacid; ciprofloxacin and lomefloxacin should be taken at least 2 hours before or 6 hours after the antacid; and norfloxacin and ofloxacin should be taken at least 2 hours before or after the antacid)	✓		✓	✓	
Folic acid (prolonged use of aluminum- and/or magnesium-containing antacids may decrease folic acid absorption by raising the pH of the small intestine; patients should be advised to take antacids at least 2 hours after folic acid)	✓		✓	✓	
Histamine H₂-receptor antagonists (concurrent use with antacids may be indicated in the treatment of peptic ulcer to relieve pain; however, simultaneous administration of medium to high doses [80 to 150mmol] of antacids is not recommended since absorption of histamine H₂-receptor antagonists may be decreased; patients should be advised not to take any antacids within 1/2 to 1 hour of histamine H₂-receptor antagonists)	✓	✓	✓	✓	✓
Iron preparations, oral (absorption may be decreased when these preparations are used concurrently with magnesium trisilicate or antacids containing carbonate; spacing the doses of the iron preparation as far as possible from doses of the antacid is recommended)	✓	✓		✓	✓
◆ **Isoniazid, oral** (concurrent use with aluminum-containing antacids may delay and decrease absorption of oral isoniazid; concurrent use should be avoided or the patient should be advised to take oral isoniazid at least 1 hour before the antacid)	✓		✓		
◆ **Ketoconazole** (antacids may cause increased gastrointestinal pH; concurrent administration with antacids may result in a marked reduction in absorption of ketoconazole; patients should be advised to take antacids at least 3 hours after ketoconazole)	✓	✓	✓	✓	✓
Lithium (sodium bicarbonate enhances lithium excretion, possibly resulting in decreased efficacy; this may be partly due to the sodium content)					✓
Mexiletine (marked alkalinization of the urine caused by sodium bicarbonate may slow renal excretion of mexiletine)					✓
◆ **Mecamylamine** (alkalinization of the urine may slow excretion and prolong the effects of mecamylamine; concurrent use is not recommended)	✓	✓	✓	✓	✓
◆ **Methenamine** (concurrent use with antacids that cause the urine to become alkaline may reduce the effectiveness of methenamine by inhibiting its conversion to formaldehyde; concurrent use is not recommended)	✓	✓	✓	✓	✓
Milk or milk products (concurrent and prolonged use with calcium carbonate or sodium bicarbonate may result in the milk-alkali syndrome)		✓			✓
Misoprostol (concurrent use with magnesium-containing antacids may aggravate misoprostol-induced diarrhea)			✓	✓	
Pancrelipase (concurrent administration of antacids may be required to prevent inactivation of pancrelipase [except enteric-coated dosage forms] by gastric pepsin and acid pH; however, calcium carbonate- and/or magnesium-containing antacids are not recommended since they may decrease the effectiveness of pancrelipase)		✓	✓	✓	

Drug Interactions for Antacids (cont.)

	Al	Ca	MGL	Mg	NaHCO₃
Penicillamine (absorption may be reduced when penicillamine is administered concurrently with aluminum- or magnesium-containing antacids; although more studies are needed to establish the significance of this interaction, it is recommended that doses of antacids and penicillamine be separated by 2 hours)	✓		✓	✓	
Phenothiazines, especially chlorpromazine, oral (absorption may be inhibited when these medications are used concurrently with aluminum- or magnesium-containing antacids; although more studies are needed to establish the significance of this interaction, simultaneous administration should be avoided)	✓		✓	✓	
Phenytoin (concurrent use with aluminum-, magnesium-, and/or calcium carbonate-containing antacids may decrease absorption of phenytoin, thus reducing serum phenytoin concentrations; although more studies are needed to establish the significance of this interaction, it is recommended that doses of antacids and phenytoin be separated by about 2 to 3 hours)	✓	✓	✓	✓	
Phosphates, oral (concurrent use with aluminum- or magnesium-containing antacids may bind the phosphate and prevent its absorption; concurrent use with calcium-containing antacids may increase potential of deposition of calcium in soft tissues if serum-ionized calcium is high)	✓	✓	✓	✓	
Quinidine (urinary excretion may be inhibited when quinidine is used concurrently with antacids in doses that cause the urine to become alkaline, possibly resulting in toxicity; dosage adjustment may be needed when therapy with these antacids is initiated or discontinued or if dosage is changed)	✓	✓	✓	✓	✓
Quinine (concurrent use with aluminum-containing antacids may decrease or delay the absorption of quinine)	✓		✓		
Salicylates (alkalinization of the urine may increase renal salicylate excretion and lower serum salicylate levels; dosage adjustments of salicylates may be necessary when chronic high-dose antacid therapy is started or stopped, especially in patients receiving large doses of the salicylate, such as patients with rheumatoid arthritis or rheumatic fever)	✓	✓	✓	✓	✓
Sodium bicarbonate, vitamin D (concurrent and prolonged use with calcium carbonate may result in the milk-alkali syndrome)		✓			
Sodium fluoride (concurrent use with aluminum hydroxide may decrease absorption and increase fecal excretion of fluoride; calcium ions may complex with and inhibit absorption of fluoride)	✓	✓	✓		
♦ **Sodium polystyrene sulfonate resin (SPSR)** (neutralization of gastric acid may be impaired when SPSR is used concurrently with calcium- or magnesium-containing antacids, possibly resulting in systemic alkalosis; concurrent use is not recommended)		✓	✓	✓	
Sucralfate (concurrent use with antacids may be indicated in the treatment of duodenal ulcer to relieve pain; however, simultaneous administration is not recommended since antacids may interfere with binding of sucralfate to the mucosa; patients should be advised not to take any antacids within 1/2 hour before or after sucralfate; concurrent use with aluminum-containing antacids may cause aluminum toxicity in patients with chronic renal failure)	✓	✓	✓	✓	✓
♦ **Tetracyclines, oral** (absorption may be decreased when oral tetracyclines are used concurrently with antacids because of possible formation of nonabsorbable complexes and/or increase in intragastric pH; patients should be advised not to take antacids within 3 to 4 hours of tetracyclines)	✓	✓	✓	✓	✓
Vitamin D, including calcifediol and calcitriol (concurrent use with magnesium-containing antacids may result in hypermagnesemia, especially in patients with chronic renal failure; concurrent use with calcium-containing antacids may result in hypercalcemia)		✓	✓	✓	

Adverse Reactions of Antacids

Al = Aluminum-containing
Ca = Calcium-containing
MGL = Magaldrate
Mg = Magnesium-containing
NaHCO₃ = Sodium-bicarbonate-containing

	Al	Ca	MGL	Mg	NaHCO$_3$
Medical attention needed*					
With long-term use in chronic renal failure in dialysis patients **Neurotoxicity** (mood or mental changes)	✓		✓		
With large doses **Fecal impaction** (continuing severe constipation)	✓	✓			
Swelling of feet or lower legs					✓
With large doses or in renal insufficiency **Metabolic alkalosis** (mood or mental changes; muscle pain or twitching; nervousness or restlessness; slow breathing; unpleasant taste; unusual tiredness or weakness)		✓			✓
With long-term or prolonged use **Hypercalcemia associated with milk-alkali syndrome** (frequent urge to urinate; continuing headache; continuing loss of appetite; nausea or vomiting; unusual tiredness or weakness)		†			✓
Osteomalacia and osteoporosis due to phosphate depletion (bone pain; swelling of wrists or ankles)	✓		‡		
With overuse or prolonged use **Renal calculi** (difficult or painful urination)		✓		§	
With prolonged use or large doses **Phosphorus depletion syndrome** (continuing feeling of discomfort; continuing loss of appetite; muscle weakness; unusual weight loss)	✓		✓		
With prolonged use or large doses and/or in renal disease **Hypermagnesemia or other electrolyte imbalance** (dizziness or lightheadedness; irregular heartbeat; mood or mental changes; unusual tiredness or weakness)			✓	✓	
Medical attention needed only if continuing or bothersome*					
Chalky taste	M	M	M	M	U
Constipation, mild	M	L	U	U	U
Diarrhea or laxative effect—with overdose	U	U	U	M	U
Increased thirst	U	U	U	U	L
Nausea or vomiting	L	U	U	L	U
Speckling or whitish discoloration of stools (concentrations of fatty acids due to aluminum salts)	L	U	U	U	U
Stomach cramps	M	U	U	L	L

M = more frequent; L = less frequent; U = unknown.

* Differences in frequency of occurrence may reflect either lack of clinical-use data or actual pharmacologic distinctions among agents (although their pharmacologic similarity suggests that side effects occurring with one may occur with the others).

† May also occur with large doses and/or in chronic renal failure with calcium carbonate.

‡ Osteomalacia and osteoporosis have been reported after chronic ingestion of large doses of aluminum hydroxide-containing antacids. Since magaldrate is converted to aluminum and magnesium hydroxides in vivo, it is likely that osteomalacia and osteoporosis may occur with excessive use of magaldrate.

§ Chronic administration of magnesium trisilicate may infrequently produce silica renal stones.

ALUMINUM HYDROXIDE/MAGNESIUM CARBONATE PRODUCTS	
Brand Name	**Dosage Form**
Gaviscon Extra Strength (GSK)	**Liquid:** 254mg-237.5mg/5mL **Tablet:** 160mg-105mg
Gaviscon Original (GSK)	**Tablet:** 80mg-20mg
ALUMINUM HYDROXIDE/MAGNESIUM CARBONATE SIMETHICONE PRODUCTS	
Brand Name	**Dosage Form**
Gelusil (GSK)	**Tablet:** 200mg-200mg-25mg
Maalox Max (Novartis)	**Liquid:** 400mg-400mg-40mg/5mL
Maalox Regular Strength (Novartis)	**Tablet:** 200mg-200mg-20mg/5mL
Mylanta Maximum Strength (J&J/Merck)	**Liquid:** 400mg-400mg-40mg/5mL
Mylanta Regular Strength (J&J/Merck)	**Liquid:** 200mg-200mg-20mg/5mL

CALCIUM CARBONATE PRODUCTS	
Brand Name	**Dosage Form**
Alka-Mints (Bayer)	**Tablet:** 850mg
Maalox Quick Dissolve (Novartis)	**Tablet:** 600mg
Rolaids Extra Strength (Pfizer)	**Tablet:** 1177mg
Titralac (3M)	**Tablet:** 420mg
Titralac Extra Stength (3M)	**Tablet:** 750mg
Tums (GSK)	**Tablet:** 500mg
Tums E-X (GSK)	**Tablet:** 750mg
Tums Lasting Effects (GSK)	**Tablet:** 500mg
Tums Smooth Dissolve (GSK)	**Tablet:** 750mg
Tums Ultra Maximum Strength (GSK)	**Tablet:** 1000mg

CALCIUM CARBONATE/MAGNESIUM HYDROXIDE PRODUCTS	
Brand Name	**Dosage Form**
Mylanta (J&J/Merck)	**Capsule:** 550mg-125mg
Mylanta Supreme (J&J/Merck)	**Liquid:** 400mg-135mg/5mL
Mylanta Ultra (J&J/Merck)	**Tablet:** 700mg-300mg
Rolaids Extra Strength (Pfizer)	**Tablet:** 675mg-135
Rolaids (Pfizer)	**Tablet:** 550mg-110mg

CALCIUM CARBONATE/MAGNESIUM HYDROXIDE/SIMETHICONE PRODUCTS	
Brand Name	**Dosage Form**
Rolaids Multi-Symptom (Pfizer)	**Tablet:** 675mg-135mg-60mg

CALCIUM CARBONATE/SIMETHICONE PRODUCTS	
Brand Name	**Dosage Form**
Gas-X w/Maalox (Novartis)	**Capsule:** 250mg-62.5mg
Maalox Max Quick Dissolve (Novartis)	**Tablet:** 1000mg-60mg
Titralac Plus (3M)	**Tablet:** 420mg-21mg

MAGNESIUM HYDROXIDE PRODUCTS	
Brand Name	**Dosage Form**
Dulcolax Milk of Magnesia (Boehringer Ingelheim)	**Liquid:** 400mg/5mL
Riopan (Wyeth)	**Liquid:** 540mg/5mL

MAGNESIUM HYDROXIDE/SIMETHICONE PRODUCTS	
Brand Name	**Dosage Form**
Riopan Plus (Wyeth)	**Suspension:** 540mg-20mg/5mL **Tablet:** 540mg-20mg
Riopan Plus Double Strength (Wyeth)	**Suspension:** 1080mg-40mg/5mL

BISMUTH SUBSALICYLATE PRODUCTS	
Brand Name	**Dosage Form**
Kaopectate (Pharmacia)	**Caplet:** 262mg **Liquid:** 262mg/15mL
Kaopectate Extra Strength (Pharmacia)	**Liquid:** 525mg/15mL
Pepto Bismol (Procter & Gamble)	**Caplet/Chewable Tablet:** 262mg **Liquid:** 262mg/15mL
Pepto Bismol Maximum Strength (Procter & Gamble)	**Liquid:** 525mg/5mL

(Continued from page 167)

For use in peptic ulcer:

In the treatment of peptic ulcer disease, to achieve adequate ant-acid effect in the stomach at the optimum time, most antacids are administered 1 and 3 hours after meals for prolonged acid-neutralizing effect and at bedtime. However, when taken at bed-time, their effect is not prolonged because of rapid gastric emptying. Additional doses of antacids may be administered to relieve pain that may occur between the regularly scheduled doses. Antacid therapy should be continued for at least 4 to 6 weeks after all symptoms have disappeared, since there is no correlation between disappearance of symptoms and actual heal-ing of the ulcer.

Aluminum hydroxide:

In the treatment of peptic ulcer, 960mg to 3.6g are given orally every 1 or 2 hours during waking hours, with dosage adjust-ments as needed. For extremely severe symptoms of peptic ulcer (hospitalized patients), 2.6 to 4.8g diluted with 2 to 3 parts of water may be given intragastrically every 30 minutes for periods of 12 or more hours a day.

For antihyperphosphatemic use:

Aluminum hydroxide:

In adults, 1.9 to 4.8g of aluminum hydroxide are given orally 3 or 4 times a day in conjunction with dietary phosphate restric-tion. In children, a dose of 50 to 150mg per kg of body weight is given in 4 to 6 divided doses in conjunction with dietary phos-phate restriction.

For antiurolithic use:

Aluminum carbonate:

In the prevention of phosphate stones, the equivalent of 1 to 3g of aluminum carbonate is given 4 times a day, 1 hour after meals and at bedtime.

For specific OTC dosing information, refer to the comprehensive product table at the end of this chapter.

BISMUTH SUBSALICYLATE

Bismuth has weak antacid properties and is indicated for the symptomatic relief of upset stomach, including heartburn, acid ingestion, and nausea.

For more information, refer to the complete monograph in "Diarrhea" under Gastrointestinal/Genitourinary System.

H₂-RECEPTOR ANTAGONISTS

PHARMACOLOGY

H₂-receptor antagonists inhibit basal and nocturnal gastric acid secretion by competitive inhibition of the action of histamine at the histamine H₂-receptors of the parietal cells. They also inhibit gastric acid secretion stimulated by food, betazole, pentagastrin, caffeine, insulin, and physiological vagal reflex.

INDICATIONS

Ulcer, duodenal (prophylaxis and treatment)—Histamine H₂-receptor antagonists are indicated for the short-term treatment of active duodenal ulcer. They are also indicated (at reduced dos-age) for the prevention of duodenal ulcer recurrence in selected patients.

Ulcer, gastric (treatment)—Cimetidine, famotidine, nizatidine, and ranitidine are indicated for the short-term treatment of active benign gastric ulcer.

Ulcer, gastric (prophylaxis)—Cimetidine and ranitidine are indi-cated (at reduced dosage) for the prevention of gastric ulcer recurrence after the healing of acute ulcers.

Heartburn, acid indigestion, and sour stomach associated with hyperacidity (prophylaxis and treatment)—Nonprescription strengths of the histamine H₂-receptor antagonists cimetidine, famotidine, and ranitidine are indicated for relief of symptoms associated with hyperacidity, including heartburn, acid indiges-tion, and sour stomach. Nonprescription strengths of cimetidine, famotidine, nizatidine, and ranitidine are also indicated in pre-vention of hyperacidity symptoms brought on by the consump-tion of food or beverages.

Hypersecretory conditions, gastric (treatment); *Zollinger-Ellison syndrome* (treatment); *mastocytosis, systemic* (treatment); *ade-noma, multiple endocrine* (treatment)—Cimetidine, famotidine, nizatidine, and ranitidine are indicated in the treatment of patho-logical gastric hypersecretion associated with Zollinger-Ellison syndrome (alone or as part of multiple endocrine neoplasia Type 1), systemic mastocytosis, and multiple endocrine adenoma.

Gastroesophageal reflux disease (GERD) (treatment)—Cimetidine, famotidine, nizatidine, and ranitidine are indicated in

Pharmacology/Pharmacokinetics of H₂-Receptor Antagonists

Drug	Mean serum concentration resulting in 50% inhibition* (ng/mL)	Time to peak concentration after oral dose (hr)	Time to peak effect (hr)	Duration of action (hr)	Elimination † (% excreted unchanged)
Cimetidine	500	0.75-1.5	Oral: 1-2	Nocturnal: 6-8 Basal: 4-5	Primarily renal (48% of oral dose; 75% of parenteral dose)‡
Famotidine	13	1-3	Oral: 1-3 Parenteral: 0.5	Nocturnal and basal: 10-12 (oral and IV)	Primarily renal (30%-35% of oral dose; 65%-70% of parenteral dose)
Nizatidine	295	0.5-3	Oral: 0.5-3	Nocturnal: Up to 12 Basal: Up to 8	Primarily renal (60% of oral dose)
Ranitidine	100	2-3	Oral: 1-3	Nocturnal: 13 Basal: 4	Primarily renal (30% of oral dose; 70% of parenteral dose)

* Refers to inhibition of pentagastrin-stimulated acid secretion.

† Trace amounts of H₂-receptor antagonists are removable by hemodialysis and peritoneal dialysis.

‡ In burn patients with thermal injury ranging from 6% to 80% of the body surface, and with normal renal function, total clearance of cimetidine has been found to be significantly increased.

the treatment of acute gastroesophageal reflux disease, which may or may not cause erosive or ulcerative esophagitis.

Pancreatic insufficiency (treatment adjunct)—Cimetidine is used to enhance pancreatic replacement by reducing peptic acid deactivation and to enhance the efficacy of orally administered pancreatic enzymes in patients with pancreatic insufficiency by reducing the secretion of hydrochloric acid. However, the efficacy of cimetidine in acute pancreatitis has not been established, and some studies have demonstrated that cimetidine may increase and prolong hyperamylasemia.

Bleeding, upper gastrointestinal (treatment)—Cimetidine, famotidine, and ranitidine are used to treat upper gastrointestinal bleeding secondary to gastric ulcer, duodenal ulcer, or hemorrhagic gastritis.

Stress-related mucosal damage (prophylaxis and treatment)—Parenteral cimetidine is indicated to prevent (and has been used to treat) upper gastrointestinal, stress-induced ulceration and bleeding, especially in intensive care patients. Parenteral ranitidine has also been used to prevent and treat this condition. However, the efficacy of histamine H_2-receptor antagonists in treating hemorrhage in critically ill patients has not been established.

Pneumonitis, aspiration (prophylaxis)—Cimetidine, ranitidine, and famotidine also are used before anesthesia induction for the prophylaxis of aspiration pneumonitis.

Arthritis, rheumatoid (treatment adjunct)—Cimetidine and ranitidine are used for the relief of gastrointestinal symptoms associated with the use of nonsteroidal anti-inflammatory drugs in the treatment of rheumatoid arthritis.

Urticaria, acute (treatment adjunct)—Cimetidine is used in combination with an antihistamine to treat acute urticaria.

CONTRAINDICATIONS

Except under special circumstances, this medication should not be used when the following medical problem exists:

- Hypersensitivity to any of the histamine H_2-receptor antagonists

Risk-benefit should be considered when the following medical problems exist:

- Acute porphyria, history of (ranitidine should be avoided in these patients)
- Cirrhosis, with history of portal systemic encephalopathy; hepatic function impairment; renal function impairment (decreased hepatic or renal clearance of histamine H_2-receptor antagonists may result in increased plasma concentrations, thus increasing the risk of side effects, especially CNS effects; dosage reduction of histamine H_2-receptor antagonists or longer intervals between doses are recommended with renal function impairment and may be necessary with hepatic function impairment)
- Immunocompromised patients (decreased gastric acidity may increase the possibility of a hyperinfection of strongyloidiasis)
- Phenylketonuria (PKU) (the chewable tablet form and the oral disintegrating tablet form of Pepcid brand of famotidine, and the effervescent granule form and the effervescent tablet form of Zantac brand of ranitidine contain aspartame, which is metabolized to phenylalanine and must be used with caution in patients with PKU)

WARNINGS/PRECAUTIONS

Patients sensitive to one of the histamine H_2-receptor antagonists may be sensitive to the other histamine H_2-receptor antagonists also.

Pregnancy: FDA Category B (cimetidine, famotidine, nizatidine, ranitidine).

Breastfeeding: Cimetidine, famotidine, nizatidine, and ranitidine appear in breast milk and could possibly suppress gastric acidity, inhibit drug metabolism, and cause CNS stimulation in the nursing infant.

ADVERSE REACTIONS

Those indicating need for medical attention: Incidence rare

For all histamine H_2-receptor antagonists:

Cardiac arrhythmias (including bradycardia, tachycardia, and atrioventricular block); dermatologic reactions (including erythema multiforme, exfoliative dermatitis, pruritus, Stevens-Johnson syndrome, and toxic epidermal necrolysis); fever; hematologic effects (including aplastic anemia, leukopenia, neutropenia, pancytopenia, thrombocytopenia, and immune hemolytic anemia—extremely rare); hepatic effects (including hepatitis and jaundice); hypersensitivity reactions (including anaphylaxis, angioedema, eosinophilia, laryngeal edema, skin rash, urticaria, vasculitis); mood or mental changes (including anxiety, agitation, confusion, hallucinations, mental depression, nervousness, psychosis); myalgia.

For cimetidine:

Agranulocytosis, arthralgia, pancreatitis.

For famotidine:

Agranulocytosis, arthralgia, asthenia, bronchospasm, fatigue, palpitations.

For nizatidine:

Amblyopia; anemia; asthenia; bronchospasm; hyperuricemia that is not associated with gout or nephrolithiasis; increased cough; infection (including pharnygitis and sinusitis); pain (including chest pain and back pain); serum sickness.

For ranitidine:

Agranulocytosis, arthralgia, blurred vision, bronchospasm, pancreatitis, premature ventricular beats.

Those indicating need for medical attention only if they continue or are bothersome: Incidence less frequent or rare

For all histamine H_2-receptor antagonists:

Decreased libido, diarrhea, dizziness, gynecomastia, headache, impotence, somnolence.

For cimetidine:

Alopecia, interstitial nephritis, polymyositis, urinary retention.

For famotidine:

Abdominal pain, alopecia, anorexia, constipation, dryness of mouth, dryness of skin, insomnia, nausea, tinnitus, vomiting.

For nizatidine:

Abdominal pain, constipation, dryness of mouth, increased sweating, insomnia, nausea, rhinitis, vomiting.

For ranitidine:

Abdominal pain, alopecia, constipation, insomnia, nausea, vomiting.

ADMINISTRATION AND DOSAGE (OTC TREATMENT)

For heartburn, acid indigestion, and sour stomach:
Cimetidine
Adults/Pediatrics ≥12 years of age: 200mg qd, max of 400mg qd.
Famotidine
Adults/Pediatrics ≥12 years of age: 10-20mg qd, max of 40mg qd.
Nizatidine
Adults/Pediatrics ≥12 years of age: 75mg qd, max of 150mg qd.
Ranitidine
Adults/Pediatrics ≥12 years of age: 75-150mg qd, max of 300mg qd.

Drug Interactions for H₂-Receptor Antagonists

Precipitant Drug	Object Drug	Effect On Object Drug	Description
Antacids	H₂-Antagonists	↓	Simultaneous administration of antacids of medium to high potency (80mmol to 150mmol HCl) is not recommended since absorption of histamine H₂-receptor antagonists may be decreased; patients should be advised not to take any antacids within 1/2 to 1 hour of taking histamine H₂-receptor antagonists.
H₂-Antagonists	Bone marrow depressants	↑	Concurrent use may increase the risk of neutropenia or other blood dyscrasias.
H₂-Antagonists	Itraconazole	↓	May increase gastrointestinal pH, which may result in a marked reduction in absorption of itraconazole or ketoconazole; patients should be advised to take histamine H₂-receptor antagonists at least 2 hours after itraconazole or ketoconazole.
H₂-Antagonists	Ketoconazole	↓	May increase gastrointestinal pH, which may result in a marked reduction in absorption of itraconazole or ketoconazole; patients should be advised to take histamine H₂-receptor antagonists at least 2 hours after itraconazole or ketoconazole.
Sucralfate	H₂-Antagonists	↓	Concurrent use may decrease the absorption of any H₂-receptor antagonist; patients should be advised to take an H₂-receptor antagonist 2 hours before sucralfate.
Cimetidine	Alcohol	↑	Some studies in humans have found increased blood alcohol levels when oral cimetidine was given in conjunction with alcohol.
Cimetidine	Anticoagulants (coumarin or indandione derivatives)	↑	Inhibition of the cytochrome P450 enzyme system by cimetidine may cause a decrease in the hepatic metabolism, which may result in delayed elimination and increased blood concentrations, when these medications are used concurrently.
Cimetidine	Benzodiazepines (chlordiazepoxide, diazepam, midazolam)	↑	Inhibition of the cytochrome P450 enzyme system by cimetidine may cause a decrease in the hepatic metabolism, which may result in delayed elimination and increased blood concentrations, when these medications are used concurrently.
Cimetidine	Calcium channel blockers (CCBs)	↑	Concurrent use may result in accumulation of the CCB as a result of inhibition of first-pass metabolism; caution and careful titration of the CCB dose is recommended.
Cimetidine	Cyclosporine	↑	Cimetidine has been reported to increase plasma concentrations of cyclosporine and may increase the risk of nephrotoxicity.
Cimetidine	Glipizide	↑	Inhibition of the cytochrome P450 enzyme system by cimetidine may cause a decrease in the hepatic metabolism, which may result in delayed elimination and increased blood concentrations, when these medications are used concurrently.
Cimetidine	Glyburide	↑	Inhibition of the cytochrome P450 enzyme system by cimetidine may cause a decrease in the hepatic metabolism, which may result in delayed elimination and increased blood concentrations, when these medications are used concurrently.
Cimetidine	Lidocaine	↑	Concurrent administration may result in reduced hepatic clearance of lidocaine, possibly resulting in delayed elimination and increased blood concentrations; lower doses of lidocaine may be required.
Cimetidine	Metoprolol	↑	Inhibition of the cytochrome P450 enzyme system by cimetidine may cause a decrease in the hepatic metabolism, which may result in delayed elimination and increased blood concentrations, when these medications are used concurrently.
Cimetidine	Metronidazole	↑	Inhibition of the cytochrome P450 enzyme system by cimetidine may cause a decrease in the hepatic metabolism, which may result in delayed elimination and increased blood concentrations, when these medications are used concurrently.
Cimetidine	Paroxetine	↑	In one study, steady-state plasma concentrations of paroxetine were increased by approximately 50% during concurrent administration.
Cimetidine	Phenytoin	↑	Inhibition of the cytochrome P450 enzyme system by cimetidine may cause a decrease in the hepatic metabolism, which may result in delayed elimination and increased blood concentrations, when these medications are used concurrently. Increased risk of ataxia due to increased blood concentrations.

Drug Interactions for H₂-Receptor Antagonists (cont.)

Precipitant Drug	Object Drug	Effect On Object Drug	Description
Cimetidine	Procainamide	↑	Renal elimination of procainamide may be decreased due to competition for active tubular secretion, resulting in increased blood concentration of procainamide.
Cimetidine	Propanolol	↑	Inhibition of the cytochrome P450 enzyme system by cimetidine may cause a decrease in the hepatic metabolism, which may result in delayed elimination and increased blood concentrations, when these medications are used concurrently.
Cimetidine	Quinine	↑	Concurrent use may reduce the clearance of quinine.
Cimetidine	Tricyclic antidepressants	↑	Inhibition of the cytochrome P450 enzyme system by cimetidine may cause a decrease in the hepatic metabolism, which may result in delayed elimination and increased blood concentrations, when these medications are used concurrently.
Cimetidine	Xanthines (aminophylline, caffeine, oxtriphylline, theophylline)	↑	Inhibition of the cytochrome P450 enzyme system by cimetidine may cause a decrease in the hepatic metabolism, which may result in delayed elimination and increased blood concentrations, when these medications are used concurrently.
Ranitidine	Alcohol	↑	Some studies in humans have found increased blood alcohol levels when oral ranitidine was given in conjunction with alcohol.
Ranitidine	Glipizide	↑	Ranitidine is a weak inhibitor of hepatic drug metabolism.
Ranitidine	Glyburide	↑	Ranitidine is a weak inhibitor of hepatic drug metabolism.
Ranitidine	Metoprolol	↑	Ranitidine is a weak inhibitor of hepatic drug metabolism.
Ranitidine	Midazolam	↑	Ranitidine is a weak inhibitor of hepatic drug metabolism.
Ranitidine	Nifedipine	↑	Ranitidine is a weak inhibitor of hepatic drug metabolism.
Ranitidine	Phenytoin	↑	Ranitidine is a weak inhibitor of hepatic drug metabolism. Increased risk of ataxia.
Ranitidine	Procainamide	↑	Renal elimination of procainamide may be decreased due to competition for active tubular secretion, resulting in increased blood concentration of procainamide.
Ranitidine	Theophylline	↑	Ranitidine is a weak inhibitor of hepatic drug metabolism.
Ranitidine	Warfarin	↑	Ranitidine is a weak inhibitor of hepatic drug metabolism.

CIMETIDINE PRODUCTS	
Brand Name	**Dosage Form**
Tagamet HB (GSK)	**Tablet:** 200mg
FAMOTIDINE PRODUCTS	
Brand Name	**Dosage Form**
Pepcid AC (J&J/Merck)	**Tablet:** 10mg **Capsule:** 10mg
Pepcid AC Maximum Strength (J&J/Merck)	**Tablet:** 20mg
NIZATIDINE PRODUCTS	
Brand Name	**Dosage Form**
Axid AR (Wyeth)	**Tablet:** 75mg
RANITIDINE PRODUCTS	
Brand Name	**Dosage Form**
Zantac 150 (Pfizer)	**Tablet:** 150mg
Zantac 75 (Pfizer)	**Tablet:** 75mg

PROTON PUMP INHIBITORS (OMEPRAZOLE)

PHARMACOLOGY

Omeprazole is a selective and irreversible proton pump inhibitor. Omeprazole suppresses gastric acid secretion by specific inhibition of the hydrogen-potassium adenosinetriphosphatase (H+, K+-ATPase) enzyme system found at the secretory surface of parietal cells. It inhibits the final transport of hydrogen ions (via exchange with potassium ions) into the gastric lumen. Since the H+, K+-ATPase enzyme system is regarded as the acid (proton) pump of the gastric mucosa, omeprazole is known as a gastric acid pump inhibitor. The inhibitory effect is dose related. Omeprazole inhibits both basal and stimulated acid secretion irrespective of the stimulus. Omeprazole does not have anticholinergic or histamine H_2-receptor antagonist properties.

INDICATIONS

Dyspepsia (treatment)—Omeprazole is indicated for the treatment of a complex of symptoms that may be caused by any of the conditions where a reduction in gastric acid secretion is required (eg, duodenal ulcer, gastric ulcer, nonsteroidal anti-inflammatory drug [NSAID]-induced gastric and duodenal ulcer, reflux esophagitis, gastroesophageal reflux disease) or when no identifiable organic cause is found (ie, functional dyspepsia).

Gastroesophageal reflux disease (GERD) (prophylaxis and treatment)—Omeprazole is indicated for the treatment of *heartburn* and other symptoms associated with gastroesophageal reflux disease. Omeprazole is indicated for the short-term treatment of erosive esophagitis (associated with GERD) that has been diagnosed by endoscopy. Omeprazole also is indicated to maintain healing of erosive esophagitis.

Hypersecretory conditions, gastric (treatment); *Zollinger-Ellison syndrome* (treatment); *mastocytosis, systemic* (treatment); *adenoma, multiple endocrine* (treatment)—Omeprazole is indicated for the long-term treatment of pathologic gastric hypersecretion associated with Zollinger-Ellison syndrome (alone or as part of multiple endocrine neoplasia Type 1), systemic mastocytosis, and multiple endocrine adenoma.

Ulcer, peptic (treatment); *ulcer, duodenal* (treatment)—Omeprazole is indicated for the short-term treatment of active duodenal ulcer and active benign gastric ulcer.

Ulcer, peptic, Helicobacter pylori-associated (treatment adjunct)—Omeprazole is indicated in combination with clarithromycin (and amoxicillin or metronidazole) for the treatment of

Drug Interactions for Omeprazole

Precipitant Drug	Object Drug	Effect On Object Drug	Description
Omeprazole	Ampicillin esters	↓	Omeprazole may increase gastrointestinal pH; concurrent use may result in reduced absorption.
Omeprazole	Iron salts	↓	Omeprazole may increase gastrointestinal pH; concurrent use may result in reduced absorption.
Omeprazole	Itraconazole	↓	Omeprazole may increase gastrointestinal pH; concurrent use may result in reduced absorption.
Omeprazole	Ketoconazole	↓	Omeprazole may increase gastrointestinal pH; concurrent use may result in reduced absorption.
Omeprazole	Anticoagulants (coumarin or indandione derivative)	↑	Inhibition of the cytochrome P450 enzyme system by omeprazole, especially in high doses, may cause a decrease in hepatic metabolism, which may result in delayed elimination and increased blood concentrations.
Omeprazole	Diazepam	↑	Inhibition of the cytochrome P450 enzyme system by omeprazole, especially in high doses, may cause a decrease in hepatic metabolism, which may result in delayed elimination and increased blood concentrations.
Omeprazole	Phenytoin	↑	Inhibition of the cytochrome P450 enzyme system by omeprazole, especially in high doses, may cause a decrease in the hepatic metabolism, which may result in delayed elimination and increased blood concentrations.
Omeprazole	Warfarin	↑	Inhibition of the cytochrome P450 enzyme system by omeprazole, especially in high doses, may cause a decrease in the hepatic metabolism, which may result in delayed elimination and increased blood concentrations.
Omeprazole	Benzodiazepines	↑	Clinical reports of interaction with these drugs metabolized via the cytochrome P450 system.
Omeprazole	Cyclosporine	↑	Clinical reports of interaction with these drugs metabolized via the cytochrome P450 system.
Omeprazole	Disulfiram	↑	Clinical reports of interaction with these drugs metabolized via the cytochrome P450 system.
Omeprazole	Bone marrow depressants	↑	Concurrent use may increase the leukopenic and/or thrombocytopenic effects of both these medications.
Omeprazole	Clarithromycin	↑	Concomitant use has resulted in plasma level increases of omeprazole, clarithromycin, and 14-hydroxy-clarithromycin.

duodenal and gastric ulcer associated with *H pylori* infection. Eradication of *H pylori* has been shown to reduce the risk of ulcer recurrence.

Ulcer, peptic, NSAID-induced (treatment)—Omeprazole is indicated for the treatment of duodenal or gastric ulcers associated with the use of NSAIDs.

CONTRAINDICATIONS

Except under special circumstances, this medication should not be used when the following medical problem exists:

● Hypersensitivity to omeprazole or any of its components

Risk-benefit should be considered when the following medical problem exists:

● Hepatic disease—chronic, current, or history of (dosage reduction may be required due to increased half-life in chronic hepatic disease)

WARNINGS/PRECAUTIONS

Pregnancy category C; caution in nursing. Appropriate studies on the relationship of age to the effects of omeprazole have not been performed in the pediatric population. Safety and efficacy have not been established in patients less than 18 years old.

ADVERSE REACTIONS

Those indicating need for medical attention: Incidence rare

Generalized skin reactions (including toxic epidermal necrolysis—sometimes fatal, Stevens-Johnson syndrome, erythema multiforme); hematologic abnormalities (specifically, anemia, agranulocytosis—sometimes fatal, hemolytic anemia, leukocytosis, neutropenia, pancytopenia or thrombocytopenia, hematuria); proteinuria; urinary tract infection

Those indicating need for medical attention only if they continue or are bothersome:

Incidence more frequent: Abdominal pain or colic.

Incidence less frequent:

Asthenia; back pain; CNS disturbances (specifically, dizziness, headache, somnolence, unusual tiredness); chest pain; cough; gastrointestinal disturbances (specifically, acid regurgitation, constipation, diarrhea or loose stools, flatulence, nausea and vomiting); skin rash or itching; upper respiratory infection.

ADMINISTRATION AND DOSAGE (OTC TREATMENT)

Adults: 20mg qd for 14 days; may repeat 14-day course every 4 months.

OMEPRAZOLE PRODUCTS	
Brand Name	**Dosage Form**
Prilosec OTC	**Capsule:** 20mg

DOSING INFORMATION FOR ANTACID AND HEARTBURN PRODUCTS

The following table provides a quick comparison of the ingredients and dosages of common brand-name OTC drugs. Products are listed alphabetically by drug category and generic ingredient.

BRAND NAME	INGREDIENT/STRENGTH	DOSE
ANTACID		
Alka-Mints chewable tablets *(Bayer Healthcare)*	Calcium Carbonate 850mg	**Adults & Peds ≥12 yo:** 1-2 tabs q2h. **Max:** 9 tabs q24h.
Alka-Seltzer Gold tablets *(Bayer Healthcare)*	Citric Acid/Potassium Bicarbonate/Sodium Bicarbonate 1000mg-344mg-1050mg	**Adults ≥60 yo:** 2 tabs q4h prn. **Max:** 7 tabs q24h. **Adults & Peds ≥12 yo:** 2 tabs q4h prn. **Max:** 8 tabs q24h. **Peds <12 yo:** 1 tab q4h prn. **Max:** 4 tabs q24h.
Alka-Seltzer Heartburn Relief tablets *(Bayer Healthcare)*	Citric Acid/Sodium Bicarbonate 1000mg-1940mg	**Adults ≥60 yo:** 2 tabs q4h prn. **Max:** 4 tabs q24h. **Adults & Peds ≥12 yo:** 2 tabs q4h prn. **Max:** 8 tabs q24h.
Alka-Seltzer Tablets, Antacid & Pain Relief *(Bayer Healthcare)*	Aspirin/Sodium Bicarbonate/Citric Acid 325 mg-1916 mg-1000 mg	**Adults ≥60 yo:** 2 tabs q4h prn. **Max:** 4 tabs q24h. **Adults & Peds ≥12 yo:** 2 tabs q4h prn. **Max:** 8 tabs q24h.
Brioschi powder *(Brioschi)*	Sodium Bicarbonate/Tartaric Acid 2.69g-2.43g/dose	**Adults & Peds ≥12 yo:** 1 capful (6g) dissolved in 4-6 oz water q1h. **Max:** 6 doses q24h.
Dulcolax Milk of Magnesia liquid *(Boehringer Ingelheim Consumer Healthcare)*	Magnesium Hydroxide 400mg/5mL	**Adults & Peds ≥12 yo:** 1-3 tsp (5-15mL) qd-qid.

DOSING INFORMATION FOR ANTACID AND HEARTBURN PRODUCTS (cont.)

BRAND NAME	INGREDIENT/STRENGTH	DOSE
Gaviscon Extra Strength liquid (GlaxoSmithKline Consumer Healthcare)	Aluminum Hydroxide/Magnesium Carbonate 254mg-237.5mg/5mL	**Adults:** 2-4 tsp (10-20mL) qid.
Gaviscon Extra Strength tablets (GlaxoSmithKline Consumer Healthcare)	Aluminum Hydroxide/Magnesium Carbonate 160mg-105mg	**Adults:** 2-4 tabs qid.
Gaviscon Original chewable tablets (GlaxoSmithKline Consumer Healthcare)	Aluminum Hydroxide/Magnesium Trisilicate 80mg-20mg	**Adults:** 2-4 tabs qid.
Gaviscon Regular Strength Liquid (GlaxoSmithKline Consumer Healthcare)	Aluminum Hydroxide/Magnesium Carbonate 95mg-358mg/5ml	**Adults:** 2-4 tsp (10-20mL) qid.
Maalox Quick Dissolve Regular Strength chewable tablets (Novartis Consumer Health)	Calcium Carbonate 600mg	**Adults:** 1-2 tabs prn. **Max:** 12 tabs q24h.
Mylanta—Children's (Johnson & Johnson/ Merck Consumer)	Calcium Carbonate 400 mg	**Peds 6-11 yo (48-95 lbs):** Take 2 tab prn. **Peds 2-5 yo (24-47 lbs):** Take 1 tab prn
Mylanta gelcaps (Johnson & Johnson/Merck Consumer)	Calcium Carbonate/Magnesium Hydroxide 550mg-125mg	**Adults:** 2-4 caps prn. **Max:** 12 caps q24h.
Mylanta Supreme Antacid liquid (Johnson & Johnson/Merck Consumer)	Calcium Carbonate/Magnesium Hydroxide 400mg-135mg/5mL	**Adults:** 2-4 tsp (10-20mL) qid. **Max:** 18 tsp (90mL) q24h.
Mylanta Ultra chewable tablets (Johnson & Johnson/Merck Consumer)	Calcium Carbonate/Magnesium Hydroxide 700mg-300mg	**Adults:** 2-4 tabs qid. **Max:** 10 tabs q24h.
Phillips Milk of Magnesia liquid (Bayer Healthcare)	Magnesium Hydroxide 400mg/5mL	**Adults & Peds ≥12 yo:** 30-60mL qd. **Peds 6-11 yo:** 15-30mL qd. **2-5 yo:** 5-15mL qd.
Riopan suspension (Wyeth Consumer Healthcare)	Magaldrate 540mg/5mL	**Adults:** 1-4 tsp (5-20mL) qid.
Rolaids Extra Strength Softchews (Pfizer Consumer Healthcare)	Calcium Carbonate 1177mg	**Adults:** 2-3 chews q1h prn. **Max:** 6 chews q24h.
Rolaids Extra Strength tablets (Pfizer Consumer Healthcare)	Calcium Carbonate/Magnesium Hydroxide 675mg-135mg	**Adults:** 2-4 tabs q1h prn. **Max:** 10 tabs q24h.
Rolaids tablets (Pfizer Consumer Healthcare)	Calcium Carbonate/Magnesium Hydroxide 550mg-110mg	**Adults:** 2-4 tabs q1h prn. **Max:** 12 tabs q24h.
Titralac chewable tablets (3M Consumer Healthcare)	Calcium Carbonate 420mg	**Adults:** 2 tabs q2-3h prn. **Max:** 19 tabs q24h.
Titralac Extra Strength chewable tablets (3M Consumer Healthcare)	Calcium Carbonate 750mg	**Adults:** 1-2 tabs q2-3h prn. **Max:** 10 tabs q24h.
Tums chewable tablets (GlaxoSmithKline Consumer Healthcare)	Calcium Carbonate 500mg	**Adults:** 2-4 tabs q1h prn. **Max:** 15 tabs q24h.
Tums E-X chewable tablets (GlaxoSmithKline Consumer Healthcare)	Calcium Carbonate 750mg	**Adults:** 2-4 tabs prn. **Max:** 10 tabs q24h.
Tums Lasting Effects chewable tablets (GlaxoSmithKline Consumer Healthcare)	Calcium Carbonate 500mg	**Adults:** 2 tabs prn. **Max:** 15 tabs q24h.
Tums Smooth Dissolve tablets (GlaxoSmithKline Consumer Healthcare)	Calcium Carbonate 750mg	**Adults:** 2-4 tabs prn. **Max:** 10 tabs q24h.
Tums Ultra Maximum Strength chewable tablets (GlaxoSmithKline Consumer Healthcare)	Calcium Carbonate 1000mg	**Adults:** 2-3 tabs prn. **Max:** 7 tabs q24h.
ANTACID/ANTIFLATULENT		
Gas-X with Maalox capsules (Novartis Consumer Health)	Calcium Carbonate/Simethicone 250mg-62.5mg	**Adults:** 2-4 caps prn. **Max:** 8 caps q24h.
Gelusil chewable tablets (Pfizer Consumer Healthcare)	Aluminum Hydroxide/Magnesium Hydroxide/ Simethicone 200mg-200mg-20mg	**Adults:** 2-4 tabs qid.
Maalox Max liquid (Novartis Consumer Health)	Aluminum Hydroxide/Magnesium Hydroxide/ Simethicone 400mg-400mg-40mg/5mL	**Adults & Peds ≥12 yo:** 2-4 tsp (10-20mL) qid. **Max:** 12 tsp (60mL) q24h.
Maalox Max Quick Dissolve Maximum Strength tablets (Novartis Consumer Health)	Calcium Carbonate/Simethicone 1000mg-60mg	**Adults:** 1-2 tabs prn. **Max:** 8 tabs q24h.
Maalox Regular Strength liquid (Novartis Consumer Health)	Aluminum Hydroxide/Magnesium Hydroxide/ Simethicone 200mg-200mg-20mg/5mL	**Adults & Peds ≥12 yo:** 2-4 tsp (10-20mL) qid. **Max:** 16 tsp (80mL) q24h.
Mylanta Maximum Strength liquid (Johnson & Johnson/Merck Consumer)	Aluminum Hydroxide/Magnesium Hydroxide/ Simethicone 400mg-400mg-40mg/5mL	**Adults & Peds ≥12 yo:** 2-4 tsp (10-20mL) qid. **Max:** 12 tsp (60mL) q24h.

DOSING INFORMATION FOR ANTACID AND HEARTBURN PRODUCTS (cont.)

Brand Name	Ingredient/Strength	Dose
Mylanta Regular Strength liquid *(Johnson & Johnson/Merck Consumer)*	Aluminum Hydroxide/Magnesium Hydroxide/Simethicone 200mg-200mg-20mg/5mL	**Adults & Peds ≥12 yo:** 2-4 tsp (10-20mL) qid. **Max:** 24 tsp (120mL) q24h.
Riopan Plus Double Strength suspension *(Wyeth Consumer Healthcare)*	Magaldrate/Simethicone 1080mg-40mg/5mL	**Adults:** 2-4 tsp (5-20mL) qid.
Riopan Plus suspension *(Wyeth Consumer Healthcare)*	Magaldrate/Simethicone 540mg-20mg/5mL	**Adults:** 2-4 tsp (5-20mL) qid.
Riopan Plus tablets *(Wyeth Consumer Healthcare)*	Magaldrate/Simethicone 540mg-20mg	**Adults:** 2-4 tabs qid.
Rolaids Multi-Symptom chewable tablets *(Pfizer Consumer Healthcare)*	Calcium Carbonate/Magnesium Hydroxide/Simethicone 675mg-135mg-60mg	**Adults:** 2 tabs qid prn. **Max:** 8 tabs q24h.
Titralac Plus chewable tablets *(3M Consumer Healthcare)*	Calcium Carbonate/Simethicone 420mg-21mg	**Adults:** 2 tabs q2-3h prn. **Max:** 19 tabs q24h.
BISMUTH SUBSALICYLATE		
Maalox Total Stomach Relief Maximum Strength liquid *(Novartis Consumer Health)*	Bismuth Subsalicylate 525mg/15mL	**Adults & Peds ≥12 yo:** 2 tbl (30mL) q1/2-1h. **Max:** 8 tbl (120mL) q24h.
Pepto Bismol chewable tablets *(Procter & Gamble)*	Bismuth Subsalicylate 262mg	**Adults & Peds ≥12 yo:** 2 tabs q1/2-1h. **Max:** 8 doses q24h.
Pepto Bismol caplets *(Procter & Gamble)*	Bismuth Subsalicylate 262mg	**Adults & Peds ≥12 yo:** 2 tabs q1/2-1h. **Max:** 8 doses q24h.
Pepto Bismol liquid *(Procter & Gamble)*	Bismuth Subsalicylate 262mg/15mL	**Adults & Peds ≥12 yo:** 2 tbl (30mL) q1/2-1h. **Max:** 8 doses (240mL) q24h.
Pepto Bismol Maximum Strength liquid *(Procter & Gamble)*	Bismuth Subsalicylate 525mg/15mL	**Adults ≥12 yo:** 2 tbl (30mL) q1h. **Peds 9-12 yo:** 1 tbl (15mL) q1h. **6-9 yo:** 2 tsp (10mL) q1h. **3-6 yo:** 1 tsp (5mL). **Max:** of 8 doses (240mL) q24h.
H₂-RECEPTOR ANTAGONIST		
Tagamet HB tablets *(GlaxoSmithKline Consumer Healthcare)*	Cimetidine 200mg	**Adults & Peds ≥12 yo:** 1 tab qd. **Max:** 2 tabs q24h.
Axid AR tablets *(Wyeth Consumer Healthcare)*	Nizatidine 75mg	**Adults:** 1 tab qd. **Max:** 2 tabs q24h.
Pepcid AC chewable tablets *(Johnson & Johnson/Merck Consumer)*	Famotidine 10mg	**Adults & Peds ≥12 yo:** 1 tab qd. **Max:** 2 tabs q24h.
Pepcid AC gelcaps *(Johnson & Johnson/Merck Consumer)*	Famotidine 10mg	**Adults & Peds ≥12 yo:** 1 cap qd. **Max:** 2 caps q24h.
Pepcid AC Maximum Strength tablets *(Johnson & Johnson/Merck Consumer)*	Famotidine 20mg	**Adults & Peds ≥12 yo:** 1 tab qd. **Max:** 2 tabs q24h.
Pepcid AC tablets *(Johnson & Johnson/Merck Consumer)*	Famotidine 10mg	**Adults & Peds ≥12 yo:** 1 tab qd. **Max:** 2 tabs q24h.
Zantac 150 tablets *(Pfizer Consumer Healthcare)*	Ranitidine 150mg	**Adults & Peds ≥12 yo:** 1 tab qd. **Max:** 2 tabs q24h.
Zantac 75 tablets *(Pfizer Consumer Healthcare)*	Ranitidine 75mg	**Adults & Peds ≥12 yo:** 1 tab qd. **Max:** 2 tabs q24h.
H₂-RECEPTOR ANTAGONIST/ANTACID		
Pepcid Complete chewable tablets *(Johnson & Johnson/Merck Consumer)*	Famotidine/Calcium Carbonate/Magnesium Hydroxide 10mg-800mg-165mg	**Adults & Peds ≥12 yo:** 1 tab qd. **Max:** 2 tabs q24h.
PROTON PUMP INHIBITOR		
Prilosec OTC tablets *(Procter & Gamble)*	Omeprazole 20mg	**Adults:** 1 tab qd × 14 days. May repeat 14 day course q 4 months.

Hemorrhoids

Hemorrhoids are common in both men and women, affecting about half of the US population by age 50. They are also common among pregnant women. The pressure of the fetus in the abdomen, as well as hormonal changes, cause the hemorrhoidal vessels to enlarge. These vessels are also placed under severe pressure during childbirth. For most women, however, hemorrhoids caused by pregnancy are a temporary problem.

Although anorectal symptoms usually aren't serious, they can occasionally indicate life-threatening malignancies or other disease processes for which early intervention is crucial. Almost every anorectal complaint labeled as hemorrhoids by a patient can signal a host of problems. Any patient with suspected disease of the perianus, anus, or rectum should be rigorously evaluated, including a detailed history followed by a thorough physical examination. Immunocompromised persons, including patients undergoing therapy for leukemia, lymphoma, or other malignancies, are at particular risk for developing anorectal complications and should be monitored closely.

Most researchers believe that hemorrhoids represent prolapsed submucosal vascular "cushions." It is postulated that regular straining during evacuation causes engorgement of the hemorrhoidal plexus within the cushions. With continued straining, the normal supports of the vascular cushions are stretched and the cushions begin to prolapse. Depending on their location, hemorrhoids are classified as either external or internal. External hemorrhoids arise from the external hemorrhoidal plexus at the anal margin. The plexus is subject to distention during defecation. As a result, a vessel may rupture and form a perianal hematoma or thrombosis within one of the veins in the plexus. Internal hemorrhoids arise from the internal hemorrhoidal plexus. They are classified by the degree of prolapse and by their ability to be reduced. Classification and treatment options are based on severity.

External tags or skin tabs are deformities of the skin of the external anal margin and occur as redundant folds. These may be the sequelae of prior thrombosed external hemorrhoids that have become organized into fibrous appendages. External anal tags can also arise after hemorrhoidectomy or de novo in the case of inflammatory bowel disease. Although external tags do not cause symptoms, they may be uncomfortable when swelling occurs or may interfere with proper hygiene. They can be excised in the office under local anesthesia as long as vascular cushions are absent in the surrounding area.

There are several OTC products available to alleviate the symptoms of hemorrhoids; many of them contain hydrocortisone, phenylephrine, or a topical anesthetic.

BULK-FORMING LAXATIVES

PHARMACOLOGY

Bulk-forming laxatives absorb water and expand to provide increased bulk and moisture content to the stool. The increased bulk encourages normal peristalsis and bowel motility.

INDICATIONS

Constipation (prophylaxis)—Oral bulk-forming laxative are indicated prophylactically in patients who should not strain during defecation, such as those with an episiotomy wound, painful thrombosed hemorrhoids, fissures or perianal abscesses, body wall and diaphragmatic hernias, anorectal stenosis, or post myocardial infarction.

Constipation (treatment)—Oral laxatives are indicated for the short-term relief of constipation. Oral bulk-forming laxatives are indicated to facilitate defecation in geriatric patients with diminished colonic motor response. Oral bulk-forming laxatives and stool softener laxatives are preferred to treat constipation that may occur during pregnancy and postpartum to help re-establish normal bowel function or to avoid straining if hemorrhoids are present.

CONTRAINDICATIONS

Except under special circumstances, this medication should not be used when the following medical problems exist:

- Appendicitis, or symptoms of
- Bleeding, rectal, undiagnosed
- Congestive heart failure
- Hypertension
- Diabetes mellitus
- Intestinal obstruction
- Sensitivity to the bulk-forming laxatives
- Dysphagia (esophageal obstruction may occur)

WARNINGS/PRECAUTIONS

Pregnancy: FDA Category B.

ADVERSE REACTIONS

Those indicating need for medical attention: Incidence less frequent

- Allergies to some vegetable components (difficulty breathing; skin rash or itching)
- Esophageal blockage or intestinal impaction

ADMINISTRATION AND DOSAGE

General Dosing Information

Bulk-forming laxatives are suitable for long-term therapy, if necessary.

For specific OTC dosing information, refer to the comprehensive product table at the end of this section.

DOCUSATE

PHARMACOLOGY

Docusate is a stool softener that reduces surface film tension of interfacing liquid contents of the bowel, promoting permeation of additional liquid into the stool to form a softer mass.

INDICATIONS

Constipation (prophylaxis)—Stool softener laxatives are indicated prophylactically in patients who should not strain during defecation, such as those with an episiotomy wound, painful thrombosed hemorrhoids, fissures or perianal abscesses, body wall and diaphragmatic hernias, anorectal stenosis, or post myocardial infarction.

Constipation (treatment)—Oral laxatives are indicated for the short-term relief of constipation. Oral bulk-forming laxatives and stool softener laxatives are preferred to treat constipation that may occur during pregnancy and postpartum to help re-establish normal bowel function or to avoid straining if hemorrhoids are present.

CONTRAINDICATIONS

Except under special circumstances, this medication should not be used when the following medical problems exist:

- Appendicitis, or symptoms of
- Bleeding, rectal, undiagnosed
- Congestive heart failure
- Hypertension
- Diabetes mellitus
- Intestinal obstruction
- Sensitivity to the class of laxative being used

WARNINGS/PRECAUTIONS

Pregnancy: FDA Category C.

ADVERSE REACTIONS

Those indicating need for medical attention: Incidence rare

- Allergies, undetermined (skin rash)

  Those indicating need for medical attention only if they continue or are bothersome: Incidence less frequent

- Stomach and/or intestinal cramping
- Throat irritation (with liquid forms)

ADMINISTRATION AND DOSAGE

General Dosing Information

Because stool softener laxatives may increase absorption of other laxatives, including mineral oil, they are not given within 2

Drug Interactions for Laxatives

Precipitant Drug	Object Drug	Effect On Object Drug	Description
Bulk-forming Laxatives	Anticoagulants, oral Digitalis glycosides Salicylates	↓	Concurrent use with cellulose bulk-forming laxatives may reduce the desired effect because of physical binding or other absorptive hindrance; a 2-hour interval between dosage with such medication and laxative dosage is recommended.
Laxatives, all classes	Potassium-sparing diuretics Potassium supplements	↓	Chronic use or overuse of laxatives may reduce serum potassium concentrations by promoting excessive potassium loss from the intestinal tract; may interfere with potassium-retaining effects of potassium-sparing diuretics.
Stool softeners	Danthron Mineral oil	↑	Concurrent use with a stool softener laxative may enhance the systemic absorption of these agents. Although such combinations are intentionally used in some "fixed-dose" laxative preparations, the propensity for toxic effects is greatly increased. Liver injury has been reported with the danthron combination following repeated dosage.

CALCIUM POLYCARBOPHIL PRODUCTS

Brand Name	Dosage Form
Fiberall (Novartis)	**Tablets:** 1250mg
Equalactin (Numark)	**Tablets:** 625mg
Fibercon (Lederle)	**Tablets:** 625mg
Fiber-Lax (Rugby)	**Tablets:** 625mg
Konsyl Fiber (Konsyl)	**Tablets:** 625mg
Perdiem (Novartis)	**Tablets:** 625mg
Phillips' Fibercaps (Bayer)	**Tablets:** 625mg

METHYCELLULOSE PRODUCTS

Brand Name	Dosage Form
Citrucel (GSK)	**Powder:** 2g/tbl **Tablet:** 500mg

PSYLLIUM PRODUCTS

Brand Name	Dosage Form
Fiberall (Novartis)	**Powder:** 3.4g/tsp **Wafer:** 3.4g
Konsyl (Konsyl)	**Powder:** 6g/tsp
Konsyl-D (Konsyl)	**Powder:** 3.4g/tsp
Metamucil (Procter & Gamble)	**Capsules:** 0.52g **Powder:** 3.4g/tsp
	Wafers: 1.7g

hours of such preparations. Inform patients of this warning. The bitter taste of some liquid preparations of this type of laxative may be improved by diluting each dose in milk or fruit juice.

For specific OTC dosing information, refer to the comprehensive product table at the end of this section.

TOPICAL ANESTHETICS

Local anesthetics block both the initiation and conduction of nerve impulses by decreasing the neuronal membrane's permeability to sodium ions. This reversibly stabilizes the membrane and inhibits depolarization, resulting in the failure of a propagated action potential and subsequent conduction blockade.

Topical anesthetics are indicated to relieve pain, pruritus, and inflammation associated with minor skin disorders.

Hemorrhoids; inflammation, anorectal; and pain, anorectal— The following medications are effective when applied to the anal, perianal, or anorectal areas: benzocaine (ointment); dibucaine; pramoxine; tetracaine hydrochloride (cream); and tetracaine and menthol. However, they are not likely to relieve symptoms associated with conditions confined to the rectum, which lacks sensory nerve fibers.

Benzocaine/Dibucaine/Pramoxine/Tetracaine

Adults/Pediatrics ≥2 years of age: Apply to the affected area 3 or 4 times a day as needed.

For more information, refer to the complete monograph for topical anesthetics in "Burns" under Dermatological Conditions.

TOPICAL CORTICOSTEROIDS

Corticosteroids diffuse across cell membranes and complex with specific cytoplasmic receptors. These complexes then enter the cell nucleus, bind to DNA (chromatin), and stimulate transcription of messenger RNA (mRNA) and subsequent protein synthesis of various inhibitory enzymes responsible for the anti-inflammatory effects of topical corticosteroids. These anti-inflammatory effects include inhibition of early processes such as edema, fibrin deposition, capillary dilatation, movement of phagocytes into the area, and phagocytic activities. Later processes, such as capillary production, collagen deposition, and keloid formation also are inhibited by corticosteroids. The overall actions of topical corticosteroids are catabolic.

Topical corticosteroids are indicated to provide symptomatic relief of inflammation and/or pruritus associated with acute and chronic corticosteroid-responsive disorders. The location of the skin lesion to be treated should be considered in selecting a formulation.

Cream/Ointment

Adults: Apply to affected area 1 to 4 times a day.

For more information, refer to the complete monograph for topical corticosteroids in "Contact Dermatitis" under Dermatological Conditions.

WITCH HAZEL

Witch hazel is a topical astringent with anti-inflammatory properties. Witch hazel extracts contain anti-inflammatory components, possess an astringent effect, and possess significant antiviral activity against herpes simplex virus type 1 (HSV-1). The antioxidant components of witch hazel extract act as a superoxide scavenger. Witch hazel extracts contain volatile components and a variety of phenolic metabolites (tannins, flavonoids, and phenolic acids) that have vasoconstrictive qualities, reduce blood flow, and act as an anti-inflammatory to skin and mucous membranes. Thermometric measurements confirm a reduction of skin temperature.

At lower concentrations, witch hazel reduces capillary permeability and covers cell membranes; at higher concentrations, the surface skin proteins are denatured, forming a denser colloidal structure that covers the wound area. This might explain the mildly antibacterial effect. Drug and tincture preparations of witch hazel bark exert a stronger astringent effect than preparations made from leaves. When fluid extracts of witch hazel are applied to inflamed exudates and secretions (preferably on injured skin surface areas), as well as mucous membranes in the deeper layers of the skin, a protein-tannin film forms. In the deeper layers of the skin, mucous secretions are inhibited and bleeding from small capillaries is stopped through coagulation.

Witch Hazel is indicated for the temporary relief of hemorrhoids.

Cream

Adults: Apply twice daily to affected area.

DOCUSATE PRODUCTS	
Brand Name	**Dosage Form**
Colace (Purdue)	**Capsule:** 50mg, 100mg
	Liquid: 100mg/10mL
	Solution: 20mg/5mL
Dulcolaz (Boehringer Ingelheim)	**Capsule:** 100mg
Ex-Lax Stool Softener (Novartis)	**Tablet:** 100mg
Fleet Sof-Lax (CB Fleet)	**Tablet:** 100mg
Phillips' Stool Softener (Bayer)	**Capsule:** 100mg
Surfak Stool Softener (Pharmacia)	**Capsule:** 240mg
DIBUCAINE PRODUCTS	
Brand Name	**Dosage Form**
Nupercainal (Novartis)	**Cream:** 0.50% **Ointment:** 1%
PRAMOXINE PRODUCTS	
Brand Name	**Dosage Form**
Tronolane (Lee Pharma)	**Cream:** 1%

HYDROCORTISONE PRODUCTS	
Brand Name	**Dosage Form**
Anusol HC-1 (Pfizer)	**Ointment:** 1%
Preparation H Cortisone (Wyeth)	**Cream:** 1%
WITCH HAZEL PRODUCTS	
Brand Name	**Dosage Form**
Anusol HC-1 (Pfizer)	**Ointment:** 1%
Preparation H Cortisone (Wyeth)	**Cream:** 1%

DOSING INFORMATION FOR HEMORRHOIDAL PRODUCTS

The following table provides a quick comparison of the ingredients and dosages of common brand-name OTC drugs. Products are listed alphabetically by drug category and brand name.

BRAND NAME	INGREDIENT/STRENGTH	DOSE
ANESTHETICS/ANESTHETIC COMBINATIONS		
Anusol Hemorrhoidal Ointment *(Warner-Lambert Consumer Healthcare)*	Pramoxine Hydrochloride/Zinc Oxide 1%-12.5%	**Adults & Peds ≥12 yo:** Apply to affected area prn. **Max:** 5 times q24h.
Fleet Pain Relief Pre-Moistened Anorectal Pads *(CB Fleet)*	Pramoxine Hydrochloride/Glycerin 1%-12%	**Adults & Peds ≥12 yo:** Apply to affected area prn. **Max:** 5 times q24h.
Hemorid Maximum Strength Hemorrhoidal Creme with Aloe *(Pfizer Consumer Healthcare)*	Petrolatum/Mineral Oil/Pramoxine HCl/Phenylephrine HCl 30%-20%-1%-0.25%	**Adults & Peds ≥12 yo:** Apply to affected area qid.
Nupercainal ointment *(Novartis Consumer Health)*	Dibucaine 1%	**Adults & Peds ≥12 yo:** Apply to affected area tid-qid.
Preparation H Hemorrhoidal Cream, Maximum Strength Pain Relief *(Wyeth Consumer Healthcare)*	Glycerin/Phenylephrine HCl/Pramoxine HCl/White Petrolatum 14.4%-0.25%-1%-15%	**Adults & Peds ≥12 yo:** Apply to affected area qid.
Tronolane Anesthetic Hemorrhoid Cream *(Lee Pharmaceuticals)*	Pramoxine Hydrochloride 1%	**Adults:** Apply to affected area prn. **Max:** 5 times q24h.
BULK-FORMING LAXATIVES		
Citrucel caplets *(GlaxoSmithKline Consumer Healthcare)*	Methylcellulose 500mg	**Adults ≥12 yo:** 2-4 tabs qd. **Max:** 12 tabs q24h. **Peds 6-12 yo:** 1 tabs qd. **Max:** 6 tabs q24h.
Citrucel powder *(GlaxoSmithKline Consumer Healthcare)*	Methylcellulose 2g/tbl	**Adults ≥12 yo:** 1 tbl (11.5g) qd-tid. **Peds 6-12 yo:** 1/2 tbl (5.75g) qd.
Equalactin chewable tablet *(Numark Laboratories)*	Calcium Polycarbophil 625mg	**Adults & Peds ≥12 yo:** 2 tabs qd. **Max:** 8 tabs qd.
Fiberall powder *(Novartis Consumer Health)*	Psyllium 3.4g/tsp	**Adults ≥12 yo:** 1 tsp qd-tid. **Peds 6-12 yo:** 1/2 tsp qd-tid.
Fiberall tablets *(Novartis Consumer Health)*	Calcium Polycarbophil 1250mg	**Adults ≥12 yo:** 1 tabs qd. **Max:** 4 tabs qd.
Fibercon caplets *(Lederle Consumer Health)*	Calcium Polycarbophil 625mg	**Adults ≥12 yo:** 2 tabs qd. **Max:** 8 tabs qd.
Fiber-Lax tablets *(Rugby Laboratories)*	Calcium Polycarbophil 625mg	**Adults ≥12 yo:** 2 tabs qd. **Max:** 8 tabs qd.
Konsyl Easy Mix powder *(Konsyl Pharmaceuticals)*	Psyllium 6g/tsp	**Adults ≥12 yo:** 1 tsp qd-tid. **Peds 6-12 yo:** 1/2 tsp qd-tid.
Konsyl Fiber tablets *(Konsyl Pharmaceuticals)*	Calcium Polycarbophil 625mg	**Adults ≥12 yo:** 2 tabs qd. **Max:** 8 tabs qd.
Konsyl Orange powder *(Konsyl Pharmaceuticals)*	Psyllium 3.4g	**Adults ≥12 yo:** 1 tsp qd-tid. **Peds 6-12 yo:** 1/2 tsp qd-tid.
Konsyl Original powder *(Konsyl Pharmaceuticals)*	Psyllium 6g/tsp	**Adults ≥12 yo:** 1 tsp qd-tid. **Peds 6-12 yo:** 1/2 tsp qd-tid.
Konsyl-D powder *(Konsyl Pharmaceuticals)*	Psyllium 3.4g/tsp	**Adults ≥12 yo:** 1 tsp qd-tid. **Peds 6-12 yo:** 1/2 tsp qd-tid.
Metamucil capsules *(Procter & Gamble)*	Psyllium 0.52g	**Adults & Peds ≥12 yo:** 4 caps qd-tid.
Metamucil Original Texture powder *(Procter & Gamble)*	Psyllium 3.4g/tsp	**Adults ≥12 yo:** 1 tsp qd-tid. **Peds 6-12 yo:** 1/2 tsp qd-tid.

DOSING INFORMATION FOR HEMORRHOIDAL PRODUCTS (cont.)

Brand Name	Ingredient/Strength	Dose
Metamucil Smooth Texture powder (Procter & Gamble)	Psyllium 3.4g/tsp	**Adults ≥12 yo:** 1 tsp qd-tid. **Peds 6-12 yo:** 1/2 tsp qd-tid.
Metamucil wafers (Procter & Gamble)	Psyllium 1.7g/tsp	**Adults ≥12 yo:** 2 wafers qd-tid. **Peds 6-12 yo:** 1 wafer qd-tid.
Phillips Fibercaps (Bayer Healthcare)	Calcium Polycarbophil 625mg	**Adults ≥12 yo:** 2 tabs qd. **Max:** 8 tabs qd. **Peds 6-12 yo:** 1 tab qd. **Max:** 4 tabs qd.
HYDROCORTISONE		
Anusol HC Anti-Itch Ointment (Warner-Lambert Consumer Healthcare)	Hydrocortisone Acetate 1%	**Adults & Peds ≥12 yo:** Insert 1 supp tid-qid.
Cortizone 10 External Anal Itch Relief Cream with Aloe (Pfizer Consumer Healthcare)	Hydrocortisone 1%	**Adults & Peds ≥12 yo:** Apply to affected area tid-qid.
Preparation H Anti-Itch Cream (Whitehall-Robins Healthcare)	Hydrocortisone 1.0%	**Adults & Peds ≥12 yo:** Apply to affected area tid-qid.
STOOL SOFTENER		
Colace capsules (Purdue Products)	Docusate Sodium 100mg	**Adults ≥12 yo:** 1-3 caps qd. **Peds 2-12 yo:** 1 cap qd.
Colace capsules (Purdue Products)	Docusate Sodium 50mg	**Adults ≥12 yo:** 1-6 caps qd. **Peds 2-12 yo:** 1-3 caps qd.
Colace liquid (Purdue Products)	Docusate Sodium 10mg/mL	**Adults ≥12 yo:** 5-15mL qd-bid. **Peds 2-12 yo:** 5-15mL qd.
Colace syrup (Purdue Products)	Docusate Sodium 60mg/15mL	**Adults ≥12 yo:** 15-90mL qd. **Peds 2-12 yo:** 5-37.5mL qd.
Correctol Stool Softener Laxative soft-gels (Schering-Plough)	Docusate Sodium 100mg	**Adults ≥12 yo:** Take 1-3 cap qd. **Peds 6-12 yo:** Take 1 cap qd.
Doculase Constipation Relief softgels (Western Research Laboratories)	Docusate Sodium 100mg	**Adults ≥12 yo:** Take 1-3 cap qd. **Peds 6-12 yo:** Take 1 cap qd.
Doculase Constipation Relief softgels (Western Research Laboratories)	Docusate Sodium 50mg	**Adults ≥12 yo:** Take 1-3 cap qd. **Peds 6-12 yo:** Take 1 cap qd.
Docusol Constipation Relief, Mini Enemas (Western Research Laboratories)	Docusate Sodium 283mg	**Adults ≥12 yo:** Take 1-3 units qd. **Peds 6-12 yo:** Take 1 unit qd.
Dulcolax Stool Softener capsules (Boehringer Ingelheim Consumer Healthcare)	Docusate Sodium 100mg	**Adults ≥12 yo:** 1-3 caps qd. **Peds 2-12 yo:** 1 cap qd.
Ex-Lax Stool Softener tablets (Novartis Consumer Health)	Docusate Sodium 100mg	**Adults ≥12 yo:** 1-3 caps qd. **Peds 2-12 yo:** 1 cap qd.
Fleet Sof-Lax tablets (CB Fleet)	Docusate Sodium 100mg	**Adults ≥12 yo:** 1-3 caps qd. **Peds 2-12 yo:** 1 cap qd.
Kaopectate Liqui-Gels (Pharmacia Consumer Healthcare)	Docusate Sodium 240mg	**Adults & Peds ≥12 yo:** 1 cap qd until normal bowel movement.
Phillips Stool Softener capsules (Bayer Healthcare)	Docusate Sodium 100mg	**Adults ≥12 yo:** 1-3 caps qd. **Peds 2-12 yo:** 1 cap qd.
WITCH HAZEL/WITCH HAZEL COMBINATIONS		
Hemspray Hemorrhoid Relief Spray (Blairex Laboratories)	Witch Hazel/Glycerin/Phenylephrine HCl/Camphor 50%-20%-0.25%-0.15%	**Adults & Peds ≥12 yo:** Apply to affected area prn. **Max:** 5 times q24h.
Hemspray Hemorrhoid Relief Swabs (Blairex Laboratories)	Witch Hazel/Glycerin/Phenylephrine HCl/Camphor 50%-20%-0.25%-0.15%	**Adults & Peds ≥12 yo:** Apply to affected area prn. **Max:** 5 times q24h.
Preparation H Hemorrhoidal Cooling Gel (Whitehall-Robins Healthcare)	Phenylephrine HCl/Witch Hazel 0.25%-50.0%	**Adults & Peds ≥12 yo:** Apply to affected area qid.
Preparation H Medicated Wipes (Whitehall-Robins Healthcare)	Witch Hazel 50%	**Adults & Peds ≥12 yo:** Apply to affected area prn. **Max:** 6 times q24h.
T.N. Dickinson's Witch Hazel Hemorrhoidal Pads (Dickinson Brands)	Witch Hazel 50%	**Adults & Peds ≥12 yo:** Apply to affected area prn. **Max:** 6 times q24h.
Tucks Hemorrhoidal Pads with Witch Hazel (Warner-Lambert Consumer Healthcare)	Witch Hazel 50%	**Adults & Peds ≥12 yo:** Apply to affected area prn. **Max:** 6 times q24h.
Tucks Hemorrhoidal Towelettes with Witch Hazel (Warner-Lambert Consumer Healthcare)	Witch Hazel 50%	**Adults & Peds ≥12 yo:** Apply to affected area prn. **Max:** 6 times q24h.

DOSING INFORMATION FOR HEMORRHOIDAL PRODUCTS (cont.)

Brand Name	Ingredient/Strength	Dose
MISCELLANEOUS		
Anusol Hemorrhoidal Suppositories *(Warner-Lambert Consumer Healthcare)*	Topical Starch 51%	**Adults & Peds ≥12 yo:** Insert 1 supp prn. **Max:** 6 times q24h.
Preparation H Hemorrhoidal Ointment *(Whitehall-Robins Healthcare)*	Mineral Oil/Petrolatum/Phenylephrine HCl/Shark Liver Oil 14%-71.9%-0.25%-3.0%	**Adults & Peds ≥12 yo:** Apply to affected area qid.
Preparation H Hemorrhoidal Suppositories *(Whitehall-Robins Healthcare)*	Cocoa Butter/Phenylephrine HCl/Shark Liver Oil 85.5%-0.25%-3.0%	**Adults & Peds ≥12 yo:** Insert 1 supp qid.
Rectal Medicone Suppositories *(Lee Pharmaceuticals)*	Phenylephrine HCl 0.25%	**Adults & Peds ≥12 yo:** Insert 1 supp tid-qid.
Tronolane Suppositories *(Lee Pharmaceuticals)*	Zinc Oxide 5%	**Adults & Peds ≥12 yo:** Insert 1 supp tid-qid.

Lactose Intolerance

Lactose intolerance is defined as the inability to digest lactose, a type of sugar found in milk and other diary products. Normally, the small intestine produces lactase, an enzyme that converts this type of sugar into a form the body can use. Lactose intolerance occurs when the small intestine does not produce enough of this enzyme. Symptoms of lactose intolerance range from mild to severe and usually begin 30 minutes to 2 hours after eating or drinking milk or milk products. Common symptoms include abdominal cramps, bloating, flatulence, weight loss, malnutrition, slow growth, abdominal distention, abdominal fullness, diarrhea, and gurgling or rumbling sounds in the abdomen. There are a number of OTC products containing the enzyme lactase that are indicated to treat lactose intolerance.

LACTASE

PHARMACOLOGY

Lactase enzymatically breaks down the disaccharide lactose into 2 monosaccharides—glucose and galactose. Unlike lactose, glucose and galactose are readily absorbed and do not produce a hyperosmotic stat in the intestinal tract.

INDICATIONS

Lactose intolerance (treatment)—Lactase is a natural enzyme that helps the body break down lactose, the complex sugar found in dairy foods. If not properly digested, lactose can cause flatulence, bloating, cramps, or diarrhea.

CONTRAINDICATIONS

Except under special circumstances, this medication should not be used when the following medical problems exist:

• Hypersensitivity to lactase.

WARNINGS/PRECAUTIONS

Pregnancy: Problems in humans have not been documented.

Breastfeeding: Problems in humans have not been documented.

ADVERSE REACTIONS

None reported.

ADMINISTRATION AND DOSAGE

Tablets

Adults/Pediatrics: 1 to 3 tablets with the first bite of dairy food or beverage.

LACTASE PRODUCTS	
Brand Name	**Dosage Form**
Lactaid Extra Strength (McNeil)	**Tablet:** 4500 U
Lactaid Original (McNeil)	**Tablet:** 3300 U
Lactaid Ultra (McNeil)	**Tablet:** 9000 U
Lactrase (Schwarz)	**Capsule:** 250mg

DOSING INFORMATION FOR LACTASE PRODUCTS

The following table provides a quick comparison of the ingredients and dosages of common brand-name OTC drugs.

BRAND NAME	INGREDIENT/STRENGTH	DOSE
Lactaid Extra Strength caplets *(McNeil Consumer)*	Lactase Enzyme 4500 FCC	**Adults:** Take 2 tabs with every dairy meal.
Lactaid Fast Act caplets *(McNeil Consumer)*	Lactase Enzyme 9000 FCC	**Adults:** Take 1 tab with every dairy meal.
Lactaid Fast Act chewable tablet *(McNeil Consumer)*	Lactase Enzyme 9000 FCC	**Adults:** Chew 1 tab with every dairy meal.
Lactaid Original Strength caplets *(McNeil Consumer)*	Lactase Enzyme 3000 FCC	**Adults:** Take 3 tabs with every dairy meal.
Lactaid Ultra caplets *(McNeil Consumer)*	Lactase Enzyme 9000 FCC	**Adults:** Take 1 tab with every dairy meal.

Nausea and Vomiting

Nausea with or without vomiting is a common complaint that may reflect an insignificant and transient illness or herald a life-threatening disease. In an otherwise healthy individual, self-limited nausea or vomiting that lasts less than 48 hours rarely represents a major problem. Persistent or chronic nausea and vomiting indicate a more serious underlying illness and may adversely affect the patient's nutrition, fluid balance, serum electrolyte balance, and quality of life. The management of nausea and vomiting is aimed first at identifying and correcting the complications of nausea and vomiting, then at identifying the underlying disease, and finally at symptomatic relief. A patient with dehydration, hypotension, or electrolyte disturbances secondary to severe nausea and vomiting is likely to require hospitalization for management.

Nausea is defined as epigastric distress associated with the sensation of a need to vomit; it may lead to anorexia and decreased food intake. Vomiting is the ejection of matter from the stomach through the esophagus and mouth and is the result of a complex pattern of gastrointestinal (GI) motility consisting of retrograde duodenal contractions, a forceful downward thrust of the diaphragm, and relaxation of the lower esophageal sphincter. Stimulation of the area postrema activates the nucleus of the solitary tract, leading to nausea and vomiting. Although they typically occur together, nausea and vomiting can occur independently. The differential diagnosis is similar for each symptom; however, vomiting can be stimulated in the absence of nausea, especially in the patient with central nervous system (CNS) disease. Vomiting is initiated in the vomiting center, which is located in the area postrema on the dorsal surface of the medulla oblongata, a region that lacks a blood-brain diffusion barrier. Stimuli to the vomiting center come from different regions, including the chemoreceptor trigger zone in the floor of the fourth ventricle, higher regions of the brain, and the GI tract via the vagus nerve.

Drugs are a frequent cause of nausea and vomiting. Food poisoning, viral gastroenteritis, and drugs are the most common causes of nausea and vomiting not associated with abdominal pain. The inhalational anesthetic agents, particularly nitrous oxide, are significant causes of postoperative emesis, especially when compared to newer agents, such as propofol. Postoperative vomiting is a greater problem in women and children than in men. Nausea and, to some degree, vomiting may be an expected side effect of a drug (e.g., an opiate analgesic) or a sign of toxicity (digitalis). Cancer chemotherapy can cause severe nausea and vomiting acutely or after a short delay. In addition, nausea and vomiting associated with anorexia, malaise, and weight loss may occur as systemic effects of a neoplasm. Various metabolic changes can cause intermittent or chronic nausea and/or vomiting. Nausea accompanies up to 70% of uncomplicated pregnancies. Vomiting in pregnancy is generally self-limited and does not require treatment; severe vomiting (hyperemesis gravidarum) occurs in less than 1% of pregnant women but can cause significant fluid loss and electrolyte disturbances. Ketoacidosis, uremia, and adrenal insufficiency are other metabolic disorders associated with nausea and vomiting. Myocardial infarction, particularly an inferior wall or large area infarction, may produce nausea and vomiting through stimulation of vagal afferent pathways. Gastroparesis, a disorder in which weak contractions of the gastric muscles or uncoordinated contractions of the duode-

num cause poor propulsion, may be associated with chronic and disabling vomiting. Gastroparesis may be caused by primary disease of the GI tract or may be secondary to a systemic disease (e.g., scleroderma, amyloidosis, and particularly diabetes). Patients with gastroparesis often have left upper quadrant abdominal distention and a succussion splash.

There is increasing recognition that nausea and vomiting are also part of a symptom complex associated with nonspecific motility disorders of the duodenum and stomach. Patients with a gastric outlet obstruction caused by duodenal ulcer, gastric carcinoma, or pancreatic carcinoma often vomit a large volume that consists of the contents of previous meals. A succussion splash is present on examination. Rarely, peristaltic waves are seen moving across the left upper quadrant. Patients with nonobstructing mucosal diseases of the stomach also complain of nausea and vomiting, possibly due to poor accommodation of the gastric fundus to ingested food. A gastric ulcer or gastritis may increase upper GI irritability, which may cause the patient to vomit soon after eating. Generally, patients with a duodenal ulcer do not vomit but gain relief of their symptoms by frequent eating. Physical examination will not demonstrate an increased gastric volume in these patients. Nausea may be reported by patients with psychiatric disorders, such as anorexia nervosa, bulimia nervosa, and depression. Vomiting that alarms the family or close associates of a patient with an eating disorder may be the major symptom that leads to the diagnosis of bulimia following binge eating. Recognition by a dentist of accelerated destruction of a patient's tooth enamel from prolonged contact with gastric acid may aid in diagnosis. Nausea and vomiting can be the sentinel symptoms of CNS disease associated with an elevated cerebrospinal fluid pressure. The vomiting may be projectile without preceding nausea or retching. If a patient's symptoms do not point to the GI tract, consider a CNS cause. A disturbance of the vestibular system, as in motion sickness, can cause nausea and vomiting. The afferent pathway is via the eighth cranial nerve. Activation of the brainstem is mediated primarily via histamine H_1 and muscarinic cholinergic rather than dopaminergic or serotonergic pathways. Thus, antihistamines and anticholinergics are first-line therapy. Vestibular disorders cause extensive autonomic activation resulting in salivation, diaphoresis, pallor, and disturbed gastric motility. Associated vertigo or tinnitus suggests vestibular disease.

It is important to differentiate between rumination and reflux. In rumination, the gastric contents are pushed up into the esophagus because of a voluntary increase in gastric intraluminal pressure. In contrast, a decrease in lower esophageal sphincter pressure with normal variations in intragastric pressure leads to reflux (for more information, see "Heartburn/Gastroesophageal Reflux Disease" under Gastrointestinal/Genitourinary System). Regurgitation caused by a swallowing disorder may be mistaken for vomiting. However, pharyngeal dysmotility is associated with choking and oral (and/or nasal) regurgitation of food that has not been mixed with gastric juices. It is not associated with nausea. An esophageal (Zenker) diverticulum can discharge its contents hours after the patient has eaten, making it difficult to differentiate from vomiting. However, regurgitated material from a Zenker diverticulum is not mixed with gastric juices or bile. Severe reflux esophagitis may present with regurgitation of food into the back of the throat, especially while the patient is sleeping. Heartburn is common, but patients with long-standing reflux often lose this sensation. Regurgitation typically follows a recent meal and occurs more often if the patient lies down or increases the intra-abdominal pressure by lifting a heavy object or performing a Valsalva maneuver.

There are a number of OTC products used to relieve mild nausea or vomiting (e.g., bismuth subsalicylate and phosphorated carbohydrate solutions) and to prevent nausea associated with motion sickness (e.g., meclizine, dimenhydrinate).

ANTIHISTAMINES

Anti-emetic; antivertigo agent—The mechanism by which some antihistamines exert their anti-emetic, anti-motion sickness, and antivertigo effects is not precisely known but may be related to their central anticholinergic actions. They diminish vestibular stimulation and depress labyrinthine function. An action on the medullary chemoreceptive trigger zone may also be involved in the anti-emetic effect.

Motion sickness (prophylaxis and treatment); *vertigo* (treatment)—Dimenhydrinate and diphenhydramine are indicated for the prevention and treatment of the nausea, vomiting, dizziness, or vertigo related to motion sickness.

Dimenhydrinate

For anti-emetic/antivertigo use:

Adults/Pediatrics ≥12 years of age: 50 to 100mg every 4 to 6 hours.

Pediatrics 2 to 6 years of age: 12.5 to 25mg every 6 to 8 hours as needed; not to exceed 75mg/day.

Pediatrics 6 to 12 years of age: 25 to 50mg every 6 to 8 hours as needed; not to exceed 150mg/day.

For more information, refer to the complete monograph for antihistamines in "Allergic Rhinitis" under Respiratory System.

Diphenhydramine

For anti-emetic/antivertigo use:

Adults: 25 to 50mg every 4 to 6 hours as needed.

Pediatrics: 1 to1.5mg/kg of body weight every 4 to 6 hours as needed; not to exceed 300mg/day.

For more information, refer to the complete monograph for antihistamines in "Allergic Rhinitis" under Respiratory System.

BISMUTH SUBSALICYLATE

Gastric distress (treatment)—Bismuth subsalicylate is indicated for the symptomatic relief of upset stomach, including heartburn, acid indigestion, and nausea in adults and children 12 years of age and older.

Adults/Pediatrics ≥12 year of age: 524mg every 30 minutes to 1 hour as needed, up to 8 doses in 24 hours.

Pediatrics 9 to 12 years of age: 262mg every 30 minutes to 1 hour as needed, up to 8 doses in 24 hours.

Pediatrics 6 to 9 years of age: 174mg every 30 minutes to 1 hour as needed, up to 8 doses in 24 hours.

Pediatrics 3 to 6 years of age: 87mg every 30 minutes to 1 hour as needed, up to 8 doses in 24 hours.

For more information, refer to the complete monograph for bismuth subsalicylate in "Diarrhea" under Gastrointestinal/Genitourinary System.

DIMENHYDRINATE PRODUCTS	
Brand Name	**Dosage Form**
Dramamine (Pharmacia)	**Tablet:** 50mg

DIPHENHYDRAMINE PRODUCTS	
Brand Name	**Dosage Form**
Benadryl (Pfizer)	**Capsule:** 25mg **Tablet:** 25mg
Benadryl Allergy (Pfizer)	**Solution:** 12.5mg/5mL **Tablet:** 12.5mg
Benadryl Allergy Fastmelt	**Tablet:** 19mg
Nytol (GSK)	**Tablet:** 25mg
Nytol Maximum Strength (GSK)	**Tablet:** 50mg
Simply Sleep (McNeil)	**Tablet:** 25mg
Sominex (GSK)	**Tablet:** 25mg, 50mg
Unisom Maximum Strength(Pfizer)	**Tablet:** 50mg

BISMUTH SUBSALICYLATE PRODUCTS	
Brand Name	**Dosage Form**
Kaopectate (Pharmacia)	**Caplet:** 262mg **Liquid:** 262mg/15mL
Kaopectate Extra Strength (Pharmacia)	**Liquid:** 525mg/15mL
Pepto Bismol (Procter & Gamble)	**Caplet/Chewable Tablet:** 262mg **Liquid:** 262mg/15mL
Pepto Bismol Maximum Strength (Procter & Gamble)	**Liquid:** 525mg/15mL

MECLIZINE PRODUCTS	
Brand Name	**Dosage Form**
Dramamine II (Pharmacia)	**Tablet:** 25mg
Bonine (Insight)	**Tablet:** 25mg

MECLIZINE

Anti-emetic; antivertigo agent—The mechanism by which meclizine exerts its anti-emetic, anti-motion sickness, and antivertigo effects is not precisely known but may be related to its central anticholinergic actions. It diminishes vestibular stimulation and depresses labyrinthine function. An action on the medullary chemoreceptive trigger zone may also be involved in the anti-emetic effect.

Motion sickness (prophylaxis and treatment)—Meclizine is indicated for the prophylaxis and treatment of nausea, vomiting, and dizziness associated with motion sickness.

For motion sickness (prophylaxis and treatment):

Adults/Pediatrics ≥12 years of age: 25 to 50mg 1 hour before travel; may repeat every 24 hours as needed.

For more information, refer to the complete monograph for meclizine in "Motion Sickness" under Central Nervous System.

DOSING INFORMATION FOR NAUSEA/VOMITING PRODUCTS

The following table provides a quick comparison of the ingredients and dosages of common brand-name OTC drugs. Products are listed alphabetically by drug category and brand name.

BRAND NAME	INGREDIENT/STRENGTH	DOSE
BISMUTH SUBSALICYLATE		
Kaopectate caplet *(Pharmacia Consumer Healthcare)*	Bismuth Subsalicylate 262mg caplets	**Adults & Peds ≥12 yo:** 2 tabs q1/2-1h. **Max:** 8 doses q24h.
Kaopectate Extra Strength *(Pharmacia Consumer Healthcare)*	Bismuth Subsalicylate 525mg/15mL	**Adults ≥12 yo:** 2 tbl (30mL). **Peds 9-12 yo:** 1 tbl (15mL) q1h prn. **6-9 yo:** 2 tsp (10mL) q1h prn. **3-6 yo:** 1 tsp (5mL) q1h prn. **Max:** 8 doses q24h.
Kaopectate liquid *(Pharmacia Consumer Healthcare)*	Bismuth Subsalicylate 262mg/15mL	**Adults ≥12 yo:** 2 tbl (30mL). **Peds 9-12 yo:** 1 tbl (15mL) q1h prn. **6-9 yo:** 2 tsp (10mL) q1h prn. **3-6 yo:** 1 tsp (5mL) q1h prn. **Max:** 8 doses q24h.
Pepto Bismol chewable tablets *(Procter & Gamble)*	Bismuth Subsalicylate 262mg	**Adults & Peds ≥12 yo:** 2 tabs q1/2-1h. **Max:** 8 doses q24h.
Pepto Bismol caplets *(Procter & Gamble)*	Bismuth Subsalicylate 262mg	**Adults & Peds ≥12 yo:** 2 tabs q1/2-1h. **Max:** 8 doses q24h.
Pepto Bismol liquid *(Procter & Gamble)*	Bismuth Subsalicylate 262mg/15mL	**Adults & Peds ≥12 yo:** 2 tbl (30mL) q1/2-1h. **Max:** 8 doses q24h.
Pepto Bismol Maximum Strength *(Procter & Gamble)*	Bismuth Subsalicylate 525mg/15mL	**Adults ≥12 yo:** 2 tbl (30mL). **Peds 9-12 yo:** 1 tbl (15mL) q1h prn. **6-9 yo:** 2 tsp (10mL) q1h prn. **3-6 yo:** 1 tsp (5mL) q1h prn. **Max:** 8 doses q24h.
DIMENHYDRINATE		
Dramamine chewable tablets *(Pharmacia Consumer Healthcare)*	Dimenhydrinate 50mg	**Adults & Peds ≥12 yo:** 1-2 tabs q4-6h. **Max:** 8 tabs q24h. **Peds 6-12 yo:** 1/2-1 tab q6-8h. **Max:** 3 tabs q24h **Peds 2-6 yo:** 1/4-1/2 tab q6-8h. **Max:** 1/2-1 tab q24h.
Dramamine tablets *(Pharmacia Consumer Healthcare)*	Dimenhydrinate 50mg	**Adults & Peds ≥12 yo:** 1-2 tabs q4-6h. **Max:** 8 tabs q24h. **Peds 6-12 yo:** 1/2-1 tab q6-8h. **Max:** 3 tabs q24h **Peds 2-6 yo:** 1/4-1/2 tab q6-8h. **Max:** 1/2-1 tab q24h.
MECLIZINE		
Bonine chewable tablets *(Pfizer Consumer Healthcare)*	Meclizine HCl 25mg	**Adults & Peds ≥12 yo:** Take 1-2 tabs qd as directed
Dramamine Less Drowsy Formula *(Pharmacia Consumer Healthcare)*	Meclizine HCl 25mg	**Adults & Peds ≥12 yo:** Take 1-2 tabs qd as directed
MISCELLANEOUS		
Emetrol solution *(Pfizer Consumer Healthcare)*	Dextrose/Lebulose/Phosphoric Acid 1.87g-1.87g-21.5mg/5mL	**Adults ≥12 yo:** 1 or 2 tbl q15min prn. **Peds 2 to 12 yo:** 1 or 2 tsp q15min prn. Not to be taken for more than 1 hour (5 doses).
Cola syrup *(Humco)*	High Fructose Corn Syrup, Sucrose, Water, Caramel Color, Phosphoric Acid, Natural Flavors, Caffeine	**Adults ≥12 yo:** 1 or 2 tbl q15min prn. **Peds 2 to 12 yo:** 1 or 2 tsp q15min prn. Not to be take more then 4 to 6 doses/day.

Pinworm Infection

Pinworms (*Enterobius vermicularis*) are a type of parasite that infects the intestines and survives by eating nutrients from the infected person's food. Pinworms are most common in school-aged children and are spread directly from person to person or by touching bedding, food, and other items contaminated with the eggs. Common symptoms of pinworm infection include intense itching around the anus, loss of appetite, abdominal pain, difficulty sleeping due to itching, and vaginal irritation or discomfort. There are both prescription and nonprescription medications available to treat pinworms. Most OTC products contain pyrantel pamoate.

PYRANTEL PAMOATE

PHARMACOLOGY

Pyrantel is not vermicidal or ovicidal. It acts as a depolarizing neuromuscular-blocking agent, thereby causing sudden contraction, followed by paralysis, of pinworms and other parasites. This makes them incapable of maintaining their position in the intestinal lumen. The incapacitated parasites are then expelled from the body in the fecal stream by peristalsis. Pyrantel also acts as a cholinesterase inhibitor and ganglionic stimulant.

INDICATIONS

Ascariasis (treatment)—Pyrantel is indicated in the treatment of ascariasis caused by *Ascaris lumbricoides* (common roundworm).

Enterobiasis (treatment)—Pyrantel is indicated in the treatment of enterobiasis (oxyuriasis) caused by *Enterobius vermicularis* (formerly *Oxyuris vermicularis*) (pinworm).

Helminth infections, multiple (treatment)—Pyrantel is indicated in the treatment of multiple helminth infections.

Hookworm infection (treatment)—Pyrantel is used in the treatment of hookworm infection (uncinariasis) caused by *Ancylostoma duodenale* (common hookworm; Old World or European hookworm) and *Necator americanus* (American or New World hookworm).

Trichostrongyliasis (treatment)—Pyrantel is used in the treatment of trichostrongyliasis caused by *Trichostrongylus* species.

CONTRAINDICATIONS

Risk-benefit should be considered when the following medical problems exist:

• Hypersensitivity to pyrantel.

• Liver disease.

Warnings/Precautions

Pregnancy: Adequate and well-controlled studies in humans have not been done. However, the use of pyrantel during pregnancy is not recommended.

Breastfeeding: Pyrantel is poorly and incompletely absorbed from the gastrointestinal tract, and resulting maternal serum concentrations are low (0.05-0.13 mcg/mL). Therefore, it is unlikely that significant amounts of pyrantel would be excreted in breast milk. Problems in humans have not been documented. However, the Canadian manufacturer recommends discontinuing breast-feeding while on pyrantel therapy.

DRUG INTERACTIONS

Piperazine—major clinical significance: May antagonize the anthelmintic effects of pyrantel; concurrent use is not recommended.

Adverse Reactions

Those indicating need for medical attention: Incidence rare

Hypersensitivity (skin rash).

Those indicating need for medical attention only if they continue or are bothersome: Incidence less frequent

Central nervous system (CNS) effects (dizziness; drowsiness; headache; irritability; trouble in sleeping).

Gastrointestinal disturbances (abdominal or stomach cramps or pain; diarrhea; loss of appetite; nausea or vomiting).

ADMINISTRATION AND DOSING

General Dosing Information

No special preparations (eg, dietary restrictions or fasting, concurrent medications, purging, or cleansing enemas) are required before, during, or immediately after treatment with pyrantel. Pyrantel may be taken with or without food at any time of day. It may be taken alone or with milk or fruit juice.

For hookworms: In the treatment of hookworms, especially in patients who are heavily infected or have inadequate dietary intake of iron, concurrent iron therapy may be required if anemia occurs. Iron therapy may need to be continued for up to 6 months to replenish iron stores.

For pinworms: Because of the high probability of transfer of pinworms, it is usually recommended that all members of the household be treated concurrently. Retreatment of entire household is recommended 2 to 3 weeks following initial treatment.

Suspension/Tablets

For ascariasis:

Adults/Pediatrics >2 years of age: 11mg/kg of body weight as a single dose. May be repeated in 2 to 3 weeks if necessary.

For enterobiasis:

Adults/Pediatrics >2 years of age: 11mg/kg of body weight as a single dose. Repeat in 2 to 3 weeks.

For hookworm:

Adults/Pediatrics >2 years of age: 11mg/kg of body weight once a day for 3 days.

For trichostrongyliasis:

Adults/Pediatrics >2 years of age: 11mg/kg of body weight as a single dose.

Alternative Dosing for Infants and Children weighing:

- 11 to 16kg (25-37lb)—125mg (base).
- 17 to 28kg (38-62lb)—250mg (base).
- 29 to 39kg (63-87lb)—375mg (base).
- 40 to 50kg (88-112lb)—500mg (base).
- 51 to 62kg (113-137lb)—625mg (base).
- 63 to 73kg (138-162lb)—750mg (base).
- 74 to 84kg (163-187lb)—875mg (base).
- >85kg (>188 lb)—1000mg (base).

OR

- ≤11kg (≤25lb)—125mg (base).
- 12 to 23kg (26-50lb)—250mg (base).
- 24 to 45kg (51-100lb)—500mg (base).
- 46 to 68kg (101-150lb)—750mg (base).
- >69kg (>151lb)—1000mg (base).

In the treatment of ascariasis, enterobiasis, or uncinariasis (hookworm infection), pyrantel may be given in the above amounts as a single dose. Alternatively, in the treatment of uncinariasis, pyrantel may be given in the above amounts once a day for 3 days.

PYRANTEL PAMOATE PRODUCTS	
Brand Name	**Dosage Form**
Reese's Pinworm (Reese)	**Tablet:** 180mg **Suspension:** 144mg/mL
No Doz Maximum Strength (BMS)	**Tablet:** 200mg

Aches and Pains

Everyone experiences pain at some point. Pain is defined as an unpleasant sensation localized to a particular area of the body. Pain is often a sign of something wrong and is the most common reason for visits to physicians. Acute pain usually begins suddenly, is ordinarily sharp in intensity, and is often due to trauma or injury. Acute pain often results from burns or cuts, broken bones, surgery, infection, and other assaults to the body. Chronic pain is the type of pain that persists even after an injury or illness has healed. Common chronic pain complaints include headache, lower back pain, cancer pain, arthritis pain, neuropathic pain, and psychogenic pain. There are many OTC products available to treat pain. Many contain acetaminophen, salicylates (e.g., aspirin), and NSAIDs (ibuprofen, ketoprofen, naproxen).

ACETAMINOPHEN

PHARMACOLOGY

Analgesic—The mechanism of analgesic action has not been fully determined. Acetaminophen may act predominantly by inhibiting prostaglandin synthesis in the central nervous system and, to a lesser extent, through a peripheral action by blocking pain-impulse generation. The peripheral action may also be due to inhibition of prostaglandin synthesis or to inhibition of the synthesis or actions of other substances that sensitize pain receptors to mechanical or chemical stimulation.

Antipyretic—Acetaminophen probably produces antipyresis by acting centrally on the hypothalamic heat-regulating center to produce peripheral vasodilation, resulting in increased blood flow to the skin, sweating, and heat loss. The central action probably involves inhibition of prostaglandin synthesis in the hypothalamus.

INDICATIONS

Pain (treatment); *pain, arthritic, mild* (treatment); *fever* (treatment)—Acetaminophen is indicated to relieve mild to moderate pain and reduce fever. It provides symptomatic relief only; additional therapy to treat the cause of the pain or fever should be instituted when necessary. Acetaminophen has minimal anti-inflammatory activity and does not relieve redness, swelling, or stiffness due to arthritis; it cannot be used in place of aspirin or other salicylates or other nonsteroidal anti-inflammatory drugs (NSAIDs) in the treatment of rheumatoid arthritis. However, it may be used to relieve pain due to mild osteoarthritis. Acetaminophen may be used when aspirin therapy is contraindicated or inadvisable; e.g., in patients receiving anticoagulants or uricosuric agents, in patients with hemophilia or other bleeding problems, and in those with upper gastrointestinal disease or intolerance or hypersensitivity to aspirin. However, chronic, high-dose acetaminophen therapy may require adjustment of anticoagulant dosage based on increased monitoring of prothrombin time in patients receiving a coumarin- or indandione-derivative anticoagulant.

CONTRAINDICATIONS

Risk-benefit should be considered when the following medical problems exist:

- Alcoholism, active—*major clinical significance* (increased risk of hepatotoxicity).

- Hepatic disease—*major clinical significance* (increased risk of hepatotoxicity).

- Viral hepatitis—*major clinical significance* (increased risk of hepatotoxicity).

- Phenylketonuria (products that contain aspartame, which is metabolized to phenylalanine, may be hazardous to patients with phenylketonuria, especially young children; caution is recommended).

- Renal function impairment, severe (risk of adverse renal effects may be increased with prolonged use of high doses; occasional use is acceptable).

- Sensitivity to acetaminophen or aspirin (increased risk of allergic reaction).

WARNINGS/PRECAUTIONS

Patients sensitive to aspirin may not be sensitive to acetaminophen; however, mild bronchospastic reactions with acetaminophen have been reported in some aspirin-sensitive asthmatics (less than 5% of those tested)..

Pregnancy: Problems in humans have not been documented. Although controlled studies have not been done, it has been shown that acetaminophen crosses the placenta.

Breastfeeding: Problems in humans have not been documented. Although peak concentrations of 10 to 15µg/mL (66.2-99.3 µmol/L) have been measured in breast milk 1 to 2 hours following maternal ingestion of a single 650mg dose, neither acetaminophen nor its metabolites were detected in the urine of the nursing infants. The half-life in breast milk is 1.35 to 3.5 hours.

ADVERSE REACTIONS

Those indicating need for medical attention: Incidence rare

Agranulocytosis (fever with or without chills; sores, ulcers or white spots on lips or in mouth; sore throat).

Anemia (unusual tiredness or weakness).

Dermatitis, allergic (skin rash, hives, or itching).

Hepatitis (yellow eyes or skin).

Renal colic (pain, severe and/or sharp, in lower back and/or side)—with prolonged use of high doses in patients with severe renal function impairment.

Renal failure (sudden decrease in amount of urine).

Sterile pyuria (cloudy urine).

Thrombocytopenia (rarely, unusual bleeding or bruising; black, tarry stools; blood in urine or stools; pinpoint red spots on skin)—usually asymptomatic.

ADMINISTRATION AND DOSAGE

General dosing information

The dosages are based on the FDA's proposed labeling requirements for OTC internal analgesic, antipyretic, and antirheumatic products. The dosage unit of 80mg (1.23 grains) is used for pediatric dosages; the dosage unit of 325mg (5 grains) is used for adult dosages. The conversion factor of 1 grain equal to 65mg is used. The dosages recommended by manufacturers of individual products, and the strengths of individual products, may not conform to the recommended dosages. One retrospective study has suggested that long-term daily use of acetaminophen may be associated with an increased risk of chronic renal disease (analgesic nephropathy). The results of this study are not considered conclusive, and further investigation is required to establish a causal association. However, until more definitive information is available, prolonged daily administration of acetaminophen should probably be limited to patients who are receiving appropriate medical supervision.

For analgesic/antipyretic use:

Capsules/Granules/Powder/Solution/Suspension/Tablets

Adults/Pediatrics >13 years of age: 325 to 500mg every 3 hours; 325 to 650mg every 4 hours; 650 to 1000mg every 6 hours; or 1300mg every 8 hours.

Pediatrics <3 months of age: 40mg every 4 hours as needed.

Pediatrics 4 to 12 months of age: 80mg every 4 hours as needed.

Pediatrics 1 to 2 years of age: 120mg every 4 hours as needed.

Pediatrics 2 to 4 years of age: 160mg every 4 hours as needed.

Pediatrics 4 to 6 years of age: 240mg every 4 hours as needed.

Pediatrics 6 to 9 years of age: 320mg every 4 hours as needed.

Pediatrics 9 to 11 years of age: 320mg to 400mg every 4 hours as needed.

Pediatrics 11 to 12 years of age: 320mg to 480mg every 4 hours as needed.

Suppositories

Adults/Pediatrics >13 years of age: 325mg to 650mg every 4 hours or 650mg every 6 hours as needed.

Pediatrics 2 to 4 years of age: 160mg every 4 hours as needed.

Pediatrics 4 to 6 years of age: 240mg every 4 hours as needed.

Pediatrics 6 to 9 years of age: 320mg every 4 hours as needed.

Pediatrics 9 to 11 years of age: 320mg to 400mg every 4 hours as needed.

Pediatrics 11 to 12 years of age: 320mg to 480mg every 4 hours as needed.

NSAIDs (IBUPROFEN, KETOPROFEN, NAPROXEN)

PHARMACOLOGY

Nonsteroidal anti-inflammatory drugs (NSAIDs) inhibit the activity of the enzyme cyclo-oxygenase, resulting in decreased formation of precursors of prostaglandins and thromboxanes from arachidonic acid. Also, meclofenamate and mefenamic acid have been shown to inhibit competitively the actions of prosta-

Drug Interactions for Acetaminophen

Precipitant Drug	Object Drug	Effect On Object Drug	Description
Acetaminophen	◆ Alcohol ◆ Hepatic enzyme inducers ◆ Hepatotoxic medicatons	↔	Risk of hepatotoxicity with single toxic doses or prolonged use of high dosages of acetaminophen may be increased in alcoholics or in patients regularly taking other hepatotoxic medications or hepatic enzyme inducers.
Acetaminophen	Anticoagulants, coumarin- or indandione-derivative	↑	Concurrent chronic, high-dose administration may increase the anticoagulant effect, possibly by decreasing hepatic synthesis of procoagulant factors; anticoagulant dosage adjustment based on increased monitoring of prothrombin time may be necessary when chronic, high-dosage acetaminophen therapy is initiated or discontinued; however, this does not apply to occasional use, or to chronic use of dosages <2g/d, of acetaminophen.
Acetaminophen	NSAIDs Salicylates	↔	Prolonged concurrent use of acetaminophen and a salicylate is not recommended because recent evidence suggests that chronic, high-dosage administration of the combined analgesics (1.35g/d, or cumulative ingestion of 1kg annually, for 3 years or longer) significantly increases the risk of analgesic nephropathy, renal papillary necrosis, end-stage renal disease, and cancer of the kidney or urinary bladder; also, it is recommended that for short-term use, the combined dosage of acetaminophen plus salicylate not exceed that recommended for acetaminophen or a salicylate given alone. Prolonged concurrent use of acetaminophen and NSAIDs other than aspirin may also increase the risk of adverse renal effects; it is recommended that patients be under close medical supervision while receiving such combined therapy.
Barbiturates (except butalbital) Primidone	Acetaminophen	↓	Chronic use has been reported to decrease the therapeutic effects of acetaminophen, probably because of increased metabolism resulting from induction of hepatic microsomal enzyme activity; the possibility should be considered that similar effects may occur with other hepatic enzyme inducers.

◆ = Major clinical significance; NSAID = nonsteroidal anti-inflammatory drug.

glandins. Although the resultant decrease in prostaglandin synthesis and activity in various tissues may be responsible for many of the therapeutic (and adverse) effects of NSAIDs, other actions may also contribute significantly to the therapeutic effects of these medications.

Antirheumatic (nonsteroidal anti-inflammatory): NSAIDs act via analgesic and anti-inflammatory mechanisms; the therapeutic effects are not due to pituitary-adrenal stimulation. These medications do not affect the progressive course of rheumatoid arthritis.

Analgesic: NSAIDs may block pain-impulse generation via a peripheral action that may involve reduction of the activity of prostaglandins, and possibly inhibition of the synthesis or actions of other substances that sensitize pain receptors to mechanical or chemical stimulation. The antibradykinin activity of NSAIDs may also be involved in the relief of pain, since bradykinin has been shown to act together with prostaglandins to cause pain.

Antigout agent: NSAIDs act via analgesic and anti-inflammatory mechanisms. However, they do not correct hyperuricemia.

Anti-inflammatory (nonsteroidal): The exact mechanisms have not been determined. NSAIDs may act peripherally in inflamed tissue, probably by reducing prostaglandin activity in these tissues and possibly by inhibiting the synthesis and/or actions of other local mediators of the inflammatory response. Inhibition of leukocyte migration, inhibition of the release and/or actions of lysosomal enzymes, and actions on other cellular and immunological processes in mesenchymal and connective tissue may be involved. Indomethacin has been shown to inhibit phosphodiesterase, with a resultant increase in intracellular cyclic adenosine monophosphate (cAMP) concentration. NSAIDs have been shown to inhibit leukotriene synthesis, inhibit bradykinin activity, and stabilize lysosomal membranes.

Antipyretic: NSAIDs probably produce antipyresis by acting centrally on the hypothalamic heat-regulating center to produce peripheral vasodilation, resulting in increased blood flow to the skin, sweating, and heat loss. The central action probably involves reduction of prostaglandin activity in the hypothalamus.

Drug Interactions for NSAIDs

Precipitant Drug	Object Drug	Effect On Object Drug	Description
Acetaminophen	NSAIDs	↔	Prolonged concurrent use of acetaminophen with a NSAID may increase the risk of adverse renal effects; it is recommended that patients be under close medical supervision while receiving such combined therapy.
◆ Alcohol ◆ Corticosteroids ◆ Corticotropin (chronic therapeutic use) ◆ Potassium supplements	NSAIDs	↑	Concurrent use with a NSAID may increase the risk of gastrointestinal side effects, including ulceration or hemorrhage; however, concurrent use with a glucocorticoid or corticotropin in the treatment of arthritis may provide additional therapeutic benefit and permit reduction of glucocorticoid or corticotropin dosage.
◆ Cefamandole ◆ Cefoperazone ◆ Cefotetan ◆ Plicamycin ◆ Valproic acid	NSAIDs	↑	These medications may cause hypoprothrombinemia; concurrent use with a NSAID may increase the risk of bleeding because of additive interferences with platelet function and/or the potential occurrence of NSAID-induced gastrointestinal ulceration or hemorrhage.
NSAIDs	ACE inhibitors	↓	Reports suggest diminished antihypertensive effect of ACE inhibitors by NSAIDs and that NSAIDs use in patients receiving ACE inhibitors may potentiate renal disease states.
NSAIDs	◆ Anticoagulants, coumarin- or indanedione-derivative ◆ Heparin ◆ Thrombolytic agents, such as: alteplase anistreplase streptokinase urokinase or warfarin	↔	Inhibition of platelet aggregation by NSAIDs, and the possibility of NSAID-induced gastrointestinal ulceration or bleeding, may be hazardous to patients receiving anticoagulant or thrombolytic therapy.
NSAIDs	Antidiabetic agents Insulin		NSAIDs may increase the hypoglycemic effect of these medications because prostaglandins are directly involved in regulatory mechanisms of glucose metabolism and possibly because of displacement of the oral antidiabetics from serum proteins; dosage adjustments of the antidiabetic agent may be necessary; glipizide and glyburide, due to their nonionic binding characteristics, may not be affected as much as the other oral antidiabetic agents; however, caution with concurrent use is recommended.

Drug Interactions for NSAIDs (cont.)

Precipitant Drug	Object Drug	Effect On Object Drug	Description
NSAIDs	Antihypertensives Diuretics, especially triamterene ◆	↓	Increased monitoring of the response to an antihypertensive agent may be advisable when any NSAID is used concurrently because NSAIDs have been shown to reduce or reverse the effects of antihypertensives, possibly by inhibiting renal prostaglandin synthesis and/or by causing sodium and fluid retention. NSAIDs may decrease the diuretic, natriuretic, and antihypertensive effects of diuretics, probably by inhibiting renal prostaglandin synthesis.
NSAIDs	◆ Aspirin	↑	Concurrent use of aspirin with other NSAIDs may increase the risk of bleeding at sites other than the gastrointestinal tract because of additive inhibition of platelet aggregation.
NSAIDs	Bone marrow depressants	↑	Leukopenic and/or thrombocytopenic effects of these medications may be increased with concurrent or recent therapy if an NSAID causes the same effects; dosage adjustment of the bone marrow depressant, if necessary, should be based on blood counts.
NSAIDs	Colchicine	↔	Concurrent use with an NSAID may increase the risk of gastrointestinal ulceration or hemorrhage.
NSAIDs	◆ Cyclosporine Gold compounds Nephrotoxic medications	↑	Inhibition of renal prostaglandin activity by NSAIDs may increase the plasma concentration of cyclosporine and/or the risk of cyclosporine-induced nephrotoxicity; patients should be carefully monitored during concurrent use.
NSAIDs	Digitalis glycosides	↑	NSAIDs may increase digoxin concentrations, leading to an increased risk of digitalis toxicity; increased monitoring and dosage adjustments of the digitalis glycoside may be necessary during and following concurrent NSAID therapy.
NSAIDs	◆ Lithium	↑	NSAIDs may increase the steady-state concentration of lithium, possibly by decreasing its renal clearance.
NSAIDs	◆ Methotrexate	↑	NSAIDs may decrease protein binding and/or renal elimination of methotrexate, resulting in increased and prolonged methotrexate plasma concentrations and an increased risk of toxicity, especially during high-dose methotrexate infusion therapy.
NSAIDs	Photosensitizing medications	↑	Concurrent use with photosensitizing NSAIDs may cause additive photosensitizing effects.
Platelet aggregation inhibitors	NSAIDs	↑	Concurrent use may increase the risk of bleeding because of additive inhibition of platelet aggregation, as well as the potential for NSAID-induced gastrointestinal ulceration or hemorrhage.
◆ Probenecid	Ketoprofen	↑	Concurrent use is not recommended; probenecid decreases ketoprofen's renal clearance (by approximately 66%) and protein binding (by 28%), and inhibits formation and renal clearance of ketoprofen conjugates, leading to greatly increased ketoprofen plasma concentration and risk of toxicity.
◆ Probenecid	NSAIDs	↑	Probenecid may decrease excretion and increase serum concentrations of other NSAIDs, possibly enhancing effectiveness and/or increasing the potential for toxicity; a decrease in dosage of the NSAID may be necessary if adverse effects occur.

◆ = Major clinical significance.

Antidysmenorrheal: By inhibiting the synthesis and activity of intrauterine prostaglandins (which are thought to be responsible for the pain and other symptoms of primary dysmenorrhea), NSAIDs decrease uterine contractility and uterine pressure, increase uterine perfusion, and relieve ischemic as well as spasmodic pain. The antibradykinin activity of NSAIDs may also be involved in relief of dysmenorrhea, since bradykinin has been shown to induce uterine contractions and act together with prostaglandins to cause pain. Also, NSAIDs may relieve, to some extent, extrauterine symptoms (such as headache, nausea, and vomiting) that may be associated with excessive prostaglandin production.

Vascular headache prophylactic and suppressant: Analgesic actions may be involved in the relief of headache. Also, by reducing prostaglandin activity, NSAIDs may directly prevent or relieve certain types of headache thought to be caused by prostaglandin-induced dilation or constriction of cerebral blood vessels.

Prostaglandin synthesis inhibitor, renal: Inhibition of renal prostaglandin synthesis probably is responsible for the beneficial effect of indomethacin (a prescription NSAID) in patients with Bartter's syndrome, which is thought to be caused by excessive production of renal prostaglandins.

INDICATIONS

Rheumatic disease (treatment), such as:

Arthritis, rheumatoid—Ibuprofen, ketoprofen, and naproxen are indicated for the treatment of acute or chronic rheumatoid arthritis.

Osteoarthritis—Ibuprofen, ketoprofen, and naproxen are indicated for relief of acute or chronic osteoarthritis.

Ankylosing spondylitis—Naproxen is indicated for relief of acute or chronic ankylosing spondylitis.

Arthritis, juvenile—Ibuprofen and naproxen are indicated for relief of acute or chronic juvenile arthritis.

Pain (treatment)—Ibuprofen, ketoprofen, and naproxen are indicated for relief of mild to moderate pain, especially when antiinflammatory actions may also be desired, e.g., following dental, obstetric, or orthopedic surgery, and for relief of musculoskeletal pain due to soft tissue athletic injuries (strains or sprains). Those NSAIDs indicated for relief of pain are also recommended for relief of mild to moderate bone pain caused by metastatic neoplastic disease. However, careful patient selection is necessary, especially in patients receiving chemotherapy, because of the potential gastrointestinal or renal toxicity and the platelet aggregation-inhibiting actions of these medications.

Gouty arthritis, acute (treatment)—Naproxen is indicated for relief of the pain and inflammation associated with acute gouty arthritis.

Inflammation, nonrheumatic (treatment)—Most of the NSAIDs are indicated (or used) in the treatment of painful nonrheumatic inflammatory conditions, such as athletic injuries, bursitis, capsulitis, synovitis, tendinitis, or tenosynovitis. Naproxen is indicated for treatment of bursitis and/or tendinitis of any joint.

Fever (treatment)—Ibuprofen and naproxen are indicated for reduction of fever.

Dysmenorrhea (treatment)—Ibuprofen, ketoprofen, and naproxen are indicated for relief of the pain and other symptoms of primary dysmenorrhea.

Headache, vascular (prophylaxis); *headache, vascular* (treatment)—Ibuprofen, ketoprofen,. and naproxen are used to relieve (when taken at the first sign of onset) migraine headache or other vascular headaches.

CONTRAINDICATIONS

Except under special circumstances, this medication should not be used when the following medical problems exist:

For all NSAIDs:

- Allergic reaction, severe, such as anaphylaxis or angioedema, induced by aspirin or other NSAIDs, history of or
- Nasal polyps associated with bronchospasm, aspirin-induced (high risk of severe allergic reactions because of cross-sensitivity)

Risk-benefit should be considered when the following medical problems exist:

For all NSAIDs:

- Allergic reaction, mild, such as allergic rhinitis, urticaria, or skin rash, induced by aspirin or other NSAIDs, history of (possibility of cross-sensitivity)
- Anemia or
- Asthma (may be exacerbated)
- Conditions predisposing to and/or exacerbated by fluid retention, such as: compromised cardiac function; congestive heart disease; edema, pre-existing hypertension; renal function impairment or failure (NSAIDs may cause fluid retention and edema)
- Conditions predisposing to gastrointestinal toxicity, such as: alcoholism, active; gastrointestinal bleeding (GI), history of; inflammatory or ulcerative disease of the upper or lower gastrointestinal tract, including Crohn's disease, diverticulitis, peptic ulcer disease, or ulcerative colitis, active or history of; or tobacco use or recent history of use (Patients with prior history of peptic ulcer disease or GI bleeding and who use NSAIDs have a greater than 10-fold risk for developing a GI bleed. NSAIDs should preferably not be given to patients with active peptic ulcer disease or gastrointestinal bleeding. If NSAID administration is considered essential, extreme caution should be used and an antiulcer regimen should be administered concurrently; caution and close supervision are also recommended for other patients in whom there is a significant risk of gastrointestinal toxicity. Misoprostol or sucralfate should be considered as prophylaxis for those at high risk.)
- Congestive heart failure; diabetes mellitus; edema, pre-existing; extracellular volume depletion; sepsis (increased risk of renal failure)
- Hemophilia or other bleeding problems including coagulation or platelet function disorders (increased risk of bleeding because most NSAIDs inhibit platelet aggregation and may cause gastrointestinal ulceration or hemorrhage)
- Hepatic cirrhosis or hepatic function impairment (Risk of renal failure is increased in patients with hepatic function impairment, since most NSAIDs are metabolized hepatically. Liver function impairment, especially if associated with chronic alcoholic cirrhosis, produces variability in ketoprofen pharmacokinetics and reduces ketoprofen protein binding. The concentration of unbound ketoprofen may be doubled; caution and careful monitoring are recommended. Also, only immediate-release ketoprofen dosage forms should be used if the patient's serum albumin is lower than 3.5 grams per deciliter. In addition, hepatic cirrhosis, especially if associated with chronic alcoholism, increases the concentration of unbound naproxen, even though the total plasma concentration may be decreased. The lowest effective dose should be administered and the patient carefully monitored. If systemic manifestations [eosinophilia, rash, etc], liver or renal disease symptoms, or persistent or worsening abnormal liver tests occur, NSAIDs should be discontinued.)

- Renal function impairment (Increased risk of hyperkalemia and of adverse renal effects, including acute renal failure; especially careful monitoring of the patient is recommended. NSAIDs and/or their metabolites are excreted primarily via the kidneys. A reduction in dosage may be required to prevent accumulation.)
- Renal function impairment.
- Stomatitis (may be induced by NSAIDs; this symptom of possible NSAID-induced blood dyscrasias may be masked by pre-existing stomatitis).
- Systemic lupus erythematosus (SLE) (patient may be predisposed to NSAID-induced central nervous system and/or renal adverse effects).

PRECAUTIONS TO CONSIDER

Patients sensitive to one of the nonsteroidal anti-inflammatory drugs (NSAIDs), including aspirin, ketorolac, and NSAIDs no longer commercially available (such as oxyphenbutazone, suprofen, and zomepirac) may also be sensitive to any of the other NSAIDs. NSAIDs may cause bronchoconstriction or anaphylaxis in aspirin-sensitive asthmatics, especially those with aspirin-induced nasal polyps, asthma, and other allergic reactions (the "aspirin triad"). Patients with bronchospastic reactions to aspirin may be desensitized to this effect by administration of initially small and gradually increasing doses of aspirin. Desensitization must be carried out by physicians who are experienced with the technique, in a facility having personnel, equipment, and medications immediately available for treatment of any adverse reaction to the medication (especially anaphylaxis or severe bronchospasm). Desensitization to aspirin also desensitizes the patient to other NSAIDs. However, unless aspirin or another NSAID is then administered on a daily basis, sensitivity to these medications redevelops within a few days.

Pregnancy: In general, NSAIDs are not recommended for use in the third trimester. *Ibuprofen*: Not recommended in pregnancy. *Ketoprofen*: FDA Category B. *Naproxen*: FDA Category C.

Breastfeeding: Problems in humans have not been documented with most NSAIDs; however, their use is generally not recommended. *Ibupofen, ketoprofen, and naproxen*: Not recommended for use in nursing.

Geriatrics: Whether geriatric patients are at increased risk of serious gastrointestinal toxicity during NSAID therapy has not been established. However, NSAID-induced gastrointestinal ulceration and/or bleeding may be more likely to cause serious consequences, including fatalities, in geriatric patients than in younger adults. In addition, elderly patients are more likely to have age-related renal function impairment, which may increase the risk of NSAID-induced hepatic or renal toxicity and may also require dosage reduction to prevent accumulation of the medication. Some clinicians recommend that geriatric patients, especially those 70 years of age or older, be given one half of the usual adult dose initially. Also, careful monitoring of the patient is recommended.

ADMINISTRATION AND DOSAGE

General Dosing Information

Patients who do not respond to one NSAID may respond to another. In responsive patients, partial symptomatic relief of arthritic symptoms usually occurs within 1 or 2 weeks, although maximum effectiveness may occur only after several weeks of therapy.

A reduction of initial dosage, possibly to as low as one-half the usual adult dose, is recommended for geriatric patients, especially those 70 years of age or older. However, if the reduced

dose fails to produce an adequate clinical response and the medication is well tolerated, dosage may be increased as required and tolerated. A reduction of dosage may also be required to prevent accumulation of NSAIDs and/or their metabolites (some of which may be unstable and may be hydrolyzed to the parent compound when their excretion is delayed) in patients with renal function impairment.

Long-term use of NSAIDs in doses that approach or exceed maximum dosage recommendations should be considered only if the clinical benefit is increased sufficiently to offset the higher risk of gastrointestinal toxicity or other adverse effects. To minimize the potential risk for an adverse gastrointestinal event, the lowest effective NSAID dose should be used for the shortest possible duration. For high-risk patients, alternate therapies that do not involve NSAIDs should be considered. In the treatment of primary dysmenorrhea, maximum benefit is achieved by initiating NSAID therapy as rapidly as possible after the onset of menses. Prophylactic therapy (ie, starting NSAID administration a few days prior to the expected onset of the menstrual period) has not been found to provide additional therapeutic benefit.

Concurrent use of a NSAID with an opioid analgesic provides additive analgesia and may permit lower doses of the opioid analgesic to be utilized. The analgesic activity of non-opioid analgesics is subject to a ceiling effect. Therefore, administration of a NSAID in higher-than-recommended analgesic doses may not provide additional therapeutic benefit in the treatment of pain not associated with inflammation. In the treatment of arthritis, most of these agents have been shown to provide additional symptomatic relief when administered concurrently with gold compounds or glucocorticoids. NSAIDs may permit reduction of glucocorticoid dosage; however, reductions of glucocorticoid dosage, especially following long-term use, should be gradual to avoid symptoms associated with adrenal insufficiency or other manifestations of too-sudden withdrawal.

IBUPROFEN

Suspension/Tablet

For analgesic (mild to moderate pain)/antidysmenorrheal use:

Adults: 200 to 400mg every 4 to 6 hours as needed.

For antipyretic use:

Adults/Pediatrics ≥*12 years of age*: 200 to 400mg every 4 to 6 hours as needed.

Pediatric 6 months to 12 years of age: 5mg/kg for fevers less than 102.5°F (39.17°C) and 10mg/kg for fevers higher. Dosage may be repeated, if necessary, every 4 to 6 hours.

For antirheumatic use:

Adults/Pediatrics ≥*12 years of age*: 1200 to 3200mg/day in 3 or 4 divided doses. Max: 3600mg/day.

Pediatric 6 months to 12 years of age: 30 to 40mg/kg/day in 3 or 4 divided doses.

KETOPROFEN

Capsules/Tablets

For analgesic (mild to moderate pain)/antidysmenorrheal use:

Adults: 25 to 50mg every 6 to 8 hours as needed.

For antirheumatic use:

Adults: 150 to 300mg/day in 3 or 4 divided doses. Max: 300mg/day.

(Continued on page 204)

Adverse Reactions of NSAIDs

	Ibuprofen	Ketoprofen	Naproxen
Note: Differences in frequency of occurrence may reflect either lack of clinical-use data or actual pharmacologic distinctions among agents (although their pharmacologic similarity suggests that side effects occurring with one may occur with the others). M = more frequent (3%-9%); L = less frequent (1%-3%); R = rare (<1%); U = unknown.			
Medical attention needed			
Cardiovascular effects **Note:** Many of these cardiovascular effects may occur secondary to NSAID-induced renal function impairment.			
Angina pectoris or exacerbation of (chest pain)	U	U	U
Bleeding, other than gastrointestinal, including:			
Hemoptysis (spitting blood)	U	R	U
Nosebleeds, unexplained	R *	R	U
Cardiac arrhythmias	R *	R *	U
Chest pain	U	U	U
Congestive heart failure or exacerbation of (chest pain; shortness of breath; troubled breathing, tightness in chest, and/or wheezing; decrease in amount of urine; swelling of face, fingers, feet, or lower legs; unusual tiredness; weight gain)	R	R	R
Edema, pulmonary (shortness of breath, troubled breathing, tightness in chest, and/or wheezing)	U	U	U
Increased blood pressure—may reach hypertensive levels	R	R	U
Pericarditis (chest pain; fever with or without chills; shortness of breath, troubled breathing, and/or tightness in chest)	U	U	U
Central nervous system effects			
Confusion	R	R	R
Convulsions	U	U	U
Dysarthria (trouble in speaking)	U	U	U
Forgetfulness	U	R	U
Hallucinations	R *	R *	U
Headache, severe, especially in the morning	U	U	U
Meningitis, aseptic (severe headache, drowsiness, confusion, stiff neck and/or back, general feeling of illness, nausea)	R	U	R *
Migraine (headache, severe and throbbing, sometimes with nausea or vomiting)	U	R	U
Neuropathy, peripheral (numbness, tingling, pain, or weakness in hands or feet)	R *	R	R *
Dermatologic effects			
Dermatitis, allergic:			
Bullous eruption/blisters	R	R	U
Eczema	U	U	U
Hives	R	R	M
Itching	L	R	R*
Skin rash	M	L	M
Dermatitis, exfoliative (fever with or without chills; red, thickened, or scaly skin; swollen and/or painful glands; unusual bruising)	U	R	R
Desquamation (peeling of skin)	U	U	U
Erythema (reddening of skin) *or other skin discoloration*	U	R	U
Erythema multiforme (fever with or without chills; muscle cramps or pain; skin rash; sores, ulcers, or white spots on lips or in mouth)	R	U	R *
Erythema nodosum (fever with or without chills; skin rash)	U	U	U
Photosensitivity reactions resembling porphyria cutanea tarda and epidermyolysis bullosa (blistering, scarring, darkening, or lightening of skin color)	U	U	R
Stevens-Johnson syndrome (bleeding or crusting sores on lips; chest pain; fever with or without chills; muscle cramps or pain; skin rash; sores, ulcers, or white spots in mouth; sore throat)	R	U	R *

Adverse Reactions of NSAIDs (cont.)

	Ibuprofen	Ketoprofen	Naproxen
Toxic epidermal necrolysis (redness, tenderness, itching, burning, or peeling of skin; sore throat; fever with or without chills)	R *	U	R *
Digestive system effects			
Abdominal distention (swelling of abdomen)	U	U	U
Bleeding from rectum—with rectal dosage forms	—	M	R
Colitis or exacerbation of or	U	U	R
Enterocolitis or	U	U	U
Regional enteritis or exacerbation of (abdominal pain, cramping, or discomfort; bloody stools; diarrhea)	U	U	U
Dysphagia (difficulty in swallowing)	U	U	U
Esophagitis (burning feeling in throat or chest, difficulty in swallowing)	U	U	U
Gastritis (burning feeling in chest or stomach, indigestion, tenderness in stomach area)	R	R	U
Gastroenteritis (severe abdominal pain, diarrhea, loss of appetite, nausea, weakness)	U	U	U
Gastrointestinal bleeding or hemorrhage—reported independently of gastrointestinal ulceration or perforation, including **melena** (bloody stools) and **hematemesis** (vomiting blood or material that looks like coffee grounds) †	R	R	R
Gastrointestinal perforation‡ and/or	R	R	R
Gastrointestinal ulceration‡, including esophageal, gastric, or peptic ulceration, multiple gastrointestinal ulcerations, and perforation of pre-existing sigmoid lesions, e.g., diverticula, carcinoma (severe pain, cramping, or burning; bloody or black, tarry stools; vomiting of blood or material that looks like coffee grounds; severe and continuing nausea, heartburn, and/or indigestion) **Note:** Intestinal ulceration may lead to stenosis and obstruction. Also, paralytic ileus has been reported with meclofenamate, but a causal relationship has not been established.	R	R	R
Pancreatitis (abdominal pain, fever with or without chills, swelling and/or tenderness in upper abdominal or stomach area)	R	R*	U
Genitourinary effects			
Bladder pain	U	U	U
Bleeding from vagina, unexplained, unexpected, and/or unusually heavy menstrual bleeding	R *	R	R
Blood in urine	R	R	R
Crystalluria, renal calculi, or ureteral obstruction (blood in urine; difficult, burning, or painful urination; severe pain in lower back, side, or abdomen)—with phenylbutazone, may be composed of uric acid crystals and with sulindac, may be composed of sulindac metabolites	U	U	U
Cystitis or	R	L	R
Urethritis or	U	U	U
Urinary tract infection (bloody or cloudy urine; difficult, burning, or painful urination; frequent urge to urinate)	U	U	U
Dysuria (burning, painful, or difficult urination)	U	U	U
Frequent urge to urinate	U	U	U
Incontinence (loss of bladder control)	U	U	U
Proteinuria (cloudy urine)	U	U	U
Strong-smelling urine	U	U	U
Hematologic effects			
Agranulocytosis (granulocytopenia) (fever with or without chills; sores, ulcers, or white spots on lips or in mouth; sore throat)	R	R	R
Anemia (unusual tiredness or weakness)—may be associated with gastrointestinal bleeding or microbleeding or with hemodilution caused by fluid retention	R	R	U

Adverse Reactions of NSAIDs (cont.)

	Ibuprofen	Ketoprofen	Naproxen
Aplastic anemia (pancytopenia) (shortness of breath, troubled breathing, tightness in chest, and/or wheezing; sores, ulcers, or white spots on lips or in mouth; sore throat)	R	U	R *
Bone marrow depression—signs and symptoms are listed under individual entries for *Aplastic anemia* and *Thrombocytopenia*	U	U	U
Disseminated intravascular coagulation	U	U	U
Ecchymosis/bruising	U	U	L
Eosinophilia	R	U	R
Hemolytic anemia (troubled breathing, exertional; unusual tiredness or weakness)	R	R	R *
Hypocoagulability (bleeding from cuts or scratches that lasts longer than usual)	U	R	U
Leukopenia (neutropenia) (usually asymptomatic; rarely, fever or chills, cough or hoarseness, lower back or side pain, painful or difficult urination)	R	U	R
Petechia (pinpoint red spots on skin)	U	U	U
Thrombocytopenia with or without purpura (usually asymptomatic; rarely, unusual bleeding or bruising; black, tarry stools; blood in urine or stools; pinpoint red spots on skin)	R	R	R
Hepatic effects, including			
Cholestatic hepatitis or jaundice (dark urine; fever; itching; light-colored stools; pain, tenderness, and/or swelling in upper abdominal area; skin rash; swollen glands)	U	U	U
Hepatitis or jaundice, toxic (loss of appetite, nausea, vomiting, yellow eyes or skin, swelling in upper abdominal area)	R	R	R
Hypersensitivity reactions			
See also *Dermatologic effects*			
Anaphylaxis or anaphylactoid reactions (changes in facial skin color; skin rash, hives, and/or itching; fast or irregular breathing; puffiness or swelling of the eyelids or around the eyes; shortness of breath, troubled breathing, tightness in chest, and/or wheezing)—may include anaphylactic shock with sudden, severe decrease in blood pressure and collapse	R	R	R
Angiitis (vasculitis) (muscle pain, cramps, and/or weakness; shortness of breath, troubled breathing, tightness in chest, and/or wheezing; skin rash; spitting blood; unusual tiredness or weakness)	R *	U	R *
Angioedema (large, hive-like swellings on face, eyelids, mouth, lips, and/or tongue)	R *	U	R *
Bronchospastic allergic reactions (shortness of breath, troubled breathing, tightness in chest, and/or wheezing)	R	R	U
Fever with or without chills	U	U	R
Laryngeal edema (shortness of breath or troubled breathing)	U	R	U
Loeffler's syndrome (eosinophilic pneumonitis) (chest pain; fever with or without chills; shortness of breath, troubled breathing, tightness in chest, and/or wheezing; unusual weakness)	U	U	R
Rhinitis, allergic (unexplained runny nose or sneezing)	R	R	U
Serum sickness-like reaction (fever with or without chills; muscle cramps, pain, and/or weakness; skin rash, hives, and/or itching; shortness of breath, troubled breathing, tightness in chest, and/or wheezing; swollen and/or painful glands)	R *	U	U
Systemic lupus erythematosus (SLE)-like syndrome (bloody or cloudy urine; chest pain; fever with or without chills; shortness of breath, troubled breathing, tightness in chest, and/or wheezing; skin rash, hives, and/or itching; sudden decrease in amount of urine; swelling of face, fingers, feet, and/or lower legs; swollen and/or painful glands; unusual weakness; rapid weight gain)	R *	U	U
Loosening or splitting of fingernails or other nail disorder	U	R	U
Lymphadenopathy (swollen and/or painful glands)	U	U	U
Muscle cramps or pain—not present before treatment and not related to condition being treated	U	R	R
Mood or mental changes			
Disorientation	U	U	U

Adverse Reactions of NSAIDs (cont.)

	Ibuprofen	Ketoprofen	Naproxen
Feelings of depersonalization	U	U	U
Mental depression	R	L	R
Psychotic reaction	U	U	U
Syncope (fainting)	U	U	U
Ocular effects			
Amblyopia, toxic, or	R	U	U
Corneal opacity or	U	U	U
Retinal or macular disturbances (blurred vision or other vision change)	U	U	U
Blurred or double vision or any change in vision	R	L	L
Conjunctivitis (eye pain, redness, irritation, and/or swelling)	R	R	U
Corneal deposits	U	U	U
Dry, irritated, or swollen eyes	R	R	U
Eye pain	U	R	U
Palpebral edema (swollen eyelids)	U	U	U
Retinal hemorrhage (red eyes)	U	R	U
Scotomata (change in vision)	R	U	U
Oral/perioral effects			
Gingival ulceration or	R	U	U
Stomatitis, aphthous (sores, ulcers, or white spots on lips or in mouth)	R	L	L
Glossitis (irritated tongue)	U	U	U
Swelling of lips and tongue	U	U	U
Otic effects			
Decreased hearing or any change in hearing	R	R	L
Ringing or buzzing in ears	L	L	M
Renal effects			
Fluid retention/edema (increased blood pressure; decrease in amount of urine; swelling of face, fingers, feet, and/or lower legs; rapid weight gain)	L	M	M
Glomerulitis or glomerulonephritis	U	U	U
Hyperkalemia (difficulty in speaking, low blood pressure, slow or irregular heartbeat, troubled breathing, severe weakness in arms or legs)	U	U	U
Interstitial nephritis (bloody or cloudy urine; increased blood pressure; sudden decrease in amount of urine; swelling of face, fingers, feet, and/or lower legs; rapid weight gain)—may be hypersensitivity-mediated	U	R	R
Nephrosis (sudden decrease in amount of urine; swelling of face, fingers, feet, and/or lower legs; rapid weight gain)	U	U	U
Nephrotic syndrome (cloudy urine, swelling of face)	U	R	R
Oliguria/anuria (cessation of urination)—reported independently of renal impairment or failure	U	U	U
Polyuria (sudden, large increase in frequency and quantity of urine)	R	U	U
Renal impairment or failure (increased blood pressure; shortness of breath, troubled breathing, tightness in chest, and/or wheezing; sudden decrease in amount of urine; swelling of face, fingers, feet, and/or lower legs; continuing thirst; unusual tiredness or weakness; weight gain)	R	R	R
Renal papillary or tubular necrosis	R *	U	R
Shortness of breath or troubled breathing	R	R	M
Thirst, continuing	U	R	L
Medical attention needed only if continuing or bothersome			
Cardiovascular effects			
Fast heartbeat	R *	R	U
Flushing or hot flashes	R	U	U
Increased sweating	U	L	L

Adverse Reactions of NSAIDs (cont.)

	Ibuprofen	Ketoprofen	Naproxen
Pounding heartbeat	R	R	L
Central nervous system effects			
Anxiety	U	U	U
Dizziness	M	L	M
Drowsiness	R	L	M
Headache, mild to moderate	L	M	M
Lightheadedness/vertigo	U	R	L
Nervousness or irritability	L	M	U
Trembling or twitching	U	U	U
Trouble in sleeping	R	L	R
Unusual weakness with no other signs or symptoms	U	U	R
Dermatologic effects			
Photosensitive or photoallergic dermatologic reaction (severe sunburn; skin rash, redness, itching, and/or discoloration after exposure to sunlight)	R *	R	R
Gastrointestinal effects			
Abdominal cramps, pain, or discomfort, mild to moderate	M	M	M
Bitter taste or other taste change	U	R	U
Bloated feeling or gas	L	M	U
Constipation	L	M	M
Decreased appetite or loss of appetite	L	L	U
Diarrhea	L	M	L
Epigastric pain or discomfort (stomach pain or discomfort, mild to moderate)	M	U	U
Heartburn	M	U	M
Indigestion	L	M§	L
Nausea	M	M	M
Rectal irritation—with rectal dosage forms	—	M	—
Vomiting	L	L	R
General feeling of discomfort or illness	U	L	R
Irritation, dryness, or soreness of mouth	R	R	U
Muscle weakness	U	U	R
Photophobia (increased sensitivity of eyes to light)	U	U	U
Weight loss, unexplained	U	R	U

* Has been reported, but a causal relationship has not been established.

† See also dermatologic effects, hematologic effects, hepatic effects, and renal effects for signs and symptoms of many of the reported components of this syndrome.

‡ Serious gastrointestinal effects, including ulceration, perforation, and/or bleeding, may occur at any time, with or without warning signs and/or symptoms, during chronic therapy with NSAIDs. The risk of NSAID-induced gastrointestinal toxicity may increase with the duration of therapy as well as with dosage. In clinical trials with nabumetone, peptic ulceration occurred in approximately 0.3%, 0.5%, and 0.8% of patients treated for 6 months, 1 year, and 2 years, respectively. In clinical trials with other NSAIDs, upper gastrointestinal tract ulceration, bleeding, or perforation occurred in approximately 1% of patients treated for 3 to 6 months and in approximately 2% to 4% of patients treated for 1 year. Risk factors that may increase the risk of NSAID-induced gastrointestinal toxicity, other than those associated with an increased risk of peptic ulcer disease in any patient, have not been identified.

§ Frequency of occurrence is 10% or higher.

(Continued from page 199)

NAPROXEN

Tablets

For antigout use:

Adults: 750mg initially, then 250mg every 8 hours until attack subsides.

For anti-inflammatory/analgesic (mild to moderate pain)/antidysmenorrheal use:

Adults: 500mg initially, then 250mg every 6 to 8 hours as needed.

For antipyretic use:

Adults/Pediatrics ≥12 years of age: 200 to 400mg every 4 to 6 hours as needed.

Pediatric 6 months to 12 years of age: 5mg/kg for fevers less than 102.5°F (39.17°C) and 10mg/kg for fevers higher. Dosage may be repeated, if necessary every 4 to 6 hours.

For antirheumatic use:

Adults/Pediatrics ≥12 years of age: 250 to 500mg twice daily.

Pediatrics: 10mg/kg/day in 2 divided doses.

IBUPROFEN PRODUCTS	
Brand Name	**Dosage Form**
Advil (Wyeth)	**Capsule:** 200mg **Tablet:** 200mg
Advil Children's (Wyeth)	**Tablet:** 50mg
Advil Junior (Wyeth)	**Tablet:** 100mg
Midol Cramp Formula (Bayer)	**Tablet:** 200mg
Motrin IB (McNeil)	**Tablet:** 200mg
Motrin Children's (McNeil)	**Suspension:** 100mg/5mL
Motrin Infants' (McNeil)	**Suspension:** 50mg/1.25mL
Motrin Junior (McNeil)	**Tablet:** 100mg
Motrin Migraine Pain (McNeil)	**Tablet:** 200mg
KETOPROFEN PRODUCTS	
Brand Name	**Dosage Form**
Orudis KT (Wyeth)	**Tablet:** 12.5mg
NAPROXEN PRODUCTS	
Brand Name	**Dosage Form**
Aleve (Bayer)	**Capsule:** 220mg **Tablet:** 220mg
Aleve Arthritis (Bayer)	**Tablet:** 220mg
Midol Extended Relief (Bayer)	**Tablet:** 220mg

SALICYLATES

PHARMACOLOGY

The analgesic, antipyretic, and anti-inflammatory effects of aspirin are due to actions by both the acetyl and the salicylate portions of the intact molecule as well as by the active salicylate metabolite. The actions of other salicylates are due only to the salicylate portion of the molecule. Aspirin directly inhibits the activity of the enzyme cyclo-oxygenase to decrease the formation of precursors of prostaglandins and thromboxanes from arachidonic acid. Salicylate may competitively inhibit prostaglandin formation. Although many of the therapeutic and adverse effects of these medications may result from inhibition of prostaglandin synthesis (and consequent reduction of prostaglandin activity) in various tissues, other actions may also contribute significantly to the therapeutic effects.

Analgesic: Salicylates: Produce analgesia through a peripheral action by blocking pain impulse generation and via a central action, possibly in the hypothalamus. The peripheral action may predominate and probably involves inhibition of the synthesis of prostaglandins, and possibly inhibition of the synthesis and/or actions of other substances, which sensitize pain receptors to mechanical or chemical stimulation.

Anti-inflammatory (nonsteroidal): Exact mechanisms have not been determined. Salicylates may act peripherally in inflamed tissue, probably by inhibiting the synthesis of prostaglandins and possibly by inhibiting the synthesis and/or actions of other mediators of the inflammatory response. Inhibition of leukocyte migration, inhibition of the release and/or actions of lysosomal enzymes, and actions on other cellular and immunological processes in mesenchymal and connective tissues may be involved.

Antipyretic: May produce antipyresis by acting centrally on the hypothalamic heat-regulating center to produce peripheral vasodilation resulting in increased cutaneous blood flow, sweating, and heat loss. The central action may involve inhibition of prostaglandin synthesis in the hypothalamus; however, there is some evidence that fevers caused by endogenous pyrogens that do not act via a prostaglandin mechanism may also respond to salicylate therapy.

Antirheumatic (nonsteroidal anti-inflammatory): Act via analgesic and anti-inflammatory mechanisms; the therapeutic effects are not due to pituitary-adrenal stimulation.

Platelet aggregation inhibitor: The platelet aggregation-inhibiting effect of aspirin specifically involves the compound's ability to act as an acetyl donor to the platelet membrane; the nonacetylated salicylates have no clinically significant effect on platelet aggregation. Aspirin affects platelet function by inhibiting the enzyme prostaglandin cyclooxygenase in platelets, thereby preventing the formation of the aggregating agent thromboxane A_2. This action is irreversible; the effects persist for the life of the platelets exposed. Aspirin may also inhibit formation of the platelet aggregation inhibitor prostacyclin (prostaglandin I_2) in blood vessels; however, this action is reversible. These actions may be dose-dependent. Although there is some evidence that doses lower than 100mg per day may not inhibit prostacyclin synthesis, optimum dosage that will suppress thromboxane A_2 formation without suppressing prostacyclin generation has not been determined.

INDICATIONS

Pain (treatment) or *Fever* (treatment)—Salicylates are indicated to relieve mild to moderate pain such as headache, toothache, and menstrual cramps and to reduce fever. These medications provide only symptomatic relief; additional therapy to treat the cause of the pain or fever should be instituted when necessary. However, the presence of an illness that may predispose toward Reye's syndrome (ie, an acute febrile illness, especially influenza or varicella) should be ruled out before salicylate therapy is initiated in a pediatric or adolescent patient.

Salicylates are recommended for relief of mild to moderate bone pain caused by metastatic neoplastic disease. However, careful patient selection is necessary, especially in patients receiving chemotherapy, because of the platelet aggregation-inhibiting effect of aspirin and because salicylates may cause hypoprothrombinemia or gastrointestinal or renal toxicity.

Delayed-release formulations containing aspirin or sodium salicylate may not be as useful as immediate-release formulations for single-dose administration for analgesia or antipyresis because the delayed absorption prolongs the onset of action.

Drug Interactions for Salicylates

Precipitant Drug	Object Drug	Effect On Object Drug	Description
Acetaminophen	Salicylates	↔	Prolonged concurrent use of acetaminophen with a salicylate is not recommended because chronic, high-dose administration of the combined analgesics (1.35g daily, or cumulative ingestion of 1kg annually, for 3 years or longer) significantly increases the risk of analgesic nephropathy, renal papillary necrosis, end-stage renal disease, and cancer of the kidney or urinary bladder.
Acidifiers, urinary (ammonium chloride, ascorbic acid [vitamin C], potassium or sodium phosphates)	Salicylates	↑	Acidification of the urine by these medications decreases salicylate excretion, leading to increased salicylate plasma concentrations; initiation of therapy with these medications in patients stabilized on a salicylate may lead to toxic salicylate concentrations.
Alcohol ♦ NSAIDs	Salicylates	↔	Concurrent use of these medications with a salicylate may increase the risk of gastrointestinal side effects, including ulceration and gastrointestinal blood loss; also, concurrent use of a salicylate with an NSAID may increase the risk of severe gastrointestinal side effects without providing additional symptomatic relief and is therefore not recommended.
♦ Alkalizers, urinary, such as: carbonic anhydrase inhibitors; citrates; sodium bicarbonate; antacids, chronic high-dose use (especially calcium- and/or magnesium-containing)	Salicylates	↓	Alkalinization of the urine by these medications increases salicylate excretion, leading to decreased salicylate plasma concentrations, reduced effectiveness, and shortened duration of action; also, withdrawal of a urinary alkalizer from a patient stabilized on a salicylate may increase the plasma salicylate concentration to a toxic level; however, the antacids present in buffered aspirin formulations may not be present in sufficient quantity to alkalinize the urine.
Antacids Histamine H$_2$-receptor antagonists	Enteric-coated salicylate formulations	↔	Concurrent administration of these medications, which increase intragastric pH, with an enteric-coated medication may cause premature dissolution, and loss of the protective effect, of the enteric coating.
Antiemetics (including antihistamines and phenothiazines)	Salicylates	↔	Antiemetics may mask the symptoms of salicylate-induced ototoxicity, such as dizziness, vertigo, and tinnitus.
♦ Aspirin	NSAIDs	↓	Aspirin may decrease the bioavailability of many NSAIDs, including diflunisal, fenoprofen, indomethacin, meclofenamate, piroxicam (to 80% of the usual plasma concentration), and the active sulfide metabolite of sulindac; aspirin has also been shown to decrease the protein binding and increase the plasma clearance of ketoprofen, and to decrease the formation and excretion of ketoprofen conjugates.
Bismuth subsalicylate	Salicylates	↑	Ingestion of large repeated doses as for traveler's diarrhea may produce substantial plasma salicylate concentrations; concurrent use with large doses of analgesic salicylates may increase the risk of salicylate toxicity.
Buffered salicylate formulations	Ciprofloxacin Enoxacin Itraconazole Ketoconazole Lomefloxacin Norfloxacin Ofloxacin Tetracyclines	↓	Antacids present in buffered aspirin formulations, and the magnesium in choline and magnesium salicylates or magnesium salicylate, interfere with absorption of these medications; if used concurrently, the interacting salicylate should be taken at least 6 hours before or 2 hours after ciprofloxacin or lomefloxacin, 8 hours before or 2 hours after enoxacin, 2 hours after itraconazole, 3 hours before or after ketoconazole, 2 hours before or after norfloxacin or ofloxacin, and 3 to 4 hours before or after a tetracycline.

♦ = Major clinical significance.

Drug Interactions for Salicylates (cont.)

Precipitant Drug	Object Drug	Effect On Object Drug	Description
◆ Cefamandole ◆ Cefoperazone ◆ Cefotetan ◆ Plicamycin ◆ Valproic aci	Salicylates	↔	These medications may cause hypoprothrombinemia; in addition, plicamycin or valproic acid may inhibit platelet aggregation; concurrent use with aspirin may increase the risk of bleeding because of additive interferences with blood clotting.
Corticosteroids Corticotropin (ACTH)	Salicylates	↓	May increase salicylate excretion, resulting in lower plasma concentrations and increased salicylate dosage requirements; salicylism may result when corticosteroids or corticotropin dosage is subsequently decreased or discontinued, especially in patients receiving large (antirheumatic) doses of salicylate; also, the risk of gastrointestinal side effects, including ulceration and gastrointestinal blood loss, may be increased; however, concurrent use in the treatment of arthritis may provide additive therapeutic benefit and permit reduction of corticosteroid or corticotropin dosage.
Furosemide	Salicylates	↑	In addition to increasing the risk of ototoxicity, concurrent use of furosemide with high doses of salicylate may lead to salicylate toxicity because of competition for renal excretory sites.
Laxatives, cellulose-containing	Salicylates	↓	Concurrent use may reduce the salicylate effect because of physical binding or other absorptive hindrance; medications should be administered 2 hours apart.
Salicylates	◆ Anticoagulants, coumarin- or indandione-derivative ◆ Heparin ◆ Thrombolytic agents, such as: alteplase, anistreplase, streptokinase, urokinase	↑	Salicylates may displace a coumarin- or indandione-derivative anticoagulant from its protein-binding sites, and, in high doses, may cause hypoprothrombinemia, leading to increased anticoagulation and risk of bleeding. The potential occurrence of gastrointestinal ulceration or hemorrhage during salicylate therapy, especially aspirin, may cause increased risk to patients receiving anticoagulant or thrombolytic therapy.
Salicylates	Anticonvulsants, hydantoin	↑	Salicylates may decrease hydantoin metabolism, leading to increases in hydantoin plasma concentrations, efficacy, and/or toxicity; adjustment of hydantoin dosage may be required when chronic salicylate therapy is initiated or discontinued.
Salicylates	◆ Antidiabetic agents, oral Insulin	↑	Effects of these medications may be increased by large doses of salicylates; dosage adjustments may be necessary; potentiation of oral antidiabetic agents may be caused partially by displacement from serum proteins; glipizide and glyburide, because of their nonionic binding characteristics, may not be affected as much as the other oral agents; however, caution in concurrent use is recommended.
Salicylates	◆ Methotrexate	↓	Salicylates may displace methotrexate from its binding sites and decrease its renal clearance, leading to toxic methotrexate plasma concentrations; if they are used concurrently, methotrexate dosage should be decreased, the patient observed for signs of toxicity, and/or methotrexate plasma concentration monitored; also, it is recommended that salicylate therapy be discontinued 24 to 48 hours prior to administration of a high-dose methotrexate infusion, and not resumed until the plasma methotrexate concentration has decreased to a nontoxic level (usually at least 12 hours postinfusion).

Drug Interactions for Salicylates (cont.)

Precipitant Drug	Object Drug	Effect On Object Drug	Description
Salicylates	♦ Ototoxic medications (especially vancomycin)	↔	Concurrent or sequential administration of these medications with a salicylate should be avoided because the potential for ototoxicity may be increased; hearing loss may occur and may progress to deafness even after discontinuation of the medication; these effects may be reversible, but usually are permanent.
Salicylates	♦ Probenecid ♦ Sulfinpyrazone	↓	Concurrent use is not recommended when these medications are used to treat hyperuricemia or gout, because the uricosuric effect of these medications may be decreased by doses of salicylates that produce serum salicylate concentrations above 5mg per 100mL; also, these medications may inhibit the uricosuric effect achieved when serum salicylate concentrations are above 10 to 15mg per 100mL.
Salicylates	Zidovudine	↑	In theory, aspirin may competitively inhibit the hepatic glucuronidation and decrease the clearance of zidovudine, leading to potentiation of zidovudine toxicity; the possibility must be considered that aspirin toxicity may also be increased.

Inflammation, nonrheumatic (treatment)—Salicylates are indicated to relieve myalgia, musculoskeletal pain, and other symptoms of nonrheumatic inflammatory conditions such as athletic injuries, bursitis, capsulitis, tendinitis, and nonspecific acute tenosynovitis.

Arthritis, rheumatoid (treatment), *Arthritis, juvenile* (treatment), or *Osteoarthritis* (treatment)—Salicylates are indicated for the symptomatic relief of acute and chronic rheumatoid arthritis, juvenile arthritis, osteoarthritis, and related rheumatic diseases. Aspirin is usually the first agent to be used and may be the drug of choice in patients able to tolerate prolonged therapy with high doses. These agents do not affect the progressive course of rheumatoid arthritis.

Concurrent treatment with a glucocorticoid or a disease-modifying antirheumatic agent may be needed, depending on the condition being treated and patient response.

Rheumatic fever (treatment)—Salicylates are indicated to reduce fever and inflammation in rheumatic fever. However, they do not prevent cardiac or other complications associated with this condition. Sodium salicylate should be avoided in rheumatic fever if congestive cardiac complications are present because of its sodium content. Also, large doses of any salicylate should be avoided in rheumatic fever if severe carditis is present because of possible adverse cardiovascular effects.

Platelet aggregation (prophylaxis)—Aspirin (tablets, chewable tablets, delayed-release capsules or tablets, and buffered formulations) is indicated as a platelet aggregation inhibitor in the following: *Ischemic attacks, transient, in males* (prophylaxis); *Thromboembolism, cerebral* (prophylaxis); or *Thromboembolism, cerebral, recurrence* (prophylaxis)—Aspirin is indicated in the treatment of men who have had transient brain ischemia due to fibrin platelet emboli to reduce the recurrence of transient ischemic attacks (TIAs) and the risk of stroke and death. Aspirin is also used in the treatment of women with transient brain ischemia due to fibrin platelet emboli. However, its efficacy in preventing stroke and death in female patients has not been established.

Myocardial infarction (prophylaxis) or *Myocardial reinfarction* (prophylaxis)—Aspirin is indicated to prevent myocardial infarction in patients with unstable angina pectoris and to prevent recurrence of myocardial infarction in patients with a history of myocardial infarction.

Thromboembolism (prophylaxis)—Aspirin is used in low doses to decrease the risk of thromboembolism following orthopedic (hip) surgery (especially total hip replacement) and in patients with arteriovenous shunts. Platelet aggregation inhibitors, although not as consistently effective as an anticoagulant or an anticoagulant plus dipyridamole, may provide some protection against the development of thromboembolic complications in patients with mechanical prosthetic heart valves. Therefore, administration of aspirin, alone or in combination with dipyridamole, may be considered if anticoagulant therapy is contraindicated for these patients. Patients with bioprosthetic cardiac valves who are in normal sinus rhythm generally do not require prolonged antithrombotic therapy, but long-term aspirin administration may be considered on an individual basis.

Aspirin is also indicated, alone or in combination with dipyridamole, to reduce the risk of thrombosis and/or reocclusion of saphenous vein aortocoronary bypass grafts following coronary bypass surgery.

Aspirin is also indicated, alone or in combination with dipyridamole, to reduce the risk of thrombosis and/or reocclusion of prosthetic or saphenous vein femoral popliteal bypass grafts.

Because the patient may be at risk for thromboembolic complications, including myocardial infarction and stroke, long-term aspirin therapy may also be indicated for maintaining patency following coronary or peripheral vascular angioplasty and for treating patients with peripheral vascular insufficiency caused by arteriosclerosis.

Prolonged antithrombotic therapy is generally not needed to maintain vessel patency following vascular reconstruction procedures in high-flow, low-resistance arteries larger than 6mm in diameter. However, long-term aspirin therapy may be indicated, because patients requiring such procedures may be at risk for other thrombotic complications.

CONTRAINDICATIONS

Except under special circumstances, this medication should not be used when the following medical problems exist:

For all salicylates:

- Bleeding ulcers or
- Hemorrhagic states, other active (may be exacerbated, especially by aspirin).
- Hemophilia or other bleeding problems, including coagulation or platelet function disorders (increased risk of hemorrhage, especially with aspirin).

For aspirin only (in addition to the contraindications listed above for all salicylates):

- Angioedema, anaphylaxis, or other severe sensitivity reaction induced by aspirin or other NSAIDs, history of or
- Nasal polyps associated with asthma, induced or exacerbated by aspirin (high risk of severe sensitivity reaction to aspirin).
- Thrombocytopenia (increased risk of bleeding because aspirin inhibits platelet aggregation).

For choline and magnesium salicylates and for magnesium salicylate only (in addition to the contraindications listed above for all salicylates):

- Renal insufficiency, chronic advanced (risk of hypermagnesemic toxicity).

Risk-benefit should be considered when the following medical problems exist:

For all salicylates:

- Anemia (may be exacerbated by gastrointestinal blood loss during salicylate, especially aspirin, therapy; also, salicylate-induced peripheral vasodilation may lead to pseudoanemia).
- Conditions predisposing to fluid retention, such as:
- Compromised cardiac function or
- Hypertension (in patients with carditis, high doses of salicylates may precipitate congestive heart failure or pulmonary edema; patients with congestive heart disease may be more susceptible to adverse renal effects; sodium content of sodium salicylate may be detrimental to these patients when large doses are administered chronically).

Gastritis, erosive or

Peptic ulcer (may be exacerbated because of ulcerogenic effects, especially with aspirin; risk of gastrointestinal bleeding is increased).

Gout (salicylates may increase serum uric acid concentrations and may interfere with efficacy of uricosuric agents).

Hepatic function impairment (salicylates metabolized hepatically; also, patients with decompensated hepatic cirrhosis may be more susceptible to adverse renal effects; in severe hepatic impairment, inhibition of platelet function by aspirin may increase the risk of hemorrhage).

Hypoprothrombinemia or

Vitamin K deficiency (increased risk of bleeding because of antiplatelet action of aspirin and the hypoprothrombinemic effect of high doses of salicylates).

Renal function impairment (salicylate elimination may be reduced; also, the risk of renal adverse effects may be increased; choline and magnesium salicylates or magnesium salicylate should be used with caution in patients with mild or moderate renal impairment because of the risk of hypermagnesemic toxicity; however, as stated above, these medications should not be used if chronic advanced renal insufficiency is present).

Sensitivity reaction, mild, to aspirin or other NSAIDs, history of (risk of sensitivity reaction, especially with aspirin).

Symptoms of nasal polyps associated with bronchospasm, or angioedema, anaphylaxis, or other severe allergic reactions induced by aspirin or other NSAIDs (although cross-sensitivity leading to severe reactions occurs very rarely with the nonacetylated salicylates, caution is recommended; however, as indicated above, aspirin should not be used).

Thyrotoxicosis (may be exacerbated by large doses).

For aspirin only (in addition to those listed above for all salicylates):

- Asthma (increased risk of bronchospastic sensitivity reaction).
- Glucose-6-phosphate dehydrogenase (G6PD) deficiency (rarely, aspirin has caused hemolytic anemia in these patients).

For formulations containing caffeine:

- Cardiac disease, severe (high doses of caffeine may increase risk of tachycardia or extrasystoles, which may lead to heart failure).
- Sensitivity to caffeine, history of (risk of allergic reaction).

PRECAUTIONS TO CONSIDER

Patients sensitive to one salicylate, including methyl salicylate (oil of wintergreen), or to other nonsteroidal anti-inflammatory drugs (NSAIDs) may be sensitive to other salicylates also. Patients sensitive to aspirin may not necessarily be sensitive to nonacetylated salicylates. Patients sensitive to tartrazine dye may be sensitive to aspirin also, and vice versa. Cross-sensitivity between aspirin and other NSAIDs that results in bronchospastic or cutaneous reactions may be eliminated if the patient undergoes a desensitization procedure.

Possible Adverse/Toxic Effects of Chronic Salicylate Use

Note: Adverse effects are more likely to occur at serum salicylate concentrations of 300mcg per mL (30mg per 100mL) or above; however, they may also occur at lower serum concentrations, especially in patients 60 years of age or older. Serum concentrations at which adverse or toxic effects have been reported during chronic therapy are listed below.

Salicylate Concentration (mcg per mL/ mg per 100mL)	Effect
195-210/19.5-21	Mild toxicity (tinnitus, decreased hearing)
250/25	Hepatotoxicity (abnormal liver function tests)
250/25	Decreased renal function
300/30	Decreased prothrombin time
310/31	Deafness
350/35	Hyperventilation
>400/40	Metabolic acidosis, other signs of severe toxicity

Pregnancy—First trimester: Salicylates readily cross the placenta. Although it has been reported that salicylate use during pregnancy may increase the risk of birth defects in humans, controlled studies using aspirin have not shown proof of teratogenicity. Studies in humans with other salicylates have not been done. *Aspirin extended-release tablets*: FDA Category D. *Magnesium salicylate and salsalate*: FDA Category C. *Third trimester*: Chronic, high-dose salicylate therapy may result in prolonged gestation, increased risk of postmaturity syndrome (fetal damage or death due to decreased placental function if pregnancy is greatly prolonged), and increased risk of maternal antenatal hemorrhage. Also, ingestion of salicylates, especially aspirin, during the last 2 weeks of pregnancy may increase the risk of fetal or neonatal hemorrhage. The possibility that regular use late in pregnancy may result in constriction or premature closure of the fetal ductus arteriosus, possibly leading to persistent pulmonary hypertension and heart failure in the neonate, must also be considered. Overuse or abuse of aspirin late in pregnancy has been reported to increase the risk of stillbirth or neonatal death, possibly because of antenatal hemorrhage or premature ductus arteriosus closure, and to decreased birth weight; however, studies using therapeutic doses of aspirin have not shown these adverse effects.

Breastfeeding: Problems in humans with usual analgesic doses have not been documented. However, salicylate is distributed into breast milk; with chronic, high-dose use, intake by the infant may be high enough to cause adverse effects.

Pediatrics: Aspirin use may be associated with the development of Reye's syndrome in children and teenagers with acute febrile illnesses, especially influenza and varicella. It is recommended that salicylate therapy not be initiated in febrile pediatric or adolescent patients until after the presence of such an illness has been ruled out. Also, it is recommended that chronic salicylate therapy in these patients be discontinued if a fever occurs, and not resumed until it has been determined that an illness that may predispose to Reye's syndrome is not present or has run its course. Other forms of salicylate toxicity may also be more prevalent in pediatric patients, especially children who have a fever or are dehydrated. Especially careful monitoring of the serum salicylate concentration is recommended in pediatric patients with Kawasaki disease. Absorption of aspirin is impaired during the early febrile stage of the disease; therapeutic anti-inflammatory plasma salicylate concentrations may be extremely difficult to achieve. Also, as the febrile stage passes, absorption is improved; salicylate toxicity may occur if dosage is not readjusted.

Geriatrics: Geriatric patients may be more susceptible to the toxic effects of salicylates, possibly because of decreased renal function. Lower doses than those usually recommended for adults, especially for long-term use or for use of long-acting salicylates (such as choline and magnesium salicylates and salsalate), may be required.

ADVERSE REACTIONS

Those indicating need for medical attention

Incidence less frequent or rare:

Anaphylactoid reaction (bluish discoloration or flushing or redness of skin; coughing; difficulty in swallowing; dizziness or feeling faint, severe; skin rash, hives [may include giant urticaria], and/or itching; stuffy nose; swelling of eyelids, face, or lips; tightness in chest, troubled breathing, and/or wheezing, especially in asthmatic patients); anemia (unusual tiredness or weakness)—for aspirin or buffered aspirin only; may occur secondary to gastrointestinal microbleeding; anemia, hemolytic (troubled breathing, exertional; unusual tiredness or weakness)— reported with aspirin only, almost always in patients with glu-

cose-6-phosphate (G6PD) deficiency; bronchospastic allergic reaction (shortness of breath, troubled breathing, tightness in chest, and/or wheezing); dermatitis, allergic (skin rash, hives, or itching); gastrointestinal ulceration, possibly with bleeding (bloody or black, tarry stools; stomach pain, severe; vomiting of blood or material that looks like coffee grounds).

Incidence unknown:

Rectal irritation—for aspirin suppository dosage form.

Those indicating need for medical attention only if they continue or are bothersome:

Incidence more frequent with aspirin; less frequent with enteric-coated or buffered formulations and with other salicylates:

Gastrointestinal irritation (mild stomach pain; heartburn or indigestion; nausea with or without vomiting).

ADMINISTRATION AND DOSAGE

General Dosing Information

A reduction in initial dosage is recommended for geriatric patients, especially those receiving long-acting salicylates (e.g., choline and magnesium salicylates, salsalate) or prolonged therapy. These patients may be more susceptible to salicylate toxicity, especially if accumulation occurs because of impaired renal function. If the reduced dosage is not effective, dosage may gradually be increased as tolerated.

For treatment of arthritis, dosage is usually increased gradually until symptoms are relieved, therapeutic plasma concentrations are achieved, or signs of toxicity, such as tinnitus or headache, occur. If these signs should appear, dosage should be reduced. However, tinnitus is not a reliable index of maximum salicylate tolerance, especially in very young or geriatric patients or those with impaired hearing. For treatment of arthritis, dosage adjustments should not be made more frequently than once weekly, unless a reduction in dosage is required because of side effects, because up to 7 days may be required to achieve steady-state plasma concentrations.

The risk of Reye's syndrome must be considered when salicylates are administered to children and teenagers. It is recommended that salicylates be withheld from pediatric and adolescent patients with a fever or other symptoms of an illness that may predispose to Reye's syndrome until it has been determined that such an illness is not present or has run its course.

Dosage should be reduced if fever or illness causes fluid depletion, especially in children. In general, it is recommended that aspirin therapy be discontinued 5 days before surgery to prevent possible occurrence of bleeding problems.

For oral dosage forms only:

These medications (except enteric-coated formulations) should be administered after meals or with food to lessen gastric irritation. It is recommended that tablet and capsule dosage forms of these medications always be administered with a full glass (240mL) of water and that the patient remain in an upright position for 15 to 30 minutes after administration. These measures may reduce the risk of the medication becoming lodged in the esophagus, which has been reported to cause prolonged esophageal irritation and difficulty in swallowing in some patients receiving NSAIDs.

It is recommended that aspirin or buffered aspirin products not be chewed before swallowing for at least 7 days following tonsillectomy or oral surgery because of possible injury to oral tissues from prolonged contact with aspirin. Aspirin or buffered aspirin tablets should not be placed directly on a tooth or gum surface because of possible injury to tissues.

Concurrent use of an antacid and/or a histamine H_2-receptor antagonist (cimetidine, famotidine, or ranitidine) may protect against salicylate-induced gastric irritation or ulceration. However, the fact that chronic, high-dose antacid use may alkalinize the urine and increase salicylate excretion must be considered. Also, because these medications may cause premature dissolution, and loss of the protective effect, of enteric coatings, they will not provide additive protection against gastric irritation when administered concurrently with enteric-coated dosage forms.

ASPIRIN

Chewing gum tablet

For analgesic use:

Adults/Pediatrics ≥12 years of age: 454 to 650mg every 4 hours as needed.

Pediatrics 3 to 6 years of age: 227mg up to 3 times a day as needed. Maximim: No more than 5 doses each 24 hours, unless directed otherwise by a physician.

Pediatrics 6 to 12 years of age: 227 to 454mg up to 4 times a day as needed. Maximim: No more than 5 doses each 24 hours, unless directed otherwise by a physician.

Suppositories

For analgesic/antipyretic use:

Adults/Pediatrics ≥12 years of age: 325 to 650mg every 4 hours as needed.

Pediatrics 2 to 4 years of age: 160mg every 4 hours as needed.

Pediatrics 4 to 6 years of age: 240mg every 4 hours as needed.

Pediatrics 6 to 9 years of age: 325mg every 4 hours as needed.

Pediatrics 9 to 11 years of age: 325 to 400mg every 4 hours as needed.

Pediatric 11 to 12 years of age: 325 to 480mg every 4 hours as needed.

For antirheumatic use:

Adults: 3.6 to 5.4g/day in divided doses. Maximum: 7.8g/day.

Pediatrics: 80 to 100mg/kg of body weight a day in divided doses.

Tablet

For analgesic/antipyretic use:

Adults/Pediatrics ≥12 years of age: 325 to 500mg every 3 hours; or 325 to 650mg every 4 hours; 650 to 1000mg every 6 hours as needed.

Pediatrics 2 to 4 years of age: 160mg every 4 hours as needed.

Pediatrics 4 to 6 years of age: 240mg every 4 hours as needed.

Pediatrics 6 to 9 years of age: 320 to 325mg every 4 hours as needed.

Pediatrics 9 to 11 years of age: 320 to 400mg every 4 hours as needed.

Pediatric 11 to 12 years of age: 320 to 480mg every 4 hours as needed.

For antirheumatic use:

Adults: 3.6 to 5.4g/day in divided doses. Max: 7.8g/day.

Pediatrics: 80 to 100mg/kg of body weight a day in divided doses.

For ischemic attacks, transient:

Adults: 1g/day in divided doses.

For platelet aggregation inhibition:

Adults/Pediatrics ≥12 years of age: 80 to 325mg/day.

MAGNESIUM SALICYLATE

Tablet

For analgesic/antipyretic/antirheumatic use:

Adults: 607.4mg every 4 hours as needed; or 934mg every 6 hours as needed.

ASPIRIN PRODUCTS	
Brand Name	**Dosage Form**
Ascriptin (Novartis)	**Tablet:** 81mg
Aspergum (Schering-Plough)	**Gum:** 227mg
Bayer Aspirin Regimen (Bayer)	**Tablet:** 81mg, 325mg
Bayer Children's Aspirin (Bayer)	**Tablet:** 81mg
Bayer Extra Strength (Bayer)	**Tablet:** 500mg
Bayer Genuine Aspirin (Bayer)	**Tablet:** 325mg
Ecotrin (GSK)	**Tablet:** 325mg
Ecotrin Adult Low Strength (GSK)	**Tablet:** 81mg
Ecotrin Maximum Strength (GSK)	**Tablet:** 500mg
Halfprin (Kramer)	**Tablet:** 81mg, 162mg
St. Joseph (McNeil)	**Tablet:** 81mg

BUFFERED ASPIRIN PRODUCTS

Brand Name	Dosage Form
Alka-Seltzer (Bayer)	**Tablet:** 325mg
Alka-Seltzer Extra Strength (Bayer)	**Tablet:** 500mg
Ascriptin (Novartis)	**Tablet:** 325mg
Ascriptin Arthritis Pain (Novartis)	**Tablet:** 325mg
Ascriptin Maximum Strength (Novartis)	**Tablet:** 500mg
Bayer Plus Extra Strength (Bayer)	**Tablet:** 500mg
Bufferin (BMS)	**Tablet:** 325mg
Bufferin Extra Strength (BMS)	**Tablet:** 500mg

MAGNESIUM SALICYLATE PRODUCTS

Brand Name	Dosage Form
Doan's Extra Strength (Novartis)	**Tablet:** 500mg
Doan's Regular Strength (Novartis)	**Tablet:** 325mg
Momentum (Medtech)	**Tablet:** 467mg

DOSING INFORMATION FOR ANALGESIC PRODUCTS

The following table provides a quick comparison of the ingredients and dosages of common brand-name OTC drugs. Products are listed alphabetically by drug category and brand name.

BRAND NAME	INGREDIENT/STRENGTH	DOSE
ACETAMINOPHEN		
Anacin Aspirin Free tablets (*Insight Pharmaceuticals*)	Acetaminophen 500mg	**Adults & Peds ≥12 yo:** 2 tabs q6h. **Max:** 8 tabs q24h.
Feverall Childrens' suppositories (*Alpharma*)	Acetaminophen 120mg	**Peds 3-6 yo:** 1 supp. q4-6h. **Max:** 6 supp. q24h.
Feverall Infants' suppositories (*Alpharma*)	Acetaminophen 80mg	**Peds 3-11 months:** 1 supp. q6h. **12-36 months:** 1 supp. q4h. **Max:** 6 supp. q24h.
Feverall Jr. Strength suppositories (*Alpharma*)	Acetaminophen 120mg	**Peds 6-12 yo:** 1 supp. q4-6h. **Max:** 6 supp. q24h.
Tylenol 8 Hour caplets (*McNeil Consumer*)	Acetaminophen 650mg	**Adults & Peds ≥12 yo:** 2 tabs q8h prn. **Max:** 6 tabs q24h.
Tylenol 8 Hour geltabs (*McNeil Consumer*)	Acetaminophen 650mg	**Adults & Peds ≥12 yo:** 2 tabs q8h prn. **Max:** 6 tabs q24h.
Tylenol Arthritis caplets (*McNeil Consumer*)	Acetaminophen 650mg	**Adults:** 2 tabs q8h prn. **Max:** 6 tabs q24h.
Tylenol Arthritis geltabs (*McNeil Consumer*)	Acetaminophen 650mg	**Adults:** 2 tabs q8h prn. **Max:** 6 tabs q24h.
Tylenol Children's Meltaways tablets (*McNeil Consumer*)	Acetaminophen 80mg	**Peds 2-3 yo (24-35 lbs):** 2 tabs. **4-5 yo (36-47 lbs):** 3 tabs. **6-8 yo (48-59 lbs):** 4 tabs. **9-10 yo (60-71 lbs):** 5 tabs. **11 yo (72-95 lbs):** 6 tabs. May repeat q4h. **Max:** 5 doses q24h.
Tylenol Children's suspension (*McNeil Consumer*)	Acetaminophen 160mg/5mL	**Peds 2-3 yo (24-35 lbs):** 1 tsp (5mL). **4-5 yo (36-47 lbs):** 1.5 tsp (7.5mL). **6-8 yo (48-59 lbs):** 2 tsp (10mL). **9-10 yo (60-71 lbs):** 2.5 tsp (12.5mL). **11 yo (72-95 lbs):** 3 tsp (15mL). May repeat q4h. **Max:** 5 doses q24h.
Tylenol Extra Strength caplets (*McNeil Consumer*)	Acetaminophen 500mg	**Adults & Peds ≥12 yo:** 2 tabs q4-6h prn. **Max:** 8 tabs q24h.
Tylenol Extra Strength Cool caplets (*McNeil Consumer*)	Acetaminophen 500mg	**Adults & Peds ≥12 yo:** 2 tabs q4-6h prn. **Max:** 8 tabs q24h.
Tylenol Extra Strength gelcaps (*McNeil Consumer*)	Acetaminophen 500mg	**Adults & Peds ≥12 yo:** 2 caps q4-6h prn. **Max:** 8 caps q24h.
Tylenol Extra Strength liquid (*McNeil Consumer*)	Acetaminophen 1000mg/30mL	**Adults & Peds ≥12 yo:** 2 tbl (30mL) q4-6h prn. **Max:** 8 tbl (120mL) q24h.
Tylenol Extra Strength tablets (*McNeil Consumer*)	Acetaminophen 500mg	**Adults & Peds ≥12 yo:** 2 tabs q4-6h prn. **Max:** 8 tabs q24h.

DOSING INFORMATION FOR ANALGESIC PRODUCTS (cont.)

BRAND NAME	INGREDIENT/STRENGTH	DOSE
Tylenol Infants' suspension *(McNeil Consumer)*	Acetaminophen 80mg/0.8mL	**Peds 2-3 yo (24-35 lbs):** 1.6 mL q4h prn. **Max:** 5 doses (8mL) q24h.
Tylenol Junior Meltaways tablets *(McNeil Consumer)*	Acetaminophen 160mg	**Peds 6-8 yo (48-59 lbs):** 2 tabs. **9-10 yo (60-71 lbs):** 2.5 tabs. **11 yo (72-95 lbs):** 3 tabs. **12 yo (≥96 lbs):** 4 tabs. May repeat q4h. **Max:** 5 doses q24h.
Tylenol Regular Strength tablets *(McNeil Consumer)*	Acetaminophen 325mg	**Adults & Peds ≥12 yo:** 2 tabs q4-6h prn. **Max:** 12 tabs q24h. **Peds 6-11 yo:** 1 tab q4-6h. **Max:** 5 tabs q24h.
ACETAMINOPHEN COMBINATION		
Excedrin Extra Strength caplets *(Bristol-Myers Squibb)*	Acetaminophen/Aspirin/Caffeine 250mg-250mg-65mg	**Adults & Peds ≥12 yo:** 2 tabs q6h. **Max:** 8 tabs q24h.
Excedrin Extra Strength geltabs *(Bristol-Myers Squibb)*	Acetaminophen/Aspirin/Caffeine 250mg-250mg-65mg	**Adults & Peds ≥12 yo:** 2 tabs q6h. **Max:** 8 tabs q24h.
Excedrin Extra Strength tablets *(Bristol-Myers Squibb)*	Acetaminophen/Aspirin/Caffeine 250mg-250mg-65mg	**Adults & Peds ≥12 yo:** 2 tabs q6h. **Max:** 8 tabs q24h.
Excedrin Migraine caplets *(Bristol-Myers Squibb)*	Acetaminophen/Aspirin/Caffeine 250mg-250mg-65mg	**Adults:** 2 tabs prn. **Max:** 2 tabs q24h.
Excedrin Migraine geltabs *(Bristol-Myers Squibb)*	Acetaminophen/Aspirin/Caffeine 250mg-250mg-65mg	**Adults:** 2 tabs prn. **Max:** 2 tabs q24h.
Excedrin Migraine tablets *(Bristol-Myers Squibb)*	Acetaminophen/Aspirin/Caffeine 250mg-250mg-65mg	**Adults:** 2 tabs prn. **Max:** 2 tabs q24h.
Excedrin Quicktabs tablets *(Bristol-Myers Squibb)*	Acetaminophen/Caffeine 500mg-65mg	**Adults & Peds ≥12 yo:** 2 tabs q6h. **Max:** 8 tabs q24h.
Excedrin Sinus Headache caplets *(Bristol-Myers Squibb)*	Acetaminophen/Phenylephrine HCl 325mg-5mg	**Adults & Peds ≥12 yo:** 2 tabs q4h. **Max:** 12 tabs q24h.
Excedrin Sinus Headache tablets *(Bristol-Myers Squibb)*	Acetaminophen/Phenylephrine HCl 325mg-5mg	**Adults & Peds ≥12 yo:** 2 tabs q4h. **Max:** 12 tabs q24h.
Excedrin Tension Headache caplets *(Bristol-Myers Squibb)*	Acetaminophen/Caffeine 500mg-65mg	**Adults & Peds ≥12 yo:** 2 tabs q6h. **Max:** 8 tabs q24h.
Excedrin Tension Headache geltabs *(Bristol-Myers Squibb)*	Acetaminophen/Caffeine 500mg-65mg	**Adults & Peds ≥12 yo:** 2 tabs q6h. **Max:** 8 tabs q24h.
Excedrin Tension Headache tablets *(Bristol-Myers Squibb)*	Acetaminophen/Caffeine 500mg-65mg	**Adults & Peds ≥12 yo:** 2 tabs q6h. **Max:** 8 tabs q24h.
Goody's Headache Powders *(GlaxoSmtihKline Consumer Healthcare)*	Acetaminophen/Aspirin/Caffeine 260mg-520mg-32.5mg	**Adults & Peds ≥12 yo:** 1 powder q4-6h. **Max:** 4 powders q24h.
Midol Menstrual Complete caplets *(Bayer Healthcare)*	Acetaminophen/Caffeine/Pyrilamine Maleate 500mg-60mg-15mg	**Adults & Peds ≥12 yo:** 2 tabs q6h. **Max:** 8 tabs q24h.
Midol Menstrual Complete caplets *(Bayer Healthcare)*	Acetaminophen/Caffeine/Pyrilamine Maleate 500mg-60mg-15mg	**Adults & Peds ≥12 yo:** 2 tabs q6h. **Max:** 8 tabs q24h.
Midol PMS caplets *(Bayer Healthcare)*	Acetaminophen/Pamabrom/Pyrilamine 500mg-25mg-15mg	**Adults & Peds ≥12 yo:** 2 tabs q6h. **Max:** 8 tabs q24h.
Midol Teen caplets *(Bayer Healtcare)*	Acetaminophen/Pamabrom 500mg-25mg	**Adults & Peds ≥12 yo:** 2 tabs q6h. **Max:** 8 tabs q24h.
Pamprin Multi-Symptom caplets *(Chattem Consumer Products)*	Acetaminophen/Pamabrom/Pyrilamine 500mg-25mg-15mg	**Adults & Peds ≥12 yo:** 2 tabs q4-6h. **Max:** 8 tabs q24h.
Premsyn PMS caplets *(Chattem Consumer Products)*	Acetaminophen/Pamabrom/Pyrilamine 500mg-25mg-15mg	**Adults & Peds ≥12 yo:** 2 tabs q4-6h. **Max:** 8 tabs q24h.
Tylenol Women's caplets *(McNeil Consumer)*	Acetaminophen/Pamabrom 500mg-25mg	**Adults & Peds ≥12 yo:** 2 tabs q4-6h. **Max:** 8 tabs q24h.
Vanquish caplets *(Bayer Healthcare)*	Acetaminophen/Aspirin/Caffeine 194mg-227mg-33mg	**Adults & Peds ≥12 yo:** 2 tabs q6h. **Max:** 8 tabs q24h.
ACETAMINOPHEN/SLEEP AID		
Excedrin PM caplets *(Bristol-Myers Squibb)*	Acetaminophen/Diphenhydramine 500mg-38mg	**Adults & Peds ≥12 yo:** 2 tabs qhs.
Excedrin PM geltab *(Bristol-Myers Squibb)*	Acetaminophen/Diphenhydramine citrate 500mg-38 mg	**Adults & Peds ≥12 yo:** 2 tabs qhs.

DOSING INFORMATION FOR ANALGESIC PRODUCTS (cont.)

Brand Name	Ingredient/Strength	Dose
Excedrin PM tablet *(Bristol-Myers Squibb)*	Acetaminophen/Diphenhydramine citrate 500mg-38 mg	**Adults & Peds ≥12 yo:** 2 tabs qhs.
Goody's PM Powders *(GlaxoSmithKline Consumer Healthcare)*	Acetaminophen/Diphenhydramine 1000mg-76mg/dose	**Adults & Peds ≥12 yo:** 1 packet (2 powders) qhs.
Tylenol PM caplets *(McNeil Consumer)*	Acetaminophen/Diphenhydramine 500mg-25mg	**Adults & Peds ≥12 yo:** 2 tabs qhs.
Tylenol PM gelcaps *(McNeil Consumer)*	Acetaminophen/Diphenhydramine 500mg-25mg	**Adults & Peds ≥12 yo:** 2 caps qhs.
Tylenol PM geltabs *(McNeil Consumer)*	Acetaminophen/Diphenhydramine 500mg-25mg	**Adults & Peds ≥12 yo:** 2 tabs qhs.
NSAIDs		
Advil caplets *(Wyeth Consumer Healthcare)*	Ibuprofen 200mg	**Adults & Peds ≥12 yo:** 1-2 tabs q4-6h. **Max:** 6 tabs q24h.
Advil Children's Chewables tablets *(Wyeth Consumer Healthcare)*	Ibuprofen 50mg	**Peds 2-3 yr (24-35 lb):** 2 tabs q6-8h. **4-5 yr (36-47 lb):** 3 tabs q6-8h. **6-8 yr (45-89 lb):** 4 tabs q6-8h. **9-10 yr (60-71 lb):** 5 tabs q6-8h. **11 yr (72-95 lb):** 6 tabs q6-8h. **Max:** 4 doses q24h
Advil Children's suspension *(Wyeth Consumer Healthcare)*	Ibuprofen 100mg/5mL	**Peds 2-3 yo (24-35 lbs):** 1 tsp (5mL). **4-5 yo (36-47 lbs):** 1.5 tsp (7.5mL). **6-8 yo (48-59 lbs):** 2 tsp (10mL). **9-10 yo (60-71 lbs):** 2.5 tsp (12.5mL). **11 yo (72-95 lbs):** 3 tsp (15mL). May repeat q6-8h. **Max:** 4 doses q24h.
Advil gelcaps *(Wyeth Consumer Healthcare)*	Ibuprofen 200mg	**Adults & Peds ≥12 yo:** 1-2 caps q4-6h. **Max:** 6 caps q24h.
Advil Infants' Drops *(Wyeth Consumer Healthcare)*	Ibuprofen 50mg/1.25mL	**Peds 6-11 months (12-17 lbs):** 1.25mL. **12-23 months (18-23 lbs):** 1.875mL. May repeat q6-8h. **Max:** 4 doses q24h.
Advil Junior Strength tablets *(Wyeth Consumer Healthcare)*	Ibuprofen 100mg	**Peds 6-10 yo (48-71 lbs):** 2 tabs. **11 yo (72-95 lbs):** 3 tabs. May repeat q6-8h. **Max:** 4 doses q24h.
Advil Junior Strength tablets *(Wyeth Consumer Healthcare)*	Ibuprofen 100mg	**Peds 6-10 yo (48-71 lbs):** 2 tabs. **11 yo (72-95 lbs):** 3 tabs. May repeat q6-8h. **Max:** 4 doses q24h.
Advil liqui-gels *(Wyeth Consumer Healthcare)*	Ibuprofen 200mg	**Adults & Peds ≥12 yo:** 1-2 caps q4-6h. **Max:** 6 caps q24h.
Advil Migraine capsules *(Wyeth Consumer Healthcare)*	Ibuprofen 200mg	**Adults:** 2 caps prn. **Max:** 2 caps q24h.
Advil tablets *(Wyeth Consumer Healthcare)*	Ibuprofen 200mg	**Adults & Peds ≥12 yo:** 1-2 tabs q4-6h. **Max:** 6 tabs q24h.
Aleve caplets *(Bayer Healthcare)*	Naproxen Sodium 220mg	**Adults ≥65 yo:** 1 tab q12h. **Max:** 2 tabs q24h. **Adults & Peds ≥12 yo:** 1 tab q8-12h. **Max:** 3 tabs q24h.
Aleve gelcaps *(Bayer Healthcare)*	Naproxen Sodium 220mg	**Adults ≥65 yo:** 1 cap q12h. **Max:** 2 caps q24h. **Adults & Peds ≥12 yo:** 1 cap q8-12h. **Max:** 3 caps q24h.
Aleve tablets *(Bayer Healthcare)*	Naproxen Sodium 220mg	**Adults ≥65 yo:** 1 tab q12h. **Max:** 2 tabs q24h. **Adults & Peds ≥12 yo:** 1 tab q8-12h. **Max:** 3 tabs q24h.
Midol Cramps and Body Aches tablets *(Bayer Healthcare)*	Ibuprofen 200mg	**Adults & Peds ≥12 yo:** 1-2 tabs q4-6h. **Max:** 6 tabs q24h.
Midol Extended Relief caplets *(Bayer Healthcare)*	Naproxen Sodium 220mg	**Adults & Peds ≥12 yo:** 1 tabs q8-12h. **Max:** 3 tabs q24h.

DOSING INFORMATION FOR ANALGESIC PRODUCTS (cont.)

BRAND NAME	INGREDIENT/STRENGTH	DOSE
Motrin Children's suspension *(McNeil Consumer)*	Ibuprofen 100mg/5mL	**Peds 2-3 yo (24-35 lbs):** 1 tsp (5mL). **4-5 yo (36-47 lbs):** 1.5 tsp (7.5mL). **6-8 yo (48-59 lbs):** 2 tsp (10mL). **9-10 yo (60-71 lbs):** 2.5 tsp (12.5mL). **11 yo (72-95 lbs):** 3 tsp (15mL). May repeat q6-8h. **Max:** 4 doses q24h.
Motrin IB caplets *(McNeil Consumer)*	Ibuprofen 200mg	**Adults & Peds ≥12 yo:** 1-2 tabs q4-6h. **Max:** 6 tabs q24h.
Motrin IB gelcaps *(McNeil Consumer)*	Ibuprofen 200mg	**Adults & Peds ≥12 yo:** 1-2 tabs q4-6h. **Max:** 6 tabs q24h.
Motrin IB tablets *(McNeil Consumer)*	Ibuprofen 200mg	**Adults & Peds ≥12 yo:** 1-2 tabs q4-6h. **Max:** 6 tabs q24h.
Motrin Infants' Drops *(McNeil Consumer)*	Ibuprofen 50mg/1.25mL	**Peds 6-11 months (12-17 lbs):** 1.25mL. **12-23 months (18-23 lbs):** 1.875mL. May repeat q6-8h. **Max:** 4 doses q24h.
Motrin Junior Strength chewable tablets *(McNeil Consumer)*	Ibuprofen 100mg	**Peds 6-8 yo (48-59 lbs):** 2 tabs. **9-10 yo (60-71 lbs):** 2.5 tabs. **11 yo (72-95 lbs):** 3 tabs. May repeat q6-8h. **Max:** 4 doses q24h.
Nuprin caplets *(Bristol-Myers Squibb)*	Ibuprofen 200mg	**Adults & Peds ≥12 yo:** 1-2 tabs q4-6h. **Max:** 6 tabs q24h.
Nuprin tablets *(Bristol-Myers Squibb)*	Ibuprofen 200mg	**Adults & Peds ≥12 yo:** 1-2 tabs q4-6h. **Max:** 6 tabs q24h.
Orudis KT tablets *(Wyeth Consumer Healthcare)*	Ketoprofen Magnesium 12.5mg	**Adults:** 1-2 tabs q4-6h. **Max:** 6 tabs q24h.
SALICYLATES		
Anacin 81 tablets *(Insight Pharmaceuticals)*	Aspirin 81mg	**Adults & Peds ≥12 yo:** 4-8 tabs q4h. **Max:** 48 tabs q24h.
Aspergum chewable tablets *(Schering-Plough)*	Aspirin 227mg	**Adults & Peds ≥12 yo:** 2 tabs q4h. **Max:** 16 tabs q24h.
Bayer Aspirin Extra Strength caplets *(Bayer Healthcare)*	Aspirin 500mg	**Adults & Peds ≥12 yo:** 1-2 tabs q4-6h. **Max:** 8 tabs q24h.
Bayer Aspirin safety coated caplets *(Bayer Healthcare)*	Aspirin 325mg	**Adults & Peds ≥12 yo:** 1-2 tabs q4h or 3 tabs q6h. **Max:** 12 tabs q24h.
Bayer Children's Aspirin chewable tablets *(Bayer Healthcare)*	Aspirin 81mg	**Adults & Peds ≥12 yo:** 4-8 tabs q4h. **Max:** 48 tabs q24h.
Bayer Low Dose Aspirin tablets *(Bayer Healthcare)*	Aspirin 81mg	**Adults & Peds ≥12 yo:** 4-8 tabs q4h. **Max:** 48 tabs q24h.
Bayer Original Aspirin tablets *(Bayer Healthcare)*	Aspirin 325mg	**Adults & Peds ≥12 yo:** 1-2 tabs q4h or 3 tabs q6h. **Max:** 12 tabs q24h.
Doan's Extra Strength caplets *(Novartis Consumer Health)*	Magnesium Salicylate Tetrahydrate 580mg	**Adults & Peds ≥12 yo:** 2 tabs q6h. **Max:** 8 tabs q24h.
Doan's Regular Strength caplets *(Novartis Consumer Health)*	Magnesium Salicylate Tetrahydrate 377mg	**Adults & Peds ≥12 yo:** 2 tabs q4h. **Max:** 12 tabs q24h.
Ecotrin Adult Low Strength tablets *(GlaxoSmithKline Consumer Healthcare)*	Aspirin 81mg	**Adults:** 4-8 tabs q4h. **Max:** 48 tabs q24h.
Ecotrin Enteric Low Strength tablets *(GlaxoSmithKline Consumer Healthcare)*	Aspirin 81mg	**Adults:** 4-8 tabs q4h. **Max:** 48 tabs q24h.
Ecotrin Enteric Regular Strength tablets *(GlaxoSmtihKline Consumer Healthcare)*	Aspirin 325mg	**Adults & Peds ≥12 yo:** 1-2 tabs q4h. **Max:** 12 tabs q24h.
Ecotrin Maximum Strength tablets *(GlaxoSmithKline Consumer Healthcare)*	Aspirin 500mg	**Adults & Peds ≥12 yo:** 2 tabs q6h. **Max:** 8 tabs q24h.
Ecotrin Regular Strength tablets *(GlaxoSmithKline Consumer Healthcare)*	Aspirin 325mg	**Adults & Peds ≥12 yo:** 1-2 tabs q4h. **Max:** 12 tabs q24h.
Halfprin 162mg tablets *(Kramer Laboratories)*	Aspirin 162mg	**Adults & Peds ≥12 yo:** 2-4 tabs q4h. **Max:** 24 tabs q24h.
Halfprin 81mg tablets *(Kramer Laboratories)*	Aspirin 81mg	**Adults & Peds ≥12 yo:** 4-8 tabs q4h. **Max:** 48 tabs q24h.

DOSING INFORMATION FOR ANALGESIC PRODUCTS (cont.)

Brand Name	Ingredient/Strength	Dose
St. Joseph Adult Low Strength chewable tablets *(McNeil Consumer)*	Aspirin 81mg	**Adults & Peds ≥12 yo:** 4-8 tabs q4h. **Max:** 48 tabs q24h.
St. Joseph Adult Low Strength tablets *(McNeil Consumer)*	Aspirin 81mg	**Adults & Peds ≥12 yo:** 4-8 tabs q4h. **Max:** 48 tabs q24h.
SALICYLATES, BUFFERED		
Ascriptin Maximum Strength tablets *(Novartis Consumer Health)*	Aspirin Buffered with Maalox/Calcium Carbonate 500mg	**Adults & Peds ≥12 yo:** 2 tabs q4h. **Max:** 8 tabs q24h.
Ascriptin Regular Strength tablets *(Novartis Consumer Health)*	Aspirin Buffered with Maalox/Calcium Carbonate 325mg	**Adults & Peds ≥12 yo:** 2 tabs q4h. **Max:** 12 tabs q24h.
Bayer Extra Strength Plus caplets *(Bayer Healthcare)*	Aspirin Buffered with Calcium Carbonate 500mg	**Adults & Peds ≥12 yo:** 1-2 tabs q4-6h. **Max:** 8 tabs q24h.
Bufferin Extra Strength tablets *(Bristol-Myers Squibb)*	Aspirin Buffered with Calcium Carbonate/ Magnesium Oxide/Magnesium Carbonate 500mg	**Adults & Peds ≥12 yo:** 2 tabs q6h. **Max:** 8 tabs q24h.
Bufferin tablets *(Bristol-Myers Squibb)*	Aspirin Buffered with Calcium Carbonate/ Magnesium Oxide/Magnesium Carbonate 325mg	**Adults & Peds ≥12 yo:** 2 tabs q4h. **Max:** 12 tabs q24h.
SALICYLATE COMBINATION		
Alka-Seltzer effervescent tablets *(Bayer Healthcare)*	Aspirin/Citric Acid/Sodium Bicarbonate/ Sodium 325mg-1000mg-1916mg-567mg	**Adults & Peds ≥12 yo:** 2 tabs q4h. **Max:** 8 tabs q24h.
Alka-Seltzer Extra Strength effervescent tablets *(Bayer Healthcare)*	Aspirin/Citric Acid/Sodium Bicarbonate/ Sodium 500mg-1000mg-1985mg-588mg	**Adults & Peds ≥12 yo:** 2 tabs q6h. **Max:** 7 tabs q24h.
Alka-Seltzer Morning Relief effervescent tablets *(Bayer Healthcare)*	Aspirin/Caffeine 500mg-65mg	**Adults & Peds ≥12 yo:** 2 tabs q6h. **Max:** 8 tabs q24h.
Anacin Pain Reliever caplets *(Insight Pharmaceuticals)*	Aspirin/Caffeine 400mg-32mg	**Adults & Peds ≥12 yo:** 2 tabs q6h. **Max:** 8 tabs q24h.
Anacin Extra Strength tablets *(Insight Pharmaceuticals)*	Aspirin/Caffeine 500mg-32mg	**Adults & Peds ≥12 yo:** 2 tabs q6h. **Max:** 8 tabs q24h.
Anacin tablets *(Insight Pharmaceuticals)*	Aspirin/Caffeine 400mg-32mg	**Adults & Peds ≥12 yo:** 2 tabs q6h. **Max:** 8 tabs q24h.
Bayer Back & Body Pain caplets *(Bayer Healthcare)*	Aspirin/Caffeine 500mg-32.5mg	**Adults & Peds ≥12 yo:** 2 tabs q6h. **Max:** 8 tabs q24h.
Bayer Rapid Headache Relief caplets *(Bayer Healthcare)*	Aspirin/Caffeine 500mg-65 mg	**Adults & Peds ≥12 yo:** 2 tabs q6h. **Max:** 8 tabs q24h.
BC Arthritis Strength powders *(GlaxoSmtihKline Consumer Healthcare)*	Aspirin/Caffeine/Salicylamide 742mg-38mg-222mg	**Adults & Peds ≥12 yo:** 1 powder q3-4h. **Max:** 4 powders q24h.
BC Original powders *(GlaxoSmithKline Consumer Healthcare)*	Aspirin/Caffeine/Salicylamide 650mg-33.3mg-195mg	**Adults & Peds ≥12 yo:** 1 powder q 3-4 h.
SALICYLATE/SLEEP AID		
Alka-Seltzer PM Pain Reliever & Sleep Aid, effervescent tablets *(Bayer Healthcare)*	Aspirin/Diphenhydramine Citrate 325mg-38 mg	**Adults & Peds ≥12 yo:** 2 tabs qpm.
Bayer Extra Strength Night Time Relief caplets *(Bayer Healthcare)*	Aspirin/Diphenhydramine 500mg-38.3mg	**Adults & Peds ≥12 yo:** 2 tabs qhs.
Doan's Extra Strength PM caplets *(Novartis Consumer Health)*	Magnesium Salicylate Tetrahydrate/ Diphenhydramine 580mg-25mg	**Adults & Peds ≥12 yo:** 2 tabs qhs.

Arthralgia

Arthralgia is defined as pain and/or stiffness in a joint. Arthralgia can be caused by injury to any of the ligaments, bursae, or tendons surrounding the joint. Arthralgia is also a feature of arthritis, or joint inflammation. Causes of arthralgia include arthritis, aseptic necrosis, bursitis, osteochondritis dissecans, sickle cell anemia, steroid withdrawal, cartilage tears, fractures, septic arthritis, sprains, and tendinitis. There are many OTC products available to treat arthralgia including acetaminophen, salicylates (e.g., aspirin), and NSAIDs (ibuprofen, ketoprofen, naproxen).

ACETAMINOPHEN

Analgesic—The mechanism of analgesic action has not been fully determined. Acetaminophen may act predominantly by inhibiting prostaglandin synthesis in the central nervous system and, to a lesser extent, through a peripheral action by blocking pain-impulse generation. The peripheral action may also be due to inhibition of prostaglandin synthesis or to inhibition of the synthesis or actions of other substances that sensitize pain receptors to mechanical or chemical stimulation.

Capsule/Granules/Powder/Solution/Suspension/Tablet

For analgesic use:

Adults/Pediatrics ≥13 years of age: 325mg to 500mg every 3 hours, 325mg to 650mg every 4 hours, or 650 to 1000mg every 6 hours, or 1300mg every 8 hours.

Pediatrics ≤3 months of age: 40mg every 4 hours as needed.

Pediatrics 4 to 12 months of age: 80mg every 4 hours as needed.

Pediatrics 1 to 2 years of age: 120mg every 4 hours as needed.

Pediatrics 2 to 4 years of age: 160mg every 4 hours as needed.

Pediatrics 4 to 6 years of age: 240mg every 4 hours as needed.

Pediatrics 6 to 9 years of age: 320mg every 4 hours as needed.

Pediatrics 9 to 11 years of age: 320mg to 400mg every 4 hours as needed.

Pediatrics 11 to 12 years of age: 320mg to 480mg every 4 hours as needed.

SUPPOSITORIES

For analgesic use:

Adults/Pediatrics ≥13 years of age: 325mg to 650mg every 4 hours or 650mg every 6 hours as needed.

Pediatrics 2 to 4 years of age: 160mg every 4 hours as needed.

Pediatrics 4 to 6 years of age: 240mg every 4 hours as needed.

Pediatrics 6 to 9 years of age: 320mg every 4 hours as needed.

Pediatrics 9 to 11 years of age: 320mg to 400mg every 4 hours as needed.

Pediatrics 11 to 12 years of age: 320mg to 480mg every 4 hours as needed.

For more information, refer to the complete monograph for acetaminophen in "Aches and Pains" under Musculoskeletal System.

ASPIRIN

Analgesic—Salicylates produce analgesia through a peripheral action by blocking pain impulse generation and via a central action, possibly in the hypothalamus. The peripheral action may predominate and probably involves inhibition of the synthesis of prostaglandins, and possibly inhibition of the synthesis and/or actions of other substances, which sensitize pain receptors to mechanical or chemical stimulation.

SUPPOSITORIES

For analgesic use:

Adults/Pediatrics ≥12 years of age: 325 to 650mg every 4 hours as needed.

Pediatrics 2 to 4 years of age: 160mg every 4 hours as needed.

Pediatrics 4 to 6 years of age: 240mg every 4 hours as needed.

Pediatrics 6 to 9 years of age: 325mg every 4 hours as needed.

Pediatrics 9 to 11 years of age: 325 to 400mg every 4 hours as needed.

Pediatric 11 to 12 years of age: 325 to 480mg every 4 hours as needed.

ACETAMINOPHEN PRODUCTS	
Brand Name	**Dosage Form**
Anacin Aspirin Free (Insight)	**Tablet:** 500mg
FeverAll (Alpharma)	**Suppositories:** 80mg, 120mg 325mg, 650mg
Tylenol 8 Hour (McNeil)	**Tablet:** 650mg
Tylenol Arthritis (McNeil)	**Tablet:** 650mg
Tylenol Children's Meltaways (McNeil)	**Tablet:** 80mg
Tylenol Children's (McNeil)	**Suspension:** 160mg/5mL
Tylenol Extra Strength (McNeil)	**Capsule:** 500mg **Liquid:** 1000mg/30mL
	Tablet: 500mg
Tylenol Infants'	**Suspension:** 80mg/0.8mL
Tylenol Junior Meltaways (McNeil)	**Tablet:** 160mg
Tylenol Regular Strength (McNeil)	**Tablet:** 325mg

Tablet

For analgesic use:

Adults/Pediatrics ≥12 years of age: 325 to 500mg every 3 hours; or 325 to 650mg every 4 hours; 650 to 100mg every 6 hours as needed.

Pediatrics 2 to 4 years of age: 160mg every 4 hours as needed.

Pediatrics 4 to 6 years of age: 240mg every 4 hours as needed.

Pediatrics 6 to 9 years of age: 320 to 325mg every 4 hours as needed.

Pediatrics 9 to 11 years of age: 320 to 400mg every 4 hours as needed.

Pediatric 11 to 12 years of age: 320 to 480mg every 4 hours as needed.

For more information, refer to the complete monograph for salicylates in "Aches and Pains" under Musculoskeletal System.

CAFFEINE

Analgesia adjunct—Caffeine constricts cerebral vasculature with an accompanying decrease in cerebral blood flow and in the

ASPIRIN PRODUCTS	
Brand Name	**Dosage Form**
Ascriptin (Novartis)	**Tablet:** 81mg
Aspergum (Schering)	**Gum:** 227mg
Bayer Aspirin Regimen (Bayer)	**Tablet:** 81mg, 325mg
Bayer Children's Aspirin	**Tablet:** 81mg
Bayer Extra Strength (Bayer)	**Tablet:** 500mg
Bayer Genuine Aspirin (Bayer)	**Tablet:** 325mg
Ecotrin (GSK)	**Tablet:** 325mg
Ecotrin Adult Low Strength (GSK)	**Tablet:** 81mg
Ecotrin Maximum Strength (GSK)	**Tablet:** 500mg
Halfprin (Kramer)	**Tablet:** 81mg, 162mg
St. Joseph (McNeil)	**Tablet:** 81mg
BUFFERED ASPIRIN PRODUCTS	
Brand Name	**Dosage Form**
Alka-Seltzer (Bayer)	**Tablet:** 325mg
Alka-Seltzer Extra Strength (Bayer)	**Tablet:** 500mg
Ascriptin (Novartis)	**Tablet:** 325mg
Ascriptin Arthritis Pain (Novartis)	**Tablet:** 325mg
Ascriptin Maximum Strength (Novartis)	**Tablet:** 500mg
Bayer Plus Extra Strength (Bayer)	**Tablet:** 500mg
Bufferin (BMS)	**Tablet:** 325mg
Bufferin Extra Strength (BMS)	**Tablet:** 500mg

ACETAMINOPHEN/CAFFEINE PRODUCTS	
Brand Name	**Dosage Form**
Excedrin Tension Headache (BMS)	**Tablet:** 500mg-65mg
ACETAMINOPHEN/ASPIRIN/CAFFEINE PRODUCTS	
Brand Name	**Dosage Form**
Excedrin Extra Strength (BMS)	**Tablet:** 250mg-250mg-65mg
Excedrin Migraine (BMS)	**Tablet:** 250mg-250mg-65mg
Goody's Fast Pain Relief (GSK)	**Tablet:** 130mg-260mg-16.25mg
Goody's Headache Powder (GSK)	**Tablet:** 260mg-520mg-32.5mg
ASPIRIN/CAFFEINE PRODUCTS	
Brand Name	**Dosage Form**
Alka-Seltzer Morning Relief (Bayer)	**Tablet:** 500mg-65mg
Anacin (Wyeth)	**Tablet:** 400mg-32mg
Anacin Maximum Strength (Wyeth)	**Tablet:** 500mg-32mg
Bayer Rapid Headache Relief (Bayer)	**Tablet:** 500mg-65mg
ASPIRIN/CAFFEINE/SALICYLAMIDE PRODUCTS	
Brand Name	**Dosage Form**
BC Head Powder (GSK)	**Tablet:** 650mg-33.3mg-195mg
BC Head Powder (GSK)	**Tablet:** 742mg-36mg-222mg

oxygen tension of the brain. It has been suggested that the addition of caffeine to aspirin or to aspirin/acetaminophen combinations may help to relieve headache by providing a more rapid onset of action and/or enhanced pain relief with a lower dose of the analgesic. In some patients, caffeine may reduce headache pain by reversing caffeine withdrawal symptoms. Recent studies with ergotamine indicate that the enhancement of effect by the addition of caffeine may be due to improved gastrointestinal absorption of ergotamine when administered with caffeine.

For more information, refer to the complete monograph for caffeine in "Drowsiness/Lethargy" under Central Nervous System.

CAPSAICIN

PHARMACOLOGY

The precise mechanism of action has not been fully elucidated. Capsaicin is a neuropeptide-active agent that affects the synthesis, storage, transport, and release of substance P. Substance P is thought to be the principal chemical mediator of pain impulses from the periphery to the central nervous system. In addition, substance P has been shown to be released into joint tissues where it activates inflammatory intermediates that are involved with the development of rheumatoid arthritis. Capsaicin renders skin and joints insensitive to pain by depleting and preventing reaccumulation of substance P in peripheral sensory neurons. With the depletion of substance P in the nerve endings, local pain impulses cannot be transmitted to the brain.

INDICATIONS

Neuralgia (treatment)—Capsaicin is indicated for the treatment of neuralgias, such as the pain following herpes zoster (shingles) and painful diabetic neuropathy.

Osteoarthritis (treatment); *rheumatoid arthritis* (treatment)— Capsaicin is indicated for the treatment of pain from osteoarthritis and rheumatoid arthritis.

Pain, neurogenic, other (treatment)—Capsaicin is used to treat the pain associated with postmastectomy pain syndrome (PMPS) and reflex sympathetic dystrophy syndrome (RSDS, causalgia).

Pruritus, aquagenic (treatment); *pruritus, hemodialysis-induced* (treatment)—Capsaicin is used in the treatment of pruritus associated with hemodialysis and exposure to water (aquagenic).

CONTRAINDICATIONS

Except under special circumstances, this medication should not be used when the following medical problem exists:

- Broken or irritated skin on area to be treated—major clinical significance (will cause pain and further irritation of skin).

Risk-benefit should be considered when the following medical problem exists:

- Sensitivity to capsaicin or to the fruits of Capsicum plants (e.g., hot peppers).

WARNINGS/PRECAUTIONS

Pregnancy: Problems in humans have not been documented.

Breastfeeding: It is not known whether capsaicin, applied topically, is distributed into breast milk. However, problems in humans have not been documented.

ADVERSE REACTIONS

Those indicating need for medical attention only if they continue or are bothersome:

Incidence more frequent

Warm, stinging, or burning sensation at the site of application.

ADMINISTRATION AND DOSING

General Dosing Information

The cream should be applied sparingly and rubbed well into the affected area so that little or no cream is left on the surface of the skin. During the first 1 or 2 weeks of treatment, application of a topical lidocaine product before capsaicin application may reduce initial discomfort. A therapeutic pain response is usually achieved within 2 to 4 weeks. Most patients with arthritis notice an initial response within 1 or 2 weeks. Most patients with neuralgia pain begin to respond within 2 to 4 weeks, although patients with pain from head and neck neuralgias may take 4 to 6 weeks to respond. Continued application of capsaicin 3 or 4 times daily is necessary to sustain pain relief. If the medicine is discontinued and pain recurs, capsaicin treatment may be restarted. Persons using capsaicin to treat arthritis in their hands should avoid washing their hands for at least 30 minutes after application. When capsaicin is used for the treatment of neuralgia due to herpes zoster, it should not be applied to the skin until after the zoster lesions have healed. If a bandage is being used on the treated area, it should not be applied tightly.

Cream

Adults/Pediatrics >2 years of age: Apply to affected area 3 to 4 times a day.

IBUPROFEN

Analgesic—Ibuprofen may block pain-impulse generation via a peripheral action that may involve reduction of the activity of prostaglandins, and possibly inhibition of the synthesis or actions of other substances that sensitize pain receptors to mechanical or chemical stimulation. The antibradykinin activity of ibuprofen may also be involved in relief of pain, since bradykinin has been shown to act together with prostaglandins to cause pain.

Capsule/Suspension/Tablet

For analgesic use (mild to moderate pain):

Adults: 200 to 400mg every 4 to 6 hours as needed.

For more information, refer to the complete monograph for NSAIDs in "Aches and Pains" under Musculoskeletal System.

CAPSAICIN PRODUCTS	
Brand Name	**Dosage Form**
Capsin (Pryde)	**Lotion:** 0.03%, 0.08%
Icy Hot Arthritis Therapy (Chattem)	**Gel:** 0.03%
Zostrix (Rodlen)	**Cream:** 0.03% **Stick:** 0.03%
Zostrix High Potency (Rodlen)	**Stick:** 0.08%
Zostrix Sports (Rodlen)	**Cream:** 0.08%

KETOPROFEN

Analgesic—Ketoprofen may block pain-impulse generation via a peripheral action that may involve reduction of the activity of prostaglandins, and possibly inhibition of the synthesis or actions of other substances that sensitize pain receptors to mechanical or chemical stimulation. The antibradykinin activity of ketoprofen may also be involved in relief of pain, since bradykinin has been shown to act together with prostaglandins to cause pain.

Capsules/Tablets

For analgesic use (mild to moderate pain):

Adults: 25 to 50mg every 6 to 8 hours as needed.

MAGNESIUM SALICYLATE

Analgesic—Salicylates produce analgesia through a peripheral action by blocking pain impulse generation and via a central action, possibly in the hypothalamus. The peripheral action may predominate and probably involves inhibition of the synthesis of prostaglandins, and possibly inhibition of the synthesis and/or actions of other substances, which sensitize pain receptors to mechanical or chemical stimulation.

Tablets

For analgesic use:

Adults: 607.4mg every 4 hours as needed; or 934mg every 6 hours as needed.

NAPROXEN

Analgesic—Naproxen may block pain-impulse generation via a peripheral action that may involve reduction of the activity of prostaglandins, and possibly inhibition of the synthesis or actions of other substances that sensitize pain receptors to mechanical or chemical stimulation. The antibradykinin activity of naproxen may also be involved in relief of pain, since bradykinin has been shown to act together with prostaglandins to cause pain.

Capsule/Tablet

For analgesic use (mild to moderate pain):

Adults: 500mg initially, then 250mg every 6 to 8 hours as needed.

For more information, refer to the complete monograph for NSAIDs in "Aches and Pains" under Musculoskeletal System.

IBUPROFEN PRODUCTS	
Brand Name	**Dosage Form**
Advil (Wyeth)	**Capsule:** 200mg **Tablet:** 200mg
Advil Children's (Wyeth)	**Tablet:** 50mg
Advil Junior (Wyeth)	**Tablet:** 100mg
Midol Cramp Formula (Bayer)	**Tablet:** 200mg
Motrin IB (McNeil)	**Tablet:** 200mg
Motrin Children's (McNeil)	**Suspension:** 100mg/5mL
Motrin Infants' (McNeil)	**Suspension:** 50mg/1.25mL
Motrin Junior (McNeil)	**Tablet:** 100mg
Motrin Migraine Pain (McNeil)	**Tablet:** 200mg
KETOPROFEN PRODUCTS	
Brand Name	**Dosage Form**
Orudis KT (Wyeth)	**Tablet:** 12.5mg
MAGNESIUM SALICYLATE PRODUCTS	
Brand Name	**Dosage Form**
Doan's Extra Strength (Novartis)	**Tablet:** 500mg
Doan's Regular Strength (Novartis)	**Tablet:** 325mg
Momentum (Medtech)	**Tablet:** 467mg
NAPROXEN PRODUCTS	
Brand Name	**Dosage Form**
Aleve (Bayer)	**Capsule:** 220mg **Tablet:** 220mg
Aleve Arthritis (Bayer)	**Tablet:** 220mg
Midol Extended Relief (Bayer)	**Tablet:** 220mg

DOSING INFORMATION FOR ARTHRALGIA PRODUCTS

The following table provides a quick comparison of the ingredients and dosages of common brand-name OTC drugs. Products are listed alphabetically by drug category and brand name.

BRAND NAME	INGREDIENT/STRENGTH	DOSE
ACETAMINOPHEN		
Anacin Aspirin Free tablets *(Insight Pharmaceuticals)*	Acetaminophen 500mg	**Adults & Peds** ≥12 yo: 2 tabs q6h. **Max:** 8 tabs q24h.
Tylenol 8 Hour caplets *(McNeil Consumer)*	Acetaminophen 650mg	**Adults & Peds** ≥12 yo: 2 tabs q8h prn. **Max:** 6 tabs q24h.
Tylenol 8 Hour geltabs *(McNeil Consumer)*	Acetaminophen 650mg	**Adults & Peds** ≥12 yo: 2 tabs q8h prn. **Max:** 6 tabs q24h.
Tylenol Arthritis caplets *(McNeil Consumer)*	Acetaminophen 650mg	**Adults:** 2 tabs q8h prn. **Max:** 6 tabs q24h.
Tylenol Arthritis geltabs *(McNeil Consumer)*	Acetaminophen 650mg	**Adults:** 2 tabs q8h prn. **Max:** 6 tabs q24h.
Tylenol Children's Meltaways tablets *(McNeil Consumer)*	Acetaminophen 80mg	**Peds 2-3 yo (24-35 lbs):** 2 tabs. **4-5 yo (36-47 lbs):** 3 tabs. **6-8 yo (48-59 lbs):** 4 tabs. **9-10 yo (60-71 lbs):** 5 tabs. **11 yo (72-95 lbs):** 6 tabs. May repeat q4h. **Max:** 5 doses q24h.
Tylenol Children's suspension *(McNeil Consumer)*	Acetaminophen 160mg/5mL	**Peds 2-3 yo (24-35 lbs):** 1 tsp (5mL). **4-5 yo (36-47 lbs):** 1.5 tsp (7.5mL). **6-8 yo (48-59 lbs):** 2 tsp (10mL). **9-10 yo (60-71 lbs):** 2.5 tsp (12.5mL). **11 yo (72-95 lbs):** 3 tsp (15mL). May repeat q4h. **Max:** 5 doses q24h.
Tylenol Extra Strength caplets *(McNeil Consumer)*	Acetaminophen 500mg	**Adults & Peds** ≥12 yo: 2 tabs q4-6h prn. **Max:** 8 tabs q24h.
Tylenol Extra Strength Cool caplets *(McNeil Consumer)*	Acetaminophen 500mg	**Adults & Peds** ≥12 yo: 2 tabs q4-6h prn. **Max:** 8 tabs q24h.
Tylenol Extra Strength gelcaps *(McNeil Consumer)*	Acetaminophen 500mg	**Adults & Peds** ≥12 yo: 2 caps q4-6h prn. **Max:** 8 caps q24h.
Tylenol Extra Strength liquid *(McNeil Consumer)*	Acetaminophen 1000mg/30mL	**Adults & Peds** ≥12 yo: 2 tbl (30mL) q4-6h prn. **Max:** 8 tbl (120mL) q24h.
Tylenol Extra Strength tablets *(McNeil Consumer)*	Acetaminophen 500mg	**Adults & Peds** ≥12 yo: 2 tabs q4-6h prn. **Max:** 8 tabs q24h.
Tylenol Infants' suspension *(McNeil Consumer)*	Acetaminophen 80mg/0.8mL	**Peds 2-3 yo (24-35 lbs):** 1.6 mL q4h prn. **Max:** 5 doses (8mL) q24h.
Tylenol Junior Meltaways tablets *(McNeil Consumer)*	Acetaminophen 160mg	**Peds 6-8 yo (48-59 lbs):** 2 tabs. **9-10 yo (60-71 lbs):** 2.5 tabs. **11 yo (72-95 lbs):** 3 tabs. **12 yo (≥96 lbs):** 4 tabs. May repeat q4h. **Max:** 5 doses q24h.
Tylenol Regular Strength tablets *(McNeil Consumer)*	Acetaminophen 325mg	**Adults & Peds** ≥12 yo: 2 tabs q4-6h prn. **Max:** 12 tabs q24h. **Peds 6-11 yo:** 1 tab q4-6h. **Max:** 5 tabs q24h.
NSAIDs		
Advil caplets *(Wyeth Consumer Healthcare)*	Ibuprofen 200mg	**Adults & Peds** ≥12 yo: 1-2 tabs q4-6h. **Max:** 6 tabs q24h.
Advil Children's Chewables tablets *(Wyeth Consumer Healthcare)*	Ibuprofen 50mg	**Peds 2-3 yr (24-35 lb):** 2 tabs q6-8h. **4-5 yr (36-47 lb):** 3 tabs q6-8h. **6-8 yr (45-89 lb):** 4 tabs q6-8h. **9-10 yr (60-71 lb):** 5 tabs q6-8h. **11 yr (72-95 lb):** 6 tabs q6-8h. **Max:** 4 doses q24h
Advil Children's suspension *(Wyeth Consumer Healthcare)*	Ibuprofen 100mg/5mL	**Peds 2-3 yo (24-35 lbs):** 1 tsp (5mL). **4-5 yo (36-47 lbs):** 1.5 tsp (7.5mL). **6-8 yo (48-59 lbs):** 2 tsp (10mL). **9-10 yo (60-71 lbs):** 2.5 tsp (12.5mL). **11 yo (72-95 lbs):** 3 tsp (15mL). May repeat q6-8h. **Max:** 4 doses q24h.
Advil gelcaps *(Wyeth Consumer Healthcare)*	Ibuprofen 200mg	**Adults & Peds** ≥12 yo: 1-2 caps q4-6h. **Max:** 6 caps q24h.
Advil Infants' Drops *(Wyeth Consumer Healthcare)*	Ibuprofen 50mg/1.25mL	**Peds 6-11 months (12-17 lbs):** 1.25mL. **12-23 months (18-23 lbs):** 1.875mL. May repeat q6-8h. **Max:** 4 doses q24h.

DOSING INFORMATION FOR ARTHRALGIA PRODUCTS (cont.)

BRAND NAME	INGREDIENT/STRENGTH	DOSE
Advil Junior Strength tablets (*Wyeth Consumer Healthcare*)	Ibuprofen 100mg	**Peds 6-10 yo (48-71 lbs):** 2 tabs. **11 yo (72-95 lbs):** 3 tabs. May repeat q6-8h. **Max:** 4 doses q24h.
Advil Junior Strength tablets (*Wyeth Consumer Healthcare*)	Ibuprofen 100mg	**Peds 6-10 yo (48-71 lbs):** 2 tabs. **11 yo (72-95 lbs):** 3 tabs. May repeat q6-8h. **Max:** 4 doses q24h.
Advil liqui-gels (*Wyeth Consumer Healthcare*)	Ibuprofen 200mg	**Adults & Peds ≥12 yo:** 1-2 caps q4-6h. **Max:** 6 caps q24h.
Advil Migraine capsules (*Wyeth Consumer Healthcare*)	Ibuprofen 200mg	**Adults:** 2 caps prn. **Max:** 2 caps q24h.
Advil tablets (*Wyeth Consumer Healthcare*)	Ibuprofen 200mg	**Adults & Peds ≥12 yo:** 1-2 tabs q4-6h. **Max:** 6 tabs q24h.
Aleve caplets (*Bayer Healthcare*)	Naproxen Sodium 220mg	**Adults ≥65 yo:** 1 tab q12h. **Max:** 2 tabs q24h. **Adults & Peds ≥12 yo:** 1 tab q8-12h. **Max:** 3 tabs q24h.
Aleve gelcaps (*Bayer Healthcare*)	Naproxen Sodium 220mg	**Adults ≥65 yo:** 1 cap q12h. **Max:** 2 caps q24h. **Adults & Peds ≥12 yo:** 1 cap q8-12h. **Max:** 3 caps q24h.
Aleve tablets (*Bayer Healthcare*)	Naproxen Sodium 220mg	**Adults ≥65 yo:** 1 tab q12h. **Max:** 2 tabs q24h. **Adults & Peds ≥12 yo:** 1 tab q8-12h. **Max:** 3 tabs q24h.
Motrin Children's suspension (*McNeil Consumer*)	Ibuprofen 100mg/5mL	**Peds 2-3 yo (24-35 lbs):** 1 tsp (5mL). **4-5 yo (36-47 lbs):** 1.5 tsp (7.5mL). **6-8 yo (48-59 lbs):** 2 tsp (10mL). **9-10 yo (60-71 lbs):** 2.5 tsp (12.5mL). **11 yo (72-95 lbs):** 3 tsp (15mL). May repeat q6-8h. **Max:** 4 doses q24h.
Motrin IB caplets (*McNeil Consumer*)	Ibuprofen 200mg	**Adults & Peds ≥12 yo:** 1-2 tabs q4-6h. **Max:** 6 tabs q24h.
Motrin IB gelcaps (*McNeil Consumer*)	Ibuprofen 200mg	**Adults & Peds ≥12 yo:** 1-2 tabs q4-6h. **Max:** 6 tabs q24h.
Motrin IB tablets (*McNeil Consumer*)	Ibuprofen 200mg	**Adults & Peds ≥12 yo:** 1-2 tabs q4-6h. **Max:** 6 tabs q24h.
Motrin Infants' Drops (*McNeil Consumer*)	Ibuprofen 50mg/1.25mL	**Peds 6-11 months (12-17 lbs):** 1.25mL. **12-23 months (18-23 lbs):** 1.875mL. May repeat q6-8h. **Max:** 4 doses q24h.
Motrin Junior Strength chewable tablets (*McNeil Consumer*)	Ibuprofen 100mg	**Peds 6-8 yo (48-59 lbs):** 2 tabs. **9-10 yo (60-71 lbs):** 2.5 tabs. **11 yo (72-95 lbs):** 3 tabs. May repeat q6-8h. **Max:** 4 doses q24h.
Nuprin caplets (*Bristol-Myers Squibb*)	Ibuprofen 200mg	**Adults & Peds ≥12 yo:** 1-2 tabs q4-6h. **Max:** 6 tabs q24h.
Nuprin tablets (*Bristol-Myers Squibb*)	Ibuprofen 200mg	**Adults & Peds ≥12 yo:** 1-2 tabs q4-6h. **Max:** 6 tabs q24h.
Orudis KT tablets (*Wyeth Consumer Healthcare*)	Ketoprofen Magnesium 12.5mg	**Adults:** 1-2 tabs q4-6h. **Max:** 6 tabs q24h.
RUBS & LINIMENTS		
Absorbine Jr Deep Pain Relief patches (*W.F. Young*)	Menthol 5.0%	**Adults & Peds ≥12 yo:** Apply to affected area bid.
Absorbine Jr liquid (*W.F. Young*)	Menthol 1.27%	**Adults & Peds ≥2 yo:** Apply to affected area tid-qid.
Absorbine Jr patches (*W.F. Young*)	Menthol 1.3%	**Adults & Peds ≥12 yo:** Apply to affected area bid.
Arthricare Women Extra Moisturizing (*Del Pharmaceuticals*)	Capsaicin 0.025%	**Adults & Peds ≥12 yo:** Apply to affected area tid-qid.
Arthricare Women Multi-Action (*Del Pharmaceuticals*)	Capsaicin/Menthol/Methyl nicotinate 0.025%-1.25%-0.25%	**Adults & Peds ≥12 yo:** Apply to affected area tid-qid.
Arthricare Women Quick Dry Rub (*Del Pharmaceuticals*)	Capsaicin 0.025%	**Adults & Peds ≥12 yo:** Apply to affected area tid-qid.

DOSING INFORMATION FOR ARTHRALGIA PRODUCTS (cont.)

BRAND NAME	INGREDIENT/STRENGTH	DOSE
Arthricare Women Ultra-Strength (Del Pharmaceuticals)	Capsaicin/Menthol 0.075%-2%	**Adults & Peds ≥12 yo:** Apply to affected area tid-qid.
Arthritis Hot cream (Chattem)	Methyl Salicylate/Menthol 15%-10%	**Adults:** Apply to affected area prn up to qid.
BenGay Pain Relieving Patch (Pfizer Consumer Healthcare)	Menthol 1.4%	**Adults & Peds ≥12 yo:** Apply to affected area tid-qid.
BenGay Ultra Strength cream (Pfizer Consumer Healthcare)	Methyl Salicylate/Menthol/Camphor 30%-10%-4%	**Adults & Peds ≥12 yo:** Apply to affected area qd-tid.
BenGay Ultra Strength Pain Relieving Patch (Pfizer Consumer Healthcare)	Menthol 5%	**Adults & Peds ≥12 yo:** Apply to affected area tid-qid.
BenGay Vanishing sent gel (Pfizer Consumer Healthcare)	Menthol 2.5%	**Adults & Peds ≥12 yo:** Apply to affected area tid-qid.
Bodyglide Maximum Strength WarmFX (Sternoff)	Methyl Salicylate/Menthol 30%-15%	**Adults:** Apply to affected area prn.
Boericke & Tafel Triflora Arthritis gel (Boericke & Tafel)	Symphytum Officinale/Rhus Toxicodendron/Ledum Palustre 10%-5%-2.5%	**Adults & Peds ≥12 yo:** Apply to affected area qd-qid.
Capzasin-HP Arthritis Pain Relief cream (Chattem)	Capsaicin 0.075%	**Adults:** Apply to affected area tid-qid.
Capzasin-P Arthritis Pain Relief cream (Chattem)	Capsaicin 0.025%	**Adults:** Apply to affected area tid-qid.
Emu Lifestyle Active Lifestyle cream (Emu Lifestyle)	Menthol 3%	**Adults & Peds ≥10 yo:** Apply to affected area qd-qid.
Emu Lifestyle Active Lifestyle Cream, for Arthritis and Joints (Emu Lifestyle)	Trolamine Salicylate 10%	**Adults & Peds ≥10 yo:** Apply to affected area qd-qid.
Flexall Maximum Strength gel (Chattem)	Menthol 16%	**Adults & Peds ≥12 yo:** Apply to affected area prn up to qid.
Flexall Maximum Strength gel pump (Chattem)	Menthol 16%	**Adults & Peds ≥12 yo:** Apply to affected area prn up to qid.
Heet Pain Relieving Liniment (Medtech)	Methyl Salicylate/Camphor/Oleoresin Capsicum 17%-3.6%-.025%	**Adults:** Apply to affected area prn.
Icy Hot balm (Chattem)	Methyl Salicyalte/Menthol 29%-7.6%	**Adults:** Apply to affected area prn.
Icy Hot Chill Stick (Chattem)	Methyl Salicyalte/Menthol 30%-10%	**Adults:** Apply to affected area prn.
Icy Hot cream (Chattem)	Methyl Salicyalte/Menthol 30%-10%	**Adults:** Apply to affected area prn.
Icy Hot Patch Extra Stength (Arm, Neck, Leg) (Chattem)	Menthol 5%	**Adults & Peds ≥12 yo:** Apply to affected area prn up to qid.
Icy Hot Patch Extra Stength (Back) (Chattem)	Menthol 5%	**Adults & Peds ≥12 yo:** Apply to affected area prn up to qid.
Icy Hot Sleeve (Ankles, Elbows, Knees, Wrist) (Chattem)	Menthol 16%	**Adults & Peds ≥12 yo:** Apply to affected area prn up to qid.
Icy Hot Sleeve (Wrists, Small Ankles, and Elbows) (Chattem)	Menthol 16%	**Adults & Peds ≥12 yo:** Apply to affected area prn up to qid.
Mobisyl Maximum Strength Arthritis cream (B.F. Ascher & Company)	Trolamine Salicylate 10%	**Adults & Peds ≥12 yo:** Apply to affected area tid-qid
Nuprin Arthritis High Potency cream (Bristol-Myers Squibb)	Capsaicin 0.075%	**Adults & Peds ≥12 yo:** Apply to affected area tid-qid.
Nuprin Arthritis High Potency patch (Bristol-Myers Squibb)	Capsaicin 0.025%	**Adults & Peds ≥4 yo:** Apply to affected area bid.
Nuprin Arthritis Maximum Strength gel (Bristol-Myers Squibb)	Capsaicin/Menthol 0.075%-8%	**Adults & Peds ≥2 yo:** Apply to affected area tid-qid.
Nuprin Arthritis Maximum Strength gel (Bristol-Myers Squibb)	Capsaicin/Menthol 0.075%-8%	**Adults & Peds ≥12 yo:** Apply to affected area tid-qid.
Super Blue Pain Relief cream (Spring)	Menthol 2.75%	**Adults & Peds ≥12 yo:** Apply to affected area tid-qid.
Thera-gesic Maximum Strength cream (Mission Pharmacal)	Mehtyl Salicylate/Menthol 15%-1%	**Adults & Peds ≥12 yo:** Apply to affected area tid-qid.
Thera-gesic Plus cream (Mission Pharmacal)	Mehtyl Salicylate/Menthol 25%-4%	**Adults & Peds ≥12 yo:** Apply to affected area tid-qid.

DOSING INFORMATION FOR ARTHRALGIA PRODUCTS (cont.)

Brand Name	Ingredient/Strength	Dose
Ultra Blue Topical Analgesic gel (BNG Enterprises)	Menthol 4%	**Adults & Peds ≥2 yo:** Apply to affected area tid-qid.
Watkins Liniment Pain Relief Spray (Watkins)	Camphor/Menthol 3.5%-2.5%	**Adults & Peds ≥2 yo:** Apply to affected area tid-qid.
WellPatch Arthritis Patch, Pain Relieving Pad (Mentholatum)	Methyl Salicylate 10%	**Adults & Peds ≥12 yo:** Apply to affected area qd-bid
Zostrix cream (Rodlen)	Capsaicin 0.025%	**Adults:** Apply to affected area tid-qid.
Zostrix HP cream (Rodlen)	Capsaicin 0.075%	**Adults:** Apply to affected area tid-qid.
SALICYLATES		
Anacin 81 tablets (Insight Pharmaceuticals)	Aspirin 81mg	**Adults & Peds ≥12 yo:** 4-8 tabs q4h. **Max:** 48 tabs q24h.
Aspergum chewable tablets (Schering-Plough)	Aspirin 227mg	**Adults & Peds ≥12 yo:** 2 tabs q4h. **Max:** 16 tabs q24h.
Bayer Aspirin Extra Strength caplets (Bayer Healthcare)	Aspirin 500mg	**Adults & Peds ≥12 yo:** 1-2 tabs q4-6h. **Max:** 8 tabs q24h.
Bayer Aspirin safety coated caplets (Bayer Healthcare)	Aspirin 325mg	**Adults & Peds ≥12 yo:** 1-2 tabs q4h or 3 tabs q6h. **Max:** 12 tabs q24h.
Bayer Children's Aspirin chewable tablets (Bayer Healthcare)	Aspirin 81mg	**Adults & Peds ≥12 yo:** 4-8 tabs q4h. **Max:** 48 tabs q24h.
Bayer Low Dose Aspirin tablets (Bayer Healthcare)	Aspirin 81mg	**Adults & Peds ≥12 yo:** 4-8 tabs q4h. **Max:** 48 tabs q24h.
Bayer Original Aspirin tablets (Bayer Healthcare)	Aspirin 325mg	**Adults & Peds ≥12 yo:** 1-2 tabs q4h or 3 tabs q6h. **Max:** 12 tabs q24h.
Doan's Extra Strength caplets (Novartis Consumer Health)	Magnesium Salicylate Tetrahydrate 580mg	**Adults & Peds ≥12 yo:** 2 tabs q6h. **Max:** 8 tabs q24h.
Doan's Regular Strength caplets (Novartis Consumer Health)	Magnesium Salicylate Tetrahydrate 377mg	**Adults & Peds ≥12 yo:** 2 tabs q4h. **Max:** 12 tabs q24h.
Ecotrin Adult Low Strength tablets (GlaxoSmithKline Consumer Healthcare)	Aspirin 81mg	**Adults:** 4-8 tabs q4h. **Max:** 48 tabs q24h.
Ecotrin Enteric Low Strength tablets (GlaxoSmithKline Consumer Healthcare)	Aspirin 81mg	**Adults:** 4-8 tabs q4h. **Max:** 48 tabs q24h.
Ecotrin Enteric Regular Strength tablets (GlaxoSmithKline Consumer Healthcare)	Aspirin 325mg	**Adults & Peds ≥12 yo:** 1-2 tabs q4h. **Max:** 12 tabs q24h.
Ecotrin Maximum Strength tablets (GlaxoSmithKline Consumer Healthcare)	Aspirin 500mg	**Adults & Peds ≥12 yo:** 2 tabs q6h. **Max:** 8 tabs q24h.
Ecotrin Regular Strength tablets (GlaxoSmithKline Consumer Healthcare)	Aspirin 325mg	**Adults & Peds ≥12 yo:** 1-2 tabs q4h. **Max:** 12 tabs q24h.
Halfprin 162mg tablets (Kramer Laboratories)	Aspirin 162mg	**Adults & Peds ≥12 yo:** 2-4 tabs q4h. **Max:** 24 tabs q24h.
Halfprin 81mg tablets (Kramer Laboratories)	Aspirin 81mg	**Adults & Peds ≥12 yo:** 4-8 tabs q4h. **Max:** 48 tabs q24h.
St. Joseph Adult Low Strength chewable tablets (McNeil Consumer)	Aspirin 81mg	**Adults & Peds ≥12 yo:** 4-8 tabs q4h. **Max:** 48 tabs q24h.
St. Joseph Adult Low Strength tablets (McNeil Consumer)	Aspirin 81mg	**Adults & Peds ≥12 yo:** 4-8 tabs q4h. **Max:** 48 tabs q24h.
SALICYLATES, BUFFERED		
Ascriptin Maximum Strength tablets (Novartis Consumer Health)	Aspirin Buffered with Maalox/Calcium Carbonate 500mg	**Adults & Peds ≥12 yo:** 2 tabs q4h. **Max:** 8 tabs q24h.
Ascriptin Regular Strength tablets (Novartis Consumer Health)	Aspirin Buffered with Maalox/Calcium Carbonate 325mg	**Adults & Peds ≥12 yo:** 2 tabs q4h. **Max:** 12 tabs q24h.
Bayer Extra Strength Plus caplets (Bayer Healthcare)	Aspirin Buffered with Calcium Carbonate 500mg	**Adults & Peds ≥12 yo:** 1-2 tabs q4-6h. **Max:** 8 tabs q24h.
Bufferin Extra Strength tablets (Bristol-Myers Squibb)	Aspirin Bufferred with Calcium Carbonate/Magnesium Oxide/Magnesium Carbonate 500mg	**Adults & Peds ≥12 yo:** 2 tabs q6h. **Max:** 8 tabs q24h.
Bufferin tablets (Bristol-Myers Squibb)	Aspirin Buffered with Calcium Carbonate/Magnesium Oxide/Magnesium Carbonate 325mg	**Adults & Peds ≥12 yo:** 2 tabs q4h. **Max:** 12 tabs q24h.

Myalgia

Myalgia is defined as muscle pain, although it can also involve ligaments, tendons, and fascia as well as the muscle itself. The most common causes are physical tension or stress, overuse, and injury or trauma such as sprains and strains. Muscle pain can also be due to polymyositis, dermatomyositis, lupus, fibromyalgia, polymyalgia rheumatica, infections, electrolyte imbalances, rhabdomyolysis, and drugs such as statins. There are numerous OTC medications used to treat myalgia, including acetaminophen, salicylates, NSAIDs (e.g., ibuprofen, ketoprofen, naproxen), and rubs or liniments.

ACETAMINOPHEN

Analgesic—The mechanism of analgesic action has not been fully determined. Acetaminophen may act predominantly by inhibiting prostaglandin synthesis in the central nervous system and, to a lesser extent, through a peripheral action by blocking pain-impulse generation. The peripheral action may also be due to inhibition of prostaglandin synthesis or to inhibition of the synthesis or actions of other substances that sensitize pain receptors to mechanical or chemical stimulation.

Capsule/Granules/Powder/Solution/Suspension/Tablet

For analgesic use:

Adults/Pediatrics ≥13 years of age: 325g to 500mg every 3 hours; 325 to 650mg every 4 hours; 650 to 1000mg every 6 hours; or 1300mg every 8.hours.

Pediatrics ≤3 months of age: 40mg every 4 hours as needed.

Pediatrics 4 to 12 months of age: 80mg every 4 hours as needed.

Pediatrics 1 to 2 years of age: 120mg every 4 hours as needed.

Pediatrics 2 to 4 years of age: 160mg every 4 hours as needed.

Pediatrics 4 to 6 years of age: 240mg every 4 hours as needed.

Pediatrics 6 to 9 years of age: 320mg every 4 hours as needed.

Pediatrics 9 to 11 years of age: 320mg to 400mg every 4 hours as needed.

Pediatrics 11 to 12 years of age: 320mg to 480mg every 4 hours as needed.

Suppositories

For analgesic use:

Adults/Pediatrics ≥13 years of age: 325 to 650mg every 4 hours or 650mg every 6 hours as needed.

Pediatrics 2 to 4 years of age: 160mg every 4 hours as needed.

Pediatrics 4 to 6 years of age: 240mg every 4 hours as needed.

Pediatrics 6 to 9 years of age: 320mg every 4 hours as needed.

Pediatrics 9 to 11 years of age: 320 to 400mg every 4 hours as needed.

Pediatrics 11 to 12 years of age: 320 to 480mg every 4 hours as needed.

For more information, refer to the complete monograph for acetaminophen in "Aches and Pains" under Musculoskeletal System

ASPIRIN

Analgesic—Salicylates produce analgesia through a peripheral action by blocking pain-impulse generation and via a central action, possibly in the hypothalamus. The peripheral action may predominate and probably involves inhibition of the synthesis of prostaglandins, and possibly inhibition of the synthesis and/or actions of other substances, which sensitize pain receptors to mechanical or chemical stimulation.

Suppositories

For analgesic use:

Adults/Pediatrics ≥12 years of age: 325 to 650mg every 4 hours as needed.

Pediatrics 2 to 4 years of age: 160mg every 4 hours as needed.

Pediatrics 4 to 6 years of age: 240mg every 4 hours as needed.

Pediatrics 6 to 9 years of age: 325mg every 4 hours as needed.

Pediatrics 9 to 11 years of age: 325 to 400mg every 4 hours as needed.

Pediatric 11 to 12 years of age: 325 to 480mg every 4 hours as needed.

ACETAMINOPHEN PRODUCTS	
Brand Name	**Dosage Form**
Anacin Aspirin Free (Insight)	**Tablet:** 500mg
Feverall (Alpharma)	**Suppositories:** 80mg, 120mg 325mg, 650mg
Tylenol 8 Hour (McNeil)	**Tablet:** 650mg
Tylenol Arthritis (McNeil)	**Tablet:** 650mg
Tylenol Children's Meltaways (McNeil)	**Tablet:** 80mg
Tylenol Children's (McNeil)	**Suspension:** 160mg/5mL
Tylenol Extra Strength (McNeil)	**Capsule:** 500mg **Liquid:** 1000mg/30mL
	Tablet: 500mg
Tylenol Infants' (McNeil)	**Suspension:** 80mg/0.8mL
Tylenol Junior Meltaways (McNeil)	**Tablet:** 160mg
Tylenol Regular Strength (McNeil)	**Tablet:** 325mg

Tablet

For analgesic use:

Adults/Pediatrics ≥12 years of age: 325 to 500mg every 3 hours' 325 to 650mg every 4 hours; or 650 to 1000mg every 6 hours as needed.

Pediatrics 2 to 4 years of age: 160mg every 4 hours as needed.

Pediatrics 4 to 6 years of age: 240mg every 4 hours as needed.

Pediatrics 6 to 9 years of age: 320 to 325mg every 4 hours as needed.

Pediatrics 9 to 11 years of age: 320 to 400mg every 4 hours as needed.

Pediatric 11 to 12 years of age: 320 to 480mg every 4 hours as needed.

For more information, refer to the complete monograph for salicylates in "Aches and Pains" under Musculoskeletal System.

CAFFEINE

Analgesia adjunct—Caffeine constricts cerebral vasculature, resulting in decreased cerebral blood flow as well as a decrease in the oxygen tension of the brain. It has been suggested that the addition of caffeine to aspirin or aspirin/acetaminophen combinations may help to relieve headache by providing a more rapid onset of action and/or enhanced pain relief with a lower dose of the analgesic. In some patients, caffeine may reduce headache pain by reversing caffeine withdrawal symptoms. Recent studies with ergotamine indicate that the enhanced effect by the addition of caffeine may be due to improved gastrointestinal absorption of ergotamine when administered with caffeine.

For more information, refer to the complete monograph for caffeine in "Drowsiness/Lethargy" under Central Nervous System.

ASPIRIN PRODUCTS	
Brand Name	**Dosage Form**
Ascriptin (Novartis)	**Tablet:** 81mg
Aspergum (Schering)	**Gum:** 227mg
Bayer Aspirin Regimen (Bayer)	**Tablet:** 81mg, 325mg
Bayer Children's Aspirin (Bayer)	**Tablet:** 81mg
Bayer Extra Strength (Bayer)	**Tablet:** 500mg
Bayer Genuine Aspirin (Bayer)	**Tablet:** 325mg
Ecotrin (GSK)	**Tablet:** 325mg
Ecotrin Adult Low Strength (GSK)	**Tablet:** 81mg
Ecotrin Maximum Strength (GSK)	**Tablet:** 500mg
Halfprin (Kramer)	**Tablet:** 81mg; 162mg
St. Joseph (McNeil)	**Tablet:** 81mg

BUFFERED ASPIRIN PRODUCTS	
Brand Name	**Dosage Form**
Alka-Seltzer (Bayer)	**Tablet:** 325mg
Alka-Seltzer Extra Strength (Bayer)	**Tablet:** 500mg
Ascriptin (Novartis)	**Tablet:** 325mg
Ascriptin Arthritis Pain (Novartis)	**Tablet:** 325mg
Ascriptin Maximum Strength (Novartis)	**Tablet:** 500mg
Bayer Plus Extra Strength (Bayer)	**Tablet:** 500mg
Bufferin (BMS)	**Tablet:** 325mg
Bufferin Extra Strength (BMS)	**Tablet:** 500mg

ACETAMINOPHEN/ CAFFEINE PRODUCTS	
Brand Name	**Dosage Form**
Excedrin Tension Headache (BMS)	**Tablet:** 500mg-65mg

ACETAMINOPHEN/ ASPIRIN/ CAFFEINE PRODUCTS	
Brand Name	**Dosage Form**
Excedrin Extra Strength (BMS)	**Tablet:** 250mg-250mg-65mg
Excedrin Migraine (BMS)	**Tablet:** 250mg-250mg-65mg
Goody's Fast Pain Relief (GSK)	**Tablet:** 130mg-260mg-16.25mg
Goody's Headache Powders (GSK)	**Tablet:** 260mg-520mg-32.5mg

CAPSAICIN

Capsaicin's precise mechanism of action has not been fully elucidated. It is a neuropeptide-active agent that affects the synthesis, storage, transport, and release of substance P. Substance P is thought to be the principal chemical mediator of pain impulses from the periphery to the central nervous system. In addition, substance P has been shown to be released into joint tissues where it activates inflammatory intermediates that are involved in the development of rheumatoid arthritis. Capsaicin renders skin and joints insensitive to pain by depleting and preventing reaccumulation of substance P in peripheral sensory neurons. With the depletion of substance P in the nerve endings, local pain impulses cannot be transmitted to the brain.

Cream

Adults/Pediatrics ≥2 *years of age*: Apply to affected area 3 to 4 times a day.

For more information, refer to the complete monograph for capsaicin in "Arthralgia" under Musculoskeletal System.

IBUPROFEN

Analgesic—Ibuprofen may block pain-impulse generation via a peripheral action that may involve reduction of the activity of prostaglandins, and possibly inhibition of the synthesis or actions of other substances that sensitize pain receptors to mechanical or chemical stimulation. The antibradykinin activity of ibuprofen may also be involved in relief of pain, since bradykinin has been shown to act together with prostaglandins to cause pain.

Capsule/Suspension/Tablet

For analgesic use (mild to moderate pain):

Adults: 200 to 400mg every 4 to 6 hours as needed.

For more information, refer to the complete monograph for NSAIDs in "Aches and Pains" under Musculoskeletal System.

KETOPROFEN

Analgesic—Ketoprofen may block pain-impulse generation via a peripheral action that may involve reduction of the activity of prostaglandins, and possibly inhibition of the synthesis or actions of other substances that sensitize pain receptors to mechanical or chemical stimulation. The antibradykinin activity of ketoprofen may also be involved in relief of pain, since bradykinin has been shown to act together with prostaglandins to cause pain.

Capsules/Tablets

For analgesic use (mild to moderate pain):

Adults: 25 to 50mg every 6 to 8 hours as needed.

For more information, refer to the complete monograph for NSAIDs in "Aches and Pains" under Musculoskeletal System.

ASPIRIN/ CAFFEINE PRODUCTS	
Brand Name	**Dosage Form**
Alka-Seltzer Morning Relief (Bayer)	**Tablet:** 500mg-65mg
Anacin (Wyeth)	**Tablet:** 400mg-32mg
Anacin Maximum Strength (Wyeth)	**Tablet:** 500mg-32mg
Bayer Rapid Headache Relief (Bayer)	**Tablet:** 500mg-65mg

ASPIRIN/ CAFFEINE/ SALICYLAMIDE PRODUCTS	
Brand Name	**Dosage Form**
BC Powder Original (GSK)	**Tablet:** 650mg-33.3mg-195mg
BC Powder Arthritis Strength (GSK)	**Tablet:** 742mg-38mg-222mg

CAPSAICIN PRODUCTS	
Brand Name	**Dosage Form**
Capsin (Pryde)	**Lotion:** 0.03%, 0.08%
Icy Hot Arthritis Therapy (Chattem)	**Gel:** 0.03%
Zostrix (Rodlen)	**Cream:** 0.03% **Stick:** 0.03%
Zostrix High Potency (Rodlen)	**Stick:** 0.08mg
Zostrix Sports (Rodlen)	**Cream:** 0.08%

IBUPROFEN PRODUCTS	
Brand Name	**Dosage Form**
Advil (Wyeth)	**Capsule:** 200mg **Tablet:** 200mg
Advil Junior (Wyeth)	**Tablet:** 100mg
Midol Cramp Formula (Bayer)	**Tablet:** 200mg
Motrin IB (McNeil)	**Tablet:** 200mg
Motrin Children's (McNeil)	**Suspension:** 100mg/ 5mL
Motrin Infants' (McNeil)	**Suspension:** 50mg/ 1.25mL
Motrin Junior (McNeil)	**Tablet:** 100mg
Motrin Migraine Pain (McNeil)	**Tablet:** 200mg

MAGNESIUM SALICYLATE

Analgesic—Salicylates produce analgesia through a peripheral action by blocking pain-impulse generation and via a central action, possibly in the hypothalamus. The peripheral action may predominate and probably involves inhibition of the synthesis of prostaglandins, and possibly inhibition of the synthesis and/or actions of other substances, which sensitize pain receptors to mechanical or chemical stimulation.

Tablets

For analgesic use:

Adults: 607.4mg every 4 hours as needed; or 934mg every 6 hours as needed.

For more information, refer to the complete monograph for salicylates in "Aches and Pains" under Musculoskeletal System.

NAPROXEN

Analgesic—Naproxen may block pain-impulse generation via a peripheral action that may involve reduction of the activity of prostaglandins, and possibly inhibition of the synthesis or actions of other substances that sensitize pain receptors to mechanical or chemical stimulation. The antibradykinin activity of naproxen may also be involved in relief of pain, since bradykinin has been shown to act together with prostaglandins to cause pain.

Capsule/Tablet

For analgesic use (mild to moderate pain):

Adults: 500mg initially, then 250mg every 6 to 8 hours as needed.

For more information, refer to the complete monograph for NSAIDs in "Aches and Pains" under Musculoskeletal System.

KETOPROFEN PRODUCTS	
Brand Name	**Dosage Form**
Orudis KT (Wyeth)	**Tablet:** 12.5mg

MAGNESIUM SALICYLATE PRODUCTS	
Brand Name	**Dosage Form**
Doan's Extra Strength (Novartis)	**Tablet:** 500mg
Doan's Regular Strength (Novartis)	**Tablet:** 325mg
Momentum (Medtech)	**Tablet:** 467mg

NAPROXEN PRODUCTS	
Brand Name	**Dosage Form**
Aleve (Bayer)	**Capsule:** 220mg **Tablet:** 220mg
Aleve Arthritis (Bayer)	**Tablet:** 220mg
Midol Extended Relief (Bayer)	**Tablet:** 220mg

DOSING INFORMATION FOR MYALGIA PRODUCTS

The following table provides a quick comparison of the ingredients and dosages of common brand-name OTC drugs. Products are listed alphabetically by generic ingredient and brand name.

BRAND NAME	INGREDIENT/STRENGTH	DOSE
ACETAMINOPHEN		
Anacin Aspirin Free tablets *(Insight Pharmaceuticals)*	Acetaminophen 500mg	**Adults & Peds ≥12 yo:** 2 tabs q6h. **Max:** 8 tabs q24h.
Tylenol 8 Hour caplets *(McNeil Consumer)*	Acetaminophen 650mg	**Adults & Peds ≥12 yo:** 2 tabs q8h prn. **Max:** 6 tabs q24h.
Tylenol 8 Hour geltabs *(McNeil Consumer)*	Acetaminophen 650mg	**Adults & Peds ≥12 yo:** 2 tabs q8h prn. **Max:** 6 tabs q24h.
Tylenol Arthritis caplets *(McNeil Consumer)*	Acetaminophen 650mg	**Adults:** 2 tabs q8h prn. **Max:** 6 tabs q24h.
Tylenol Arthritis geltabs *(McNeil Consumer)*	Acetaminophen 650mg	**Adults:** 2 tabs q8h prn. **Max:** 6 tabs q24h.
Tylenol Children's Meltaways tablets *(McNeil Consumer)*	Acetaminophen 80mg	**Peds 2-3 yo (24-35 lbs):** 2 tabs. **4-5 yo (36-47 lbs):** 3 tabs. **6-8 yo (48-59 lbs):** 4 tabs. **9-10 yo (60-71 lbs):** 5 tabs. **11 yo (72-95 lbs):** 6 tabs. May repeat q4h. **Max:** 5 doses q24h.
Tylenol Children's suspension *(McNeil Consumer)*	Acetaminophen 160mg/5mL	**Peds 2-3 yo (24-35 lbs):** 1 tsp (5mL). **4-5 yo (36-47 lbs):** 1.5 tsp (7.5mL). **6-8 yo (48-59 lbs):** 2 tsp (10mL). **9-10 yo (60-71 lbs):** 2.5 tsp (12.5mL). **11 yo (72-95 lbs):** 3 tsp (15mL). May repeat q4h. **Max:** 5 doses q24h.

DOSING INFORMATION FOR MYALGIA PRODUCTS (cont.)

BRAND NAME	INGREDIENT/STRENGTH	DOSE
Tylenol Extra Strength caplets *(McNeil Consumer)*	Acetaminophen 500mg	**Adults & Peds ≥12 yo:** 2 tabs q4-6h prn. **Max:** 8 tabs q24h.
Tylenol Extra Strength Cool caplets *(McNeil Consumer)*	Acetaminophen 500mg	**Adults & Peds ≥12 yo:** 2 tabs q4-6h prn. **Max:** 8 tabs q24h.
Tylenol Extra Strength gelcaps *(McNeil Consumer)*	Acetaminophen 500mg	**Adults & Peds ≥12 yo:** 2 caps q4-6h prn. **Max:** 8 caps q24h.
Tylenol Extra Strength liquid *(McNeil Consumer)*	Acetaminophen 1000mg/30mL	**Adults & Peds ≥12 yo:** 2 tbl (30mL) q4-6h prn. **Max:** 8 tbl (120mL) q24h.
Tylenol Extra Strength tablets *(McNeil Consumer)*	Acetaminophen 500mg	**Adults & Peds ≥12 yo:** 2 tabs q4-6h prn. **Max:** 8 tabs q24h.
Tylenol Infants' suspension *(McNeil Consumer)*	Acetaminophen 80mg/0.8mL	**Peds 2-3 yo (24-35 lbs):** 1.6 mL q4h prn. **Max:** 5 doses (8mL) q24h.
Tylenol Junior Meltaways tablets *(McNeil Consumer)*	Acetaminophen 160mg	**Peds 6-8 yo (48-59 lbs):** 2 tabs. **9-10 yo (60-71 lbs):** 2.5 tabs. **11 yo (72-95 lbs):** 3 tabs. **12 yo (≥96 lbs):** 4 tabs. May repeat q4h. **Max:** 5 doses q24h.
Tylenol Regular Strength tablets *(McNeil Consumer)*	Acetaminophen 325mg	**Adults & Peds ≥12 yo:** 2 tabs q4-6h prn. **Max:** 12 tabs q24h. **Peds 6-11 yo:** 1 tab q4-6h. **Max:** 5 tabs q24h.

NSAIDs

BRAND NAME	INGREDIENT/STRENGTH	DOSE
Advil caplets *(Wyeth Consumer Healthcare)*	Ibuprofen 200mg	**Adults & Peds ≥12 yo:** 1-2 tabs q4-6h. **Max:** 6 tabs q24h.
Advil Children's Chewables tablets *(Wyeth Consumer Healthcare)*	Ibuprofen 50mg	**Peds 2-3 yr (24-35 lb):** 2 tabs q6-8h. **4-5 yr (36-47 lb):** 3 tabs q6-8h. **6-8 yr (45-89 lb):** 4 tabs q6-8h. **9-10 yr (60-71 lb):** 5 tabs q6-8h. **11 yr (72-95 lb):** 6 tabs q6-8h. **Max:** 4 doses q24h
Advil Children's suspension *(Wyeth Consumer Healthcare)*	Ibuprofen 100mg/5mL	**Peds 2-3 yo (24-35 lbs):** 1 tsp (5mL). **4-5 yo (36-47 lbs):** 1.5 tsp (7.5mL). **6-8 yo (48-59 lbs):** 2 tsp (10mL). **9-10 yo (60-71 lbs):** 2.5 tsp (12.5mL). **11 yo (72-95 lbs):** 3 tsp (15mL). May repeat q6-8h. **Max:** 4 doses q24h.
Advil gelcaps *(Wyeth Consumer Healthcare)*	Ibuprofen 200mg	**Adults & Peds ≥12 yo:** 1-2 caps q4-6h. **Max:** 6 caps q24h.
Advil Infants' Drops *(Wyeth Consumer Healthcare)*	Ibuprofen 50mg/1.25mL	**Peds 6-11 months (12-17 lbs):** 1.25mL. **12-23 months (18-23 lbs):** 1.875mL. May repeat q6-8h. **Max:** 4 doses q24h.
Advil Junior Strength tablets *(Wyeth Consumer Healthcare)*	Ibuprofen 100mg	**Peds 6-10 yo (48-71 lbs):** 2 tabs. **11 yo (72-95 lbs):** 3 tabs. May repeat q6-8h. **Max:** 4 doses q24h.
Advil Junior Strength tablets *(Wyeth Consumer Healthcare)*	Ibuprofen 100mg	**Peds 6-10 yo (48-71 lbs):** 2 tabs. **11 yo (72-95 lbs):** 3 tabs. May repeat q6-8h. **Max:** 4 doses q24h.
Advil liqui-gels *(Wyeth Consumer Healthcare)*	Ibuprofen 200mg	**Adults & Peds ≥12 yo:** 1-2 caps q4-6h. **Max:** 6 caps q24h.
Advil Migraine capsules *(Wyeth Consumer Healthcare)*	Ibuprofen 200mg	**Adults:** 2 caps prn. **Max:** 2 caps q24h.
Advil tablets *(Wyeth Consumer Healthcare)*	Ibuprofen 200mg	**Adults & Peds ≥12 yo:** 1-2 tabs q4-6h. **Max:** 6 tabs q24h.
Aleve caplets *(Bayer Healthcare)*	Naproxen Sodium 220mg	**Adults ≥65 yo:** 1 tab q12h. **Max:** 2 tabs q24h. **Adults & Peds ≥12 yo:** 1 tab q8-12h. **Max:** 3 tabs q24h.
Aleve gelcaps *(Bayer Healthcare)*	Naproxen Sodium 220mg	**Adults ≥65 yo:** 1 cap q12h. **Max:** 2 caps q24h. **Adults & Peds ≥12 yo:** 1 cap q8-12h. **Max:** 3 caps q24h.
Aleve tablets *(Bayer Healthcare)*	Naproxen Sodium 220mg	**Adults ≥65 yo:** 1 tab q12h. **Max:** 2 tabs q24h. **Adults & Peds ≥12 yo:** 1 tab q8-12h. **Max:** 3 tabs q24h.

DOSING INFORMATION FOR MYALGIA PRODUCTS (cont.)

Brand Name	Ingredient/Strength	Dose
Motrin Children's suspension (McNeil Consumer)	Ibuprofen 100mg/5mL	**Peds 2-3 yo (24-35 lbs):** 1 tsp (5mL). **4-5 yo (36-47 lbs):** 1.5 tsp (7.5mL). **6-8 yo (48-59 lbs):** 2 tsp (10mL). **9-10 yo (60-71 lbs):** 2.5 tsp (12.5mL). **11 yo (72-95 lbs):** 3 tsp (15mL). May repeat q6-8h. **Max:** 4 doses q24h.
Motrin IB caplets (McNeil Consumer)	Ibuprofen 200mg	**Adults & Peds ≥12 yo:** 1-2 tabs q4-6h. **Max:** 6 tabs q24h.
Motrin IB gelcaps (McNeil Consumer)	Ibuprofen 200mg	**Adults & Peds ≥12 yo:** 1-2 tabs q4-6h. **Max:** 6 tabs q24h.
Motrin IB tablets (McNeil Consumer)	Ibuprofen 200mg	**Adults & Peds ≥12 yo:** 1-2 tabs q4-6h. **Max:** 6 tabs q24h.
Motrin Infants' Drops (McNeil Consumer)	Ibuprofen 50mg/1.25mL	**Peds 6-11 months (12-17 lbs):** 1.25mL. **12-23 months (18-23 lbs):** 1.875mL. May repeat q6-8h. **Max:** 4 doses q24h.
Motrin Junior Strength chewable tablets (McNeil Consumer)	Ibuprofen 100mg	**Peds 6-8 yo (48-59 lbs):** 2 tabs. **9-10 yo (60-71 lbs):** 2.5 tabs. **11 yo (72-95 lbs):** 3 tabs. May repeat q6-8h. **Max:** 4 doses q24h.
Nuprin caplets (Bristol-Myers Squibb)	Ibuprofen 200mg	**Adults & Peds ≥12 yo:** 1-2 tabs q4-6h. **Max:** 6 tabs q24h.
Nuprin tablets (Bristol-Myers Squibb)	Ibuprofen 200mg	**Adults & Peds ≥12 yo:** 1-2 tabs q4-6h. **Max:** 6 tabs q24h.
Orudis KT tablets (Wyeth Consumer Healthcare)	Ketoprofen Magnesium 12.5mg	**Adults:** 1-2 tabs q4-6h. **Max:** 6 tabs q24h.
RUBS & LINIMENTS		
Absorbine Jr Deep Pain Relief patches (W.F. Young)	Menthol 5.0%	**Adults & Peds ≥12 yo:** Apply to affected area bid.
Absorbine Jr liquid (W.F. Young)	Menthol 1.27%	**Adults & Peds ≥2 yo:** Apply to affected area tid-qid.
Absorbine Jr patches (W.F. Young)	Menthol 1.3%	**Adults & Peds ≥12 yo:** Apply to affected area bid.
Arthricare Women Extra Moisturizing cream (Del Pharmaceuticals)	Capsaicin 0.025%	**Adults & Peds ≥2 yo:** Apply to affected area tid-qid.
Arthricare Women Multi-Action cream (Del Pharmaceuticals)	Capsaicin/Menthol/Methyl nicotinate 0.025%-1.25%-0.25%	**Adults & Peds ≥2 yo:** Apply to affected area tid-qid.
Arthricare Women Quick Dry Rub (Del Pharmaceuticals)	Capsaicin 0.025%	**Adults & Peds ≥2 yo:** Apply to affected area tid-qid.
Arthricare Women Ultra-Strength cream (Del Pharmaceuticals)	Capsaicin/Menthol 0.075%-2%	**Adults & Peds ≥2 yo:** Apply to affected area tid-qid.
Arthritis Hot cream (Chattem)	Methyl Salicylate/Menthol 15%-10%	**Adults:** Apply to affected area prn up to qid.
BenGay Pain Relieving Patch (Pfizer Consumer Healthcare)	Menthol 1.4%	**Adults & Peds ≥12 yo:** Apply to affected area tid-qid.
BenGay Ultra Strength cream (Pfizer Consumer Healthcare)	Methyl Salicylate/Menthol/Camphor 30%-10%-4%	**Adults & Peds ≥12 yo:** Apply to affected area qd-tid.
BenGay Ultra Strength Pain Relieving Patch (Pfizer Consumer Healthcare)	Menthol 5%	**Adults & Peds ≥12 yo:** Apply to affected area tid-qid.
BenGay Vanishing Scent gel (Pfizer Consumer Healthcare)	Menthol 2.5%	**Adults & Peds ≥12 yo:** Apply to affected area tid-qid.
Bodyglide Maximum Strength WarmFX (Sternoff)	Methyl Salicylate/Menthol 30%-15%	**Adults:** Apply to affected area prn.
Boericke & Tafel Triflora Arthritis gel (Boericke & Tafel)	Symphytum Officinale/Rhus Toxicodendron/Ledum Palustre 10%-5%-2.5%	**Adults & Peds ≥2 yo:** Apply to affected area qd-qid.
Capzasin-HP cream (Chattem)	Capsaicin 0.075%	**Adults:** Apply to affected area tid-qid.
Capzasin-P cream (Chattem)	Capsaicin 0.025%	**Adults:** Apply to affected area tid-qid.
Emu Lifestyle Active Lifestyle cream (Emu Lifestyle)	Menthol 3%	**Adults & Peds ≥10 yo:** Apply to affected area qd-qid.

DOSING INFORMATION FOR MYALGIA PRODUCTS (cont.)

Brand Name	Ingredient/Strength	Dose
Emu Lifestyle Active Lifestyle Cream, for Arthritis and Joints (Emu Lifestyle)	Trolamine Salicylate 10%	**Adults & Peds ≥10 yo:** Apply to affected area qd-qid.
Flexall Maximum Strength gel (Chattem)	Menthol 16%	**Adults & Peds ≥12 yo:** Apply to affected area prn up to qid.
Flexall Maximum Strength gel pump (Chattem)	Menthol 16%	**Adults & Peds ≥12 yo:** Apply to affected area prn up to qid.
Heet Pain Relieving Liniment (Medtech)	Methyl Salicylate/Camphor/Oleoresin Capsicum 17%-3.6%- .025%	**Adults:** Apply to affected area prn.
Icy Hot balm (Chattem)	Methyl Salicyalte/Menthol 29%-7.6%	**Adults:** Apply to affected area prn.
Icy Hot Chill Stick (Chattem)	Methyl Salicyalte/Menthol 30%-10%	**Adults:** Apply to affected area prn.
Icy Hot cream (Chattem)	Methyl Salicyalte/Menthol 30%-10%	**Adults:** Apply to affected area prn.
Icy Hot Patch Extra Stength (Arm, Neck, Leg) (Chattem)	Menthol 5%	**Adults & Peds ≥12 yo:** Apply to affected area prn up to qid.
Icy Hot Patch Extra Stength (Back) (Chattem)	Menthol 5%	**Adults & Peds ≥12 yo:** Apply to affected area prn up to qid.
Icy Hot Sleeve (Ankles, Elbows, Knees, Wrist) (Chattem)	Menthol 16%	**Adults & Peds ≥12 yo:** Apply to affected area prn up to qid.
Icy Hot Sleeve (Wrists, Small Ankles, and Elbows) (Chattem)	Menthol 16%	**Adults & Peds ≥12 yo:** Apply to affected area prn up to qid.
Mobisyl Maximum Strength Arthritis cream (B.F. Ascher & Company)	Trolamine Salicylate 10%	**Adults & Peds ≥12 yo:** Apply to affected area tid-qid
Nuprin Arthritis High Potency cream (Bristol-Myers Squibb)	Capsaicin 0.075%	**Adults & Peds ≥12 yo:** Apply to affected area tid-qid.
Nuprin Arthritis High Potency patch (Bristol-Myers Squibb)	Capsaicin 0.025%	**Adults & Peds ≥4 yo:** Apply to affected area bid.
Nuprin Arthritis Maximum Strength gel (Bristol-Myers Squibb)	Capsaicin/Menthol 0.075%-8%	**Adults & Peds ≥2 yo:** Apply to affected area tid-qid.
Nuprin Arthritis Maximum Strength gel (Bristol-Myers Squibb)	Capsaicin/Menthol 0.075%-8%	**Adults & Peds ≥2 yo:** Apply to affected area tid-qid.
Super Blue Pain Relief cream (Spring)	Menthol 2.75%	**Adults & Peds ≥12 yo:** Apply to affected area tid-qid.
Thera-gesic Maximum Strength cream (Mission Pharmacal)	Mehtyl Salicylate/Menthol 15%-1%	**Adults & Peds ≥12 yo:** Apply to affected area tid-qid.
Thera-gesic Plus cream (Mission Pharmacal)	Mehtyl Salicylate/Menthol 25%-4%	**Adults & Peds ≥12 yo:** Apply to affected area tid-qid.
Ultra Blue Topical Analgesic gel (BNG Enterprises)	Menthol 4%	**Adults & Peds ≥2 yo:** Apply to affected area tid-qid.
Watkins Liniment Pain Relief Spray (Watkins)	Camphor/Menthol 3.5%-2.5%	**Adults & Peds ≥2 yo:** Apply to affected area tid-qid.
WellPatch Arthritis Patch, Pain Relieving Pad (Mentholatum)	Methyl Salicylate 10%	**Adults & Peds ≥12 yo:** Apply to affected area qd-bid
Zostrix cream (Rodlen)	Capsaicin 0.025%	**Adults:** Apply to affected area tid-qid.
Zostrix HP cream (Rodlen)	Capsaicin 0.075%	**Adults:** Apply to affected area tid-qid.
SALICYLATES		
Anacin 81 tablets (Insight Pharmaceuticals)	Aspirin 81mg	**Adults & Peds ≥12 yo:** 4-8 tabs q4h. **Max:** 48 tabs q24h.
Aspergum chewable tablets (Schering-Plough)	Aspirin 227mg	**Adults & Peds ≥12 yo:** 2 tabs q4h. **Max:** 16 tabs q24h.
Bayer Aspirin Extra Strength caplets (Bayer Healthcare)	Aspirin 500mg	**Adults & Peds ≥12 yo:** 1-2 tabs q4-6h. **Max:** 8 tabs q24h.
Bayer Aspirin safety coated caplets (Bayer Healthcare)	Aspirin 325mg	**Adults & Peds ≥12 yo:** 1-2 tabs q4h or 3 tabs q6h. **Max:** 12 tabs q24h.
Bayer Children's Aspirin chewable tablets (Bayer Healthcare)	Aspirin 81mg	**Adults & Peds ≥12 yo:** 4-8 tabs q4h. **Max:** 48 tabs q24h.
Bayer Low Dose Aspirin tablets (Bayer Healthcare)	Aspirin 81mg	**Adults & Peds ≥12 yo:** 4-8 tabs q4h. **Max:** 48 tabs q24h.

DOSING INFORMATION FOR MYALGIA PRODUCTS (cont.)

BRAND NAME	INGREDIENT/STRENGTH	DOSE
Bayer Original Aspirin tablets *(Bayer Healthcare)*	Aspirin 325mg	**Adults & Peds ≥12 yo:** 1-2 tabs q4h or 3 tabs q6h. **Max:** 12 tabs q24h.
Doan's Extra Strength caplets *(Novartis Consumer Health)*	Magnesium Salicylate Tetrahydrate 580mg	**Adults & Peds ≥12 yo:** 2 tabs q6h. **Max:** 8 tabs q24h.
Doan's Regular Strength caplets *(Novartis Consumer Health)*	Magnesium Salicylate Tetrahydrate 377mg	**Adults & Peds ≥12 yo:** 2 tabs q4h. **Max:** 12 tabs q24h.
Ecotrin Adult Low Strength tablets *(GlaxoSmithKline Consumer Healthcare)*	Aspirin 81mg	**Adults:** 4-8 tabs q4h. **Max:** 48 tabs q24h.
Ecotrin Enteric Low Strength tablets *(GlaxoSmithKline Consumer Healthcare)*	Aspirin 81mg	**Adults:** 4-8 tabs q4h. **Max:** 48 tabs q24h.
Ecotrin Enteric Regular Strength tablets *(GlaxoSmithKline Consumer Healthcare)*	Aspirin 325mg	**Adults & Peds ≥12 yo:** 1-2 tabs q4h. **Max:** 12 tabs q24h.
Ecotrin Maximum Strength tablets *(GlaxoSmithKline Consumer Healthcare)*	Aspirin 500mg	**Adults & Peds ≥12 yo:** 2 tabs q6h. **Max:** 8 tabs q24h.
Ecotrin Regular Strength tablets *(GlaxoSmithKline Consumer Healthcare)*	Aspirin 325mg	**Adults & Peds ≥12 yo:** 1-2 tabs q4h. **Max:** 12 tabs q24h.
Halfprin 162mg tablets *(Kramer Laboratories)*	Aspirin 162mg	**Adults & Peds ≥12 yo:** 2-4 tabs q4h. **Max:** 24 tabs q24h.
Halfprin 81mg tablets *(Kramer Laboratories)*	Aspirin 81mg	**Adults & Peds ≥12 yo:** 4-8 tabs q4h. **Max:** 48 tabs q24h.
St. Joseph Adult Low Strength chewable tablets *(McNeil Consumer)*	Aspirin 81mg	**Adults & Peds ≥12 yo:** 4-8 tabs q4h. **Max:** 48 tabs q24h.
St. Joseph Adult Low Strength tablets *(McNeil Consumer)*	Aspirin 81mg	**Adults & Peds ≥12 yo:** 4-8 tabs q4h. **Max:** 48 tabs q24h.
SALICYLATES, BUFFERED		
Ascriptin Maximum Strength tablets *(Novartis Consumer Health)*	Aspirin Buffered with Maalox/ Calcium Carbonate 500mg	**Adults & Peds ≥12 yo:** 2 tabs q4h. **Max:** 8 tabs q24h.
Ascriptin Regular Strength tablets *(Novartis Consumer Health)*	Aspirin Buffered with Maalox/ Calcium Carbonate 325mg	**Adults & Peds ≥12 yo:** 2 tabs q4h. **Max:** 12 tabs q24h.
Bayer Extra Strength Plus caplets *(Bayer Healthcare)*	Aspirin Buffered with Calcium Carbonate 500mg	**Adults & Peds ≥12 yo:** 1-2 tabs q4-6h. **Max:** 8 tabs q24h.
Bufferin Extra Strength tablets *(Bristol-Myers Squibb)*	Aspirin Bufferred with Calcium Carbonate/ Magnesium Oxide/ Magnesium Carbonate 500mg	**Adults & Peds ≥12 yo:** 2 tabs q6h. **Max:** 8 tabs q24h.
Bufferin tablets *(Bristol-Myers Squibb)*	Aspirin Bufferred with Calcium Carbonate/ Magnesium Oxide/ Magnesium Carbonate 325mg	**Adults & Peds ≥12 yo:** 2 tabs q4h. **Max:** 12 tabs q24h.

Osteoporosis

Osteoporosis is a condition of low bone mass and microarchitectural disruption that results in fractures with minimal trauma. Common sites of osteoporotic fracture include the vertebral bodies, the distal forearm, and the proximal femur. Because the skeletons of patients with osteoporosis are diffusely fragile, other sites, such as the ribs and long bones, also fracture with high frequency. The term *primary osteoporosis* denotes reduced bone mass and fractures found in menopausal women (postmenopausal osteoporosis) or in older men and women (senile osteoporosis). *Secondary osteoporosis* refers to bone loss resulting from specific clinical disorders, such as thyrotoxicosis or hyperadrenocorticism. States of estrogen-dependent bone loss, such as exercise-related amenorrhea or prolactin-secreting tumors, are conventionally treated as special cases of primary osteoporosis.

Eighty percent of the skeleton, the so-called cortical bone, consists of bony plates organized around central nutrient Haversian canals. Much of the remaining skeleton consists of trabecular bone, a honeycomb of vertical and horizontal bars that reside in marrow and fat. Most trabecular bone is located in the axial, or central, skeleton, particularly the vertebral bodies, pelvis, and proximal femur. Because bone turnover takes place only on bone surfaces, the high surface-to-volume ratio of trabecular bone compared with cortical bone underlies its earlier and more impressive response to altered turnover. Conditions that produce diffusely decreased bone mineral density (osteopenia) and bone strength are termed metabolic bone diseases. The most common metabolic bone disease is osteoporosis, which is characterized by decreases in both bone matrix and bone mineral. In contrast, the less common osteomalacia (rickets in children) is characterized by decreased bone mineral but intact bone matrix. Although osteomalacia is typically associated with vitamin D deficiency or resistance, calcium or phosphate deficiency, and serum biochemical abnormalities, clinical features of osteoporosis and osteomalacia tend to overlap. Sometimes the two disorders are only distinguishable (if necessary) by bone biopsy. Notably, the term *osteopenia* refers to decreased calcification or density of bone but does not imply causality.

The amount of skeletal bone at any time in adult life reflects its maximal amount at skeletal maturity (peak bone mass), minus what has been subsequently lost. Bone gained during adolescence accounts for about 60% of final adult values. Bone acquisition is almost complete by age 17 years in girls and by age 20 years in boys. Heredity accounts for most of the variance in bone acquisition. Other factors include circulating reproductive steroids, physical activity, and dietary calcium. The adolescent growth spurt represents a window of opportunity during which adequate exposure to key nutrients, physical activity, and reproductive hormone concentrations permit one to achieve the maximum bone mass permitted by genetic endowment. It also represents a window of vulnerability during which dietary insufficiency, immobilization, and failure of reproductive function may constrain bone acquisition, resulting in a lower peak bone mass and less reserve to accommodate future losses. Recent trends in habitual physical activity and calcium intake for North American teenagers, particularly girls, are unfortunately not encouraging in regard to optimal bone mass acquisition during this critical period of life.

Bone lost during adult life reflects inefficiencies in bone remodeling, a lifelong process of bone destruction and renewal that constitutes the final common pathway through which diet, hormones, and physical activity affect the rate of bone loss. Remodeling begins when marrow-derived precursor cells cluster on the bone surface where they fuse into multinucleated osteoclasts, which in turn dig a cavity into the bone (resorption). This process releases embedded chemical mediators from the bone matrix that recruit osteoblastic cells into the resorption cavity. Osteoblasts replace missing bone by secreting new bone matrix, which later mineralizes. A single remodeling cycle normally takes up to 6 months. If remodeling were efficient, each cycle would completely replace the resorbed bone and there would be no net change in bone mass. Remodeling, however, is not entirely efficient, and the replaced bone does not always equal the amount previously removed, leaving a small bone deficit after each cycle. Remodeling imbalance is minuscule for any given remodeling event, and the accumulation of bone deficits may be detected only after many years. Its occurrence, however, underlies the process of age-related bone loss. Any increase in the overall rate of bone remodeling will increase the rate of bone loss. Even though bone densitometry suggests that bone mass in both men and women remains stable until about age 50 years, bone biopsies reveal remodeling inefficiencies as early as the third decade of life. Primary regulators of adult bone mass include physical activity, reproductive endocrine status, and calcium nutriture. Optimal maintenance of bone requires sufficiency in all areas, and deficiency in one area is not compensated by attention to others. For example, amenorrheic athletes lose bone despite frequent, high-intensity physical activity and supplemental calcium intake.

There are many dietary supplements available OTC to aid in the prevention and management of osteoporosis, most of which contain calcium and/or vitamin D.

CALCIUM SUPPLEMENTS

PHARMACOLOGY

Calcium is essential for the functional integrity of the nervous, muscular, and skeletal systems. It plays a role in normal cardiac function, renal function, respiration, blood coagulation, and cell membrane and capillary permeability. Also, calcium helps to regulate the release and storage of neurotransmitters and hormones, the uptake and binding of amino acids, absorption of vitamin B_{12}, and gastrin secretion.

The major fraction (99%) of calcium is in the skeletal structure primarily as hydroxyapatite, $Ca_{10}(PO_4)_6(OH)_2$; small amounts of calcium carbonate and amorphous calcium phosphates are also present. The calcium of bone is in a constant exchange with the calcium of plasma. Since the metabolic functions of calcium are essential for life, when there is a disturbance in the calcium balance because of dietary deficiency or other causes, the stores of calcium in bone may be depleted to fill the body's more acute needs. Therefore, on a chronic basis, normal mineralization of bone depends on adequate amounts of total body calcium.

INDICATIONS

Hypocalcemia, acute (treatment)—Parenteral calcium salts (ie, acetate, chloride, gluceptate, and gluconate) are indicated in the treatment of hypocalcemia in conditions that require a rapid increase in serum calcium-ion concentration, such as in neonatal hypocalcemic tetany; tetany due to parathyroid deficiency; hypocalcemia due to hungry bones syndrome (remineralization hypocalcemia) following surgery for hyperparathyroidism; vitamin D deficiency; and alkalosis. Calcium salts have been used as adjunctive therapy for insect bites or stings, such as black widow spider bites, and for sensitivity reactions, especially when characterized by urticaria, and as an aid in the management of acute symptoms of lead colic. Parenteral calcium gluconate and calcium glucepetate are also used for the prevention of hypocalcemia during exchange transfusions.

Electrolyte depletion (treatment)—Calcium acetate, parenteral calcium chloride, calcium gluconate, and calcium glucepetate are used in conditions that require an increase in calcium ions for electrolyte adjustment.

Cardiac arrest (treatment adjunct)—Parenteral calcium chloride or calcium gluconate may also be used as an adjunct in cardiac resuscitation, particularly after open-heart surgery, to strengthen myocardial contractions, as after defibrillation or when there is an inadequate response to catecholamines.

Hyperkalemia (treatment)—Calcium chloride and parenteral calcium gluconate are used to decrease or reverse the cardiac depressant effects of hyperkalemia on electrocardiographic (ECG) function.

Hypermagnesemia (treatment adjunct)—Calcium chloride, calcium glucepetate, and calcium gluconate injections have also been used as an aid in the treatment of central nervous system (CNS) depression due to overdosage of magnesium sulfate.

Hypocalcemia, chronic (treatment)—Oral calcium supplements provide a source of calcium ions for treating calcium depletion occurring in conditions such as chronic hypoparathyroidism, pseudohypoparathyroidism, osteomalacia, rickets, chronic renal failure, and hypocalcemia secondary to the administration of anticonvulsant medications. When chronic hypocalcemia is due to vitamin D deficiency, oral calcium salts may be administered concomitantly with vitamin D analogs. However, calcium phosphate should *not* be used in patients with hypoparathyroidism or renal failure, since phosphate levels may be too high and giving more phosphate would exacerbate the condition. Calcium supplements should not be used in hyperparathyroidism, unless the need for a calcium supplement is high and the patient is carefully monitored. For treatment of hypocalcemia, supplementation is preferred.

Calcium deficiency (prophylaxis)—Oral calcium salts are used as dietary supplemental therapy for persons who may not get enough calcium in their regular diet. However, for prophylaxis of calcium deficiency, dietary improvement, rather than supplementation, is preferred. Due to increased needs, children and pregnant women are at greatest risk. Pre- and postmenopausal women, adolescents, especially girls, and the elderly may not receive adequate calcium in their diets. However, studies have shown that supplemental calcium in postmenopausal women without functioning ovaries does not lead to increases in bone density, even in the presence of supplemental vitamin D. Calcium supplements are used as part of the prevention and treatment of osteoporosis in patients with an inadequate calcium intake. The use of calcium citrate may reduce the risk of kidney stones in susceptible patients. The use of water-soluble salts of calcium (i.e., citrate, gluconate, and lactate) may be preferable to acid-soluble salts (i.e., carbonate and phosphate) for patients with reduced stomach acid or for patients taking acid-inhibiting medication, such as the histamine H_2-receptor antagonists.

—Some unusual diets (e.g., reducing diets that drastically restrict food selection) may not supply minimum daily requirements of calcium. Supplementation is necessary in patients receiving total parenteral nutrition (TPN) or undergoing rapid weight loss or in those with malnutrition, because of inadequate dietary intake.

—Recommended intakes for all vitamins and most minerals are increased during pregnancy. Many physicians recommend that pregnant women receive multivitamin and mineral supplements, especially those pregnant women who do not consume an adequate diet and those in high-risk categories (ie, women carrying more than one fetus, heavy cigarette smokers, and alcohol and drug abusers). Taking excessive amounts of a multivitamin and mineral supplement may be harmful to the mother and/or fetus and should be avoided.

—Recommended intakes for all vitamins and most minerals are increased during breastfeeding.

Hyperacidity (treatment)—Calcium carbonate is an antacid used to treat hyperacidity.

Hyperphosphatemia (treatment)—Calcium carbonate is used in patients with end-stage renal failure (renal osteodystrophy) to lower serum phosphate concentrations. However, it should be used with caution in patients on chronic hemodialysis. Calcium citrate is also used in renal failure as a phosphate binder.

CONTRAINDICATIONS

Except under special circumstances, these medications should not be used when the following medical problems exist:

For all calcium supplements:

- Hypercalcemia, primary or secondary—*major clinical significance.*

- Hypercalciuria or renal calculi, calcium—*major clinical significance.*

- Sarcoidosis—*major clinical significance* (may potentiate hypercalcemia).

For calcium phosphate, dibasic or tribasic, only:

- Hypoparathyroidism—*major clinical significance.*

- Renal insufficiency—*major clinical significance* (may increase risk of hyperphosphatemia).

For parenteral calcium salts only:

- Digitalis toxicity—*major clinical significance* (increased risk of arrhythmias).

Risk-benefit should be considered when the following medical problems exist:

For all calcium supplements:

- Dehydration—*major clinical significance.*

- Electrolyte imbalance, other—*major clinical significance* (may increase risk of hypercalcemia).

- Diarrhea.

- Malabsorption, gastrointestinal, chronic (fecal excretion of calcium may be increased, although patients with chronic diarrhea or malabsorption commonly need calcium supplements).

- Renal calculi, history of—*major clinical significance* (risk of recurrent stone formation).

- Renal function impairment, chronic—*major clinical significance* (may increase risk of hypercalcemia; however, calcium carbonate or calcium citrate may be used as a phosphate binder in renal failure; also, some patients with renal failure have symptomatic hypocalcemia and need cautious treatment with calcium salts).

For calcium carbonate and calcium phosphate only:

- Achlorhydria or hypochlorhydria (calcium absorption may be decreased unless the calcium carbonate or phosphate is taken with meals).

For parenteral calcium salts only:

- Cardiac function impairment—*major clinical significance.*
- Ventricular fibrillation during cardiac resuscitation—*major clinical significance* (increased risk of arrhythmias; however, calcium may increase strength of myocardial contraction, make fibrillation coarser, and help in electrical defibrillation, especially with concomitant hyperkalemia).

WARNINGS/PRECAUTIONS

Pregnancy: Pregnancy studies have not been done in humans. However, problems have not been documented with intake of normal daily recommended amounts. *Second and third trimesters*: Some studies have shown that calcium supplementation begun in the second trimester may be effective in lowering blood pressure in pregnant women with pregnancy-induced hypertension or preeclampsia, both of which may possibly be associated with increased calcium demand of the fetus during the last trimester. During pregnancy, there is an increased need for calcium to calcify fetal bones and to increase the maternal skeletal mass in preparation for lactation. This need is normally met by enhanced intestinal absorption of calcium, increased vitamin D production, and a concurrent increase in calcitonin secretion, which prevents unwanted bone resorption in the maternal skeleton. The maternal parathyroid glands undergo hyperplasia, producing greater amounts of parathyroid hormone, which acts indirectly to increase intestinal absorption of calcium, reabsorption at the distal renal tubules, and bone calcium mobilization. However, the prescribing of calcium supplements during pregnancy may be necessary since standard prenatal vitamins along with normal intake of dairy products may not provide sufficient elemental calcium for the average pregnant woman.

Calcium acetate, calcium chloride, calcium gluceptate, calcium gluconate injection—FDA Category C.

Other calcium salts—FDA pregnancy categories not currently included in product labeling.

Breastfeeding: Problems in nursing babies have not been documented with intake of normal daily recommended amounts. Although some oral supplemental calcium may be distributed into breast milk, the concentration is not sufficient to produce an adverse effect in the neonate. It is not known whether calcium chloride or calcium gluconate is distributed into breast milk.

Pediatrics: Parenteral calcium preparations, especially calcium chloride: The extreme irritation and possibility of tissue necrosis and sloughing caused by intravenous (IV) injection of calcium preparations usually restrict its use in pediatric patients because of the small vasculature of this patient group.

For calcium gluceptate injection only: It is not recommended that calcium gluceptate be administered intramuscularly to infants and children except in emergencies when the IV route is technically impossible, because of the possibility of severe tissue necrosis or sloughing.

ADVERSE REACTIONS

Those indicating need for medical attention: Incidence more frequent

With parenteral dosage forms only:

Hypotension (dizziness); flushing and/or sensation of warmth or heat; irregular heartbeat; nausea or vomiting; skin redness, rash, pain, or burning at injection site; sweating; tingling sensation; decrease in blood pressure, moderate —with calcium chloride only.

Incidence rare:

Hypercalcemic syndrome, acute (drowsiness; continuing nausea and vomiting; weakness); renal calculi, calcific (difficult or painful urination)—with oral dosage forms.

Early symptoms of hypercalcemia:

Constipation, severe; dryness of mouth; headache, continuing; increased thirst; irritability; loss of appetite; mental depression; metallic taste; unusual tiredness or weakness.

Late symptoms of hypercalcemia:

Confusion; drowsiness; high blood pressure; increased sensitivity of eyes or skin to light, especially in hemodialysis patients; irregular, fast, or slow heartbeat; nausea and vomiting; unusually large amount of urine or increased frequency of urination.

ADMINISTRATION AND DOSAGE

General Dosing Information

The action of calcium supplements depends upon their content of calcium ions. The various calcium salts contain the following amounts of elemental calcium:

Calcium salt	Calcium (mg/g)	Calcium (mEq/g)	Percentage of calcium
Calcium acetate	253	12.2	25.3
Calcium carbonate	400	20	40
Calcium chloride	272	13.6	27.2
Calcium citrate	211	10.5	21.1
Calcium glubionate	65	3.2	6.5
Calcium gluceptate	82	4.1	8.2
Calcium gluconate	90	4.5	9
Calcium lactate	130	6.5	13
Calcium phosphate, dibasic	230	11.5	23
Calcium phosphate, tribasic	380	19	38

(Continued on page 237)

Drug Interactions for Calcium

Precipitant Drug	Object Drug	Effect On Object Drug	Description
Alcohol Caffeine	Calcium	↓	Concurrent use of excessive amounts of these substances has been reported to decrease calcium absorption.
Calcium	Aluminum-containing antacids	↑	Concurrent use with calcium citrate may enhance aluminum absorption.
Calcium	Calcitonin	↓	Concurrent use may antagonize the effect of calcitonin in the treatment of hypercalcemia; however, when calcitonin is prescribed for osteoporosis or Paget's disease of the bone, calcium intake should be generous to prevent hypocalcemia, which might generate secondary hyperparathyroidism; calcium-containing preparations may be given 4 hours after calcitonin.
Calcium	Calcium channel blockers	↓	Concurrent use of these medications in quantities sufficient to raise serum calcium concentrations above normal may reduce the response to verapamil and probably other calcium channel blockers.
◆ Calcium	Cellulose sodium phosphate	↓	Concurrent use may decrease effectiveness of cellulose sodium phosphate in preventing hypercalciuria.
◆ Calcium	Digitalis glycosides	↔	Concurrent use of parenteral calcium salts with digitalis glycosides may increase the risk of cardiac arrhythmias; therefore, when the parenteral administration of calcium salts to digitalized patients is deemed necessary, caution and close ECG monitoring are recommended.
◆ Calcium	Etidronate	↓	Concurrent use with calcium supplements may prevent absorption of etidronate; patients should be advised not to take etidronate within 2 hours of calcium supplements.
Calcium	Fluoroquinolones	↓	Concurrent use may reduce absorption by chelation of fluoroquinolones, resulting in lower serum and urine concentrations of fluoroquinolones; therefore, concurrent use is not recommended.
◆ Calcium	Gallium nitrate	↓	Concurrent use with calcium supplements may antagonize the effect of gallium nitrate.
Calcium	Iron supplements	↓	Concurrent use with calcium carbonate and calcium phosphate will decrease the absorption of iron; iron supplements should not be taken within 1-2 hours of calcium carbonate or phosphate.
◆ Calcium	Magnesium-containing preparations Other calcium-containing preparations	↑	Concurrent use may increase serum magnesium or calcium concentrations in susceptible patients, mainly patients with impaired renal function, leading to hypermagnesemia or hypercalcemia.
Calcium	Milk	↔	Concurrent excessive and prolonged use with calcium supplements may result in the milk-alkali syndrome.
Calcium	Neuromuscular blocking agents, except succinylcholine	↔	Concurrent use with parenteral calcium salts usually reverses the effects of nondepolarizing neuromuscular blocking agents; also, concurrent use with calcium salts has been reported to enhance or prolong the neuromuscular blocking action of tubocurarine.
◆ Calcium	Phenytoin	↓	Concurrent use decreases the bioavailability of both phenytoin and calcium because of possible formation of a nonabsorbable complex; patients should be advised not to take calcium supplements within 1-3 hours of taking phenytoin.
Calcium	Sodium bicarbonate	↔	Concurrent and prolonged use with calcium supplements may result in milk-alkali syndrome.
◆ Calcium	Tetracyclines, oral	↓	Concurrent use may decrease absorption of tetracyclines because of possible formation of nonabsorbable complexes and increase in intragastric pH; patients should be advised not to take calcium supplements within 1-3 hours of taking tetracyclines.

Drug Interactions for Calcium (cont.)

Precipitant Drug	Object Drug	Effect On Object Drug	Description
Estrogens	Calcium	↑	Concurrent use may increase calcium absorption, which is used to therapeutic advantage when estrogens are prescribed for the treatment of postmenopausal osteoporosis.
Fiber Phytates	Calcium	↓	Concurrent use of large amounts of fiber or phytates with calcium supplements, especially in patients being treated for hypocalcemia, may reduce calcium absorption by formation of nonabsorbable complexes.
Potassium phosphates Potassium and sodium phosphates	Calcium	↔	Concurrent use with calcium supplements may increase potential for deposition of calcium in soft tissues if serum ionized calcium is high.
Sodium fluoride	Calcium	↓	Concurrent use may cause the calcium ions to complex with fluoride and inhibit absorption of both fluoride and calcium; however, if sodium fluoride is used with calcium supplements to treat osteoporosis, a 1- to 2-hour interval should elapse between doses.
Thiazide diuretics	Calcium	↑	Concurrent use with large doses of calcium supplements may result in hypercalcemia because of reduced calcium excretion.
Vitamin A	Calcium	↓	Excessive intake ($\geq$7500 RE or 25,000 IU/d) may stimulate bone loss and counteract the effects of calcium supplements and may cause hypercalcemia.
Vitamin D (especially calcifediol and calcitriol)	Calcium	↑	Concurrent use of large doses of vitamin D with calcium supplements may excessively increase intestinal absorption of calcium, increasing the risk of chronic hypercalcemia in susceptible patients; monitoring of serum calcium concentrations is essential during long-term therapy.

♦ = Major clinical significance. ECG = electrocardiogram; IU = International Unit; RE = Retinol Equivalent.

The following table includes the number of tablets of each calcium salt required to provide 1000mg of elemental calcium:

Calcium supplement	Salt per tablet (mg)	Calcium per tablet (mg)	Tablets to provide 1000mg of calcium
Calcium carbonate	625	250	4
	650	260	4
	750	300	4
	835	334	3
	1250	500	2
	1500	600	2
Calcium citrate	950	200	5
Calcium gluconate	500	45	22
	650	58	17
	1000	90	11
Calcium lactate	325	42	24
	650	84	12
Calcium phosphate, dibasic	500	115	9
Calcium phosphate, tribasic	800	304	4
	1600	608	2

Administration of calcium supplements should not preclude the use of other measures intended to correct the underlying cause of calcium depletion. In the prevention of osteoporosis, postmenopausal women are sometimes also given estrogens to prevent bone resorption and/or small doses of vitamin D (usually 400IU/d) to enhance calcium absorption. If estrogens are prescribed, either cyclically or continuously for women who have not undergone a hysterectomy, it is recommended that a progestin such as medroxyprogesterone acetate also be given to reduce or prevent the possibility of adverse endometrial changes from occurring. The Food and Drug Administration (FDA) has issued warnings that bonemeal and dolomite (sometimes used as sources of calcium) may contain lead in sufficient quantities to be dangerous.

For parenteral dosage forms only:

The injection should be warmed to body temperature prior to administration, unless precluded by an emergency situation. Following injection, the patient should remain recumbent for a short period of time to prevent dizziness. Parenteral calcium salts are administered by *slow* IV injection (excepting calcium glycerophosphate and calcium lactate combination, which is given by intramuscular injection) to prevent a high concentration of calcium from reaching the heart and causing cardiac syncope. Side effects experienced by the conscious patient are often the result of too rapid a rate of IV administration of calcium salts. Administration should be temporarily discontinued with the appearance of abnormal electrocardiogram (ECG) readings or with patient complaints of discomfort; administration may be resumed when the abnormal reading or the discomfort has disappeared. Severe necrosis, requiring skin grafting, and calcification can occur at the site of infiltration after IV injection, especially after push injection. Transient increases in blood pressure, especially in the elderly or patients with hypertension, may occur during IV administration of calcium salts.

Diet/nutrition:

Oral calcium supplements are best taken 1 to 1 1/2 hours after meals in 3 to 4 daily doses. However, calcium glubionate syrup should be administered before meals to enhance absorption. In the elderly, who may be more prone than younger patients to impaired stomach acid production, calcium absorption may be increased by the use of a more soluble calcium salt, such as calcium citrate, gluconate, or lactate. The poor solubility of carbonate and phosphate salts makes them less desirable as antihypocalcemic agents in patients with known achlorhydria or hypochlorhydria.

Recommended dietary intakes for calcium:

The Recommended Dietary Allowances (RDAs) for vitamins and minerals are determined by the Food and Nutrition Board of the National Research Council and are intended to provide adequate nutrition in most healthy persons under usual environmental stresses. In addition, a different designation may be used by the FDA for food and dietary supplement labeling purposes, as with Daily Value (DV). DVs replace the previous labeling terminology, United States Recommended Daily Allowances (USRDAs).

Daily recommended intakes for calcium are generally defined as follows:

Population Group	RDA (mg)
Birth to 3 years of age	400-800
Children 4 to 6 years of age	800
Children 7 to 10 years of age	800
Adolescent and adult males	800-1200
Adolescent and adult females	800-1200
Pregnant females	1200
Breastfeeding females	1200

The following table indicates the calcium content of selected foods:

Food	Amount of calcium (mg)
Nonfat dry milk, reconstituted (1 cup)	375
Low-fat, skim, or whole milk (1 cup)	290 to 300
Yogurt (1 cup)	275 to 400
Sardines with bones (3oz)	370
Ricotta cheese, part skim (1/2 cup)	340
Salmon, canned, with bones (3oz)	285
Cheese, Swiss (1oz)	272
Cheese, cheddar (1oz)	204
Cheese, American (1oz)	174
Cottage cheese, low-fat (1 cup)	154
Tofu (4oz)	154
Shrimp (1 cup)	147
Ice milk (3/4 cup)	132

Calcium Capsules/Suspension/Tablets:

For hypocalcemia (prophylaxis):

Usual adult and adolescent dosage:

Oral, amount based on normal daily recommended intakes:

Population Group	RDA (mg)
Adolescent and adult males	800-1200
Adolescent and adult females	800-1200
Pregnant females	1200
Breastfeeding females	1200

Usual pediatric dosage:

Oral, amount based on normal daily recommended intakes:

Population Group	RDA (mg)
Infants and children	
Birth to 3 years of age	400-800
4 to 6 years of age	800
7 to 10 years of age	800

VITAMIN D

PHARMACOLOGY

Vitamin D is essential for promoting absorption and utilization of calcium and phosphate and for normal calcification of bone. Along with parathyroid hormone and calcitonin, it regulates serum calcium concentrations by increasing serum calcium and phosphate concentrations as needed. Vitamin D stimulates calcium and phosphate absorption from the small intestine and mobilizes calcium from bone.

Exposure of the skin to ultraviolet rays in sunlight results in formation of cholecalciferol (vitamin D_3). Ergocalciferol (calciferol, vitamin D_2) is found in commercial vitamin preparations and is used as a food additive; cholecalciferol is found in vitamin D-fortified milk. Cholecalciferol and ergocalciferol are transferred to the liver where they are converted to calcifediol (25-hydroxycholecalciferol), which is then transferred to the kidneys and converted to calcitriol (1,25-dihydroxycholecalciferol, thought to be the most active form) and 24,25-dihydroxycholecalciferol (physiologic role not determined). Dihydrotachysterol is a synthetic reduction product of ergocalciferol; it has only weak antirachitic activity and is metabolically activated by 25-hydroxylation in the liver. Alfacalcidol is rapidly converted to 1,25-dihydroxycholecalciferol in the liver. Doxercalciferol is activated by CYP 27 in the liver to form 1-alpha, 25-dihydroxyvitamin D_2 (major metabolite); activation does not require involvement of the kidneys.

Calcitriol appears to act by binding to a specific receptor in the cytoplasm of the intestinal mucosa and subsequently being incorporated into the nucleus, probably leading to formation of the calcium-binding protein that results in increased absorption of calcium from the intestine. Also, calcitriol may regulate the transfer of calcium ions from bone and stimulate reabsorption of calcium in the distal renal tubule, thereby effecting calcium homeostasis in the extracellular fluid.

Vitamin D, doxercalciferol, and paricalcitol have been shown to reduce parathyroid hormone levels.

INDICATIONS

Hypocalcemia, chronic (treatment); *hypophosphatemia* (treatment); *osteodystrophy* (treatment); *rickets* (prophylaxis and treatment)—Therapeutic doses of specific vitamin D analogs are used in the treatment of chronic hypocalcemia, hypophosphatemia, rickets, and osteodystrophy associated with various medical conditions, including chronic renal failure, familial hypophosphatemia, and hypoparathyroidism (postsurgical or idiopathic, or pseudohypoparathyroidism). Some analogs have been found to reduce elevated parathyroid hormone concentrations in patients with renal osteodystrophy associated with hyperparathyroidism.

Theoretically, any of the vitamin D analogs may be used for the above conditions. However, because of their pharmacologic properties, some may be more useful in certain situations than others. Alfacalcidol, calcitriol, and dihydrotachysterol are usually preferred in patients with renal failure since these patients have impaired ability to synthesize calcitriol from cholecalciferol and ergocalciferol; therefore, the response is more predictable. In addition, the shorter half-lives of these agents may make toxicity easier to manage (hypercalcemia reverses more quickly). Ergocalciferol may not be the preferred agent in the treatment of familial hypophosphatemia or hypoparathyroidism because the large dosages needed are associated with a risk of overdose and hypercalcemia; dihydrotachysterol and calcitriol may be preferred.

Secondary hyperparathyroidism (prophylaxis and treatment)—Paricalcitol is indicated for the prevention and treatment of secondary hyperparathyroidism associated with chronic renal failure.

CALCIUM CARBONATE PRODUCTS	
Brand Name	**Dosage Form**
Alka-mints (Bayer)	**Tablet:** 850mg
Caltrate 600 (Lederle)	**Tablet:** 600mg
Mylanta Children's (J & J/Merck)	**Tablet:** 400mg
Os-cal 500 (GSK)	**Tablet:** 500mg
Oystercal 500 (Nature's Bounty)	**Tablet:** 500mg
Rolaids (Pfizer)	**Tablet:** 220mg
Rolaids Softchews (Pfizer)	**Tablet:** 1177mg
Titralac (3M)	**Tablet:** 420mg
Titralac Extra Strength (3M)	**Tablet:** 750mg
Tums (GSK)	**Tablet:** 500mg
Tums Calcium for Life Bone Health (GSK)	**Tablet:** 500mg
Tums E-X (GSK)	**Tablet:** 750mg
Tums Ultra (GSK)	**Tablet:** 1000mg
CALCIUM CARBONATE/VITAMIN D PRODUCTS	
Brand Name	**Dosage Form**
Caltrate 600 + D (Lederle)	**Tablet:** 600mg-200IU
Os-cal 250 + D (GSK)	**Tablet:** 250mg-125IU
Os-cal 500 + D (GSK)	**Tablet:** 500mg-200IU
Oystercal 500 + D (Nature's Bounty)	**Tablet:** 500mg-125IU
Viactiv (McNeil)	**Tablet:** 500mg-100IU
CALCIUM CITRATE PRODUCTS	
Brand Name	**Dosage Form**
Citracal (Mission)	**Tablet:** 200mg
Citracel Liquitab (Mission)	**Tablet:** 500mg
CALCIUM CITRATE/VITAMIN D PRODUCTS	
Brand Name	**Dosage Form**
Citracal + D (Mission)	**Tablet:** 250mg-200IU; 265mg-200IU
CALCIUM GLUBIONATE PRODUCTS	
Brand Name	**Dosage Form**
Calcionate (Hi-Tech)	**Syrup:** 1.8g/5mL
Calciquid (Breckenridge)	**Syrup:** 1.8g/5mL
Cal-G (Key Company)	**Tablet:** 700mg
CALCIUM PHOSPHATE PRODUCTS	
Brand Name	**Dosage Form**
Posture (Inverness)	**Tablet:** 600mg
CALCIUM PHOSPHATE/VITAMIN D PRODUCTS	
Brand Name	**Dosage Form**
Posture-D (Inverness)	**Tablet:** 600mg-125IU

Doxercalciferol is indicated for the treatment of elevated intact parathyroid hormone (iPTH) levels in the management of secondary hyperparathyroidism in patients undergoing chronic renal dialysis.

Tetany (prophylaxis and treatment)—Dihydrotachysterol is indicated for (and ergocalciferol and calcitriol are used for) treatment of chronic and latent forms of postoperative tetany and idiopathic tetany.

Vitamin D deficiency (prophylaxis and treatment)—Ergocalciferol is indicated for prevention and treatment of vitamin D deficiency states. Vitamin D deficiency may occur as a result of inadequate nutrition, intestinal malabsorption, or lack of exposure to sunlight, but it does not occur in healthy individuals receiving an adequate balanced diet and exposure to sunlight. Vitamin D therapy, alone, as treatment for osteoporosis is not generally recommended; however, vitamin D supplements in doses of 400 to 800 Units may be used as part of the prevention and treatment of osteoporosis in patients with an inadequate vitamin D and/or calcium intake. For prophylaxis of vitamin D deficiency, dietary improvement, rather than supplementation, is advisable. For treatment of vitamin D deficiency, supplementation is preferred. Deficiency of vitamin D may lead to rickets and osteomalacia.

Recommended intakes may be increased and/or supplementation may be necessary in the following persons or conditions (based on documented vitamin D deficiency):

- Alcoholism.
- Dark-skinned individuals.
- Hepatic-biliary tract disease—hepatic function impairment, cirrhosis, obstructive jaundice.
- Infants, breastfed, with inadequate exposure to sunlight.
- Intestinal diseases—celiac, tropical sprue, regional enteritis, persistent diarrhea.
- Lack of exposure to sunlight combined with reduced vitamin D intake.
- Renal function impairment.
- In general, vitamin D absorption will be impaired in any condition in which fat malabsorption (steatorrhea) occurs.

Some unusual diets (eg, strict vegetarian diets with no milk intake, such as vegan vegetarian or macrobiotic, or reducing diets that drastically restrict food selection) may not supply minimum daily requirements of vitamin D. Supplementation may be necessary in patients receiving total parenteral nutrition (TPN) or undergoing rapid weight loss or in those with malnutrition, because of inadequate dietary intake.

Recommended intakes for all vitamins and most minerals are increased during pregnancy. Many physicians recommend that pregnant women receive multivitamin and mineral supplements, especially those pregnant women who do not consume an adequate diet and those in high-risk categories (ie, women carrying more than one fetus, heavy cigarette smokers, and alcohol and drug abusers). Taking excessive amounts of a multivitamin and mineral supplement may be harmful to the mother and/or fetus and should be avoided.

Pregnant women who are strict vegetarians (vegan vegetarians) and/or have minimal exposure to sunlight may need vitamin D supplementation.

Congenital rickets has been reported in newborns whose mothers had low serum levels of vitamin D.

Recommended intakes for all vitamins and most minerals are increased during breastfeeding.

Recommended intakes may be increased by the following medications: Barbiturates, cholestyramine, colestipol, hydantoin anticonvulsants, mineral oil, and primidone.

CONTRAINDICATIONS

Except under special circumstances, this medication should not be used when the following medical problems exist:

- Hypercalcemia—*major clinical significance.*
- Hypervitaminosis D—*major clinical significance.*
- Renal osteodystrophy with hyperphosphatemia—*major clinical significance* (risk of metastatic calcification; however, vitamin D therapy can begin once serum phosphate levels have stabilized).

Risk-benefit should be considered when the following medical problems exist:

- Arteriosclerosis; cardiac function impairment—*major clinical significance* (conditions may be exacerbated due to possibility of hypercalcemia and elevated serum cholesterol concentrations).
- Hyperphosphatemia—*major clinical significance* (risk of metastatic calcification; dietary phosphate restriction or administration of intestinal phosphate binders is recommended to produce normal serum phosphorus concentrations).
- Hypersensitivity to effects of vitamin D—*major clinical significance* (may be involved in causing idiopathic hypercalcemia in infants).
- Renal function impairment—*major clinical significance* (toxicity may occur in patients receiving vitamin D for nonrenal problems, although toxicity is also possible during treatment of renal osteodystrophy because of increased requirements and decreased renal function).
- Sarcoidosis and possibly other granulomatous diseases (increased sensitivity to effects of vitamin D).

WARNINGS/PRECAUTIONS

Drug Interactions: See chart on page 242.

Pregnancy: FDA Category C (except for doxercalciferol, which is Category B). Problems in humans have not been documented with intake of normal daily recommended amounts. There are insufficient data on acute and chronic vitamin D toxicity in pregnant women. Maternal hypercalcemia during pregnancy in humans may be associated with increased sensitivity to effects of vitamin D, suppression of parathyroid function, or a syndrome of peculiar (elfin) facies, mental retardation, and congenital aortic stenosis in infants.

Overdosage of vitamin D has been associated with fetal abnormalities in animals. Animal studies have shown calcitriol to be teratogenic when given in doses 4 to 15 times the dosage recommended for human use. Excessive doses of dihydrotachysterol are also teratogenic in animals. Animal studies have also shown calcifediol to be teratogenic when given in doses of 6 to 12 times the human dose.

Breastfeeding: Only small amounts of vitamin D metabolites appear in human milk. Infants who are totally breastfed and have little exposure to the sun may require vitamin D supplementation. It is not known whether paricalcitol or doxercalciferol is excreted in human milk. Because many drugs are excreted in human milk, caution should be exercised when paricalcitol or doxercalciferol are administered to a nursing woman.

ADVERSE REACTIONS

Those indicating need for medical attention:

Early symptoms of vitamin D toxicity associated with hypercalcemia:

Bone pain; constipation—usually more frequent in children and adolescents; diarrhea; drowsiness; dryness of mouth; headache, continuing; increased thirst; increase in frequency of urination, especially at night, or in amount of urine; irregular heartbeat; loss of appetite; metallic taste; muscle pain; nausea or vomiting—usually more frequent in children and adolescents; pruritus; unusual tiredness or weakness.

Late symptoms of vitamin D toxicity associated with hypercalcemia:

Bone pain; cloudy urine; conjunctivitis (redness or discharge of the eye, eyelid, or lining of the eyelid)—calcific; decreased libido (loss of sex drive); ectopic calcification (calcium deposits in tissues other than bone); high fever; high blood pressure; increased sensitivity of eyes to light or irritation of eyes; irregular heartbeat; itching of skin; lethargy (drowsiness); loss of appetite; muscle pain; nausea or vomiting and pancreatitis (stomach pain, severe); psychosis, overt (mood or mental changes)—rare; rhinorrhea (runny nose); weight loss.

ADMINISTRATION AND DOSAGE

General Dosing Information

For use as an antihypocalcemic:

Before vitamin D therapy is begun, elevated serum phosphate concentrations must be controlled. Clinical response to vitamin D depends on adequate dietary calcium. Because of individual variation in sensitivity to its effects, dosage of vitamin D must be adjusted on the basis of clinical response. Some infants are hyperreactive to even small doses. Careful titration is necessary to avoid overdosage, which induces hypercalcemia and can cause hypercalciuria and hyperphosphatemia. Dosage of vitamin D from dietary and other sources should be evaluated in determining the therapeutic dosage. The serum calcium times phosphorus (Ca X P, in mg/dL) product should not exceed 60. To control elevated serum phosphate concentrations in patients undergoing dialysis, a phosphate-binding agent should be used. The dosage of the binding agent may need to be increased during vitamin D therapy since phosphate absorption is enhanced.

For use as a dietary supplement:

Because of the infrequency of vitamin D deficiency alone, combinations of several vitamins are commonly administered. Many commercial vitamin complexes are available.

Diet/Nutrition:

The Recommended Dietary Allowances (RDAs) for vitamins and minerals are determined by the Food and Nutrition Board of the National Research Council and are intended to provide adequate nutrition in most healthy persons under usual environmental stresses. In addition, a different designation may be used by the Food and Drug Administration (FDA) for food and dietary supplement labeling purposes, as with Daily Value (DV). DVs replace the previous labeling terminology, United States Recommended Daily Allowances (USRDAs).

Normal daily recommended intakes for vitamin D in micrograms and units are generally defined as follows:

Population Group	RDA	
	Micrograms	Units
Infants and children		
Birth to 3 years of age	7.5-10	300-400
4 to 6 years of age	10	400
7 to 10 years of age	10	400
Adolescents and adults	5-10	200-400
Pregnant and breastfeeding females	10	400

These are usually provided by adequate diets and adequate exposure to sunlight (1.5-2 hours of exposure per week is sufficient for most people). Best dietary sources of vitamin D (as cholecalciferol) include some fish and fish liver oils and vitamin D-fortified milk. The vitamin D content of foods is not affected by cooking.

For parenteral dosage forms only:

Parenteral administration may be indicated in patients with malabsorption problems. Intravenous administration may be indicated in patients undergoing hemodialysis.

Drug Interactions for Vitamin D

Precipitant Drug	Object Drug	Effect On Object Drug	Description
Anticonvulsants, hydantoin Barbiturates Primidone	Vitamin D	↓	May reduce effect of vitamin D by accelerating metabolism by hepatic microsomal enzyme induction; patients on long-term anticonvulsant therapy may require vitamin D supplementation to prevent osteomalacia.
Cholestyramine Colestipol Mineral oil	Vitamin D	↓	Concurrent use may impair intestinal absorption of vitamin D since these medications have been reported to reduce intestinal absorption of fat-soluble vitamins; requirements for vitamin D may be increased in patients receiving these medications.
Corticosteroids	Vitamin D	↓	Vitamin D supplementation may be recommended by some clinicians for prolonged corticosteroid use because corticosteroids may interfere with vitamin D action.
Vitamin D	Aluminum-containing antacids	↑	Long-term use of aluminum-containing antacids as phosphate binders in hyperphosphatemia in conjunction with vitamin D has been found to increase blood levels for aluminum and may lead to aluminum bone toxicity, especially in patients with chronic renal failure.
♦ Vitamin D	Calcium-containing preparations (high doses) Thiazide diuretics	↑	Concurrent use may increase the risk of hypercalcemia; however, it may be therapeutically advantageous in elderly and high-risk groups when it is necessary to prescribe vitamin D or its derivatives together with calcium; careful monitoring of serum calcium concentrations is essential during long-term therapy.
Vitamin D	Digitalis glycosides	↑	Caution is recommended in patients being treated with these medications since the hypercalcemia that may be caused by vitamin D may potentiate the effects of digitalis glycosides, resulting in cardiac arrhythmias.
♦ Vitamin D	Magnesium-containing antacids	↑	Concurrent use may result in hypermagnesemia, especially in patients with chronic renal failure.
Vitamin D	Phosphorus-containing preparations (high doses)	↑	Concurrent use with vitamin D may increase the potential for hyperphosphatemia because of vitamin D enhancement of phosphate absorption.

♦ = Major clinical significance.

DOSING INFORMATION FOR ANTIHYPOCALCEMIC PRODUCTS

The following table provides a quick comparison of the ingredients and dosages of common brand-name OTC supplements. Products are listed alphabetically by brand name.

BRAND NAME	INGREDIENT/STRENGTH	DOSE
Caltrate 600 Plus chewable tablets (Whitehall-Robinson Healthcare)	Vitamin D 200 IU, Calcium carbonate 600mg, Magnesium 40mg, Boron 250 mcg, Zinc 7.5mg, Copper 1 mg, Manganese 1.8mg	**Adults:** 1 tab bid.
Caltrate 600 Plus Dietary Supplement with Soy Isoflavones tablets (Whitehall-Robinson Healthcare)	Vitamin D 200 IU, Calcium carbonate 600mg	**Adults:** 1 tab bid.r
Caltrate 600 Plus tablets (Whitehall-Robinson Healthcare)	Vitamin D 200 IU, Calcium carbonate 600mg, Magnesium 40mg, Boron 250mcg, Zinc 7.5mg, Copper 1mg, Manganese 1.8mg	**Adults:** 1 tab bid.
Caltrate 600 tablets (Whitehall-Robinson Healthcare)	Calcium carbonate 600mg	**Adults:** 1 tab bid.n
Caltrate 600 + D tablets (Whitehall-Robinson Healthcare)	Vitamin D 200 IU, Calcium carbonate 600mg	**Adults:** 1 tab bid.
Citracal + D tablets (Mission Pharmacal)	Vitamin D 200 IU, Calcium citrate 265mg	**Adults:** 1-2 tab bid.
Citracal 250mg + D tablets (Mission Pharmacal)	Vitamin D 62.5 IU, Calcium citrate 250mg	**Adults:** 1-2 tab bid.
Citracal tablets (Mission Pharmacal)	Calcium citrate 200mg	**Adults:** 1-2 tab bid.
Nature Made Advanced Calcium High Absorption tablets (Nature Made Nutritional Products)	Vitamin D 200 IU, Calcium carbonate 500mg, Magnesium 250mg, Zinc 7.5mg	**Adults:** 2 tabs bid.
Nature Made Calcium 500mg with Vitamin D tablets (Pharmavite)	Vitamin D 200 IU, Calcium carbonate 500mg	**Adults:** 1 tab bid.
Nature's Bounty Calcium 600 Plus Vitamin D tablets (Nature's Bounty)	Vitamin D 200mg, Calcium carbonate 600mg	**Adults:** 1-2 tab bid.
OS-Cal 500 + D tablets (GlaxoSmithKline Consumer Healthcare)	Vitamin D 400 IU, Calcium carbonate 500mg	**Adults:** 1 tab bid.
Os-Cal 500 Chewable tablets (GlaxoSmithKline Consumer Healthcare)	Calcium carbonate 500mg	**Adults:** 1 tab bid-tid.
Os-Cal 500 tablets (GlaxoSmithKline Consumer Healthcare)	Calcium carbonate 500mg	**Adults:** 1 tab bid-tid.
OS-Cal Calcium Supplement, 500mg with Vitamin D (GlaxoSmithKline Consumer Healthcare)	Vitamin D 200 IU, Calcium cabonate 500mg	**Adults:** 2-3 tabs qd.
OS-Cal Ultra 600 Plus (GlaxoSmithKline Consumer Healthcare)	Vitamin D 200 IU, Vitamin E 5IU, Vitamin C 60mg, Calcium carbonate 600mg, Magnesium 20mg, Boron 250mg, Zinc 7.5mg, Copper 1mg, Manganese 1mg	**Adults:** 1 tab bid.
Posture-D 600mg chewable tablets (Inverness Medical)	Vitamin D 125 IU, Calcium (Tribasic Calcium Phosphate) 600mg	**Adults:** 2-3 tabs qd.
Posture-D 600mg tablets (Inverness Medical)	Vitamin D 125 IU, Calcium (Tricalcium Phosphate) 600mg, Phosphorus 266mg, Magnesium 50mg	**Adults:** 2 tabs q24h.
Sundown Calcium 500mg Plus Vitamin D tablets (Sundown)	Vitamin D 125 IU, Calcium 500mg	**Adults:** 1 tab bid-tid.
Sweet Essentials Calcium Chewable Supplement (Northwest Natural Products)	Vitamin D 200 IU, Calcium carbonate 500mg, Phosphorus 250mg, Manganese 1mg	**Adults:** 2 tabs q24h.
Sweet Essentials Calcium Soft Chews, Sugar Free (Northwest Natural Products)	Vitamin D 100mg, Calcium 500mg	**Adults:** 1 tab bid.
Tums Calcium for Life Bone Health (GlaxoSmithKline Consumer Healthcare)	Calcium carbonate 500mg	**Adults:** 1 tab bid.
Viactiv Calcium Soft Chews plus Vitamin D and K for Women (McNeil Nutritionals)	Vitamin D 100mg, Calcium 500mg, Vitamin K 40mcg	**Adults:** 1-3 chewables qd.

Sprains and Strains

A sprain is a stretch and/or tear of a ligament around a joint. Ligaments are strong, flexible fibers that hold bones together. Sprains are caused when a joint is forced to move into an unnatural position. Symptoms of sprain include joint pain, swelling, joint stiffness, and bruising. The most common site of a sprain is the ankle. A strain is an injury to either a muscle or a tendon. Tendons are fibrous cords of tissue that connect muscle to bone. Symptoms of strain include muscle pain, bruising, and swelling. There are number of OTC products available to treat pain associated sprains and strains, including acetaminophen, salicylates (e.g., aspirin), NSAIDs (e.g., ibuprofen, ketoprofen, naproxen), and rubs and liniments.

ACETAMINOPHEN

Analgesic—The mechanism of analgesic action has not been fully determined. Acetaminophen may act predominantly by inhibiting prostaglandin synthesis in the central nervous system and, to a lesser extent, through a peripheral action by blocking pain-impulse generation. The peripheral action may also be due to inhibition of prostaglandin synthesis or to inhibition of the synthesis or actions of other substances that sensitize pain receptors to mechanical or chemical stimulation.

Capsule/Granules/Powder/Solution/Suspension/Tablet

For analgesic use:

Adults/Pediatrics ≥13 years of age: 325 to 500mg every 3 hours; 325 to 650mg every 4 hours; 650 to 1000mg every 6 hours; or 1300mg every 8 hours.

Pediatrics ≤3 months of age: 40mg every 4 hours as needed.

Pediatrics 4 to 12 months of age: 80mg every 4 hours as needed.

Pediatrics 1 to 2 years of age: 120mg every 4 hours as needed.

Pediatrics 2 to 4 years of age: 160mg every 4 hours as needed.

Pediatrics 4 to 6 years of age: 240mg every 4 hours as needed.

Pediatrics 6 to 9 years of age: 320mg every 4 hours as needed.

Pediatrics 9 to 11 years of age: 320 to 400mg every 4 hours as needed.

Pediatrics 11 to 12 years of age: 320 to 480mg every 4 hours as needed.

Suppositories

For analgesic use:

Adults/Pediatrics ≥13 years of age: 325 to 650mg every 4 hours or 650mg every 6 hours as needed.

Pediatrics 2 to 4 years of age: 160mg every 4 hours as needed.

Pediatrics 4 to 6 years of age: 240mg every 4 hours as needed.

Pediatrics 6 to 9 years of age: 320mg every 4 hours as needed.

Pediatrics 9 to 11 years of age: 320 to 400mg every 4 hours as needed.

Pediatrics 11 to 12 years of age: 320 to 480mg every 4 hours as needed.

For more information, refer to the complete monograph for acetaminophen in "Aches and Pains" under Musculoskeletal System.

ASPIRIN

Analgesic—Salicylates produce analgesia through a peripheral action by blocking pain-impulse generation and via a central action, possibly in the hypothalamus. The peripheral action may predominate and probably involves inhibition of the synthesis of prostaglandins, and possibly inhibition of the synthesis and/or actions of other substances, which sensitize pain receptors to mechanical or chemical stimulation.

Suppositories

For analgesic use:

Adults/Pediatrics ≥12 years of age: 325 to 650mg every 4 hours as needed.

Pediatrics 2 to 4 years of age: 160mg every 4 hours as needed.

Pediatrics 4 to 6 years of age: 240mg every 4 hours as needed.

Pediatrics 6 to 9 years of age: 325mg every 4 hours as needed.

Pediatrics 9 to 11 years of age: 325 to 400mg every 4 hours as needed.

Pediatric 11 to 12 years of age: 325 to 480mg every 4 hours as needed.

ACETAMINOPHEN PRODUCTS	
Brand Name	**Dosage Form**
Anacin Aspirin Free (Insight)	**Tablet:** 500mg
Feverall (Alpharma)	**Suppositories:** 80mg, 120mg, 325mg, 650mg
Tylenol 8 Hour (McNeil)	**Tablet:** 650mg
Tylenol Arthritis (McNeil)	**Tablet:** 650mg
Tylenol Children's Meltaways (McNeil)	**Tablet:** 80mg
Tylenol Children's (McNeil)	**Suspension:** 160mg/5mL
Tylenol Extra Strength (McNeil)	**Capsule:** 500mg **Liquid:** 1000mg/30mL **Tablet:** 500mg
Tylenol Infants' (McNeil)	**Suspension:** 80mg/0.8mL
Tylenol Junior Meltaways (McNeil)	**Tablet:** 160mg
Tylenol Regular Strength (McNeil)	**Tablet:** 325mg

Tablet

For analgesic use:

Adults/Pediatrics ≥12 years of age: 325 to 500mg every 3 hours; 325 to 650mg every 4 hours; or 650 to 1000mg every 6 hours as needed.

Pediatrics 2 to 4 years of age: 160mg every 4 hours as needed.

Pediatrics 4 to 6 years of age: 240mg every 4 hours as needed.

Pediatrics 6 to 9 years of age: 320 to 325mg every 4 hours as needed.

Pediatrics 9 to 11 years of age: 320 to 400mg every 4 hours as needed.

Pediatric 11 to 12 years of age: 320 to 480mg every 4 hours as needed.

For more information, refer to the complete monograph for salicylates in "Aches and Pains" under Musculoskeletal System.

CAFFEINE

Analgesia adjunct—Caffeine constricts cerebral vasculature, resulting in decreased cerebral blood flow as well as a decrease in the oxygen tension of the brain. It has been suggested that the addition of caffeine to aspirin or aspirin/acetaminophen combinations may help to relieve headache by providing a more rapid onset of action and/or enhanced pain relief with a lower dose of the analgesic. In some patients, caffeine may reduce headache pain by reversing caffeine withdrawal symptoms. Recent studies with ergotamine indicate that the enhanced effect by the addition of caffeine may be due to improved gastrointestinal absorption of ergotamine when administered with caffeine.

For more information, refer to the complete monograph for caffeine in "Drowsiness/Lethargy" under Central Nervous System.

ASPIRIN PRODUCTS	
Brand Name	**Dosage Form**
Ascriptin (Novartis)	**Tablet:** 81mg
Aspergum (Schering)	**Gum:** 227mg
Bayer Aspirin Regimen (Bayer)	**Tablet:** 81mg, 325mg
Bayer Children's Aspirin (Bayer)	**Tablet:** 81mg
Bayer Extra Strength (Bayer)	**Tablet:** 500mg
Bayer Genuine Aspirin (Bayer)	**Tablet:** 325mg
Ecotrin (GSK)	**Tablet:** 325mg
Ecotrin Adult Low Strength (GSK)	**Tablet:** 81mg
Ecotrin Maximum Strength (GSK)	**Tablet:** 500mg
Halfprin (Kramer)	**Tablet:** 81mg, 162mg
St. Joseph (McNeil)	**Tablet:** 81mg
BUFFERED ASPIRIN PRODUCTS	
Brand Name	**Dosage Form**
Alka-Seltzer (Bayer)	**Tablet:** 325mg
Alka-Seltzer Extra Strength (Bayer)	**Tablet:** 500mg
Ascriptin (Novartis)	**Tablet:** 325mg
Ascriptin Arthritis Pain (Novartis)	**Tablet:** 325mg
Ascriptin Maximum Strength (Novartis)	**Tablet:** 500mg
Bayer Plus Extra Strength (Bayer)	**Tablet:** 500mg
Bufferin (BMS)	**Tablet:** 325mg
Bufferin Extra Strength (BMS)	**Tablet:** 500mg

ACETAMINOPHEN/CAFFEINE PRODUCTS	
Brand Name	**Dosage Form**
Excedrin Tension Headache (BMS)	**Tablet:** 500mg-65mg
ACETAMINOPHEN/ASPIRIN/CAFFEINE PRODUCTS	
Brand Name	**Dosage Form**
Excedrin Extra Strength (BMS)	**Tablet:** 250mg-250mg-65mg
Excedrin Migraine (BMS)	**Tablet:** 250mg-250mg-65mg
Goody's Fast Pain Relief (GSK)	**Tablet:** 130mg-260mg-16.25mg
Goody's Headache Powders (GSK)	**Tablet:** 260mg-520mg-32.5mg

CAPSAICIN

Capsaicin's precise mechanism of action has not been fully elucidated. It is a neuropeptide-active agent that affects the synthesis, storage, transport, and release of substance P. Substance P is thought to be the principal chemical mediator of pain impulses from the periphery to the central nervous system. In addition, substance P has been shown to be released into joint tissues where it activates inflammatory intermediates that are involved in the development of rheumatoid arthritis. Capsaicin renders skin and joints insensitive to pain by depleting and preventing reaccumulation of substance P in peripheral sensory neurons. With the depletion of substance P in the nerve endings, local pain impulses cannot be transmitted to the brain.

CREAM

Adults/Pediatrics ≥2 years of age: Apply to affected area 3 to 4 times a day.

IBUPROFEN

Analgesic—Ibuprofen may block pain-impulse generation via a peripheral action that may involve reduction of the activity of prostaglandins, and possibly inhibition of the synthesis or actions of other substances that sensitize pain receptors to mechanical or chemical stimulation. The antibradykinin activity of ibuprofen may also be involved in relief of pain, since bradykinin has been shown to act together with prostaglandins to cause pain.

CAPSULE/SUSPENSION/TABLET

For analgesic use (mild to moderate pain):

Adults: 200 to 400mg every 4 to 6 hours as needed.

For more information, refer to the complete monograph for NSAIDs in "Aches and Pains" under Musculoskeletal System.

ASPIRIN/CAFFEINE PRODUCTS	
Brand Name	**Dosage Form**
Alka-Seltzer Morning Relief (Bayer)	**Tablet:** 500mg-65mg
Anacin (Wyeth)	**Tablet:** 400mg-32mg
Anacin Maximum Strength (Wyeth)	**Tablet:** 500mg-32mg
Bayer Rapid Headache Relief (Bayer)	**Tablet:** 500mg-65mg
ASPIRIN/CAFFEINE/SALICYLAMIDE PRODUCTS	
Brand Name	**Dosage Form**
BC Powder Original (GSK)	**Tablet:** 650mg-33.3mg-195mg
BC Powder Arthritis Strength (GSK)	**Tablet:** 742mg-38mg-222mg

CAPSAICIN PRODUCTS	
Brand Name	**Dosage Form**
Capsin (Pryde)	**Lotion:** 0.03%, 0.08%
Icy Hot Arthritis Therapy (Chattem)	**Gel:** 0.03%
Zostrix (Rodlen)	**Cream:** 0.03% **Stick:** 0.03%
Zostrix High Potency (Rodlen)	**Stick:** 0.08%
Zostrix Sports (Rodlen)	**Cream:** 0.08%

IBUPROFEN PRODUCTS	
Brand Name	**Dosage Form**
Advil (Wyeth)	**Capsule:** 200mg **Tablet:** 200mg
Advil Children's (Wyeth)	**Tablet:** 50mg
Advil Junior (Wyeth)	**Tablet:** 100mg
Midol Cramp Formula (Bayer)	**Tablet:** 200mg
Motrin IB (McNeil)	**Tablet:** 200mg
Motrin Children's (McNeil)	**Suspension:** 100mg/5mL
Motrin Infants' (McNeil)	**Suspension:** 50mg/1.25mL
Motrin Junior (McNeil)	**Tablet:** 100mg
Motrin Migraine Pain (McNeil)	**Tablet:** 200mg

KETOPROFEN

Analgesic—Ketoprofen may block pain-impulse generation via a peripheral action that may involve reduction of the activity of prostaglandins, and possibly inhibition of the synthesis or actions of other substances that sensitize pain receptors to mechanical or chemical stimulation. The antibradykinin activity of ketoprofen may also be involved in relief of pain, since bradykinin has been shown to act together with prostaglandins to cause pain.

Capsules/Tablets

For analgesic use (mild to moderate pain):

Adults: 25 to 50mg every 6 to 8 hours as needed.

For more information, refer to the complete monograph for NSAIDs in "Aches and Pains" under Musculoskeletal System.

MAGNESIUM SALICYLATE

Analgesic—Salicylates produce analgesia through a peripheral action by blocking pain-impulse generation and via a central action, possibly in the hypothalamus. The peripheral action may predominate and probably involves inhibition of the synthesis of prostaglandins, and possibly inhibition of the synthesis and/or actions of other substances, which sensitize pain receptors to mechanical or chemical stimulation.

Tablets

For analgesic use:

Adults: 607.4mg every 4 hours as needed; or 934mg every 6 hours as needed.

For more information, refer to the complete monograph for salicylates in "Aches and Pains" under Musculoskeletal System.

NAPROXEN

Analgesic—Naproxen may block pain-impulse generation via a peripheral action that may involve reduction of the activity of prostaglandins, and possibly inhibition of the synthesis or actions of other substances that sensitize pain receptors to mechanical or chemical stimulation. The antibradykinin activity of naproxen may also be involved in relief of pain, since bradykinin has been shown to act together with prostaglandins to cause pain.

Capsule/Tablet

For analgesic use (mild to moderate pain):

Adults: 500mg initially, then 250mg every 6 to 8 hours as needed.

For more information, refer to the complete monograph for NSAIDs in "Aches and Pains" under Musculoskeletal System.

KETOPROFEN PRODUCTS	
Brand Name	**Dosage Form**
Orudis KT (Wyeth)	**Tablet:** 12.5mg

MAGNESIUM SALICYLATE PRODUCTS	
Brand Name	**Dosage Form**
Doan's Extra Strength (Novartis)	**Tablet:** 500mg
Doan's Regular Strength (Novartis)	**Tablet:** 325mg
Momentum (Medtech)	**Tablet:** 467mg

NAPROXEN PRODUCTS	
Brand Name	**Dosage Form**
Aleve (Bayer)	**Capsule:** 220mg **Tablet:** 220mg
Aleve Arthritis (Bayer)	**Tablet:** 220mg
Midol Extended Relief (Bayer)	**Tablet:** 220mg

DOSING INFORMATION FOR ANALGESIC PRODUCTS

The following table provides a quick comparison of the ingredients and dosages of common brand-name OTC drugs. Products are listed alphabetically by drug category and brand name.

BRAND NAME	INGREDIENT/STRENGTH	DOSE
ACETAMINOPHEN		
Anacin Aspirin Free tablets *(Insight Pharmaceuticals)*	Acetaminophen 500mg	**Adults & Peds ≥12 yo:** 2 tabs q6h. **Max:** 8 tabs q24h.
Tylenol 8 Hour caplets *(McNeil Consumer)*	Acetaminophen 650mg	**Adults & Peds ≥12 yo:** 2 tabs q8h prn. **Max:** 6 tabs q24h.
Tylenol 8 Hour geltabs *(McNeil Consumer)*	Acetaminophen 650mg	**Adults & Peds ≥12 yo:** 2 tabs q8h prn. **Max:** 6 tabs q24h.
Tylenol Arthritis caplets *(McNeil Consumer)*	Acetaminophen 650mg	**Adults:** 2 tabs q8h prn. **Max:** 6 tabs q24h.
Tylenol Arthritis geltabs *(McNeil Consumer)*	Acetaminophen 650mg	**Adults:** 2 tabs q8h prn. **Max:** 6 tabs q24h.
Tylenol Children's Meltaways tablets *(McNeil Consumer)*	Acetaminophen 80mg	**Peds 2-3 yo (24-35 lbs):** 2 tabs. **4-5 yo (36-47 lbs):** 3 tabs. **6-8 yo (48-59 lbs):** 4 tabs. **9-10 yo (60-71 lbs):** 5 tabs. **11 yo (72-95 lbs):** 6 tabs. May repeat q4h. **Max:** 5 doses q24h.

DOSING INFORMATION FOR ANALGESIC PRODUCTS (cont.)

Brand Name	Ingredient/Strength	Dose
Tylenol Children's suspension (McNeil Consumer)	Acetaminophen 160mg/5mL	**Peds 2-3 yo (24-35 lbs):** 1 tsp (5mL). **4-5 yo (36-47 lbs):** 1.5 tsp (7.5mL). **6-8 yo (48-59 lbs):** 2 tsp (10mL). **9-10 yo (60-71 lbs):** 2.5 tsp (12.5mL). **11 yo (72-95 lbs):** 3 tsp (15mL). May repeat q4h. **Max:** 5 doses q24h.
Tylenol Extra Strength caplets (McNeil Consumer)	Acetaminophen 500mg	**Adults & Peds ≥12 yo:** 2 tabs q4-6h prn. **Max:** 8 tabs q24h.
Tylenol Extra Strength Cool caplets (McNeil Consumer)	Acetaminophen 500mg	**Adults & Peds ≥12 yo:** 2 tabs q4-6h prn. **Max:** 8 tabs q24h.
Tylenol Extra Strength gelcaps (McNeil Consumer)	Acetaminophen 500mg	**Adults & Peds ≥12 yo:** 2 caps q4-6h prn. **Max:** 8 caps q24h.
Tylenol Extra Strength liquid (McNeil Consumer)	Acetaminophen 1000mg/30mL	**Adults & Peds ≥12 yo:** 2 tbl (30mL) q4-6h prn. **Max:** 8 tbl (120mL) q24h.
Tylenol Extra Strength tablets (McNeil Consumer)	Acetaminophen 500mg	**Adults & Peds ≥12 yo:** 2 tabs q4-6h prn. **Max:** 8 tabs q24h.
Tylenol Infants' suspension (McNeil Consumer)	Acetaminophen 80mg/0.8mL	**Peds 2-3 yo (24-35 lbs):** 1.6 mL q4h prn. **Max:** 5 doses (8mL) q24h.
Tylenol Junior Meltaways tablets (McNeil Consumer)	Acetaminophen 160mg	**Peds 6-8 yo (48-59 lbs):** 2 tabs. **9-10 yo (60-71 lbs):** 2.5 tabs. **11 yo (72-95 lbs):** 3 tabs. **12 yo (≥96 lbs):** 4 tabs. May repeat q4h. **Max:** 5 doses q24h.
Tylenol Regular Strength tablets (McNeil Consumer)	Acetaminophen 325mg	**Adults & Peds ≥12 yo:** 2 tabs q4-6h prn. **Max:** 12 tabs q24h. **Peds 6-11 yo:** 1 tab q4-6h. **Max:** 5 tabs q24h.
NSAIDs		
Advil caplets (Wyeth Consumer Healthcare)	Ibuprofen 200mg	**Adults & Peds ≥12 yo:** 1-2 tabs q4-6h. **Max:** 6 tabs q24h.
Advil Children's Chewables tablets (Wyeth Consumer Healthcare)	Ibuprofen 50mg	**Peds 2-3 yr (24-35 lb):** 2 tabs q6-8h. **4-5 yr (36-47 lb):** 3 tabs q6-8h. **6-8 yr (45-89 lb):** 4 tabs q6-8h. **9-10 yr (60-71 lb):** 5 tabs q6-8h. **11 yr (72-95 lb):** 6 tabs q6-8h. **Max:** 4 doses q24h
Advil Children's suspension (Wyeth Consumer Healthcare)	Ibuprofen 100mg/5mL	**Peds 2-3 yo (24-35 lbs):** 1 tsp (5mL). **4-5 yo (36-47 lbs):** 1.5 tsp (7.5mL). **6-8 yo (48-59 lbs):** 2 tsp (10mL). **9-10 yo (60-71 lbs):** 2.5 tsp (12.5mL). **11 yo (72-95 lbs):** 3 tsp (15mL). May repeat q6-8h. **Max:** 4 doses q24h.
Advil gelcaps (Wyeth Consumer Healthcare)	Ibuprofen 200mg	**Adults & Peds ≥12 yo:** 1-2 caps q4-6h. **Max:** 6 caps q24h.
Advil Infants' Drops (Wyeth Consumer Healthcare)	Ibuprofen 50mg/1.25mL	**Peds 6-11 months (12-17 lbs):** 1.25mL. **12-23 months (18-23 lbs):** 1.875mL. May repeat q6-8h. **Max:** 4 doses q24h.
Advil Junior Strength tablets (Wyeth Consumer Healthcare)	Ibuprofen 100mg	**Peds 6-10 yo (48-71 lbs):** 2 tabs. **11 yo (72-95 lbs):** 3 tabs. May repeat q6-8h. **Max:** 4 doses q24h.
Advil Junior Strength tablets (Wyeth Consumer Healthcare)	Ibuprofen 100mg	**Peds 6-10 yo (48-71 lbs):** 2 tabs. **11 yo (72-95 lbs):** 3 tabs. May repeat q6-8h. **Max:** 4 doses q24h.
Advil liqui-gels (Wyeth Consumer Healthcare)	Ibuprofen 200mg	**Adults & Peds ≥12 yo:** 1-2 caps q4-6h. **Max:** 6 caps q24h.
Advil Migraine capsules (Wyeth Consumer Healthcare)	Ibuprofen 200mg	**Adults:** 2 caps prn. **Max:** 2 caps q24h.
Advil tablets (Wyeth Consumer Healthcare)	Ibuprofen 200mg	**Adults & Peds ≥12 yo:** 1-2 tabs q4-6h. **Max:** 6 tabs q24h.
Aleve caplets (Bayer Healthcare)	Naproxen Sodium 220mg	**Adults ≥65 yo:** 1 tab q12h. **Max:** 2 tabs q24h. **Adults & Peds ≥12 yo:** 1 tab q8-12h. **Max:** 3 tabs q24h.

DOSING INFORMATION FOR ANALGESIC PRODUCTS (cont.)

BRAND NAME	INGREDIENT/STRENGTH	DOSE
Aleve gelcaps *(Bayer Healthcare)*	Naproxen Sodium 220mg	**Adults ≥65 yo:** 1 cap q12h. **Max:** 2 caps q24h. **Adults & Peds ≥12 yo:** 1 cap q8-12h. **Max:** 3 caps q24h.
Aleve tablets *(Bayer Healthcare)*	Naproxen Sodium 220mg	**Adults ≥65 yo:** 1 tab q12h. **Max:** 2 tabs q24h. **Adults & Peds ≥12 yo:** 1 tab q8-12h. **Max:** 3 tabs q24h.
Motrin Children's suspension *(McNeil Consumer)*	Ibuprofen 100mg/5mL	**Peds 2-3 yo (24-35 lbs):** 1 tsp (5mL). **4-5 yo (36-47 lbs):** 1.5 tsp (7.5mL). **6-8 yo (48-59 lbs):** 2 tsp (10mL). **9-10 yo (60-71 lbs):** 2.5 tsp (12.5mL). **11 yo (72-95 lbs):** 3 tsp (15mL). May repeat q6-8h. **Max:** 4 doses q24h.
Motrin IB caplets *(McNeil Consumer)*	Ibuprofen 200mg	**Adults & Peds ≥12 yo:** 1-2 tabs q4-6h. **Max:** 6 tabs q24h.
Motrin IB gelcaps *(McNeil Consumer)*	Ibuprofen 200mg	**Adults & Peds ≥12 yo:** 1-2 tabs q4-6h. **Max:** 6 tabs q24h.
Motrin IB tablets *(McNeil Consumer)*	Ibuprofen 200mg	**Adults & Peds ≥12 yo:** 1-2 tabs q4-6h. **Max:** 6 tabs q24h.
Motrin Infants' Drops *(McNeil Consumer)*	Ibuprofen 50mg/1.25mL	**Peds 6-11 months (12-17 lbs):** 1.25mL. **12-23 months (18-23 lbs):** 1.875mL. May repeat q6-8h. **Max:** 4 doses q24h.
Motrin Junior Strength chewable tablets *(McNeil Consumer)*	Ibuprofen 100mg	**Peds 6-8 yo (48-59 lbs):** 2 tabs. **9-10 yo (60-71 lbs):** 2.5 tabs. **11 yo (72-95 lbs):** 3 tabs. May repeat q6-8h. **Max:** 4 doses q24h.
Nuprin caplets *(Bristol-Myers Squibb)*	Ibuprofen 200mg	**Adults & Peds ≥12 yo:** 1-2 tabs q4-6h. **Max:** 6 tabs q24h.
Nuprin tablets *(Bristol-Myers Squibb)*	Ibuprofen 200mg	**Adults & Peds ≥12 yo:** 1-2 tabs q4-6h. **Max:** 6 tabs q24h.
Orudis KT tablets *(Wyeth Consumer Healthcare)*	Ketoprofen Magnesium 12.5mg	**Adults:** 1-2 tabs q4-6h. **Max:** 6 tabs q24h.
RUBS & LINIMENTS		
Absorbine Jr Deep Pain Relief patches *(W.F. Young)*	Menthol 5.0%	**Adults & Peds ≥12 yo:** Apply to affected area bid.
Absorbine Jr liquid *(W.F. Young)*	Menthol 1.27%	**Adults & Peds ≥2 yo:** Apply to affected area tid-qid.
Absorbine Jr patches *(W.F. Young)*	Menthol 1.3%	**Adults & Peds ≥12 yo:** Apply to affected area bid.
Arthricare Women Extra Moisturizing *(Del Pharmaceuticals)*	Capsaicin 0.025%	**Adults & Peds ≥2 yo:** Apply to affected area tid-qid.
Arthricare Women Multi-Action *(Del Pharmaceuticals)*	Capsaicin/Menthol/Methyl nicotinate 0.025%-1.25%-0.25%	**Adults & Peds ≥2 yo:** Apply to affected area tid-qid.
Arthricare Women Quick Dry Rub *(Del Pharmaceuticals)*	Capsaicin 0.025%	**Adults & Peds ≥2 yo:** Apply to affected area tid-qid.
Arthricare Women Ultra-Strength *(Del Pharmaceuticals)*	Capsaicin/Menthol 0.075%-2%	**Adults & Peds ≥2 yo:** Apply to affected area tid-qid.
Arthritis Hot cream *(Chattem)*	Methyl Salicylate/Menthol 15%-10%	**Adults:** Apply to affected area prn up to qid.
BenGay Pain Relieving Patch *(Pfizer Consumer Healthcare)*	Menthol 1.4%	**Adults & Peds ≥12 yo:** Apply to affected area tid-qid.
BenGay Ultra Strength cream *(Pfizer Consumer Healthcare)*	Methyl Salicylate/Menthol/Camphor 30%-10%-4%	**Adults & Peds ≥12 yo:** Apply to affected area qd-tid.
BenGay Ultra Strength Pain Relieving Patch *(Pfizer Consumer Healthcare)*	Menthol 5%	**Adults & Peds ≥12 yo:** Apply to affected area tid-qid.
BenGay Vanishing sent gel *(Pfizer Consumer Healthcare)*	Menthol 2.5%	**Adults & Peds ≥12 yo:** Apply to affected area tid-qid.
Bodyglide Maximum Strength WarmFX *(Sternoff)*	Methyl Salicylate/Menthol 30%-15%	**Adults:** Apply to affected area prn.
Boericke & Tafel Triflora Arthritis gel *(Boericke & Tafel)*	Symphytum Officinale/Rhus Toxicodendron/Ledum Palustre 10%-5%-2.5%	**Adults & Peds ≥2 yo:** Apply to affected area qd-qid.

DOSING INFORMATION FOR ANALGESIC PRODUCTS (cont.)

BRAND NAME	INGREDIENT/STRENGTH	DOSE
Capzasin-HP *(Chattem)*	Capsaicin 0.075%	**Adults:** Apply to affected area tid-qid.
Capzasin-P *(Chattem)*	Capsaicin 0.025%	**Adults:** Apply to affected area tid-qid.
Emu Lifestyle Active Lifestyle cream *(Emu Lifestyle)*	Menthol 3%	**Adults & Peds ≥10 yo:** Apply to affected area qd-qid.
Emu Lifestyle Active Lifestyle Cream, for Arthritis and Joints *(Emu Lifestyle)*	Trolamine Salicylate 10%	**Adults & Peds ≥10 yo:** Apply to affected area qd-qid.
Flexall Maximum Strength gel *(Chattem)*	Menthol 16%	**Adults & Peds ≥12 yo:** Apply to affected area prn up to qid.
Flexall Maximum Strength gel pump *(Chattem)*	Menthol 16%	**Adults & Peds ≥12 yo:** Apply to affected area prn up to qid.
Heet Pain Relieving Liniment *(Medtech)*	Methyl Salicylate/Camphor/Oleoresin Capsicum 17%-3.6%-.025%	**Adults:** Apply to affected area prn.
Icy Hot balm *(Chattem)*	Methyl Salicyalte/Menthol 29%-7.6%	**Adults:** Apply to affected area prn.
Icy Hot Chill Stick *(Chattem)*	Methyl Salicyalte/Menthol 30%-10%	**Adults:** Apply to affected area prn.
Icy Hot cream *(Chattem)*	Methyl Salicyalte/Menthol 30%-10%	**Adults:** Apply to affected area prn.
Icy Hot Patch Extra Stength (Arm, Neck, Leg) *(Chattem)*	Menthol 5%	**Adults & Peds ≥12 yo:** Apply to affected area prn up to qid.
Icy Hot Patch Extra Stength (Back) *(Chattem)*	Menthol 5%	**Adults & Peds ≥12 yo:** Apply to affected area prn up to qid.
Icy Hot Sleeve (Ankles, Elbows, Knees, Wrist) *(Chattem)*	Menthol 16%	**Adults & Peds ≥12 yo:** Apply to affected area prn up to qid.
Icy Hot Sleeve (Wrists, Small Ankles, and Elbows) *(Chattem)*	Menthol 16%	**Adults & Peds ≥12 yo:** Apply to affected area prn up to qid.
Mobisyl Maximum Strength Arthritis cream *(B.F. Ascher & Company)*	Trolamine Salicylate 10%	**Adults & Peds ≥12 yo:** Apply to affected area tid-qid
Nuprin Arthritis High Potency cream *(Bristol-Myers Squibb)*	Capsaicin 0.075%	**Adults & Peds ≥12 yo:** Apply to affected area tid-qid.
Nuprin Arthritis High Potency patch *(Bristol-Myers Squibb)*	Capsaicin 0.025%	**Adults & Peds ≥4 yo:** Apply to affected area bid.
Nuprin Arthritis Maximum Strength gel *(Bristol-Myers Squibb)*	Capsaicin/Menthol 0.075%-8%	**Adults & Peds ≥2 yo:** Apply to affected area tid-qid.
Nuprin Arthritis Maximum Strength gel *(Bristol-Myers Squibb)*	Capsaicin/Menthol 0.075%-8%	**Adults & Peds ≥2 yo:** Apply to affected area tid-qid.
Super Blue Pain Relief cream *(Spring)*	Menthol 2.75%	**Adults & Peds ≥12 yo:** Apply to affected area tid-qid.
Thera-gesic Maximum Strength cream *(Mission Pharmacal)*	Mehtyl Salicylate/Menthol 15%-1%	**Adults & Peds ≥12 yo:** Apply to affected area tid-qid.
Thera-gesic Plus cream *(Mission Pharmacal)*	Mehtyl Salicylate/Menthol 25%-4%	**Adults & Peds ≥12 yo:** Apply to affected area tid-qid.
Ultra Blue Topical Analgesic gel *(BNG Enterprises)*	Menthol 4%	**Adults & Peds ≥2 yo:** Apply to affected area tid-qid.
Watkins Liniment Pain Relief Spray *(Watkins)*	Camphor/Menthol 3.5%-2.5%	**Adults & Peds ≥2 yo:** Apply to affected area tid-qid.
WellPatch Arthritis Patch, Pain Relieving Pad *(Mentholatum)*	Methyl Salicylate 10%	**Adults & Peds ≥12 yo:** Apply to affected area qd-bid
Zostrix cream *(Rodlen)*	Capsaicin 0.025%	**Adults:** Apply to affected area tid-qid.
Zostrix HP cream *(Rodlen)*	Capsaicin 0.075%	**Adults:** Apply to affected area tid-qid.
SALICYLATES		
Anacin 81 tablets *(Insight Pharmaceuticals)*	Aspirin 81mg	**Adults & Peds ≥12 yo:** 4-8 tabs q4h. **Max:** 48 tabs q24h.
Aspergum chewable tablets *(Schering-Plough)*	Aspirin 227mg	**Adults & Peds ≥12 yo:** 2 tabs q4h. **Max:** 16 tabs q24h.
Bayer Aspirin Extra Strength caplets *(Bayer Healthcare)*	Aspirin 500mg	**Adults & Peds ≥12 yo:** 1-2 tabs q4-6h. **Max:** 8 tabs q24h.
Bayer Aspirin safety coated caplets *(Bayer Healthcare)*	Aspirin 325mg	**Adults & Peds ≥12 yo:** 1-2 tabs q4h or 3 tabs q6h. **Max:** 12 tabs q24h.

DOSING INFORMATION FOR ANALGESIC PRODUCTS (cont.)

Brand Name	Ingredient/Strength	Dose
Bayer Children's Aspirin chewable tablets *(Bayer Healthcare)*	Aspirin 81mg	**Adults & Peds ≥12 yo:** 4-8 tabs q4h. **Max:** 48 tabs q24h.
Bayer Low Dose Aspirin tablets *(Bayer Healthcare)*	Aspirin 81mg	**Adults & Peds ≥12 yo:** 4-8 tabs q4h. **Max:** 48 tabs q24h.
Bayer Original Aspirin tablets *(Bayer Healthcare)*	Aspirin 325mg	**Adults & Peds ≥12 yo:** 1-2 tabs q4h or 3 tabs q6h. **Max:** 12 tabs q24h.
Doan's Extra Strength caplets *(Novartis Consumer Health)*	Magnesium Salicylate Tetrahydrate 580mg	**Adults & Peds ≥12 yo:** 2 tabs q6h. **Max:** 8 tabs q24h.
Doan's Regular Strength caplets *(Novartis Consumer Health)*	Magnesium Salicylate Tetrahydrate 377mg	**Adults & Peds ≥12 yo:** 2 tabs q4h. **Max:** 12 tabs q24h.
Ecotrin Adult Low Strength tablets *(GlaxoSmithKline Consumer Healthcare)*	Aspirin 81mg	**Adults:** 4-8 tabs q4h. **Max:** 48 tabs q24h.
Ecotrin Enteric Low Strength tablets *(GlaxoSmithKline Consumer Healthcare)*	Aspirin 81mg	**Adults:** 4-8 tabs q4h. **Max:** 48 tabs q24h.
Ecotrin Enteric Regular Strength tablets *(GlaxoSmithKline Consumer Healthcare)*	Aspirin 325mg	**Adults & Peds ≥12 yo:** 1-2 tabs q4h. **Max:** 12 tabs q24h.
Ecotrin Maximum Strength tablets *(GlaxoSmithKline Consumer Healthcare)*	Aspirin 500mg	**Adults & Peds ≥12 yo:** 2 tabs q6h. **Max:** 8 tabs q24h.
Ecotrin Regular Strength tablets *(GlaxoSmithKline Consumer Healthcare)*	Aspirin 325mg	**Adults & Peds ≥12 yo:** 1-2 tabs q4h. **Max:** 12 tabs q24h.
Halfprin 162mg tablets *(Kramer Laboratories)*	Aspirin 162mg	**Adults & Peds ≥12 yo:** 2-4 tabs q4h. **Max:** 24 tabs q24h.
Halfprin 81mg tablets *(Kramer Laboratories)*	Aspirin 81mg	**Adults & Peds ≥12 yo:** 4-8 tabs q4h. **Max:** 48 tabs q24h.
St. Joseph Adult Low Strength chewable tablets *(McNeil Consumer)*	Aspirin 81mg	**Adults & Peds ≥12 yo:** 4-8 tabs q4h. **Max:** 48 tabs q24h.
St. Joseph Adult Low Strength tablets *(McNeil Consumer)*	Aspirin 81mg	**Adults & Peds ≥12 yo:** 4-8 tabs q4h. **Max:** 48 tabs q24h.
SALICYLATES, BUFFERED		
Ascriptin Maximum Strength tablets *(Novartis Consumer Health)*	Aspirin Buffered with Maalox/Calcium Carbonate 500mg	**Adults & Peds ≥12 yo:** 2 tabs q4h. **Max:** 8 tabs q24h.
Ascriptin Regular Strength tablets *(Novartis Consumer Health)*	Aspirin Buffered with Maalox/Calcium Carbonate 325mg	**Adults & Peds ≥12 yo:** 2 tabs q4h. **Max:** 12 tabs q24h.
Bayer Extra Strength Plus caplets *(Bayer Healthcare)*	Aspirin Buffered with Calcium Carbonate 500mg	**Adults & Peds ≥12 yo:** 1-2 tabs q4-6h. **Max:** 8 tabs q24h.
Bufferin Extra Strength tablets *(Bristol-Myers Squibb)*	Aspirin Bufferred with Calcium Carbonate/Magnesium Oxide/Magnesium Carbonate 500mg	**Adults & Peds ≥12 yo:** 2 tabs q6h. **Max:** 8 tabs q24h.
Bufferin tablets *(Bristol-Myers Squibb)*	Aspirin Bufferred with Calcium Carbonate/Magnesium Oxide/Magnesium Carbonate 325mg	**Adults & Peds ≥12 yo:** 2 tabs q4h. **Max:** 12 tabs q24h.

Allergic and Non-allergic Conjunctivitis

The eye is an extension of the central nervous system that is formed from four major tissue layers: the conjunctiva, which is only present anteriorly; the cornea and sclera; the uvea; and, innermost, the retina. The anterior aspect of the eye is protected by the eyelids and by the conjunctiva, which covers the anterior ocular surface other than the cornea (i.e., the bulbar conjunctiva). The conjunctiva also lines the inner surfaces of the eyelids that lie in apposition to the surface of the eye (i.e., the palpebral, or tarsal, conjunctiva). Because it is thin, directly exposed to the environment, and immunologically active, the conjunctiva is the most common site of allergic eye disease. Although corneal involvement by severe allergic conjunctival disease is potentially vision threatening, most allergic conjunctival disorders are relatively mild. Immunologic disorders involving the uvea, the layer of the eye that includes the posterior iris, the ciliary body, and the choroids, are more likely to cause sight-threatening disease. However, these uveal disorders are not primarily the result of environmental exposures and are not within the spectrum of ocular allergy.

Ocular allergy includes several conditions that occur along a spectrum of specific immunologic changes within the conjunctiva. Mast cell-mediated and immunoglobulin E (IgE)-mediated reactions are the most common hypersensitivity responses of the eye. An increased prevalence of mast cells in the conjunctiva is characteristic of milder allergic eye conditions. In contrast, a predominantly lymphocytic immune response is characteristic of severe allergic conjunctival disease. Corneal involvement is substantially more likely in such disorders, and may pose a threat to vision.

Seasonal allergic conjunctivitis (SAC) is a typical mast cell-/IgE-mediated type I immediate hypersensitivity reaction that is the ocular counterpart to hay fever. Ragweed is the most common cause of allergic conjunctivitis and rhinitis, although grass pollens appear to be associated with more ocular symptoms than other allergens. Histologically, there is a discernible increase in the conjunctival population of mast cells and eosinophils. These and other cells interact and release a variety of allergic mediators, such as histamine, leukotrienes, and prostaglandins, in response to various airborne allergens.

Perennial allergic conjunctivitis (PAC) is a variant of SAC. PAC is caused by a constantly present allergen and is associated with a persistent increase in the number of allergy-mediating cells throughout the year, although patients may experience a seasonal exacerbation of symptoms. Dust mites, animal dander, and feathers are the most commonly implicated allergens in perennial allergic conjunctivitis.

In vernal keratoconjunctivitis (VKC), there is a seasonally recurrent increase in mast cells, eosinophils, and lymphocytes. VKC may represent a hypersensitivity reaction that is initially mediated by mast cells and IgE and then becomes more lymphocyte predominant as inflammation becomes chronic. "Vernal" refers to the frequent springtime onset of VKC. Eosinophils appear important in the pathogenesis of VKC, because degranulated eosinophils and their toxic products (e.g., major basic protein) are found in the conjunctiva and in the periphery of corneal ulcers in severe forms of VKC [1].

Giant papillary conjunctivitis (GPC) is associated with continuous contact between the conjunctiva of the upper eyelid and a foreign body such as an ocular prosthesis, exposed suture, or, most often, contact lens. In GPC, basophils, eosinophils, plasma cells, and lymphocytes infiltrate the conjunctiva, suggesting a mixed mast cell- and lymphocyte-mediated process. In contact lens-associated GPC, the polymers of the lens itself, preservatives in contact lens solutions (particularly thimerosal), and proteinaceous deposits on the surface of the lens are potential, although controversial, stimulating antigens.

Atopic keratoconjunctivitis (AKC) is mediated by a mixture of mast cell, IgE, and lymphocytic interactions, as reflected by chronic infiltrations of basophils, eosinophils, plasma cells, and lymphocytes in the conjunctiva. AKC typically occurs in individuals with atopy, ie, extensive allergic disorders, especially eczema and asthma.

There are a number of ophthalmic decongestants (naphazoline, oxymetazoline, phenylephrine, tetrahydrozoline) and ophthalmic decongestant/antihistamine combinations available OTC to treat the symptoms of allergic conjunctivitis.

NAPHAZOLINE (OPHTHALMIC)

PHARMACOLOGY

Naphazoline is a direct-acting sympathomimetic amine. It acts on alpha-adrenergic receptors in the arterioles of the conjunctiva to produce vasoconstriction, resulting in decreased conjunctival congestion.

INDICATIONS

Ocular redness (treatment)—Naphazoline is indicated for the temporary relief of redness associated with minor irritations of the eye, such as those caused by pollen-related allergies, colds, dust, smog, wind, swimming, or wearing contact lenses.

CONTRAINDICATIONS

Except under special circumstances, this medication should not be used when the following medical problem exists:

- Glaucoma, narrow-angle, or predisposition to—*major clinical significance* (naphazoline may cause significant mydriasis, which may precipitate an acute attack of narrow-angle glaucoma).

Risk-benefit should be considered when the following medical problems exist:

- Cardiovascular disease (systemic absorption of naphazoline may cause cardiac irregularities).
- Diabetes mellitus (systemic absorption of naphazoline may cause minimal hyperglycemia).
- Eye disease, serious, or infection or injury.
- Hypertension (systemic absorption of naphazoline may cause hypertension).
- Hyperthyroidism.
- Sensitivity to naphazoline.

WARNINGS/PRECAUTIONS

Patients sensitive to other nasal decongestants may be sensitive to this medication also.

Pregnancy: FDA Category C. Naphazoline may be systemically absorbed. Studies have not been done in either animals or humans.

Breastfeeding: It is not known whether naphazoline is distributed into breast milk, but problems in humans have not been documented. However, naphazoline may be systemically absorbed.

DRUG INTERACTIONS

Antidepressants, tricyclic; maprotiline: If significant systemic absorption of ophthalmic naphazoline occurs, concurrent use of tricyclic antidepressants or maprotiline may potentiate the pressor effect of naphazoline.

ADVERSE REACTIONS

Those indicating need for medical attention:

With excessive dosage and/or prolonged use:

Hyperemia, reactive (increase in eye irritation).

Symptoms of systemic absorption:

Dizziness, headache, increased sweating, nausea, nervousness, weakness.

Those indicating need for medical attention only if they continue or are bothersome: Incidence less frequent or rare:

Blurred vision, large pupils.

ADMINISTRATION AND DOSAGE

General Dosing Information

Treatment should not be continued for more than 72 hours, unless otherwise directed by a physician. Although some of the manufacturers recommend that patients not wear soft contact lenses during treatment with naphazoline ophthalmic solution, US Pharmacopeia (USP) medical experts do not believe this precaution is necessary, unless the patient has corneal epithelial problems and the medication is to be used more often than once every 1 to 2 hours. No significant problems have been documented with ophthalmic solutions containing 0.03% or less of benzalkonium chloride as a preservative when they are used as eye drops in patients with no significant corneal surface problem.

Adults: 1 drop of a 0.012% solution up to 4 times a day as needed.

OXYMETAZOLINE (OPHTHALMIC)

PHARMACOLOGY

Oxymetazoline is a direct-acting sympathomimetic amine. It acts on alpha-adrenergic receptors in the arterioles of the conjunctiva to produce vasoconstriction, resulting in decreased conjunctival congestion.

INDICATIONS

Ocular redness (treatment)—Oxymetazoline is indicated for the temporary relief of redness associated with minor irritations of the eye, such as those caused by pollen-related allergies, colds, dust, smog, wind, swimming, or wearing contact lenses.

CONTRAINDICATIONS

Risk-benefit should be considered when the following medical problems exist:

- Coronary artery disease; heart disease, including angina; hypertension (if significant systemic absorption of ophthalmic oxymetazoline occurs, condition may be exacerbated due to drug-induced cardiovascular effects).

- Eye disease, infection, or injury (may mask symptoms and delay treatment).

- Glaucoma, narrow-angle, or predisposition to (may precipitate an attack by dilating pupil).

- Hyperthyroidism (may exacerbate existing tachycardia or elevated blood pressure).

- Sensitivity to oxymetazoline.

WARNINGS/PRECAUTIONS

Patients sensitive to other nasal decongestants may be sensitive to this medication also.

Pregnancy: Oxymetazoline may be systemically absorbed. However, adequate and well-controlled studies in humans have not been done.

Breastfeeding: Oxymetazoline may be systemically absorbed. However, problems in humans have not been documented.

DRUG INTERACTIONS

Antidepressants, tricyclic; maprotiline: If significant systemic absorption of ophthalmic oxymetazoline occurs, concurrent use may potentiate the pressor effect of oxymetazoline.

ADVERSE REACTIONS

Those indicating need for medical attention:

With excessive dosage and/or prolonged use:

Hyperemia, reactive (increase in irritation or redness of eyes).

Symptoms of systemic absorption:

Fast, irregular, or pounding heartbeat; headache or lightheadedness; nervousness; trembling; trouble in sleeping.

ADMINISTRATION AND DOSAGE

General Dosing Information

Treatment should not be continued for more than 72 hours unless otherwise directed by a physician. Although the manufacturer recommends that patients remove soft contact lenses before using oxymetazoline ophthalmic solution, US Pharmacopeia (USP) medical experts do not believe this precaution is necessary unless the patient has corneal epithelial problems. No significant problems have been documented with ophthalmic solutions containing 0.03% or less of benzalkonium chloride as a preservative when they are used as eye drops in patients with no significant corneal surface problem.

Adults/Pediatrics >6 years of age: 1 drop of a 0.025% solution every 6 hours as needed.

NAPHAZOLINE PRODUCTS	
Brand Name	**Dosage Form**
All Clear (Baush & Lomb)	**Solution:** 0.012%
Clear Eyes (Medtech)	**Solution:** 0.012%
Naphcon (Alcon)	**Solution:** 0.012%
Rhoto V (Rhoto)	**Solution:** 0.012%

PHENYLEPHRINE (OPHTHALMIC)

PHARMACOLOGY

Phenylephrine is primarily a direct-acting sympathomimetic amine, which stimulates alpha-adrenergic receptors.

Mydriatic: Phenylephrine acts on alpha-adrenergic receptors in the dilator muscle of the pupil, producing contraction.

Decongestant, ophthalmic: Phenylephrine acts on alpha-adrenergic receptors in the arterioles of the conjunctiva, producing constriction.

INDICATIONS

OTC strength:

Ocular redness (treatment)—The 0.12% phenylephrine ophthalmic solution is indicated to provide temporary relief of redness associated with minor eye irritations, such as those caused by hay fever, colds, dust, wind, swimming, sun, smog, smoke, or wearing contact lenses.

Prescription strength:

Mydriasis, in diagnostic procedures—Refraction: Prior to determination of refractive errors, the 2.5% phenylephrine ophthalmic solution may be used effectively with homatropine, atropine, cyclopentolate, or tropicamide. Ophthalmoscopy: The 2.5% phenylephrine ophthalmic solution is indicated to produce mydriasis for ophthalmoscopic examination. Retinoscopy (shadow test): The 2.5% phenylephrine ophthalmic solution may be used alone when dilation of the pupil without cycloplegic action is desired for retinoscopy (shadow test). Blanching test: The 2.5% phenylephrine ophthalmic solution is indicated for the blanching test. If blanching occurs, the congestion is superficial and probably does not indicate iritis.

Mydriasis, preoperative—The 2.5% and 10% phenylephrine ophthalmic solutions are indicated to produce dilation of the pupil prior to intraocular surgery.

Uveitis with posterior synechiae (treatment); *synechiae, posterior* (prophylaxis)—The 2.5% and 10% phenylephrine ophthalmic solutions are indicated in patients with uveitis when synechiae are present or may develop. The formation of synechiae may be prevented by concurrent use of either of these concentrations with atropine to produce wide dilation of the pupil; however, the vasoconstrictor effect of phenylephrine may be antagonistic to the increase of local blood flow in uveal inflammation.

CONTRAINDICATIONS

Risk-benefit should be considered when the following medical problems exist:

For 2.5% or 10% strengths only:

- Arteriosclerotic changes, advanced.
- Cardiac disease.
- Diabetes mellitus.
- Glaucoma, angle-closure, predisposition to—*major clinical significance.*
- Hypertension.
- Idiopathic orthostatic hypotension (a marked increase in blood pressure may occur).
- Sensitivity to phenylephrine or sulfites.

PRECAUTIONS TO CONSIDER

Drug Interactions: See chart on page 256.

Pregnancy: FDA Category C. Studies have not been done in humans; however, ophthalmic phenylephrine may be systemically absorbed.

Breastfeeding: It is not known whether phenylephrine is distributed into breast milk, and problems in humans have not been documented; however, ophthalmic phenylephrine may be systemically absorbed.

Pediatrics: The recommended dosage should not be exceeded in pediatric patients, especially for the 2.5% and 10% solutions, since high doses of phenylephrine can increase blood pressure and cause irregular heartbeat. In addition, repeated use of 2.5% or 10% phenylephrine may result in rebound miosis and a reduced mydriatic effect. Moreover, the 10% phenylephrine solution is not recommended for use in infants, since a pronounced increase in blood pressure may occur. Also, the 2.5% and 10% concentrations are not recommended for use in low birth weight infants.

Geriatrics: Cardiovascular reactions, such as marked increase in blood pressure, syncope, myocardial infarction, tachycardia, arrhythmia, and fatal subarachnoid hemorrhage, have occurred primarily in elderly patients. In addition, repeated use of 2.5% or 10% phenylephrine, especially in older patients, may result in rebound miosis and a reduced mydriatic effect. Also, older patients may develop transient pigment floaters in the aqueous humor 40 to 45 minutes following administration of the 2.5% or 10% concentrations, the appearance of which may be similar to anterior uveitis or to a microscopic hyphema.

ADVERSE REACTIONS

Those indicating need for medical attention: Incidence less frequent with 10% solution; incidence rare with 2.5% or weaker solution

Dizziness; fast, irregular, or pounding heartbeat; increase in blood pressure; increase in sweating; paleness; trembling.

Those indicating need for medical attention only if they continue or are bothersome:

Incidence more frequent with 2.5% or 10% solution

Burning or stinging of eyes; headache; brow ache; sensitivity of eyes to light; watering of eyes.

Incidence less frequent:

Eye irritation not present before therapy.

ADMINISTRATION AND DOSAGE

General Dosing Information

Some manufacturers recommend a dosage of 2 drops of an ophthalmic solution at appropriate intervals, although the conjunctival sac will usually hold only 1 drop. To avoid excessive systemic absorption, the patient should apply digital pressure to the lacrimal sac during and for 2 or 3 minutes following instillation of the medication.

Although some manufacturers recommend that patients not wear soft contact lenses during treatment with phenylephrine ophthalmic solution, US Pharmacopeia (USP) medical experts do not believe this precaution is necessary unless the patient has corneal

OXYMETAZOLINE PRODUCTS	
Brand Name	**Dosage Form**
Ocuclear (Schering)	**Solution:** 0.025%
Visine L.R. (Pfizer)	**Solution:** 0.025%

epithelial problems and the medication is to be used more often than once every 1 to 2 hours. No significant problems have been documented with ophthalmic solutions containing 0.03% or less of benzalkonium chloride as a preservative that are used in patients with no significant corneal surface problems.

For the 2.5% and 10% solutions (available as prescription only): To prevent pain and subsequent lacrimation on administration, a suitable topical anesthetic may be applied a few minutes before use of phenylephrine solution. The recommended dosage should not be exceeded, especially in children and in individuals with high blood pressure or heart disease, since high doses of phenylephrine can increase blood pressure and cause irregular heartbeat. Repeated use of phenylephrine, especially in older patients, may result in rebound miosis and a reduced mydriatic effect.

Solution (OTC strength)

For ocular redness (treatment):

Adults/Pediatrics: 1 drop of a 0.12% solution to conjunctiva every 3 to 4 hours as needed.

Solution (prescription strength)

For mydriasis/vasoconstriction:

Adults: 1 drop of a 2.5% to 10% solution to conjunctiva; repeat in 1 hour if necessary.

Pediatrics: 1 drop of a 2.5% solution to conjunctiva; repeat in 1 hour if necessary.

For chronic mydriasis:

Adults: 1 drop of a 2.5% to 10% solution to conjunctiva 2 or 3 times a day.

Pediatrics: 1 drop of a 2.5% solution to conjunctiva 2 or 3 times a day.

For mydriasis, preoperative:

Adults: 1 drop of a 2.5% to 10% solution to conjunctiva 30 to 60 minutes prior to surgery.

Pediatrics: 1 drop of a 2.5% solution to conjunctiva 30 to 60 minutes prior to surgery.

For refraction:

Adults: 1 drop of a cycloplegic followed in 5 minutes by 1 drop of a 2.5% solution of phenylephrine to conjunctiva.

Pediatrics: 1 drop of a 1% solution of atropine followed in 10 to 15 minutes by 1 drop of a 2.5% solution of phenylephrine to conjunctiva, followed by a second drop of a 1% solution of atropine in 5 to 10 minutes. In 1 to 2 hours, the eyes are ready for refraction.

For uveitis with posterior synechiae (treatment) or synechiae, posterior (prophylaxis):

Adults: 1 drop of a 2.5% to 10% solution to conjunctiva; repeat in 1 hour if necessary, not to exceed 3 times a day.

Pediatrics: 1 drop of a 2.5% solution to conjunctiva; repeat in 1 hour if necessary. Treatment may be continued the following day if necessary.

For ophthalmoscopy:

Adults/Pediatrics: 1 drop of a 2.5% solution to conjunctiva 15 to 30 minutes prior to examination.

For retinoscopy (shadow test):

Adults/Pediatrics: 1 drop of a 2.5% solution to conjunctiva.

For blanching test:

Adults/Pediatrics: 1 drop of a 2.5% solution to the infected eye.

TETRAHYDROZOLINE (OPHTHALMIC)

PHARMACOLOGY

Decongestant (ophthalmic): Tetrahydrozoline acts on alpha-adrenergic receptors in the arterioles of the conjunctiva, producing constriction.

INDICATIONS

Ocular redness (treatment)—Tetrahydrozoline ophthalmic solution is indicated to provide temporary relief of redness associated with minor eye irritations, such as those caused by hay fever, colds, dust, wind, swimming, sun, smog, smoke, or wearing contact lenses.

CONTRAINDICATIONS

Risk-benefit should be considered when the following medical problems exist:

- Cardiac disease.

- Glaucoma, angle-closure, or predisposition to.

- Sensitivity to tetrahydrozoline.

PRECAUTIONS TO CONSIDER

Pregnancy: Effects are unknown.

Breastfeeding: It is not known whether phenylephrine is distributed into breast milk; problems in humans have not been documented.

ADVERSE REACTIONS

Those indicating need for medical attention only if they continue or are bothersome:

Burning or stinging of eyes; headache; browache; sensitivity of eyes to light; watering of eyes.

Incidence less frequent:

Eye irritation not present before therapy.

ADMINISTRATION AND DOSAGE

Solution

For ocular redness (treatment):

Adults/Pediatrics: 1-2 drop to the conjunctiva every 4 hours.

PHENYLEPHRINE PRODUCTS	
Brand Name	**Dosage Form**
Prefrin Liquifilm (Allergan)	Solution: 0.12%
TETRAHYDROZOLINE PRODUCTS	
Brand Name	**Dosage Form**
Visine Original (Pfizer)	Solution: 0.05%

Drug Interactions for Phenylephrine (ophthalmic; for 2.5% or 10% strengths only)

Precipitant Drug	Object Drug	Effect On Object Drug	Description
Guanadrel Guanethidine	Phenylephrine	↑	If significant systemic absorption of ophthalmic phenylephrine occurs, concurrent use of guanadrel or guanethidine may increase the mydriatic effect of phenylephrine; also, concurrent use may potentiate the pressor effect of phenylephrine, possibly resulting in hypertension and cardiac arrhythmias.
MAOIs (furazolidone, procarbazine, selegiline) Maprotiline Tricyclic antidepressants	Phenylephrine	↑	If significant systemic absorption of ophthalmic phenylephrine occurs, concurrent use of these medications may potentiate the pressor effect of phenylephrine; in addition, if ophthalmic phenylephrine is administered during or within 21 days following the administration of MAOIs, careful supervision with possible adjustment of dosage is recommended, since exaggerated adrenergic response may occur.

DOSING INFORMATION FOR OPHTHALMIC DECONGESTANT/ANTIHISTAMINE PRODUCTS

The following table provides a quick comparison of the ingredients and dosages of common brand-name OTC drugs. Products are listed alphabetically by generic ingredient.

Brand Name	Generic Ingredient/Strength	Dose
NAPHAZOLINE		
Clear Eyes drops (Prestige Brands)	Naphazoline HCl/Glycerin 0.012%-0.2%	**Adults:** Instil 1-2 drops to affected eye qid.
Clear Eyes ACR, Seasonal Relief (Prestige Brands)	Naphazoline HCl/Glycerin/Zinc Sulfate 0.012%-0.2%-0.25%	**Adults:** Instil 1-2 drops to affected eye qid
All Clear AR Maximum Redness Relief Lubricant drops (Bausch & Lomb)	Naphazoline HCl/Hydroxypropyl Methylcellulose/Benzalkonium Chloride 0.03%-0.5%-0.01%	**Adults:** Instil 1-2 drops to affected eye qid.
Clear Eyes for Dry Eyes, Plus Removes Redness (Prestige Brands)	Naphazoline HCl/Hypromellose/Glycerine 0.012%-0.8%-0.25%	**Adults:** Instil 1-2 drops to affected eye prn.
Naphcon-A Allergy Relief drops (Alcon)	Naphazoline HCl/Pheniramine Maleate 0.025%-0.3%	**Adults:** Apply 1-2 drops to affected eye qid.
Visine-A Allergy Relief drops (Pfizer Consumer Healthcare)	Naphazoline HCl/Pheniramine Maleate 0.025%-0.3%	**Adults & Peds ≥6 yo:** Instil 1-2 drops to affected eye qid.
Opcon-A Allergy Relief drops (Bausch & Lomb)	Naphazoline HCl/Pheniramine Maleate 0.03%-0.32%	**Adults & Peds ≥6 yo:** Instil 1-2 drops to affected eye qid.
All Clear Redness & Irritation Relief drops (Bausch & Lomb)	Naphazoline HCl/Polyethylene Glycol 300/Benzalkonium Chloride 0.012%-0.2%-0.01%	**Adults:** Instil 1-2 drops to affected eye qid.
Rohto V F Lubricant/Redness Reliever drops (Rohto Pharmaceutical)	Naphazoline HCl/Polysorbate 80 0.012%-0.2%	**Adults:** Instil 1-2 drops to affected eye qid.
OXYMETAZOLINE		
Visine L.R. Redness Reliever drops (Pfizer Consumer Healthcare)	Oxymetazoline HCl 0.025%	**Adults & Peds ≥6 yo:** Instil 1-2 drops to affected eye prn
PHENYLEPHRINE		
Allergan Relief Redness Reliever & Lubricant Eye Drops (Allergan)	Phenylephrine HCl/Polyvinyl Alcohol 0.12%-1.4%	**Adults:** Instil 1-2 drops to affected eye qid.
TETRAHYDROZOLINE		
Visine Original drops (Pfizer Consumer Healthcare)	Tetrahydrozoline HCl 0.05%	**Adults:** Instil 1-2 drops to affected eye qid
Visine Advanced Redness Reliever drops (Pfizer Consumer Healthcare)	Tetrahydrozoline HCl/Polyethylene Glycol 400/Povidone/Dextran 70 0.05%-1%-1%-0.1%	**Adults:** Instil 1-2 drops to affected eye qid.
Murine Plus Tears Plus Eye Drops (Prestige Brands)	Tetrahydrozoline HCl/Polyvinyl Alcohol/Povidone 0.05%-0.5%-0.6%	**Adults:** Instil 1-2 drops to affected eye qid.
Visine A.C. Astringent Redness Reliever drops (Pfizer Consumer Healthcare)	Tetrahydrozoline HCl/Zinc Sulfate 0.05%-0.25%	**Adults:** Instil 1-2 drops to affected eye qid.

Blepharitis

Blepharitis is defined as an inflammation of the lash follicles at the eyelid margins, caused by an excess growth of the bacteria normally present on the skin. Blepharitis is often caused by seborrheic dermatitis or a bacterial infection. Blepharitis is characterized by excess oil production in the glands near the eyelid, which causes bacterial overgrowth. Symptoms of blephartis included crusty, reddened, swollen, itching, and burning eyelids. Untreated blepharitis may lead to stypes, chalazia, corneal ulcers, conjunctivitis, loss of eyelashes, and scarring of the eyelids. The primary treatment is careful daily cleansing of the lid margins to remove the skin oil that bacteria need to survive. Lid scrub products are available OTC to treat blepharitis.

DOSING INFORMATION FOR LID SCRUB PRODUCTS

The following table provides a quick comparison of the ingredients and dosages of common brand-name OTC products.

BRAND NAME	INGREDIENT/STRENGTH	DOSE
Eye Scrub (*Novartis*)	Purified water, peg-200 glyceryl tallowate, disodium laureth sulfosuccinate, cocamidopropylamine oxide, peg-78 glyceryl cocoate, benzyl alcohol, edetate disodium.	**Adults:** Close the eye and gently cleanse lids using side to side strokes. Rinse lids with warm water.
OCuSOFT Lid Scrub (*Ocusoft*)	Deionized water, peg-80, sorbitan laurate, sodium trideceth sulfate, peg-150 distearate, cocamidopropyl hydroxysultaine, lauroamphocarboxyglycinate, sodium laureth-13 carboxylate, peg-15 tallow polyamine, quaternium-15.	**Adults:** Close the eye and gently cleanse lids using side to side strokes. Rinse lids with warm water.

Contact Lens Care

Contact lens care is necessary to prevent complications such as infection. There are different types of contact lenses, and they require different types of care and thus the use of specific kinds of products. The numerous OTC products available for contact lens care include surfactant cleaning solutions, saline solutions, enzymatic cleansers, chemical disinfection systems, and rewetting solutions.

DOSING INFORMATION FOR CONTENT LENS CARE PRODUCTS

The following table provides a quick comparison of the ingredients and dosages of common brand-name OTC products. Entries are listed alphabetically by category and brand name.

BRAND NAME	INGREDIENT/STRENGTH	DOSE
ENZYMATIC CLEANERS		
AMO Complete, Weekly Enzymatic Cleaner (AMO)	Subitilisin A	**Adults:** Rinse contact lens as directed
AMO ProFree/ GP Weekly Enzymatic Cleaner, Tablets (AMO)	Papain	**Adults:** Rinse contact lens as directed.
AMO Ultrazyme Enzymatic Cleaner, Tablets (AMO)	Subitilisin A	**Adults:** Rinse contact lens as directed
ReNu One Step Enzymatic Cleaner, Tablets (Bausch & Lomb)	Proteolytic Enzyme	**Adults:** Rinse contact lens as directed.
REWETTING SOLUTIONS		
Allergan Refresh Contacts drops (Allergan)	Carboxymethylcellulose sodium, sodium chloride, boric acid, sodium borate decahydrate, potassium chloride, calcium chloride, magnesium chloride, purified water, Purite 0.005%.	**Adults:** Apply 1-2 drops to affected eye prn.
AMO Complete Blink-N-Clean Lens Drops For Soft Contact Lenses (AMO)	Purified water, sodium chloride, polyhexamethylene biguanide 0.0001% tromethamine, hydroxypropyl methylcellulose, tyloxapol, edetate disodium	**Adults:** Apply 1-2 drops to affected eye qid.
AMO Complete Moisture Plus Lubricating and Rewetting Drops (AMO)	Purified water, sodium chloride, polyhexamethylene biguanide 0.0001%, tromethamine, hydroxypropyl methylcellulose, tyloxapol as a surfactant, edetate disodium	**Adults:** Apply 1-2 drops to affected eye qid.
AMO Lens Plus Rewetting Drops (AMO)	Sodium Chloride and Boric Acid	**Adults:** Apply 1-2 drops to affected eye prn.
Clear eyes CLR Contact Lens Relief Eye Drops (Abbott Laboratories)	Sodium chloride, hydroxypropyl methylcellulose, glycerin, sorbic acid, edetate disodium	**Adults:** Apply 1-2 drops to affected eye prn.
Clerz Plus Lens Drops (Alcon Laboratories)	Sodium chloride, edetate disodium 0.05%, polyquad 0.001%, Clens®-100 (PEG-11 Lauryl Ether Carboxylic Acid), tetronic 1304	**Adults:** Apply 2 drops to affected eye qid.
Opti-Free Express Rewetting Drops (Alcon)	Sodium chloride, edetate disodium 0.05%, polyquad 0.001%	**Adults:** Apply drops to affected eye qd.
ReNu MultiPlus Lubricating & Rewetting Drops (Bausch & Lomb)	Povidone, boric acid, potassium chloride, sodium borate, sodium chloride, edetate disodium, sorbic acid	**Adults:** Apply 2-3 drops to affected eye prn.
ReNu Rewetting Drops (Bausch & Lomb)	Boric acid, sorbic acid, edetate disodium	**Adults:** Apply 2-3 drops to affected eye prn.
Sensitive Eyes Drops for Rewetting Soft Lenses to Minimize Dryness (Bausch & Lomb)	Boric acid, sodium borate, sodium chloride, sorbic acid (0.1%, preservative), edetate disodium (0.025%, preservative)	**Adults:** Apply 2-3 drops to affected eye prn.
Visine for Contacts Lubricating & Rewetting Drops (Pfizer Consumer Healthcare)	Hypromellose, Glycerin, Potassium Sorbate, Edetate Disodium	**Adults:** Apply 1-2 drops to affected eye prn.

DOSING INFORMATION FOR CONTENT LENS CARE PRODUCTS (cont.)

BRAND NAME	INGREDIENT/STRENGTH	DOSE
RINSING/STORAGE/CLEANSING SOLUTIONS		
AMO Comfort Care Wetting & Soaking Solution (AMO)	Polyvinyl alcohol, edetate disodium and benzalkonium chloride 0.004%	**Adults:** Rinse contact lens as directed.
AMO Complete Moisture Plus, Multi-Purpose Solution (AMO)	Hydroxypropyl methylcellulose, propylene glycol, phosphate and taurine, polyhexamethylene biguanide 0.0001%, poloxamer 237, edetate disodium, sodium chloride, potassium chloride, purified water	**Adults:** Rinse contact lens as directed.
AMO Complete, Multi-Purpose Solution (AMO)	HPMC and propylene glycol, potassium chloride, sodium chloride, phosphate, taurine, poloxamer 237 and edetate disodium, PHMB (0.0001%), phosphate, taurine	**Adults:** Rinse contact lens as directed.
AMO Lens Plus Daily Cleaner (AMO)	Cocoamphocarboxyglycinate, sodium lauryl sulfate, hexylene glycol, sodium chloride, sodium phosphate	**Adults:** Rinse contact lens as directed.
AMO Lens Plus Sterile Saline Solution (AMO)	Sodium chloride, boric acid and nitrogen (nonflammable)	**Adults:** Rinse contact lens as directed.
AMO Resolve/GP Daily Cleaner (AMO)	Cocoamphocarboxyglycinate, sodium lauryl sulfate, hexylene glycol, alkyl ether sulfate	**Adults:** Rinse contact lens as directed.
AMO UltraCare Disinfecting Solution/ Neutralizer (AMO)	Hydrogen peroxide 3%, catalase, hydroxypropyl methylcellulose, cyanocobalamin	**Adults:** Rinse contact lens as directed.
AMO Wet-N-Soak Plus Wetting and Soaking Solution (AMO)	Polyvinyl alcohol, edetate disodium, and benzalkonium chloride 0.003% in a sterile, buffered, isotonic solution	**Adults:** Rinse contact lens as directed.
Aosept Clear Care, No Rub Cleaning & Disinfecting Solution (CIBA Vision)	Micro-filtered hydrogen peroxide (3%), sodium chloride (0.79%), stabilized with phosphonic acid, A phospate buffered system, fluronic 17R4	**Adults:** Rinse contact lens qd.
Aosept Disinfectant for Soft Contact Lenses (CIBA Vision)	Microfiltered hydrogen peroxide/sodium chloride 3%-0.85%	**Adults:** Rinse contact lens as directed.
Bausch & Lomb Concentrated Cleaner for Rigid Gas Permeable and Hard Contact Lenses (Bausch & Lomb)	Alkyl ether sulfate, ethoxylated alkyl phenol, tri-quaternary cocoa-based phospholipid silica gel	**Adults:** Rinse contact lens as directed.
Bausch & Lomb Wetting and Soaking Solution for Rigid Gas Permeable and Hard Contact Lenses (Bausch & Lomb)	Cationic cellulose derivative, edetate disodium, chlorhexidine gluconate	**Adults:** Rinse contact lens as directed.
Boston Advance Comfort Formula (Polymer Technology)	Cationic cellulose derivative polymer, cellulosic viscosifier, polyvinyl alcohol, derivatized polyethylene glycol, chlorhexidine gluconate (0.003%), polyaminopropyl biguanide, edetate disodium (0.05%), alkyl ether sulfate, ethoxylated alkyl phenol, triquaternary coca-based phospholipid, silica gel, titanium dioxide	**Adults:** Rinse contact lens as directed.
Boston Cleaner, Advance Formula (Polymer Technology)	Tri-quaternary cocoa-based phospholipid, silica gel, alkyl ether sulfate, titanium dioxide	**Adults:** Rinse contact lens as directed.
Boston Conditioning Solution, Advance Comfort Formula (Polymer Technology)	Chlorhexidine gluconate (0.003%), polyaminopropyl biguanide (0.0005%), edetate disodium (0.05%), polyethylene glycol, cellulosic visosifier, cationic cellulose derivative polymer, polyvinyl alcohol	**Adults:** Rinse contact lens as directed.
Boston Conditioning Solution, Original Formula (Polymer Technology)	Chlorhexidine gluconate (0.006%), edetate disodium (0.05%), derivatized polyethylene glycol, cellulosic viscosifier, cationic cellulose derivative polymer, polyvinyl alcohol	**Adults:** Rinse contact lens as directed.

DOSING INFORMATION FOR CONTENT LENS CARE PRODUCTS (cont.)

Brand Name	Ingredient/Strength	Dose
Boston Rewetting Drops (Polymer Technology)	Cationic cellulose derivative polymer, polyvinyl alcohol, hydroxyethylcellulose, chlorhexidine gluconate (0.0006%), edetate disodium (0.05%)	**Adults:** Apply drops to affected eye as directed.
Boston Simplicity Multi-Action Solution (Polymer Technology)	Betaine surfactant, peo sorbitan monolaurate, chlorhexidine gluconate (0.06%), polyaminopropyl biguanide (0.0005%), edetate disodium (0.05%), derivatized polyethylene glycol, cellulosic viscosifier, silicone glycol copolymer, polyvinyl alcohol	**Adults:** Rinse contact lens as directed.
Boston Simplus, Multi-Action Solution (Polymer Technology)	Poloxamine 1107, hydroxyalkyl-phosphonate, chlorhexidine gluconate 0.003%, polyaminopropyl biguanide 0.0005%, glucam 20, hydroxypropylmethyl cellulose	**Adults:** Rinse contact lens as directed.
CIBA Vision SoftWear Saline for Sensitive Eyes (CIBA Vision)	Isotonic saline, sodium chloride, antimicrobial buffer system, sodium borate, boric Acid, sodium perborate, 0.006% hydrogen peroxide, phosphonic acid 1	**Adults:** Rinse contact lens as directed.
Lobob Sterile Cleaning Solution for Hard Lenses (Lobob Laboratories)	Anionic Detergents	**Adults:** Rinse contact lens as directed.
Miraflow Extra-Strength Daily Cleaner (CIBA Vision)	Purified water, isopropyl alcohol w/w (15.7%), poloxamer 407, amphoteric 10	**Adults:** Rinse contact lens as directed.
Opti-Clean II Daily Lens Cleaner for Especially Sensitive Eyes (Alcon)	TWEEN 21 solubilizer, microclens, edetate disodium (0.1%), polyquad (polyquaternium-1), 0.001%	**Adults:** Rinse contact lens as directed.
Opti-Free Daily Cleaner (Alcon)	Edetate Disodium (.1%), Polyquaternium-1 (.001%)	**Adults:** Rinse contact lens as directed.
Opti-Free Express, Lasting Comfort No Rub, Multi-Purpose Disinfecting Solution (Alcon)	Citrate, tetronic 1304, AMP-95, tetronic 1304, sodium chloride, boric acid, sorbitol, AMP-95, edetate disodium, polyquad, aldox	**Adults:** Rinse contact lens qd.
Opti-Free Rinsing, Disinfecting and Storage Solution (Alcon)	Sodium chloride, edetate disodium 0.05% and Polyquad® 0.001%	**Adults:** Rinse contact lens as directed.
Opti-Free Supra Clens Daily Protein Remover (Alcon)	Propylene glycol, sodium borate and highly purified porcine pancreatin enzymes	**Adults:** Apply 1 drop to stored contact lenses.
Opti-One No Rub Multi-Purpose Solution for Soft Contact Lenses (Alcon, Inc)	Polyquad(polyquaternium-1) 0.0011%, Sodium Citrate Tetronic 1304 Pationic, Sodium Chloride, Borates, Mannitol and Edetate Disodium	**Adults:** Rinse contact lens as directed
Pliagel Cleaning Solution (Alcon)	Purified water, poloxamer 407, potassium chloride, sodium chloride, preserved with sorbic acid (0.25%), edetate trisodium (0.5%)	**Adults:** Rinse contact lens as directed.
Pure Eyes Disinfectant/Soaking Solution (CIBA Vision)	Sterile ophthalmic solution containing microfilter, sodium chloride (0.85%), stabilized with phosphates, phosphonic acid, buffered with phosphates	**Adults:** Rinse contact lens as directed.
Pure Eyes Dual-Action Cleaner/Rinse (CIBA Vision)	Sterile isotonic solution, sodium chloride, antimicrobial buffer system, boric acid, sodium borate, sodium perborate (generating up to 0.006% hydrogen), pluronic surfactant	**Adults:** Rinse contact lens as directed.
Quick Care 5 Minute System Contact Lens Cleaner (CIBA Vision)	Sodium borate, boric acid, sodium perborate	**Adults:** Rinse contact lens as directed.
ReNu MultiPlus Multi-Purpose Solution with Hydranate (Bausch & Lomb)	Hydroxyalkyl-phosphonate, poloxamine, polyaminopropyl biguanide, boric acid, edetate disodium, sodium borate, sodium chloride	**Adults:** Rinse contact lens as directed.

DOSING INFORMATION FOR CONTENT LENS CARE PRODUCTS (cont.)

BRAND NAME	INGREDIENT/STRENGTH	DOSE
ReNu MultiPlus Multi-Purpose Solution, No Rub Formula *(Bausch & Lomb)*	Hydroxyalkyl-phosphonate, poloxamine, polyaminopropyl Biguanide, boric acid, edetate disodium, sodium borate, sodium chloride	**Adults:** Rinse contact lens qd.
ReNu Multi-Purpose Solution *(Bausch & Lomb)*	Poloxamine, DYMED 0.00005%, boric acid, edetate disodium, sodium borate, sodium chloride	**Adults:** Rinse contact lens as directed.
ReNu Multi-Purpose Solution, with Moistureloc *(Bausch & Lomb)*	MoistureLoc™ (poloxamer, polyquartenim-10), poloxamine, hydranate, alexidine 0.00045%, boric acid, sodium chloride, sodium phosphate	**Adults:** Rinse contact lens as directed.
Sensitive Eyes Daily Cleaner For Soft Lenses *(Bausch & Lomb)*	Hydroxypropyl methylcellulose, poloxamine, sodium borate, sodium chloride, edetate disodium 0.5%, sorbic acid 0.25%	**Adults:** Rinse contact lens as directed.
Sensitive Eyes Plus Saline Solution For Soft Contact Lenses *(Bausch & Lomb)*	Boric acid, sodium borate, potassium chloride, polyaminopropyl biguanide, edetate disodium	**Adults:** Rinse contact lens as directed.
Sensitive Eyes Saline Solution For Soft Contact Lenses *(Bausch & Lomb)*	Boric acid, sodium borate, sodium chloride, sorbic acid, edetate disodium	**Adults:** Rinse contact lens as directed.
Unisol 4 Preservative Free Saline Solution *(Alcon Laboratories)*	Sodium chloride, boric acid, sodium borate	**Adults:** Rinse contact lens qd.

Dry or Irritated Eyes

Dry eyes are caused by lack of tears. The eye depends on the flow of tears to wash away particles or foreign bodies and to provide constant moisture and lubrication to maintain vision and comfort. Tears are a combination of water, for moisture; oils, for lubrication; mucus, for even spreading; and antibodies and special proteins, for resistance to infection. Symptoms of dry eyes include burning, scratching, stinging, or gritty sensations; pain; itching; redness; and blurring of vision. Common causes of dry eyes include aging, a dry environment, sun exposure, smoking or secondhand smoke, Sjögren's syndrome, long-term wearing of contact lenses, cold or allergy medicines, and eye injuries. There are many artificial tear products available OTC to treat dry eyes.

DOSING INFORMATION FOR ARTIFICIAL TEAR PRODUCTS

The following table provides a quick comparison of the ingredients and dosages of common brand-name OTC drugs. Products are listed alphabetically by brand name.

BRAND NAME	INGREDIENT/STRENGTH	DOSE
Akwa Tears Lubricant Eye Drops Hypotonic (Akorn)	Polyvinyl Alcohol/Benzalkonium Chloride 1.4%-0.005%	**Adults:** Instill 1-2 drops to affected eye prn.
Akwa Tears Lubricant Ophthalmic Ointment (Akorn)	White Petrolatum/Mineral Oil/Lanolin 83%-15%-2%	**Adults:** Place 1/4 in oint inside eyelid qd.
All Clear AR Maximum Redness Relief Lubricant Eye Drops (Bausch & Lomb)	Hydroxypropyl Methylcellulose/Naphazoline Hydrochloride/Benzalkonium Chloride	**Adults:** Instill 1-2 drops to affected eye qid.
All Clear Redness & Irritation Relief drops (Bausch & Lomb)	Polyethylene Glycol 300/Naphazoline Hydrochloride/Benzalkonium Chloride	**Adults:** Instill 1-2 drops to affected eye qid.
Allergan Lacri-Lube S.O.P. Lubricant Eye Ointment (Allergan)	Mineral Oil/White Petrolatum 42.5%-56.8%	**Adults:** Place 1/4 in oint inside eyelid qd.
Allergan Refresh Celluvisc, Lubricant Eye Drops (Allegran)	Carboxymethylcellulose Sodium 1%	**Adults:** Instil 1-2 drops to affected eye prn.
Allergan Refresh Endura, Lubricant Eye Drops (Allergan)	Glycerin/Polysorbate 80 1%-1%	**Adults:** Instil 1-2 drops to affected eye prn.
Allergan Refresh Liquigel, Lubricant Eye Drops (Allergan)	Carboxymethylcellulose Sodium 1%	**Adults:** Instill 1-2 drops to affected eye prn.
Allergan Refresh Lubricant Eye Drops (Allergan)	Polyvinyl Alcohol/Povidone 1.4%-0.6%	**Adults:** Instil 1-2 drops to affected eye prn.
Allergan Refresh Plus Lubricant Eye Drops (Allergan)	Carboxymethylcellulose Sodium 0.5%	**Adults:** Instil 1-2 drops to affected eye prn.
Allergan Refresh PM Lubricant Eye Ointment (Allergan)	White Petrolatum/Mineral Oil 57.3%-42.5%	**Adults:** Place 1/4 in oint inside eyelid.
Allergan Refresh Tears Lubricant Eye Drops (Allergan)	Carboxymethylcellulose Sodium 0.5%	**Adults:** Instil 1-2 drops to affected eye prn.
Allergan Refresh Tears, Lubricant Eye Drops (Allergan)	Carboxymethylcellulose Sodium 0.5%	**Adults:** Instil 1-2 drops to affected eye prn.
Allergan Relief Redness Reliever & Lubricant Eye Drops (Allergan)	Phenylephrine HCl/Polyvinyl Alcohol 0.12%-1.4%	**Adults:** Instil 1-2 drops to affected eye qid.
AMO Blink Contacts Lubricant Eye Drops (AMO)	Purified water, sodium hyaluronate, sodium chloride, potassium chloride, calcium chloride, magnesium chloride, boric acid	**Adults:** Instil 1-2 drops to affected eye prn.
Bausch & Lomb Eye Wash (Bausch & Lomb)	Boric acid, purified water, sodium borate, sodium chloride	**Adults:** Flush affected eye prn.
Bausch & Lomb Moisture Eyes Liquid Gel Lubricant Eye Drops (Bausch & Lomb)	Dextran 70/Hydroxypropyl Methylcellulose 2910 0.1%-0.8%	**Adults:** Instill drops as directed.
Bion Tears Lubricant Eye Drops (Alcon)	Dextran 70/Hydroxypropyl Methylcellulose 2910 0.1%-0.3%	**Adults:** Instil 1-2 drops to affected eye prn.
CIBA Vision Rewetting Drops (CIBA Vision)	Purified Water, Sodium Chloride, Borate Buffer, Ciba E.A. (carbamide), EDTA (2%), Poloxamer 407, Sorbic Acid (.15%)	**Adults:** Instil 1-2 drops to affected eye prn.

DOSING INFORMATION FOR ARTIFICIAL TEAR PRODUCTS (cont.)

Brand Name	Ingredient/Strength	Dose
Clear Eyes Eye Drops for Dry Eyes *(Prestige Brands)*	Carboxymethylcellulose Sodium/Glycerine 1.0%-0.25%	**Adults:** Instill 1-2 drops to affected eye prn.
Clear Eyes Eye Drops for Dry Eyes, Plus Removes Redness *(Prestige Brands)*	Hypromellose/ Glycerine/Naphazoline Hydrochloride 0.8%-0.25%-0.012%	**Adults:** Instill 1-2 drops to affected eye prn.
Clerz 2 Lubricating and Rewetting Drops *(Alcon)*	Purified water, sodium chloride, potassium chloride, sodium borate, edetate disodium, hydroxyethylcellulose, boric acid, sorbic acid and poloxamer 407	**Adults:** Instil 1-2 drops to affected eye 6 times daily **Max:** 12 drops q24h.
GenTeal Mild Dry Eyes drops *(Novartis)*	Hydroxypropyl Methylcellulose 0.2%	**Adults:** Instill 1-2 drops to affected eye prn.
GenTeal Moderate Dry Eye drops *(Novartis)*	Hydroxypropyl Methylcellulose 0.3%	**Adults:** Instill 1-2 drops to affected eye prn.
GenTeal PF Dry Eye drops *(Novartis)*	Hydroxypropyl Methylcellulose 0.3%	**Adults:** Instill 1-2 drops to affected eye prn.
Moisture Eyes Lubricant Eye Drops *(Bausch & Lomb)*	Propylene Glycol 1.0%	**Adults:** Instil 1-2 drops to affected eye prn.
Moisture Eyes PM Preservative Free Lubricant Eye Ointment *(Bausch & Lomb)*	White Petrolatum/Mineral Oil 80%-20%	**Adults:** Place 1/4 in oint inside eyelid as directed.
Murine Plus Tears Plus Eye Drops *(Abbott Laboratories)*	Polyvinyl Alcohol/Povidone/ Tetrahydrozoline Hydrochloride	**Adults:** Instill 1-2 drops to affected eye qid.
Murine Tears Lubricant Eye Drops *(Abbott Laboratories)*	Polyvinyl Alcohol/Povidone/Sodium Bicarbonate	**Adults:** Instill 1-2 drops to affected eye prn.
Muro 128 5% Sterile Ophthalmic Solution *(Bausch and Lomb)*	Sodium Chloride 5%	**Adults:** Instill 1-2 drops to affected eye q3-4h.
Muro 128 Sterile Ophthalmic 2% Solution *(Bausch & Lomb)*	Sodium Chloride 2%	**Adults:** Instill 1-2 drops to affected eye q3-4h.
Optics Laboratory Minidrops Eye Therapy *(Optics Laboratory)*	Polyvinylpyrrolidone/Polyvinyl Alcohol 6mg-4mg	**Adults:** Instill 1-2 drops to affected eye prn.
Rohto V For Eyes, Lubricant/Redness Reliever Eye Drops *(Rohto Pharmaceutical)*	Naphazoline Hydrochloride/Polysorbate 80 0.012%-0.2%	**Adults:** Instill 1-2 drops to affected eye qid.
Rohto Zi For Eyes Lubricant Eye Drops *(Rohto Pharmaceutical)*	Povidone 1.8%	**Adults:** Instill 1-2 drops to affected eye prn.
Systane Lubricant Eye Drops *(Alcon)*	Polyethylene Glycol 400/Propylene Glycol 0.4%-0.3%	**Adults:** Instill 1-2 drops to affected eye prn.
Tears Naturale Forte Lubricant Eye Drops *(Alcon)*	Dextran 70 0.1%, Glycerin 0.2%, Hydroxypropyl Methylcellulose 0.3%	**Adults:** Instill 1-2 drops to affected eye prn
Tears Naturale Free Lubricant Eye Drops *(Alcon)*	Dextran 70/Hydroxypropyl Methylcellulose 2910 0.1%-0.3%	**Adults:** Instil 1-2 drops to affected eye prn.
Tears Naturale II Polyquad Lubricant Eye Drops *(Alcon)*	Dextran 70/Hydroxypropyl Methylcellulose 2910 0.1%-0.3%	**Adults:** Instill 1-2 drops to affected eye prn.
Tears Naturale P.M. Lubricant Eye Ointment *(Alcon)*	White Petrolatum/Mineral Oil	**Adults:** Place 1/4 in oint inside eyelid qd.
TheraTears Liquid Gel, Lubricant Eye Gel *(Advanced Vision Research)*	Sodium Carboxymethylcellulose 1%	**Adults:** Instill 1-2 drops to affected eye prn.
TheraTears Lubricant Eye Drops *(Advanced Vision Research)*	Sodium Carboxymethylcellulose 0.25%	**Adults:** Instill 1-2 drops to affected eye prn.
Visine Pure Tears Lubricant Eye Drops *(Pfizer Consumer Healthcare)*	Glycerin/Hypromellose/ Polyethylene Glycol 400 0.2%-0.2%-1%	**Adults:** Instill 1-2 drops to affected eye prn.
Viva-Drops Lubricant Eye Drops *(Vision Pharmaceuticals)*	Polysorbate 80	**Adults:** Instill 1-2 drops to affected eye prn.

Stye

A stye (external hordeolum) is defined as an acute inflammation (usually a staphylococcal infection) of one or more sebaceous glands of the eyelid, characterized by pain, tenderness, and edema followed by the development of a red, indurated area on the eyelid margin. Styes may occur in crops. The red, tender bump of the stye usually comes to a head in about 3 days and breaks open and drains. The cause of a stye is often unknown but may be due to rubbing the eyes, which irritates the oil glands, or to the use of mascara, eyeliner, or other eye products that can irritate the eye. Styes are treated using warm, wet compresses and nonprescription eye ointments, solutions, or drops.

DOSING INFORMATION FOR STYE OINTMENT PRODUCTS

The following table provides a listing of the ingredients and dosage of a common brand-name OTC ointment.

BRAND NAME	GENERIC INGREDIENT/STRENGTH	DOSE
Stye Ophthalmic Ointment *(DEL)*	White Petrolatum/Mineral Oil 57.7%-31.9%	**Adults:** Place 1/4 in oint inside eyelid qd.

Canker Sores and Cold Sores

A canker sore (aphthous ulcer) is an open sore in the mouth, characterized as a painful white or yellow ulcer surrounded by a bright red area. Canker sores usually begin with a tingling or burning sensation, followed by a red spot or bump that ulcerates. Canker sores are most often found on the inner surface of the cheeks and lips, the tongue, and the soft palate and at the base of the gums. There are several OTC agents used to treat cankers; most contain a topical anesthetic or counterirritant to numb the pain.

A cold sore (herpes labialis), also known as a fever blister, is an infection caused by the herpes simplex virus. Cold sores are characterized by painful blisters on the skin of the lips, mouth, or gums or the skin around the mouth. Cold sores usually last for 7 to 10 days and then begin to resolve. They often reappear and are frequently triggered by menstruation, sun exposure, illness with fever, and stress. Both prescription and nonprescription medications are used to treat cold sores. Many of the OTC products contain a topical anesthetic or counterirritant to numb the pain associated with the eruptions.

TOPICAL ANESTHETICS (MUCOSAL)

PHARMACOLOGY

Local anesthetics block both the initiation and the conduction of nerve impulses by decreasing the neuronal membrane's permeability to sodium ions. This reversibly stabilizes the membrane and inhibits depolarization, resulting in the failure of a propagated action potential and subsequent conduction blockade.

INDICATIONS

Anesthesia, local—Indicated to provide topical anesthesia of accessible mucous membranes prior to examination, endoscopy or instrumentation, or other procedures involving the following:

Esophagus—Benzocaine (gel and topical solution); benzocaine, butamben, and tetracaine; dyclonine (topical solution); lidocaine hydrochloride (4% topical solution, topical spray solution, and oral topical solution); and tetracaine hydrochloride (topical solution).

Larynx—Benzocaine (gel and topical solution); benzocaine, butamben, and tetracaine; dyclonine (topical solution); lidocaine, hydrochloride (4% topical solution and topical spray solution); and tetracaine hydrochloride (topical solution).

Mouth (in dental procedures and oral surgery)—Benzocaine (gel, topical aerosol, and topical solution); benzocaine, butamben, and tetracaine; dyclonine (topical solution); lidocaine (ointment, topical aerosol, and oral topical solution); and lidocaine hydrochloride (oral topical solution and 4% topical solution).

Nasal cavity—Benzocaine (gel); benzocaine, butamben, and tetracaine; lidocaine hydrochloride (jelly and 4% topical solution); and tetracaine (topical solution).

Pharynx or throat—Benzocaine (gel, topical aerosol, and topical solution); benzocaine, butamben, and tetracaine; dyclonine (topical solution); lidocaine (ointment and topical aerosol); lidocaine hydrochloride (jelly, oral topical solution, and topical spray solution); and tetracaine (topical solution).

Rectum—Benzocaine (gel); benzocaine, butamben, and tetracaine (gel); and lidocaine hydrochloride (jelly).

Respiratory tract or trachea—Benzocaine (gel, topical aerosol, and topical solution); benzocaine, butamben, and tetracaine; dyclonine (topical solution); lidocaine (ointment); lidocaine hydrochloride (jelly, [oral topical solution], and 4% and 10% topical solution); and tetracaine (topical solution).

Urinary tract—Benzocaine (gel); dyclonine (topical solution); and lidocaine hydrochloride (jelly).

Vagina—Benzocaine (gel; benzocaine, butamben, and tetracaine (gel); and dyclonine (topical solution).

Gag reflex suppression—Indicated to suppress the gag reflex and/or other laryngeal and esophageal reflexes to facilitate dental examination or procedures (including oral surgery), endoscopy, or intubation: Benzocaine (gel, topical aerosol, and topical solution); benzocaine, butamben, and tetracaine (topical aerosol); dyclonine (0.5% topical solution); [lidocaine (topical aerosol)]; lidocaine hydrochloride (oral topical solution and 10% topical solution); and tetracaine hydrochloride (topical solution).

Anorectal disorders (treatment)—Indicated for the symptomatic relief of the following:

Hemorrhoids; inflammation, anorectal; pain, anorectal—Benzocaine (ointment); dibucaine; pramoxine; tetracaine hydrochloride (cream); and tetracaine and menthol. These medications are effective when applied to the anal, perianal, or anorectal areas. However, they are not likely to relieve symptoms associated with conditions confined to the rectum, which lacks sensory nerve fibers.

Pain, anogenital lesion-associated—Dyclonine (0.5% solution).

Pain, anogenital, external; pruritus, anogenital—Benzocaine (ointment); dibucaine; pramoxine (aerosol foam and cream); tetracaine hydrochloride (cream); tetracaine and menthol.

Oral cavity disorders (treatment); *perioral lesions* (treatment)—Indicated for relief of the following:

Canker sores; cold sores; fever blisters—Benzocaine (gel and topical solution); benzocaine and phenol (gel and topical solution); and lidocaine (2.5% topical solution).

Pain, gingival or oral mucosal (ie, pain caused by mouth or gum irritation, inflammation, lesions, or minor dental procedures)—Benzocaine (gel, dental paste, lozenges, and topical solution); dyclonine (lozenges and 0.5% topical solution); benzocaine and phenol (gel and topical solution); lidocaine (oral topical solution); and lidocaine hydrochloride (oral topical solution).

Pain, dental prosthetic (ie, pain or irritation caused by dentures or other dental or orthodontic appliances)—Benzocaine (dental paste, gel, ointment, and topical solution); benzocaine and phenol (gel and topical solution); and lidocaine (ointment).

Pain, teething—Benzocaine (7.5% and 10% gel).

Toothache—Benzocaine (10% and 20% gel and topical solution) and benzocaine and phenol (gel and topical solution).

Pain, esophageal (treatment)—Dyclonine (topical solution) and [lidocaine hydrochloride (oral topical solution)].

Pain, pharyngeal (treatment)—Benzocaine (lozenges); benzocaine and menthol (lozenges); dyclonine (lozenges); and lidocaine hydrochloride (oral topical solution).

Pain, vaginal (treatment)—Indicated to relieve pain following procedures such as episiotomy or perineorraphy: Benzocaine

Drug Interactions for Topical Anesthetics

Precipitant Drug	Object Drug	Effect On Object Drug	Description
Cholinesterase inhibitors (e.g., antimyasthenics; cyclophosphamide; demecarium; echothiophate; insecticides, neurotoxic; isoflurophate; thiotepa)	Ester derivatives Anesthetics	↑	These agents may inhibit metabolism of ester derivatives; absorption of significant quantities of ester derivatives in patients receiving a cholinesterase inhibitor may lead to increased risk of toxicity.
Beta-adrenergic blocking agents	Lidocaine	↑	Concurrent use may slow metabolism of lidocaine because of decreased hepatic blood flow, leading to increased risk of lidocaine toxicity if large quantities are absorbed.
Cimetidine	Lidocaine	↑	Cimetidine inhibits hepatic metabolism of lidocaine; concurrent use may lead to lidocaine toxicity if large quantities are absorbed.
Lidocaine	Antiarrhythmic agents (e.g., mexiletine; tocainide; lidocaine, systemic or parenteral-local)	↑	Risk of cardiotoxicity associated with additive cardiac effects, and, with systemic or parenteral-local lidocaine, the risk of overdose, may be increased in patients receiving these medications if large quantities of topically applied lidocaine are absorbed.
Topical anesthetics	Sulfonamides	↓	Metabolites of PABA-derivative topical anesthetics may antagonize antibacterial activity of sulfonamides, especially if the anesthetics are absorbed in significant quantities over prolonged periods of time.

(topical aerosol and topical solution) and dyclonine (topical solution).

Urethritis (treatment)—Indicated to relieve or control pain: Lidocaine hydrochloride (jelly).

CONTRAINDICATIONS

Risk-benefit should be considered when the following medical problems exist:

- Local infection at site of application (infection may alter the pH at the treatment site, leading to decrease or loss of local anesthetic effect).

- Sensitivity to the topical anesthetic being considered for use or to chemically related anesthetics and, for the ester derivatives, to para-aminobenzoic acid (PABA), parabens, or paraphenylenediamine, or sensitivity to other ingredients in the formulation.

- Skin disorders, severe or extensive, especially if skin is abraded or broken (increased absorption of anesthetic).

WARNINGS/PRECAUTIONS

Cross-sensitivity and/or related problems: Patients sensitive to one ester-derivative local anesthetic (especially a PABA derivative) may also be sensitive to other ester derivatives. Patients sensitive to PABA, parabens, or paraphenylenediamine (a hair dye) may also be sensitive to PABA-derivative topical anesthetics. Patients sensitive to one amide derivative may rarely be sensitive to other amide derivatives also. Cross-sensitivity between amide derivatives and ester derivatives, or between amides or esters and the chemically unrelated pramoxine, has not been reported.

Pregnancy—Lidocaine: FDA Category B. *Tetracaine*: FDA Category C. *For benzocaine, butamben, dibucaine, and pramoxine*: Studies in animals and humans have not been done. Problems with topical anesthetics have not been documented in humans.

Breastfeeding: Problems in humans have not been documented.

Pediatrics: Benzocaine should be used with caution in infants and young children because increased absorption through the skin (with excessive use) may result in methemoglobinemia. Benzocaine-containing topical formulations should not be used in children younger than 2 years of age unless prescribed by a physician.

Other topical anesthetics—No information is available on the relationship of age to the effects of these medications in pediatric patients following application to the skin. However, it is recommended that a physician be consulted before any topical local anesthetic is used in children younger than 2 years of age.

ADVERSE REACTIONS

Those indicating need for medical attention: Incidence less frequent

Angioedema (large, hivelike swellings on skin, mouth, or throat); dermatitis, contact (skin rash, redness, itching, or hives; burning, stinging, swelling, or tenderness not present before therapy)

ADMINISTRATION AND DOSAGE

Benzocaine/Dibucaine/Pramoxine/Tetracaine

Adults/Pediatrics ≥2 years of age: Apply to the affected area 3 or 4 times a day as needed.

Butamben

Adults: Apply to the affected area 3 or 4 times a day as needed.

Lidocaine

Adults: Apply to the affected area 3 or 4 times a day as needed.

Pediatrics: Dosage must be individualized, depending on the child's age, weight, and physical condition, up to a maximum of 4.5mg/kg of body weight.

BENZOCAINE PRODUCTS	
Brand Name	**Dosage Form**
Solarcaine (Schering)	**Spray:** 20%
DIBUCAINE PRODUCTS	
Brand Name	**Dosage Form**
Nupercainal (Novartis)	**Cream:** 0.5% **Ointment:** 1%
PRAMOXINE PRODUCTS	
Brand Name	**Dosage Form**
Sarna Sensitive (Stiefel)	**Lotion:** 1%

DOSING INFORMATION FOR CANKER AND COLD SORE PRODUCTS

The following table provides a quick comparison of the ingredients and dosages of common brand-name OTC drugs. Products are listed alphabetically by brand name.

BRAND NAME	INGREDIENT/STRENGTH	DOSE
Abreva Cold Sore/Fever Blister Treatment (*GlaxoSmithKline Consumer Healthcare*)	Docosanol 10%	**Adults & Peds ≥12 yo:** Use 5 times a day till healed.
Anbesol Cold Sore Therapy Ointment (*Wyeth Consumer Healthcare*)	Allantoin/Benzocaine/Camphor/White Petrolatum 1%-20%-3%-64.9%	**Adults & Peds ≥2 yo:** Apply to affected area tid-qid.
Anbesol Jr. Gel (*Wyeth Consumer Healthcare*)	Benzocaine 10%	**Adults & Peds ≥2 yo:** Apply to affected area qid.
Anbesol Maximum Strength Gel (*Wyeth Consumer Healthcare*)	Benzocaine 20%	**Adults & Peds ≥2 yo:** Apply to affected area qid.
Anbesol Regular Strength Gel (*Wyeth Consumer Healthcare*)	Benzocaine 10%	**Adults & Peds ≥2 yo:** Apply to affected area qid.
Anbesol Regular Strength Liquid (*Wyeth Consumer Healthcare*)	Benzocaine 10%	**Adults & Peds ≥2 yo:** Apply to affected area qid.
Campho-Phenique Cold Sore Cream (*Bayer Healthcare*)	Pramoxine HCl/White Petrolatum 1%-30%	**Adults & Peds ≥2 yo:** Apply to affected area tid-qid.
Campho-Phenique Cold Sore Gel (*Bayer Healthcare*)	Camphor/Phenol 10.8%-4.7%	**Adults & Peds ≥2 yo:** Apply to affected area qd-tid
Carmex Cold Sore Reliever and Lip Moisturizer (*Carma Lab*)	Menthol/Camphor/Alum/Salicylic Acid/Phenol	**Adults & Peds ≥12 yo:** Apply to affected area prn.
ChapStick Cold Sore Therapy (*Wyeth Consumer Healthcare*)	Allantoin/Benzocaine/Camphor/White Petrolatum 1%-20%-3%-64.9%	**Adults & Peds ≥2 yo:** Apply to affected area tid-qid.
Chloraseptic Mouth Pain Spray (*Prestige Brands*)	Phenol 1.4%	**Peds ≥2 yo:** Apply to affected area prn
Chloraseptic Mouth Pain Spray (*Prestige Brands*)	Phenol 1.4%	**Adults & Peds ≥2 yo:** Apply to affected area q2h.
Herpecin-L Lip Balm Stick, SPF 30 (*Chattem*)	Dimethicone/Methyl Anthranilate/Octyl Methoxycinnamate/Octyl Salicylate/Oxybenzone1%-5%-7.5%-5%-6%	**Adults & Peds ≥12 yo:** Apply prn
Kank-A Soft Brush Mouth Pain Gel (*Blistex*)	Benzocaine 20%	**Adults & Peds ≥2 yo:** Apply to affected area qid.
Kanka-A Mouth Pain Liquid (*Blistex*)	Benzocaine 20%	**Adults & Peds ≥2 yo:** Apply to affected area qid.
Novitra Cold Sore Maximum Strength Cream (*Boericke & Tafel*)	Zincum Oxydatum 2X HPUS	**Adults & Peds ≥2 yo:** Apply to affected area q2-3h, 6 to 8 times daily.
Orabase Maximum Strength Oral Pain Reliever (*Colgate Oral Pharmaceuticals*)	Benzocaine 20%	**Adults & Peds ≥2 yo:** Apply to affected area qid.
Orabase Soothe-N-Seal, Liquid Protectant for Canker Sore Pain Relief (*Colgate Oral Pharmaceuticals*)	Formulated 2-Octyl Cyanoacrylate	**Adults:** Apply prn.
Orajel Canker Sore Ultra Gel (*Del Pharmaceuticals*)	Benzocaine/Mentol 15%-2%	**Adults & Peds ≥2 yo:** Apply to affected area qid.
Orajel Maximum Strength Gel Oral Pain Reliever (*Del Pharmaceuticals*)	Benzocaine 20%	**Adults & Peds ≥2 yo:** Apply to affected area qid.

DOSING INFORMATION FOR CANKER AND COLD SORE PRODUCTS (cont.)

Brand Name	Ingredient/Strength	Dose
Orajel Mouth Sore Gel *(Del Pharmaceuticals)*	Benzocaine/Benzalkonium Chloride/Zinc Chloride 20%-0.02%-0.1%	**Adults & Peds ≥2 yo:** Apply to affected area qid.
Orajel Mouth Sore Swabs *(Del Pharmaceuticals)*	Benzocaine 20%	**Adults & Peds ≥2 yo:** Apply to affected area qid.
Releev 1-Day Cold Sore Treatment *(Heritage)*	Benzalkonium Chloride 0.13%	**Adults & Peds ≥2 yo:** Apply to clean dry affected area tid-qid.
Swabplus Mouth Pain Relief Swabs *(Swabplus)*	Benzocaine 7.5%	**Adults & Peds ≥2 yo:** Apply to affected area qid.
Swabplus Oral Pain Relief Swabs *(Swabplus)*	Benzocaine 20%	**Adults & Peds ≥2 yo:** Apply to affected area qid.
Tanac Liquid *(Del Pharmaceuticals)*	Benzalkonium Chloride/Benzocaine 0.12%-10%	**Adults & Peds ≥2 yo:** Apply to affected area tid-qid.
Zilactin Cold Sore Gel *(Zila Pharmaceuticals)*	Benzyl Alcohol 10%	**Adults & Peds ≥2 yo:** Apply to affected area qid.

Halitosis

Halitosis (bad breath) is an unpleasant, distinctive, or offensive odor emanating from the mouth, nose, sinuses, or pharynx. Halitosis is normally not a medical concern; however, certain diseases can be associated with bad breath. For example, patients with chronic kidney failure may have breath with an ammonia-like odor, and fruity breath odor is frequently associated with ketoacidosis. Halitosis is often caused by certain foods or beverages, vitamin supplements, poor dental hygiene, dentures, cavities, gingivitis, an abscessed or impacted tooth, tobacco smoking, alcoholism, throat infection, sinusitis, or lung infection. Diseases that can be associated with halitosis include acute necrotizing ulcerative gingivitis, acute necrotizing ulcerative mucositis, acute renal failure, bowel obstruction, bronchiectasis, chronic renal failure, diabetes, esophageal cancer, gastric carcinoma, gastrojejunocolic fistula, hepatic encephalopathy, diabetic ketoacidosis, lung abscess, atrophic rhinitis, periodontal disease, pharyngitis, and Zenker's diverticulum. There are a number of OTC mouthwashes available to treat halitosis.

DOSING INFORMATION FOR MOUTHWASH PRODUCTS

The following table provides a quick comparison of the ingredients and dosages of common brand-name OTC products. Entries are listed alphabetically by brand name.

BRAND NAME	INGREDIENT/STRENGTH	DOSE
Altoids Breath Strips (Callard & Bowser-Suchard)	Hydroxypropyl methylcellulose, flavor, maltodextrin, corn starch modified, hydroxypropylcellulose, triacetin, polysorbate 80, ethyl alcohol, sucralose, potassium acesulfame	**Adults & Peds ≥12 yo:** Use as directed.
Biotene Mouthwash (Laclede)	Purified water; xylitol; hydrogenated starch hydrosylate; propylene glycol; hydroxyethyl cellulose; aloe vera; natural peppermint; poloxamer 407; calcium Lactate; zinc gluconate; sodium benzoate; benzoic acid; potassium thiocyanate; natural enzymes: lactoferrin; lysozyme; lactoperoxidase; glucose oxidase	**Adults & Peds ≥12 yo:** Rinse mouth bid.
Breath Remedy Breath/Tongue Spray (DenTek)	Deionized water, polysorbate-60, polysorbate-80, stevia, sorbitol, flavor, tris amino, carbopol, sodium chlorate, potassium sorbate, benzalkonium chloride (OraSan)	**Adults:** Spray on tongue tid-qid.
Breath Remedy Mouth Rinse (DenTek)	Deionized water, sodium chlorate, potassium sorbate, stevia powder, peppermint oil, TWEEN 20, benzalkonium chloride (OraSan), glycerin	**Adults & Peds ≥6 yo:** Rinse mouth bid.
Cepacol Antibacterial Mouthwash (Combe)	Water; alcohol denat. 14% V/V; glycerin; flavors; sisodium phosphate; cetylpyridinium chloride (Ceepryn) 0.05%; polysorbate 80; saccharin; sodium phosphate; disodium EDTA	**Adults & Peds ≥12 yo:** Rinse mouth bid.
Crest Pro-Health Rinse (Procter & Gamble)	Cetylpyridinium Chloride 0.07%	**Adults & Peds ≥6 yo:** Rinse mouth bid.
Lavoris Mouthwash (CFCP Lavoris)	Water, alcohol, glycerin, sorbitol, poloxamer 407, Flavor*, zinc chloride, polysorbate 80, citric acid, sodium saccharin, zinc oxide, sodium hydroxide, cinnamal/cinnamic aldehyde, eugenia cayophyllus flower oil, menthol	**Adults & Peds ≥12 yo:** Rinse mouth bid.
Listerine Antiseptic Mouthwash, Tartar Control (Pfizer Consumer Helathcare)	Thymol/Eucalyptol/Methyl Salicylate/Menthol 0.064%-0.092%-0.06%-0.042%	**Adults & Peds ≥12 yo:** Rinse mouth bid.
Listerine PocketPaks Oral Care Strips (Pfizer Consumer Healthcare)	Pullulan, flavors, menthol, spartame, potassium acesulfame, copper gluconate, polysorbate 80, carrageenan, glyceryl oleate, eucalyptol, methyl salicylate, thymol, locust bean gum, propylene glycol, xanthan gum, phenylketonurics	**Adults & Peds ≥12 yo:** Use as directed.

DOSING INFORMATION FOR MOUTHWASH PRODUCTS (cont.)

BRAND NAME	INGREDIENT/STRENGTH	DOSE
Listermint Antiseptic Mouthwash (Pfizer Consumer Healthcare)	Water, glycerin, poloxamer 335, PEG-600, glavors, sodium lauryl sulfate, sodium benzoate, sodium saccharin, benzoic acid, zinc chloride	**Adults & Peds ≥12 yo:** Rinse mouth bid.
Scope Mouthwash (Procter & Gamble)	Water, alcohol (15 wt%), glycerin, flavor, polysorbate 80, sodium saccharin, sodium benzoate, cetylpyridinium Cl, domiphen bromide, benzoic acid	**Adults & Peds ≥12 yo:** Rinse mouth bid.
Targon Smokers' Mouthwash (GlaxoSmithKline Consumer Healthcare)	Water; alcohol (15.6 Wt%); glycerin; PEG-40 hydrogenated castor oil; sodium lauryl sulfate; flavor; disodium phosphate; benzoic acid; sodium saccharin	**Adults:** Rinse mouth bid.
TheraBreath Oral Rinse (Dr. Harold Katz & Fresh Start)	Purified water, oxyd-8 (proprietary stabilized oxychlor compund), sodium bicarbonate, PEG-40 hydrogenated castor oil, essential oil of peppermint, sodium benzoate, potassium sorbate, tetrasodium EDTA	**Adults & Peds ≥12 yo:** Rinse mouth bid.
TheraBrite Oral Rinse (Dr Harold Katz)	Water, xylitol, PEG 40 hydrogenated castor oil, sodium citrate, zinc gluconate, oxyd-8 (proprietary stabilized oxychlor compound), natural flavor, tetrasodium EDTA, sodium bicarbonate, melaleuca alternifolia leaf oil, citric acid	**Adults & Peds ≥12 yo:** Use as directed.
Viadent Advanced Care Oral Rinse (Colgate)	Cetyl pyridinium chloride 0.05%	**Adults & Peds ≥12 yo:** Rinse mouth bid.

Teething

Teething is the emergence of the primary teeth in the mouths of infants. Teething usually begins between the sixth and eighth months of life, and all the teeth of infancy and childhood are normally in place by the 30th month of life. These are known as the deciduous teeth and include 4 incisors, 2 canines, and 4 molars in each jaw for a total of 20 teeth. Signs of teething include drooling, irritability, gum swelling or sensitivity, sleeping problems, refusal of food, and biting on hard objects. The discomfort from teething is the direct result of pressure exerted on the tissue in the mouth, called the periodontal membrane, as the teeth erupt. There are a number of oral agents (acetaminophen, ibuprofen) and topical agents (topical anesthetics and counterirritants) available OTC to treat teething.

ACETAMINOPHEN

Antipyretic—Acetaminophen probably produces antipyresis by acting centrally on the hypothalamic heat-regulating center to produce peripheral vasodilation, resulting in increased blood flow to the skin, sweating, and heat loss. The central action probably involves inhibition of prostaglandin synthesis in the hypothalamus.

Capsule/Granules/Powder/Solution/Suspension/Tablet

For analgesic use:

Adults/Pediatrics ≥13 years of age: 325 to 500mg every 3 hours; 325 to 650mg every 4 hours; 650 to 1000mg every 6 hours; or 1300mg every 8 hours.

Pediatrics ≤3 months of age: 40mg every 4 hours as needed.

Pediatrics 4 to 12 months of age: 80mg every 4 hours as needed.

Pediatrics 1 to 2 years of age: 120mg every 4 hours as needed.

Pediatrics 2 to 4 years of age: 160mg every 4 hours as needed.

Pediatrics 4 to 6 years of age: 240mg every 4 hours as needed.

Pediatrics 6 to 9 years of age: 320mg every 4 hours as needed.

Pediatrics 9 to 11 years of age: 320 to 400mg every 4 hours as needed.

Pediatrics 11 to 12 years of age: 320 to 480mg every 4 hours as needed.

Suppositories

For analgesic use:

Adults/Pediatrics ≥13 years of age: 325 to 650mg every 4 hours, or 650mg every 6 hours as needed.

Pediatrics 2 to 4 years of age: 160mg every 4 hours as needed.

Pediatrics 4 to 6 years of age: 240mg every 4 hours as needed.

Pediatrics 6 to 9 years of age: 320mg every 4 hours as needed.

Pediatrics 9 to 11 years of age: 320 to 400mg every 4 hours as needed.

Pediatrics 11 to 12 years of age: 320 to 480mg every 4 hours as needed.

For more information, refer to the complete monograph for salicylates in "Aches and Pains" under Musculoskeletal System.

ASPIRIN

Analgesic—Salicylates produce analgesia through a peripheral action by blocking pain-impulse generation and via a central action, possibly in the hypothalamus. The peripheral action may predominate and probably involves inhibition of the synthesis of prostaglandins, and possibly inhibition of the synthesis and/or actions of other substances, which sensitize pain receptors to mechanical or chemical stimulation.

Chewing Gum Tablet

For analgesic use:

Adults/Pediatrics ≥12 years of age: 454 to 650mg every 4 hours as needed.

Pediatrics 3 to 6 years of age: 227mg up to 3 times a day as needed.

Pediatrics 6 to 12 years of age: 227 to 454mg up to 4 times a day as needed.

Suppositories

For analgesic use:

Adults/Pediatrics ≥12 years of age: 325 to 650mg every 4 hours as needed.

Pediatrics 2 to 4 years of age: 160mg every 4 hours as needed.

ACETAMINOPHEN PRODUCTS	
Brand Name	**Dosage Form**
Anacin Aspirin Free (Insight)	**Tablet:** 500mg
Feverall (Alpharma)	**Suppositories:** 80mg, 120mg 325mg, 650mg
Tylenol 8 Hour (McNeil)	**Tablet:** 650mg
Tylenol Arthritis (McNeil)	**Tablet:** 650mg
Tylenol Children's Meltaways (McNeil)	**Tablet:** 80mg
Tylenol Children's (McNeil)	**Suspension:** 160mg/5mL
Tylenol Extra Strength (McNeil)	**Capsule:** 500mg **Liquid:** 1000mg/30mL **Tablet:** 500mg
Tylenol Infants' (McNeil)	**Suspension:** 80mg/0.8mL
Tylenol Junior Meltaways (McNeil)	**Tablet:** 160mg
Tylenol Regular Strength (McNeil)	**Tablet:** 325mg

Pediatrics 4 to 6 years of age: 240mg every 4 hours as needed.

Pediatrics 6 to 9 years of age: 325mg every 4 hours as needed.

Pediatrics 9 to 11 years of age: 325 to 400mg every 4 hours as needed.

Pediatrics 11 to 12 years of age: 325 to 480mg every 4 hours as needed.

Tablet

For analgesic use:

Adults/Pediatrics ≥12 years of age: 325 to 500mg every 3 hours; 325 to 650mg every 4 hours; or 650 to 1000mg every 6 hours as needed.

Pediatrics 2 to 4 years of age: 160mg every 4 hours as needed.

Pediatrics 4 to 6 years of age: 240mg every 4 hours as needed.

Pediatrics 6 to 9 years of age: 320 to 325mg every 4 hours as needed.

Pediatrics 9 to 11 years of age: 320 to 400mg every 4 hours as needed.

Pediatrics 11 to 12 years of age: 320 to 480mg every 4 hours as needed.

For more information, refer to the complete monograph for NSAIDs in "Aches and Pains" under Musculoskeletal System.

IBUPROFEN

Analgesic—Ibuprofen may block pain-impulse generation via a peripheral action that may involve reduction of the activity of prostaglandins, and possibly inhibition of the synthesis or actions of other substances that sensitize pain receptors to mechanical or chemical stimulation. The antibradykinin activity of ibuprofen may also be involved in relief of pain, since brady-kinin has been shown to act together with prostaglandins to cause pain.

Capsule/Suspension/Tablet

For analgesic use:

Adults: 200 to 400mg every 4 to 6 hours as needed.

For more information, refer to the complete monograph for NSAIDs in "Aches and Pains" under Musculoskeletal System.

NAPROXEN

Analgesic—Naproxen may block pain-impulse generation via a peripheral action that may involve reduction of the activity of prostaglandins, and possibly inhibition of the synthesis or actions of other substances that sensitize pain receptors to mechanical or chemical stimulation. The antibradykinin activity of naproxen may also be involved in relief of pain, since brady-kinin has been shown to act together with prostaglandins to cause pain.

Capsule/Tablet

For analgesic use:

Adults: 500mg initially, then 250mg every 6 to 8 hours as needed.

For more information, refer to the complete monograph for NSAIDs in "Aches and Pains" under Musculoskeletal System.

ASPIRIN PRODUCTS	
Brand Name	**Dosage Form**
Ascriptin (Novartis)	**Tablet:** 81mg
Aspergum (Schering)	**Gum:** 227mg
Bayer Aspirin Regimen (Bayer)	**Tablet:** 81mg, 325mg
Bayer Children's Aspirin (Bayer)	**Tablet:** 81mg
Bayer Extra Strength (Bayer)	**Tablet:** 500mg
Bayer Genuine Aspirin (Bayer)	**Tablet:** 325mg
Ecotrin (GSK)	**Tablet:** 325mg
Ecotrin Adult Low Strength (GSK)	**Tablet:** 81mg
Ecotrin Maximum Strength (GSK)	**Tablet:** 500mg
Halfprin (Kramer)	**Tablet:** 81mg, 162mg
St. Joseph (McNeil)	**Tablet:** 81mg
BUFFERED ASPIRIN PRODUCTS	
Brand Name	**Dosage Form**
Alka-Seltzer (Bayer)	**Tablet:** 325mg
Alka-Seltzer Extra Strength (Bayer)	**Tablet:** 500mg
Ascriptin (Novartis)	**Tablet:** 325mg
Ascriptin Arthritis Pain (Novartis)	**Tablet:** 325mg
Ascriptin Maximum Strength (Novartis)	**Tablet:** 500mg
Bayer Plus Extra Strength (Bayer)	**Tablet:** 500mg
Bufferin (BMS)	**Tablet:** 325mg
Bufferin Extra Strength (BMS)	**Tablet:** 500mg

TOPICAL ANESTHETICS

Local anesthetics block both the initiation and conduction of nerve impulses by decreasing the neuronal membrane's permeability to sodium ions. This reversibly stabilizes the membrane and inhibits depolarization, resulting in the failure of a propagated action potential and subsequent conduction blockade.

Pain, teething—Benzocaine (7.5% and 10% gel).

Toothache—Benzocaine (10% and 20% gel and topical solution); and benzocaine and phenol (gel and topical solution).

BENZOCAINE

Gel (dental)

For toothache:

Adults/Pediatrics ≥2 years of age: Apply 10% to 20% gel to affected area up to 4 times a day.

For teething pain:

Pediatrics 4 months to 2 years of age: Apply 7.5% to 10% gel to affected area up to 4 times a day.

Pediatrics ≥2 years of age: Apply ≥7.5% gel to affected area up to 4 times a day.

Ointment (dental)

Adults: Apply to cleaned and dried dentures up to 4 times a day.

Dental paste

Adults: Apply to affected area as needed.

Topical solution (dental)

Adults: Apply 20% solution to affected area up to 4 times a day.

IBUPROFEN PRODUCTS	
Brand Name	**Dosage Form**
Advil (Wyeth)	**Capsule:** 200mg **Tablet:** 200mg
Advil Children's (Wyeth)	**Tablet:** 50mg
Advil Junior (Wyeth)	**Tablet:** 100mg
Midol Cramp Formula (Bayer)	**Tablet:** 200mg
Motrin IB (McNeil)	**Tablet:** 200mg
Motrin Children's (McNeil)	**Suspension:** 100mg/5mL
Motrin Infants' (McNeil)	**Suspension:** 50mg/1.25mL
Motrin Junior (McNeil)	**Tablet:** 100mg
Motrin Migraine Pain (McNeil)	**Tablet:** 200mg

NAPROXEN PRODUCTS	
Brand Name	**Dosage Form**
Aleve (Bayer)	**Capsule:** 220mg **Tablet:** 220mg
Aleve Arthritis (Bayer)	**Tablet:** 220mg
Midol Extended Relief (Bayer)	**Tablet:** 220mg

BENZOCAINE PRODUCTS	
Brand Name	**Dosage Form**
Anbesol (Lederle)	**Gel:** 6.30% **Solution:** 6.30%
Anbesol Baby (Lederle)	**Gel:** 7.50%
Anbesol Maximum Strength (Lederle)	**Gel:** 20% **Solution:** 20%
Detane (Del)	**Gel:** 7.50%
Kank-A (Blistex)	**Film:** 20%-0.5% **Liquid:** 20%-0.5%
Orabase-B (Colgate)	**Gel:** 20%
Orajel (Del)	**Gel:** 10% **Solution:** 10%
Orajel Baby (Del)	**Gel:** 7.50% **Swabs:** 7.50%
Orajel Baby Day & Night (Del)	**Gel:** 10%
Orajel Maximum Strength (Del)	**Gel:** 20% **Solution:** 20%
Orajel PM Maximum Strength (Del)	**Gel:** 20% **Solution:** 20%
Zilactin-B (Zila)	**Gel:** 10%

DOSING INFORMATION FOR DENTAL PAIN PRODUCTS

The following table provides a quick comparison of the ingredients and dosages of common brand-name OTC drugs. Products are listed alphabetically by generic ingredient and brand name.

BRAND NAME	INGREDIENT/STRENGTH	DOSE
ACETAMINOPHEN		
Anacin Aspirin Free tablets *(Insight Pharmaceuticals)*	Acetaminophen 500mg	**Adults & Peds ≥12 yo:** 2 tabs q6h. **Max:** 8 tabs q24h.
Tylenol 8 Hour caplets *(McNeil Consumer)*	Acetaminophen 650mg	**Adults & Peds ≥12 yo:** 2 tabs q8h prn. **Max:** 6 tabs q24h.
Tylenol 8 Hour geltabs *(McNeil Consumer)*	Acetaminophen 650mg	**Adults & Peds ≥12 yo:** 2 tabs q8h prn. **Max:** 6 tabs q24h.
Tylenol Children's Meltaways tablets *(McNeil Consumer)*	Acetaminophen 80mg	**Peds 2-3 yo (24-35 lbs):** 2 tabs. **4-5 yo (36-47 lbs):** 3 tabs. **6-8 yo (48-59 lbs):** 4 tabs. **9-10 yo (60-71 lbs):** 5 tabs. **11 yo (72-95 lbs):** 6 tabs. May repeat q4h. **Max:** 5 doses q24h.
Tylenol Children's suspension *(McNeil Consumer)*	Acetaminophen 160mg/5mL	**Peds 2-3 yo (24-35 lbs):** 1 tsp (5mL). **4-5 yo (36-47 lbs):** 1.5 tsp (7.5mL). **6-8 yo (48-59 lbs):** 2 tsp (10mL). **9-10 yo (60-71 lbs):** 2.5 tsp (12.5mL). **11 yo (72-95 lbs):** 3 tsp (15mL). May repeat q4h. **Max:** 5 doses q24h.
Tylenol Extra Strength caplets *(McNeil Consumer)*	Acetaminophen 500mg	**Adults & Peds ≥12 yo:** 2 tabs q4-6h prn. **Max:** 8 tabs q24h.
Tylenol Extra Strength Cool caplets *(McNeil Consumer)*	Acetaminophen 500mg	**Adults & Peds ≥12 yo:** 2 tabs q4-6h prn. **Max:** 8 tabs q24h.
Tylenol Extra Strength gelcaps *(McNeil Consumer)*	Acetaminophen 500mg	**Adults & Peds ≥12 yo:** 2 caps q4-6h prn. **Max:** 8 caps q24h.
Tylenol Extra Strength liquid *(McNeil Consumer)*	Acetaminophen 1000mg/30mL	**Adults & Peds ≥12 yo:** 2 tbl (30mL) q4-6h prn. **Max:** 8 tbl (120mL) q24h.
Tylenol Extra Strength tablets *(McNeil Consumer)*	Acetaminophen 500mg	**Adults & Peds ≥12 yo:** 2 tabs q4-6h prn. **Max:** 8 tabs q24h.
Tylenol Infants' suspension *(McNeil Consumer)*	Acetaminophen 80mg/0.8mL	**Peds 2-3 yo (24-35 lbs):** 1.6 mL q4h prn. **Max:** 5 doses (8mL) q24h.
Tylenol Junior Meltaways tablets *(McNeil Consumer)*	Acetaminophen 160mg	**Peds 6-8 yo (48-59 lbs):** 2 tabs. **9-10 yo (60-71 lbs):** 2.5 tabs. **11 yo (72-95 lbs):** 3 tabs. **12 yo (≥96 lbs):** 4 tabs. May repeat q4h. **Max:** 5 doses q24h.
Tylenol Regular Strength tablets *(McNeil Consumer)*	Acetaminophen 325mg	**Adults & Peds ≥12 yo:** 2 tabs q4-6h prn. **Max:** 12 tabs q24h. **Peds 6-11 yo:** 1 tab q4-6h. **Max:** 5 tabs q24h.
NSAIDs		
Advil caplets *(Wyeth Consumer Healthcare)*	Ibuprofen 200mg	**Adults & Peds ≥12 yo:** 1-2 tabs q4-6h. **Max:** 6 tabs q24h.
Advil Children's Chewables tablets *(Wyeth Consumer Healthcare)*	Ibuprofen 50mg	**Peds 2-3 yr (24-35 lb):** 2 tabs q6-8h. **4-5 yr (36-47 lb):** 3 tabs q6-8h. **6-8 yr (45-89 lb):** 4 tabs q6-8h. **9-10 yr (60-71 lb):** 5 tabs q6-8h. **11 yr (72-95 lb):** 6 tabs q6-8h. **Max:** 4 doses q24h
Advil Children's suspension *(Wyeth Consumer Healthcare)*	Ibuprofen 100mg/5mL	**Peds 2-3 yo (24-35 lbs):** 1 tsp (5mL). **4-5 yo (36-47 lbs):** 1.5 tsp (7.5mL). **6-8 yo (48-59 lbs):** 2 tsp (10mL). **9-10 yo (60-71 lbs):** 2.5 tsp (12.5mL). **11 yo (72-95 lbs):** 3 tsp (15mL). May repeat q6-8h. **Max:** 4 doses q24h.
Advil gelcaps *(Wyeth Consumer Healthcare)*	Ibuprofen 200mg	**Adults & Peds ≥12 yo:** 1-2 caps q4-6h. **Max:** 6 caps q24h.
Advil Infants' Drops *(Wyeth Consumer Healthcare)*	Ibuprofen 50mg/1.25mL	**Peds 6-11 months (12-17 lbs):** 1.25mL. **12-23 months (18-23 lbs):** 1.875mL. May repeat q6-8h. **Max:** 4 doses q24h.

DOSING INFORMATION FOR DENTAL PAIN PRODUCTS (cont.)

BRAND NAME	INGREDIENT/STRENGTH	DOSE
Advil Junior Strength tablets *(Wyeth Consumer Healthcare)*	Ibuprofen 100mg	**Peds 6-10 yo (48-71 lbs):** 2 tabs. **11 yo (72-95 lbs):** 3 tabs. May repeat q6-8h. **Max:** 4 doses q24h.
Advil Junior Strength tablets *(Wyeth Consumer Healthcare)*	Ibuprofen 100mg	**Peds 6-10 yo (48-71 lbs):** 2 tabs. **11 yo (72-95 lbs):** 3 tabs. May repeat q6-8h. **Max:** 4 doses q24h.
Advil liqui-gels *(Wyeth Consumer Healthcare)*	Ibuprofen 200mg	**Adults & Peds ≥12 yo:** 1-2 caps q4-6h. **Max:** 6 caps q24h.
Advil Migraine capsules *(Wyeth Consumer Healthcare)*	Ibuprofen 200mg	**Adults:** 2 caps prn. **Max:** 2 caps q24h.
Advil tablets *(Wyeth Consumer Healthcare)*	Ibuprofen 200mg	**Adults & Peds ≥12 yo:** 1-2 tabs q4-6h. **Max:** 6 tabs q24h.
Aleve caplets *(Bayer Healthcare)*	Naproxen Sodium 220mg	**Adults ≥65 yo:** 1 tab q12h. **Max:** 2 tabs q24h. **Adults & Peds ≥12 yo:** 1 tab q8-12h. **Max:** 3 tabs q24h.
Aleve gelcaps *(Bayer Healthcare)*	Naproxen Sodium 220mg	**Adults ≥65 yo:** 1 cap q12h. **Max:** 2 caps q24h. **Adults & Peds ≥12 yo:** 1 cap q8-12h. **Max:** 3 caps q24h.
Aleve tablets *(Bayer Healthcare)*	Naproxen Sodium 220mg	**Adults ≥65 yo:** 1 tab q12h. **Max:** 2 tabs q24h. **Adults & Peds ≥12 yo:** 1 tab q8-12h. **Max:** 3 tabs q24h.
Motrin Children's suspension *(McNeil Consumer)*	Ibuprofen 100mg/5mL	**Peds 2-3 yo (24-35 lbs):** 1 tsp (5mL). **4-5 yo (36-47 lbs):** 1.5 tsp (7.5mL). **6-8 yo (48-59 lbs):** 2 tsp (10mL). **9-10 yo (60-71 lbs):** 2.5 tsp (12.5mL). **11 yo (72-95 lbs):** 3 tsp (15mL). May repeat q6-8h. **Max:** 4 doses q24h.
Motrin IB caplets *(McNeil Consumer)*	Ibuprofen 200mg	**Adults & Peds ≥12 yo:** 1-2 tabs q4-6h. **Max:** 6 tabs q24h.
Motrin IB gelcaps *(McNeil Consumer)*	Ibuprofen 200mg	**Adults & Peds ≥12 yo:** 1-2 tabs q4-6h. **Max:** 6 tabs q24h.
Motrin IB tablets *(McNeil Consumer)*	Ibuprofen 200mg	**Adults & Peds ≥12 yo:** 1-2 tabs q4-6h. **Max:** 6 tabs q24h.
Motrin Infants' Drops *(McNeil Consumer)*	Ibuprofen 50mg/1.25mL	**Peds 6-11 months (12-17 lbs):** 1.25mL. **12-23 months (18-23 lbs):** 1.875mL. May repeat q6-8h. **Max:** 4 doses q24h.
Motrin Junior Strength chewable tablets *(McNeil Consumer)*	Ibuprofen 100mg	**Peds 6-8 yo (48-59 lbs):** 2 tabs. **9-10 yo (60-71 lbs):** 2.5 tabs. **11 yo (72-95 lbs):** 3 tabs. May repeat q6-8h. **Max:** 4 doses q24h.
Nuprin caplets *(Bristol-Myers Squibb)*	Ibuprofen 200mg	**Adults & Peds ≥12 yo:** 1-2 tabs q4-6h. **Max:** 6 tabs q24h.
Nuprin tablets *(Bristol-Myers Squibb)*	Ibuprofen 200mg	**Adults & Peds ≥12 yo:** 1-2 tabs q4-6h. **Max:** 6 tabs q24h.
SALICYLATES		
Anacin 81 tablets *(Insight Pharmaceuticals)*	Aspirin 81mg	**Adults & Peds ≥12 yo:** 4-8 tabs q4h. **Max:** 48 tabs q24h.
Aspergum chewable tablets *(Schering-Plough)*	Aspirin 227mg	**Adults & Peds ≥12 yo:** 2 tabs q4h. **Max:** 16 tabs q24h.
Bayer Aspirin Extra Strength caplets *(Bayer Healthcare)*	Aspirin 500mg	**Adults & Peds ≥12 yo:** 1-2 tabs q4-6h. **Max:** 8 tabs q24h.
Bayer Aspirin safety coated caplets *(Bayer Healthcare)*	Aspirin 325mg	**Adults & Peds ≥12 yo:** 1-2 tabs q4h or 3 tabs q6h. **Max:** 12 tabs q24h.
Bayer Children's Aspirin chewable tablets *(Bayer Healthcare)*	Aspirin 81mg	**Adults & Peds ≥12 yo:** 4-8 tabs q4h. **Max:** 48 tabs q24h.
Bayer Low Dose Aspirin tablets *(Bayer Healthcare)*	Aspirin 81mg	**Adults & Peds ≥12 yo:** 4-8 tabs q4h. **Max:** 48 tabs q24h.
Bayer Original Aspirin tablets *(Bayer Healthcare)*	Aspirin 325mg	**Adults & Peds ≥12 yo:** 1-2 tabs q4h or 3 tabs q6h. **Max:** 12 tabs q24h.

DOSING INFORMATION FOR DENTAL PAIN PRODUCTS (cont.)

Brand Name	Ingredient/Strength	Dose
Ecotrin Adult Low Strength tablets *(GlaxoSmithKline Consumer Healthcare)*	Aspirin 81mg	**Adults:** 4-8 tabs q4h. **Max:** 48 tabs q24h.
Ecotrin Enteric Low Strength tablets *(GlaxoSmithKline Consumer Healthcare)*	Aspirin 81mg	**Adults:** 4-8 tabs q4h. **Max:** 48 tabs q24h.
Ecotrin Enteric Regular Strength tablets *(GlaxoSmithKline Consumer Healthcare)*	Aspirin 325mg	**Adults & Peds ≥12 yo:** 1-2 tabs q4h. **Max:** 12 tabs q24h.
Ecotrin Maximum Strength tablets *(GlaxoSmithKline Consumer Healthcare)*	Aspirin 500mg	**Adults & Peds ≥12 yo:** 2 tabs q6h. **Max:** 8 tabs q24h.
Ecotrin Regular Strength tablets *(GlaxoSmithKline Consumer Healthcare)*	Aspirin 325mg	**Adults & Peds ≥12 yo:** 1-2 tabs q4h. **Max:** 12 tabs q24h.
Halfprin 162mg tablets *(Kramer Laboratories)*	Aspirin 162mg	**Adults & Peds ≥12 yo:** 2-4 tabs q4h. **Max:** 24 tabs q24h.
Halfprin 81mg tablets *(Kramer Laboratories)*	Aspirin 81mg	**Adults & Peds ≥12 yo:** 4-8 tabs q4h. **Max:** 48 tabs q24h.
St. Joseph Adult Low Strength chewable tablets *(McNeil Consumer)*	Aspirin 81mg	**Adults & Peds ≥12 yo:** 4-8 tabs q4h. **Max:** 48 tabs q24h.
St. Joseph Adult Low Strength tablets *(McNeil Consumer)*	Aspirin 81mg	**Adults & Peds ≥12 yo:** 4-8 tabs q4h. **Max:** 48 tabs q24h.

TOPICAL ANESTHETICS

Anbesol—Baby Oral Anesthetic Gel *(Wyeth Consumer Healthcare)*	Benzocaine 7.5%	**Peds ≥4 months:** Apply to affected area prn. **Max:** 4 doses q24h.
Anbesol Jr. Gel *(Wyeth Consumer Healthcare)*	Benzocaine 10%	**Adults & Peds ≥2 yo:** Apply to affected area prn. **Max:** 4 doses q24h.
Anbesol Maximum Strength Gel *(Wyeth Consumer Healthcare)*	Benzocaine 20%	**Adults & Peds ≥2 yo:** Apply to affected area prn. **Max:** 4 doses q24h.
Anbesol Regular Strength Gel *(Wyeth Consumer Healthcare)*	Benzocaine 10%	**Adults & Peds ≥2 yo:** Apply to affected area prn. **Max:** 4 doses q24h.
Anbesol Regular Strength Liquid *(Wyeth Consumer Healthcare)*	Benzocaine 10%	**Adults & Peds ≥2 yo:** Apply to affected area prn. **Max:** 4 doses q24h.
Chloraseptic Mouth Pain Spray *(Prestige Brands)*	Phenol 1.4%	**Peds ≥2 yo:** Apply to affected area prn.
Kank-A Soft Brush Mouth Pain Gel *(Blistex)*	Benzocaine 20%	**Adults & Peds ≥2 yo:** Apply to affected area prn. **Max:** 4 doses q24h.
Kanka-A Mouth Pain Liquid *(Blistex)*	Benzocaine 20%	**Adults & Peds ≥2 yo:** Apply to affected area prn. **Max:** 4 doses q24h.
Little Teethers Oral Pain Relief Gel *(Vetco)*	Benzocaine 7.5%	**Peds ≥4 months:** Apply to affected area prn. **Max:** 4 doses q24h.
Oajel Baby Teething Swabs *(Del Pharmaceuticals)*	Benzocaine 7.5%	**Peds ≥4 months:** Apply to affected area prn. **Max:** 4 doses q24h.
Oajel Toothache Swabs *(Del Pharmaceuticals)*	Benzocaine 20%	**Adults & Peds ≥2 yo:** Apply to affected area prn. **Max:** 4 doses q24h.
Orajel Baby Daytime and Nighttime *(Del Pharmaceuticals)*	Benzocaine 7.5% (daytime) Benzocaine 10% (nighttime)	**Peds ≥4 months:** Apply to affected area prn. **Max:** 4 doses q24h.
Orajel Baby Gel *(Del Pharmaceuticals)*	Benzocaine 7.5%	**Peds ≥4 months:** Apply to affected area prn. **Max:** 4 doses q24h.
Orajel Baby Liquid *(Del Pharmaceuticals)*	Benzocaine 7.5%	**Peds ≥4 months:** Apply 2-4 gtts to affected area prn. **Max:** 4 doses q24h.
Orajel Baby Nighttime *(Del Pharmaceuticals)*	Benzocaine 10%	**Peds ≥4 months:** Apply to affected area prn. **Max:** 4 doses q24h.
Orajel Maximum Strength Gel *(Del Pharmaceuticals)*	Benzocaine 20%	**Adults & Peds ≥2 yo:** Apply to affected area prn. **Max:** 4 doses q24h.
Orajel Maximum Strength Liquid *(Del Pharmaceuticals)*	Benzocaine 20%	**Adults & Peds ≥2 yo:** Apply to affected area prn. **Max:** 4 doses q24h.
Orajel PM Cream *(Del Pharmaceuticals)*	Benzocaine 20%	**Adults & Peds ≥2 yo:** Apply to affected area prn. **Max:** 4 doses q24h.
Swabplus Teething Pain Relief Swabs *(Swabplus)*	Benzocaine 7.5%	**Peds ≥4 months:** Apply to affected area prn. **Max:** 4 doses q24h.

Tooth Discoloration

Tooth discoloration is defined as abnormal tooth color that is anything other than the white to yellowish-white of normal teeth. It occurs when endogenous or exogenous factors disrupt formation of the tooth or stain the enamel. Discoloration can be uniform or appear as spots or lines on the teeth; these areas can also be more porous than normal enamel.

Factors that influence tooth color include congenital conditions, genetics, metabolic dysfunction, drug or chemical exposure, infections, and overexposure to fluoride. For example, inherited diseases can influence the thickness or calcium and protein content of enamel, and metabolic diseases can cause abnormalities of color and shape. Other causes of discoloration include high fever during childhood tooth formation; poor dental hygiene; treatment with tetracycline before 8 years of age; excessive fluoride either from environmental sources (naturally high levels in drinking water) or from excessive administration (fluoride applications, rinses, toothpaste, and fluoride supplements taken by mouth); severe neonatal jaundice caused by poor liver function; porphyria, a disease characterized by excessive production of pigmentation in the body; amelogenesis and dentinogenesis imperfecta, genetic defects that affect the enamel of both primary and permanent teeth; and eating foods or drinking fluids that temporarily stain the teeth (e.g., tea or coffee). There are many OTCs available to reverse tooth discoloration and whiten teeth.

DOSING INFORMATION FOR TOOTH WHITENING PRODUCTS

The following table provides a quick comparison of the ingredients and dosages of common brand-name OTC products. Entries are listed alphabetically by brand name.

BRAND NAME	INGREDIENT/STRENGTH	DOSE
Aquafresh Multi-Action Whitening Toothpaste (*GlaxoSmithKline Consumer Healthcare*)	Sodium Fluoride (0.15% w/v of fluoride ion)	**Adults & Peds ≥2 yo:** Brush pc or at least bid.
Aquafresh Whitening Toothpaste (*GlaxoSmithKline Consumer Healthcare*)	Sodium Fluoride (0.15% w/v of fluoride ion)	**Adults & Peds ≥2 yo:** Brush pc or at least bid.
Colgate Simply White Night Gel (*Colgate Personal Care*)	Alcohol; water; PEG 2M; PEG 12; hydrogen peroxide; glycerin; carbopol; sodium phosphate; phosphoric acid; BHT	**Adults:** Apply qpm as directed for 14 days.
Colgate Tartar Control Plus Whitening Toothpaste (*Colgate Personal Care*)	Sodium monofluorophosphate 0.76% (0.15% w/v of fluoride ion)	**Adults & Peds ≥2 yo:** Brush pc or at least bid.
Colgate Total Tootpaste Plus Whitening Gel (*Colgate Personal Care*)	Sodium Fluoride/Triclosan 0.24%-0.30%	**Adults & Peds ≥6 yo:** Brush pc or at least bid.
Crest Dual Action Whitening Toothpaste (*Procter & Gamble*)	Sodium Fluoride 0.243% (0.15% w/v fluoride ion)	**Adults & Peds ≥2 yo:** Brush pc or at least bid.
Crest Night Effects Whitening Gel for Sensitive Teeth (*Procter & Gamble*)	Trimethylsiloxysilicate; dimethicone; sodium bicarbonate; sodium carbonate peroxide; aluminum hydroxide; ethyl acetate; hydrophobic silica; MEK; flavor	**Adults:** Apply daily as directed.
Crest Night Effects Whitening System (*Procter & Gamble*)	Trimethylsiloxysilicate; dimethicone; sodium carbonate peroxide; sodium bicarbonate; aluminum hydroxide; ethyl acetate; hydrophobic silica; MEK; flavor	**Adults:** Apply daily as directed.
Crest Sensitivity Toothpaste Extra Whitening (*Procter & Gamble*)	Potassium Nitrate/Sodium Monofluorophosphate 5%-0.243%	**Adults & Peds ≥12 yo:** Brush pc or at least bid.
Crest Toothpaste Extra Whitening (*Procter & Gamble*)	Sodium Fluoride 0.243% (0.15% w/v fluoride ion)	**Adults & Peds ≥2 yo:** Brush pc or at least bid.
Crest Whitening Expressions Toothpaste (*Procter & Gamble*)	Sodium Fluoride 0.243% (0.15% w/v fluoride ion)	**Adults & Peds ≥2 yo:** Brush pc or at least bid.
Crest Whitening Expressions Toothpaste Liquid Gel (*Procter & Gamble*)	Sodium Fluoride 0.243% (0.15% w/v of fluoride ion)	**Adults & Peds ≥2 yo:** Brush pc or at least bid.
Crest Whitestrips (*Procter & Gamble*)	Purified water; glycerin; hydrogen peroxide; carbopol 956; sodium hydroxide; sodium saccharin	**Adults:** Apply daily as directed.
Listerine Whitening Pre-Brush Rinse (*Pfizer Consumer Healthcare*)	Water; alcohol (8%); hydrogen peroxide; sodium phosphate; poloxamer 407; sodium lauryl sulfate; sodium citrate; flavors; sodium saccharin; sucralose	**Adults:** Rinse for 60 seconds qam and qpm.

DOSING INFORMATION FOR TOOTH WHITENING PRODUCTS (cont.)

BRAND NAME	INGREDIENT/STRENGTH	DOSE
Mentadent Advanced Whitening Toothpaste (Church & Dwight)	Sodium fluoride 0.24%	**Adults & Peds ≥2 yo:** Brush pc or at least bid.
Plus+White 5 Minute Whitening System (CCA Industries)	Water; poloxamer 407; glycerin; hydrogen peroxide; methyl salicylate; sodium saccharin; phosphoric acid; blue 1	**Adults:** Apply bid as directed for 2 weeks.
Plus+White Coffee Drinkers' Whitening System (CCA Industries)	Sodium monofluorophosphate (0.15% w/v of fluoride ion)	**Adults ≥18 yo:** Brush pc or at least bid.
Rembrandt Plus Whitening Gel (Oral-B)	Sodium monofluorophosphate (0.15% w/v fluoride ion)	**Adults & Peds ≥6 yo:** Brush pc or at least bid.
Rembrandt Whiteing Strips (Oral-B)	PVP; PEG 8; water; acrylates copolymer; hydrogen peroxide; disodium pyrophosphate; sodium stannate; disodium EDTA	**Adults:** Apply daily, 30 minutes at a time, for 7 days.
Rembrandt Whitening Pen (Oral-B)	Petroleum; PVP; hydrogen peroxide; poloxamer 407; sodium saccharin; flavor	**Adults:** Apply dialy as directed.
Rembrandt Whitening Wand (Oral-B)	Water; hydrogen peroxide solution; PEG 40 hydrogenated castor oil; triethanolamine; flavor; carbomer; sodium saccharin	**Adults:** Apply prn as directed.
Sensodyne Extra Whitening Tootpaste (GlaxoSmithKline Consumer Healthcare)	Potassium Nitrate/Sodium Monofluorophosphate 5%-0.15%	**Adults & Peds ≥12 yo:** Brush pc or at least bid.
Swabplus Advanced Dental Whitening System (Swabplus)	Magnesium Peroxide/Aluminum Oxide	**Adults:** Apply daily as directed.

Xerostomia (Dry Mouth)

Xerostomia is caused primarily by limited or absent salivary flow due to dysfunction of the salivary glands. It can cause difficulties in tasting, chewing, swallowing, and speaking and can lead to the development of dental decay and infections of the mouth. Symptoms include a sticky, dry feeling in the mouth; trouble chewing, swallowing, tasting, or speaking; a burning feeling in the mouth; a dry feeling in the throat; cracked lips; a dry, rough tongue; mouth sores; and an infection in the mouth. Some causes of salivary gland dysfunction include side effects from medications; diseases such as Sjögren's syndrome, diabetes mellitus, Parkinson's disease, and HIV/AIDS; radiation therapy; chemotherapy; and nerve damage. There are several OTC products available that contain salivary enzymes and other ingredients used to treat xerostomia.

DOSING INFORMATION FOR XEROSTOMIA PRODUCTS

The following table provides a quick comparison of the ingredients and dosages of common brand-name OTC products. Entries are listed alphabetically by brand name.

Brand Name	Ingredient/Strength	Dose
Biotene Antibacterial Dry Mouth Toothpaste *(Laclede)*	Glucose Oxidase (10,000 Units), Lactoferrin (16mg), Lactoperoxidase (15,000 Units), Lysozyme (16mg), Sodium Monofluorophosphate (0.14% w/v fluoride ion)	**Adults & Peds ≥2 yo:** Brush daily.
Biotene Dry Mouth Gum, Sugar Free Mint *(Laclede)*	Lactoperoxidase (0.11 Units), Glucose Oxidase (0.15 Units)	**Adults:** Chew 2 pieces prn.
Biotene Oral Balance, Dry Mouth Relief Moisturizing Gel *(Laclede)*	Lactoperoxidase (6,000 units), Lysozyme (6mg), Glucose Oxidase (6,000 units), Lactoferrin (6mg)	**Adults & Peds ≥2 yo:** Apply to tongue qd.
Salivart Spray *(Gebauer Chemical)*	Purified Water, Sorbitol, Sodium Carboxymethylcellulose, Potassium Chloride, Potassium Phosphate Dibasic, Calcium Chloride Dihydrate, Magnesium Chloride Hexahydrate.	**Adults:** Spray into mouth prn.
Stoppers 4 Dry Mouth Spray *(Woodridge Labs)*	Deionized Water, Glycerin, Xylitol, Hydroxyethylcellulose, Lysozyme, Lactoferrin, Glucose Oxidase, Natural Spearmint Flavor, Sodium Benzoate	**Adults:** Spray into mouth prn.

Cerumen Impaction

Cerumen impaction is an obstruction of the external ear canal with wax (cerumen). Cerumen protects the ear by trapping dust, microorganisms, and other foreign particles, thus preventing them from entering and damaging the inner portions of the ear. Normally, this earwax makes it way to the opening of the ear, where it falls out or is removed by washing; however, in some people the glands produce more wax than can easily be excreted from the ear. The extra wax may harden in the external canal, resulting in blockage. Symptoms of blockage include partial hearing loss, tinnitus, earache, and a feeling of fullness in the ear. There are OTC products available to aid in the removal of earwax, most of which contain carbamide peroxide.

CARBAMIDE PEROXIDE

PHARMACOLOGY

Carbamide peroxide is prepared from hydrogen peroxide and urea. When it is exposed to moisture, nascent oxygen is released slowly and acts as weak antibacterial. The effervescence that occurs during this process along with urea's effect on tissue debridement helps to mechanically break down and loosen cerumen that has been softened by anhydrous glycerin.

INDICATIONS

Cerumen Impaction (treatment)—Carbamide peroxide 6.5% in anhydrous glycerin is approved as safe and effective in softening, loosening, and removing excessive earwax in adults and in children ages 12 years and older.

CONTRAINDICATIONS

Except under special circumstances, this medication should not be used when the following medical problems exist:

- Ear drainage, dizziness, or pain
- Perforated eardrum
- Ear surgery within past 6 weeks
- Hypersensitivity to carbamide peroxide

WARNINGS/PRECAUTIONS

Discontinue use if rash or irritation develops.

Pregnancy: Problems in humans have not been documented.

Breastfeeding: Problems in humans have not been documented.

ADVERSE REACTIONS

Those indicating need for medical attention only if they continue: Incidence rare

Burning, irritation, rash.

ADMINISTRATION AND DOSAGE

Adults/Pediatrics ≥12 years of age: Place 5 to 10 drops into affected ear bid for maximum of 4 days.

CARBAMIDE PEROXIDE PRODUCTS	
Brand Name	**Dosage Form**
Auro Wax Remover (Del)	**Solution:** 6.5%
Debrox Earwax Remover (GSK)	**Solution:** 6.5%
E-R-O Wax Removal (Scherer)	**Solution:** 6.5%
Mack's Wax Away (McKeon)	**Solution:** 6.5%
Murine Ear Wax Removal (Prestige Brands)	**Solution:** 6.5%
Otix Ear Wax Removal (DeWitt)	**Solution:** 6.5%

DOSING INFORMATION FOR EARWAX PRODUCTS

The following table provides a quick comparison of the ingredients and dosages of common brand-name OTC products. Entries are listed alphabetically by brand name.

BRAND NAME	INGREDIENT/STRENGTH	DOSE
Auro Wax Remover Ear Drops *(Del Pharmaceuticals)*	Carbamide Peroxide 6.5%	**Adults & Peds ≥12 yo:** 5-10 drops in affected ear bid for maxium of 4d.
Debrox Drops Earwax Removal Aid *(GlaxoSmithKline Consumer Healthcare)*	Carbamide Peroxide 6.5%	**Adults & Peds ≥12 yo:** 5-10 drops in affected ear bid for maxium of 4d.
E-R-O Ear Wax Removal Drops *(Scherer Laboratories)*	Carbamide Peroxide 6.5%	**Adults & Peds ≥12 yo:** 5-10 drops in affected ear bid for maxium of 4d.
Mack's Wax Away Earwax Removal Aid *(McKeon Products)*	Carbamide Peroxide 6.5%	**Adults & Peds ≥12 yo:** 5-10 drops in affected ear bid for maxium of 4d.
Murine Ear Wax Removal System *(Prestige Brands)*	Carbamide Peroxide 6.5%	**Adults & Peds ≥12 yo:** 5-10 drops in affected ear bid for maxium of 4d.
Otix Drops, Ear Wax Removal Aid *(DeWitt)*	Carbamide Peroxide 6.5%	**Adults & Peds ≥12 yo:** 5-10 drops in affected ear bid for maxium of 4d.

Otitis Externa

Otitis externa is defined as an inflammation of the skin lining the external auditory canal. Causes of otitis externa include infections (bacterial, fungal, or viral), reactive dermatoses (e.g., eczema, seborrheic dermatitis, contact dermatitis), or trauma, or a combination of these three. Otitis externa can be classified as acute or chronic. Acute diffuse otitis externa usually presents with pruritus, burning, and mild to severe ear pain that is made worse by manipulation of the pinna, by pressure on the tragus, and by jaw movement. Acute localized otitis externa (furunculosis) is usually caused by *Staphylococcus aureus* and presents with localized pain and pruritus with edema, erythema, and possible fluctuance suggestive of abscess development. Chronic otitis externa is characterized by a reduced lumen of the ear canal due to long-standing cutaneous and subcutaneous inflammation. Seborrheic dermatitis is the most common cause of chronic otitis externa and is usually seen in elderly patients. In children, chronic otitis externa is most often secondary to persistent drainage from a chronic middle ear infection.

Constant itching is the primary symptom of chronic otitis externa; in contrast to acute otitis externa, there is usually no pain when the auricle or tragus is manipulated, and both the ear canal and the surface of the drumhead are remarkably insensitive to the usual cleaning of the canal. The primary predisposing factors include high temperature and humidity levels, prolonged exposure to water (swimming, especially in fresh water, diving, excessive bathing), trauma or excoriation of the skin from scratching or aggressive cleaning of the ears (eg, with Q-tips or hairpins), and allergic reactions. Otitis externa often requires treatment with a prescription antibiotic; however, in mild cases OTC astringent agents can be used as an alternative to antibiotics when contraindicated. OTC drying agents are also available to prevent development of swimmer's ear, a form of otitis externa (for more information, see "Swimmer's Ear" under Otic Conditions).

DOSING INFORMATION FOR OTIC (OTITIS EXTERNA) PRODUCTS

The following table provides a quick comparison of the ingredients and dosages of common brand-name OTC products. Entries are listed alphabetically by brand name.

BRAND NAME	INGREDIENT/STRENGTH	DOSE
Auro-Dri Ear Water-Drying Aid *(Del Pharmaceuticals)*	Isopropyl Alcohol/Anhydrous Glycerin 95%-5%	**Adults & Peds:** Apply 4-5 drops in each ear when water remains in ear.
Hyland's Earache Drops *(Hyland's, Inc.)*	Pulsatilla 30C, Chamomilla 30 C, Sulphur 30C, Calcarea Carbonica 30C, Belladonna 30C, Lycopodium 30C	**Adults & Peds:** Apply 3-4 drops in each ear qid.
Similasan Earache Relief Drops *(Similasan)*	Chamomilla HPUS 10X, Mercurius Solubilis HPUS 15X, Sulphur HPUS 12X.	**Adults & Peds:** Apply 3-5 drops into each ear prn.
Similasan Earache Relief Kidz Size *(Similasan)*	Chamomila 10X, Mercurius Solubilis 15X, Sulphur 12X	**Adults & Peds:** Apply 2-3 drops into each ear prn.
Star-Otic *(Stellar Pharmacal)*	Isopropyl Alcohol/Anhydrous Glycerin 95%-5%	**Adults & Peds:** Apply 4-5 drops in each ear when water remains in ear.
Swim Ear Ear Drying Aid *(E.Fougera)*	Isopropyl Alcohol/Anhydrous Glycerin 95%-5%	**Adults & Peds:** Apply 4-5 drops in each ear when water remains in ear.

Swimmer's Ear

Swimmer's ear is an acute form of otitis externa. It is an inflammation, irritation, or infection of the outer ear and ear canal. It occurs when the protective film that covers the ear canal is removed, causing the canal to look red and swollen. Swimmer's ear is usually acute, but a small number of cases become chronic. The condition may develop when water, sand, dirt, or other debris gets into the ear canal. Swimmer's ear is fairly common and occurs more frequently in people who have a very narrow or hairy ear canal, live in a warm, humid climate, have impacted earwax, or have had a head injury that involves the ear. Symptoms of swimmer's ear include pain, itching, a feeling of fullness in the ear, and drainage from the ear. Swimmer's ear is usually preventable and can be cared for at home. There are several drying agents available to help prevent and treat swimmer's ear. In chronic cases or in cases of more severe infection, a prescription antibiotic may be necessary.

DOSING INFORMATION FOR OTIC (SWIMMER'S EAR) PRODUCTS

The following table provides a quick comparison of the ingredients and dosages of common brand-name OTC products. Entires are listed alphabetically by brand name.

Brand Name	Ingredient/Strength	Dose
Auro-Dri Ear Water-Drying Aid *(Del Pharmaceuticals)*	Isopropyl Alcohol/Anhydrous Glycerin 95%-5%	**Adults & Peds:** Apply 4-5 drops in each ear when water remains in ear.
Hyland's Earache Drops *(Hyland's, Inc.)*	Pulsatilla 30C, Chamomilla 30 C, Sulphur 30C, Calcarea Carbonica 30C, Belladonna 30C, Lycopodium 30C	**Adults & Peds:** Apply 3-4 drops in each ear qid.
Similasan Earache Relief *(Similasan)*	Chamomilla HPUS 10X, Mercurius Solubilis HPUS 15X, Sulphur HPUS 12X.	**Adults & Peds:** Apply 3-5 drops into each ear prn.
Similasan Earache Relief Kidz Size *(Similasan)*	Chamomila 10X, Mercurius Solubilis 15X, Sulphur 12X	**Adults & Peds:** Apply 2-3 drops into each ear prn.
Star-Otic *(Stellar Pharmacal)*	Isopropyl Alcohol/Anhydrous Glycerin 95%-5%	**Adults & Peds:** Apply 4-5 drops in each ear when water remains in ear.
Swim Ear Ear Drying Aid *(E. Fougera)*	Isopropyl Alcohol/Anhydrous Glycerin 95%-5%	**Adults & Peds:** Apply 4-5 drops in each ear when water remains in ear.

Allergic Rhinitis

Rhinitis is a generic term designed to refer to a group of symptoms—sneezing, anterior rhinorrhea, nasal congestion, and postnasal drainage. The use of the term does not imply any specific cause. The cause is best determined by classifying the rhinitis. There are multiple potential causes, including allergens (allergic rhinitis), respiratory irritants and weather conditions (chronic nonallergic rhinitis), viral upper respiratory tract infections, structural abnormalities (septal deviation, septal perforation, etc.), and medications (rhinitis medicamentosa). The pathophysiology differs for each form of rhinitis.

Allergic rhinitis is probably the most common form of chronic rhinitis. The symptoms of allergic rhinitis are caused by the release of mast cell and basophil mediators. There are two phases of the allergic reaction. The acute or early phase reaction begins within 5 to 10 minutes after allergen exposure and usually abates within an hour. Symptoms often recur 2 to 4 hours after remission. This recurrence is termed the *late-phase reaction*. The late-phase reaction is produced by the influx of inflammatory cells, including eosinophils, basophils, and lymphocytes. The importance of the late-phase reaction is that it produces a state of hyperirritability, making the nose more sensitive not only to allergen exposure, but also to exposure to respiratory irritants such as cold air, cigarette smoke, paint fumes, aerosols, and perfumes. This state of hyperresponsiveness is often referred to as priming, a term referring to the observation that the threshold dose of allergen or irritant required to produce symptoms is lowered after allergen exposure. This hyperirritability is an extremely important clinical phenomenon, because it can persist for days after a single allergen exposure.

Chronic nonallergic rhinitis is the second most common form of chronic rhinitis. As many as 23% of patients with chronic rhinitis may have no allergic component to their symptoms at all. In addition, probably over one half of patients who have allergic rhinitis also have a chronic nonallergic form of the condition as well. The term *chronic nonallergic rhinitis* does not refer to a specific cause, but rather is a "wastebasket" diagnostic term referring to any patient who has chronic rhinitis for which no other cause can be found; e.g., the patient is not allergic, does not have a chronic infection, etc. Thus, there is no single entity, chronic nonallergic rhinitis; rather, multiple varieties of this condition exist. Little is known about the pathophysiology of chronic nonallergic rhinitis. However, patients with this condition do exhibit a nonspecific nasal hyperreactivity that can be assayed by intranasal challenge with chemicals such as methacholine, histamine, and capsaicin. Some patients with chronic nonallergic rhinitis also have an abnormal nasal biopsy that demonstrates increased numbers of mast cells and eosinophils. In fact, as many as one third of adults with nonallergic rhinitis have an increased number of eosinophils on nasal smear.

Rhinitis may be the most common illness seen in outpatient medicine; it accounts for approximately 2.5% of all physician office visits. Approximately 40 million people in the US suffer from the allergic form of rhinitis, including 10% to 30% of adults and up to 40% of children, making allergic rhinitis the most common IgE-mediated disease, and the most common form of chronic illness in childhood. However, only a fraction (12.3%) of affected individuals seek medical treatment. Additionally, 17 million people are estimated to have chronic nonal-

lergic rhinitis—thus, approximately 57 million people probably suffer from the most common chronic forms of this condition. This, of course, does not take into consideration those persons with upper respiratory tract infections, structural abnormalities, and other causes of rhinitis.

The mean age of onset of nonseasonal allergic rhinitis is 9.1 years and of seasonal allergic rhinitis, 10.6 years. Prevalence decreases with age. However, the disease can begin in young adults, with 3.1% of asymptomatic first-year college students developing symptoms by the time of their senior year. Sixty-four percent of patients have a history of allergy in first-degree relatives. There is an equal incidence in males and females, and no known racial or ethnic differences in incidence.

There are many OTC medications indicated for the relief of symptoms associated with allergic rhinitis, including antihistamines (diphenhydramine, chlorpheniramine, brompheniramine, loratadine), nasal decongestants (pseuodephedrine, phenylephrine, naphazoline, oxymetazoline, xylometazoline), and saline nasal products.

ANTIHISTAMINES

PHARMACOLOGY

Antihistaminic (H_1-receptor)—Antihistamines used in the treatment of allergy act by competing with histamine for H_1-receptor sites on effector cells. They thereby prevent, but do not reverse, responses mediated by histamine alone. Antihistamines antagonize, in varying degrees, most of the pharmacological effects of histamine, including urticaria and pruritus. Also, the anticholinergic actions of most antihistamines provide a drying effect on the nasal mucosa.

Antidyskinetic—The actions of diphenhydramine in parkinsonism and in drug-induced dyskinesias appear to be related to a central inhibition of the actions of acetylcholine, which are mediated via muscarinic receptors (anticholinergic action), and to its sedative effects.

Antiemetic; antivertigo agent—The mechanism by which some antihistamines exert their antiemetic, antimotion sickness, and antivertigo effects is not precisely known, but may be related to their central anticholinergic actions. They diminish vestibular stimulation and depress labyrinthine function. An action on the medullary chemoreceptive trigger zone may also be involved in the antiemetic effect.

Antitussive—Diphenhydramine suppresses the cough reflex by a direct effect on the cough center in the medulla of the brain.

Sedative-hypnotic—Most antihistamines cross the blood-brain barrier and produce sedation due to inhibition of histamine N-methyltransferase and blockage of central histaminergic receptors. Antagonism of other central nervous system receptor sites, such as those for serotonin, acetylcholine, and alpha-adrenergic stimulation, may also be involved. Central depression is not significant with cetirizine (low doses), desloratadine, or loratadine because they do not readily cross the blood-brain barrier. Also, they bind preferentially to peripheral H_1-receptors rather than to central nervous system H_1-receptors.

Antiasthmatic—Cetirizine, and loratadine have been shown to cause mild bronchodilation and also to block histamine-induced bronchoconstriction in asthmatic patients. Also, loratadine, has been shown to diminish exercise-induced bronchospasm and hyperventilation-induced bronchospasm. Cetirizine has not been shown to be uniformly effective in preventing allergen- or exercise-induced bronchoconstriction; however, due to its inhibition of late-phase eosinophil recruitment after local allergen challenge, it has been shown to be more effective, in higher doses, than other antihistamines in reducing the symptoms of pollen-induced asthma.

INDICATIONS

Rhinitis, perennial and seasonal allergic or vasomotor (prophylaxis and treatment) or *Conjunctivitis, allergic* (prophylaxis and treatment)—Antihistamines are indicated in the prophylactic and symptomatic treatment of perennial and seasonal allergic rhinitis, vasomotor rhinitis, and allergic conjunctivitis due to inhalant allergens and foods.

Pruritus (treatment); *urticaria* (treatment); *angioedema* (treatment); *dermatographism* (treatment); *transfusion reactions, urticarial* (treatment)—Antihistamines are indicated for the symptomatic treatment of pruritus associated with allergic reactions and of mild, uncomplicated allergic skin manifestations of urticaria and angioedema, in dermatographism, and in urticaria associated with transfusions.

Sneezing (treatment); *rhinorrhea* (treatment)—Antihistamines are indicated for the relief of sneezing and rhinorrhea associated with the common cold. However, controlled clinical studies have not demonstrated that antihistamines are significantly more effective than placebo in relieving cold symptoms. Nonsedating (i.e., second-generation) antihistamines are unlikely to be useful in the treatment of the common cold symptoms since they do not have clinically significant anticholinergic effects (e.g., drying effects on nasal mucosa).

Anaphylactic or anaphylactoid reactions (treatment adjunct)—Antihistamines are indicated as adjunctive therapy to epinephrine and other standard measures for anaphylactic reactions after the acute manifestations have been controlled, and to ameliorate the allergic reactions to blood or plasma.

Parkinsonism (treatment); *extrapyramidal reactions, drug-induced* (treatment)—Diphenhydramine is indicated for the symptomatic treatment of parkinsonism and drug-induced extrapyramidal reactions in elderly patients unable to tolerate more potent antidyskinetic medications, for mild cases of parkinsonism in other age groups and, in combination with centrally acting anticholinergic agents, for other cases of parkinsonism.

Cough (treatment)—Diphenhydramine hydrochloride syrup is currently indicated as a non-narcotic cough suppressant for control of cough due to colds or allergy.

Motion sickness (prophylaxis and treatment); *vertigo* (treatment)—Dimenhydrinate and diphenhydramine are indicated for the prevention and treatment of the nausea, vomiting, dizziness, or vertigo of motion sickness.

Nausea or vomiting (prophylaxis and treatment)—Parenteral hydroxyzine is indicated for the control of nausea and vomiting, excluding nausea and vomiting of pregnancy.

Sedation—Diphenhydramine is indicated for its sedative and hypnotic effects and as a preoperative medication.

Insomnia (treatment)—Diphenhydramine and doxylamine are indicated as nighttime sleep aids to help reduce the time to fall asleep in patients having difficulty falling asleep.

CONTRAINDICATIONS

Except under special circumstances, this medication should not be used when the following medical problems exist:

- Hepatic function impairment
- Renal function impairment

Risk-benefit should be considered when the following medical problems exist:

- Bladder neck obstruction
- Prostatic hypertrophy, symptomatic
- Urinary retention, predisposition to (anticholinergic effects may precipitate or aggravate urinary retention)
- Glaucoma, angle-closure, or predisposition to (anticholinergic mydriatic effect resulting in increased intraocular pressure may precipitate an attack of angle-closure glaucoma)
- Glaucoma, open-angle (anticholinergic mydriatic effect may cause a slight increase in intraocular pressure; glaucoma therapy may need to be adjusted)
- Hypersensitivity to the antihistamine used
- Caution is recommended when dimenhydrinate, diphenhydramine, or hydroxyzine is used, since their antiemetic action may impede diagnosis of such conditions as appendicitis and obscure signs of toxicity from overdosage of other drugs.

WARNINGS/PRECAUTIONS

Patients sensitive to one of the antihistamines may be sensitive to others.

Pregnancy: FDA Category B. Well-controlled studies with azatadine, brompheniramine, chlorpheniramine, clemastine, cyproheptadine, dexchlorpheniramine, dimenhydrinate, and loratadine in humans have not been done. For diphenhydramine/doxylamine: FDA Category B.

Breastfeeding: First-generation antihistamines may inhibit lactation because of their anticholinergic actions. Small amounts of antihistamines are distributed into breast milk; use is not recommended in nursing mothers because of the risk of adverse effects, such as unusual excitement or irritability, in infants.

Pediatrics: Use is not recommended in newborn or premature infants because this age group has an increased susceptibility to anticholinergic side effects, such as central nervous system (CNS) excitation, and an increased tendency toward convulsions. A paradoxical reaction characterized by hyperexcitability may occur in children taking antihistamines.

Geriatrics: Dizziness, sedation, confusion, and hypotension may be more likely to occur in geriatric patients taking antihistamines. A paradoxical reaction characterized by hyperexcitability may occur in geriatric patients taking antihistamines. Geriatric patients are especially susceptible to the anticholinergic side effects of antihistamines, such as dryness of mouth and urinary retention (especially in males). If these side effects occur and continue or are severe, medication should probably be discontinued.

ADVERSE REACTIONS

Those indicating need for medical attention: Incidence less frequent or rare

Anaphylaxis (cough; difficulty swallowing; dizziness; fast heartbeat; hives; itching; puffiness or swelling of the eyelids or around the eyes, face, lips or tongue; shortness of breath; skin rash; tightness in chest; unusual tiredness or weakness; wheezing); blood dyscrasias (sore throat; fever; unusual bleeding or bruising; unusual tiredness or weakness)—with azatadine, brompheniramine, cyproheptadine, and dexchlorpheniramine; cardiac arrhythmias/palpitations/tachycardia (fast pounding or irregular heartbeat or pulse)—less frequent or rare with azatadine, cetirizine, clemastine, cyproheptadine, desloratadine, dexchlorpheniramine, diphenhydramine, or loratadine; cholestasis, hepatitis or other hepatic function abnormalities (abdominal or stomach pain; chills; clay-colored stools or dark urine; diarrhea; dizziness; fever; headache; itching); convulsions or seizures; edema (swelling).

Those indicating need for medical attention only if they continue or are bothersome:

Incidence more frequent:

Drowsiness; dryness of mouth, nose, or throat; gastrointestinal upset, stomach pain, or nausea—with azatadine and diphenhydramine.

Incidence less frequent or rare:

Blurred vision or any change in vision (azatadine, cetirizine, cyproheptadine, diphenhydramine, and loratadine); confusion (azatadine, cetirizine, cyproheptadine, diphenhydramine, and loratadine; not reported with diphenhydramine); difficult or painful urination (azatadine, cetirizine, chlorpheniramine, cyprohep-tadine, dexchlorpheniramine, and loratadine); dizziness (except with brompheniramine and hydroxyzine); drowsiness (brompheniramine, chlorpheniramine; reported with high doses of desloratadine and loratadine); dryness of mouth, nose, or throat (cetirizine and loratadine); increased appetite or weight gain (cetirizine and loratadine); increased sweating (azatadine, cetirizine, chlorpheniramine, cyproheptadine, loratadine); loss of appetite (cetirizine, chlorpheniramine, cyproheptadine, and loratadine); paradoxical reaction (azatadine, chlorpheniramine, cyproheptadine, desloratadine, hydroxyzine, and loratadine); photosensitivity (azatadine, cetirizine, cyproheptadine, and loratadine); ringing or buzzing in ears (azatadine, cetirizine, cyproheptadine, and loratadine); skin rash (azatadine, brompheniramine, cetirizine, clemastine, cyproheptadine, and loratadine); gastrointestinal upset, stomach pain, or nausea (cetirizine, clemastine, cyproheptadine, and loratadine); tachycardia (azatadine, cetirizine, cyproheptadine, and loratadine); thickening of mucus (cyproheptadine, dexchlorpheniramine and diphenhydramine); abnormal coordination (clumsiness or unsteadiness); constipation; diarrhea; early menses; fatigue; tremor.

ADMINISTRATION AND DOSAGE

Brompheniramine

Capsules/Elixir/Tablets

Adults/Pediatrics ≥12 years of age: 4mg every 4 to 6 hours as needed.

Pediatrics 2 to 6 years of age: 1mg every 4 to 6 hours as needed.

Pediatrics 6 to 12 years of age: 2mg every 4 to 6 hours as needed.

Drug Interactions for Antihistamines

Precipitant Drug	Object Drug	Effect On Object Drug	Description
♦ Antihistamines	Alcohol CNS-depressing agents	↑	Concurrent use may potentiate the CNS depressant effects of either these medications or antihistamines; also, concurrent use of maprotiline or tricyclic antidepressants may potentiate the anticholinergic effects of either antihistamines or these medications.
♦ Antihistamines	Anticholinergics	↑	Anticholinergic effects may be potentiated when these medications are used concurrently with antihistamines.
Antihistamines	Apomorphine	↓	Prior administration of dimenhydrinate, diphenhydramine, doxylamine, or hydroxyzine may decrease the emetic response to apomorphine in the treatment of poisoning.
Antihistamines	Ototoxic medications	↔	Concurrent use with antihistamines may mask the symptoms of ototoxicity such as tinnitus, dizziness, or vertigo.
Antihistamines	Photosensitizing medications	↑	Concurrent use of these medications with antihistamines may cause additive photosensitizing effects.
♦ MAOIs (furazolidone, procarbazine)	Antihistamines	↑	Concurrent use of MAO inhibitors with antihistamines may prolong and intensify the anticholinergic and CNS depressant effects of antihistamines; concurrent use is not recommended.
Potent inhibitors of the CYP450 enzyme system such as: erythromycin fluconazole itraconazole ketoconazole metronidazole miconazole	Loratadine	↑	Concurrent use of these medications may increase plasma levels of loratadine; there are no reports to date of serious ventricular arrhythmias associated with increased plasma levels of loratadine.

♦ = Major clinical significance. CNS = central nervous system; MAOI = monoamine oxidase inhibitor.

Chlorpheniramine

Capsules, extended-release/Tablets, extended-release

Adults/Pediatrics ≥12 years of age: 8 to 12mg every eight to twelve hours as needed.

Syrup/Tablets

Adults/Pediatrics ≥12 years of age: 4mg every 4 to 6 hours as needed.

Pediatrics 6 to 12 years of age: 2mg 3 or 4 times a day as needed. Max: 12mg per day.

Clemastine

Syrup/Tablets

Adults/Pediatrics ≥12 years of age: 1.34mg two times a day; or 2.68mg one to 3 times a day as needed.

Pediatrics 6 to 12 years of age: 0.67mg to 1.34mg two times a day; not to exceed 4.02mg/day.

Dimenhydrinate

For antiemetic/antivertigo use:

Solution/Syrup/Tablets

Adults/Pediatrics ≥12 years of age: 50 to 100mg every 4 to 6 hours.

Pediatrics 2 to 6 years of age: 12.5 to 25mg every 6 to eight hours as needed; not to exceed 75mg/day.

Pediatrics 6 to 12 years of age: 25 to 50mg every 6 to eight hours as needed; not to exceed 150mg/day.

Diphenhydramine

Capsules

For antihistaminic use:

Adults/Pediatrics ≥12 years of age: 25 to 50mg every 4 to 6 hours as needed.

Pediatrics up to 6 years of age: 6.25 to 12.5mg every 4 to 6 hours.

Pediatrics 6 to 12 years of age: 12.5 to 25mg every 4 to 6 hours; not to exceed 150mg/day.

For antiemetic/antivertigo use:

Adults: 25 to 50mg every 4 to 6 hours as needed.

Pediatrics: 1 to 1.5mg/kg of body weight every 4 to 6 hours as needed; not to exceed 300mg/day.

For sedative-hypnotic use:

Adults: 50mg twenty to thirty minutes before bedtime if needed.

Elixir/Tablets

For antihistaminic use:

Adults/Pediatrics ≥12 years of age: 25 to 50mg every 4 to 6 hours as needed.

Pediatrics: 1.25mg/kg of body weight or 37.5mg/m^2 of body surface, every 4 to 6 hours; not to exceed 300mg/day.

Pediatrics weighing up to 9.1kg: 6.25 to 12.5mg every 4 to 6 hours.

BROMPHENIRAMINE PRODUCTS	
Brand Name	**Dosage Form**
Dimetapp Allergy (Wyeth)	**Capsule:** 4mg **Tablet:** 4mg
Dimetapp Allergy Children's (Wyeth)	**Elixir:** 2mg/5mL
Dimetane Extentabs (Wyeth)	**Tablet:** 12mg
CHLORPHENIRAMINE PRODUCTS	
Brand Name	**Dosage Form**
Chlor-Trimeton (Schering)	**Syrup:** 2mg/5mL **Tablet:** 4mg, 8mg, 12mg
Efidac 24 (Novartis)	**Tablet:** 16mg
CLEMASTINE PRODUCTS	
Brand Name	**Dosage Form**
Tavist-1 (Novartis)	**Tablet:** 1.34mg
DIMENHYDRINATE PRODUCTS	
Brand Name	**Dosage Form**
Dramamine (Pharmacia)	**Tablet:** 50mg
DIPHENHYDRAMINE PRODUCTS	
Brand Name	**Dosage Form**
Benadryl (Pfizer)	**Capsule:** 25mg **Tablet:** 25mg
Benadryl Allergy (Pfizer)	**Solution:** 12.5mg/5mL **Tablet:** 12.5mg
Benadryl Allergy Fastmelt (Pfizer)	**Tablet:** 19mg
Nytol (GSK)	**Tablet:** 25mg
Nytol Maximum Strength (GSK)	**Tablet:** 50mg
Simply Sleep (McNeil)	**Tablet:** 25mg
Sominex (GSK)	**Tablet:** 25mg, 50mg
Unisom Maximum Strength (Pfizer)	**Tablet:** 50mg

Pediatrics weighing 9.1kg and over: 12.5 to 25mg every 4 to 6 hours.

For antiemetic/antivertigo use:

Adults: 25 to 50mg every 4 to 6 hours as needed.

Pediatrics: 1 to 1.5mg/kg of body weight every 4 to 6 hours as needed; not to exceed 300mg/day.

For antitussive use:

Pediatrics 2 to 6 years of age: 6.25mg every 4 to 6 hours as needed; not to exceed 25mg/day.

Pediatrics 6 to 12 years of age: 12.5mg every 4 to 6 hours as needed; not to exceed 75mg/day.

For sedative-hypnotic use:

Adults: 50mg twenty to thirty minutes before bedtime if needed.

Doxylamine

Tablets

For antihistaminic use:

Adults/Pediatrics ≥12 years of age: 12.5mg to 25mg every 4 to 6 hour as needed.

Pediatrics 6 to 12 years of age: 6.25 to 12.5mg every 4 to 6 hours as needed.

For sedative-hypnotic use:

Adults: 25mg thirty minutes before bedtime if needed.

Loratadine

Syrup

For antihistaminic use:

Adults/Pediatrics ≥6 years of age: 10mg once a day.

Pediatrics 2 to 6 years of age: 5mg once a day.

OXYMETAZOLINE

Oxymetazoline is a direct-acting sympathomimetic amine. It acts on alpha-adrenergic receptors in the arterioles of the nasal mucosa to produce constriction, resulting in decreased blood flow and decreased nasal congestion for up to 12 hours.

Congestion, nasal (treatment)—Oxymetazoline is indicated for temporary relief of nasal congestion up to 12 hours due to the common cold, sinusitis, hay fever, or other upper respiratory allergies (allergic rhinitis).

Congestion, sinus (treatment)—Nasal oxymetazoline is used for the relief of sinus congestion.

Topical solution

Adults/Pediatrics ≥6 years of age: 2 or 3 drops or sprays of a 0.05% solution into each nostril every 10 to 12 hours. Maximum of 2 doses in 24 hours.

For more information, refer to the complete monograph for oxymetazoline in "Nasal Congestion" under Respiratory System.

PHENYLEPHRINE

Phenylephrine is primarily a direct-acting sympathomimetic amine. It acts on alpha-adrenergic receptors in the arterioles of the nasal mucosa to produce constriction, resulting in decreased nasal congestion.

Congestion, nasal (treatment)—Nasal phenylephrine is indicated for the symptomatic relief of nasal congestion due to the common cold or hay fever , sinusitis, or other upper respiratory allergies.

Congestion, sinus (treatment)—Nasal phenylephrine is used for relief of sinus congestion.

Topical solution

Adults/Pediatrics ≥12 years of age: 2 or 3 drops or sprays of a 0.25% to 0.5% solution into each nostril every 4 hours as needed.

Pediatrics 2 to 6 years of age: 2 or 3 drops or sprays of a 0.125% to 0.16% solution into each nostril every 4 hours as needed.

DOXYLAMINE PRODUCTS	
Brand Name	**Dosage Form**
Unisom (Pfizer)	**Tablet:** 25mg

LORATADINE PRODUCTS	
Brand Name	**Dosage Form**
Alavert (Wyeth)	**Tablet:** 10mg
Claritin (Schering)	**Solution:** 5mg/5mL **Tablet:** 10mg
Claritin Hives Relief (Schering)	**Tablet:** 10mg
Claritin RediTabs (Schering)	**Tablet:** 10mg

OXYMETAZOLINE PRODUCTS	
Brand Name	**Dosage Form**
4-Way Long Lasting (BMS)	**Spray:** 0.05%
Afrin (Schering)	**Solution:** 0.05% **Spray:** 0.05%
Afrin Extra Moisturizing (Schering)	**Spray:** 0.05%
Afrin w/menthol (Schering)	**Spray:** 0.05%
Afrin Sinus (Schering)	**Spray:** 0.05%
Duration (Schering)	**Spray:** 0.05%
Neo-Synephrine 12 Hour (Bayer)	**Spray:** 0.05%
Sinarest Nasal (Novartis)	**Spray:** 0.05%
Vicks Sinex 12 Hour (Procter & Gamble)	**Spray:** 0.05%

Pediatrics 6 to 12 years of age: 2 or 3 drops or sprays of a 0.25% solution into each nostril every 4 hours as needed.

For more information, refer to the complete monograph for phenylephrine "Nasal Congestion" under Respiratory System.

PSEUODEPHEDRINE

Pseudoephedrine acts on alpha-adrenergic receptors in the mucosa of the respiratory tract, producing vasoconstriction. The medication shrinks swollen nasal mucous membranes; reduces tissue hyperemia, edema, and nasal congestion; and increases nasal airway patency. Also, drainage of sinus secretions may be increased and obstructed eustachian ostia may be opened.

Congestion, nasal (treatment), *Congestion, sinus* (treatment) or *Congestion, eustachian tube* (treatment)—Pseudoephedrine is indicated for temporary relief of congestion associated with acute coryza, acute eustachian salpingitis, serous otitis media with eustachian tube congestion, vasomotor rhinitis, and aerotitis (barotitis) media. Pseudoephedrine also may be indicated as an adjunct to analgesics, antihistamines, antibiotics, antitussives, or expectorants for optimum results in allergic rhinitis, croup, acute and subacute sinusitis, acute otitis media, and acute tracheobronchitis.

Capsules/Tablets

Adults/Pediatrics ≥*12 years of age*: 60mg every 4 to 6 hours. Max of 240mg/day.

Capsules, extended-release/Tablets, extended-release

Adults/Pediatrics ≥*12 years of age*: 120mg every 12 hours. Max of 240mg/day.

Solution/Syrup

Adults/Pediatrics ≥*12 years of age*: 60mg every 4 to 6 hours. Max of 240mg/day.

Pediatrics 4 to 12 months of age (5.4 to 7.7kg): 7.5mg 4 to 6 hours not to exceed 4 doses (30mg) in 24 hours.

Pediatrics 12 to 23 months of age (8.2 to 10.4kg): 11.25mg 4 to 6 hours not to exceed 4 doses (45mg) in 24 hours.

Pediatrics 2 to 6 years of age: 15mg every 4 to 6 hours, not to exceed 60mg in 24 hours.

Pediatrics 6 to 12 years of age: 30mg every 4 to 6 hours, not to exceed 120mg in 24 hours.

For more information, refer to the complete monograph for pseudoephedrine in "Nasal Congestion" under Respiratory System.

XYLOMETAZOLINE

Xylometazoline is a direct-acting sympathomimetic amine. It acts on alpha-adrenergic receptors in the nasal mucosa to produce vasoconstriction, resulting in decreased blood flow and decreased nasal congestion.

Congestion, nasal (treatment)—Xylometazoline is indicated for the temporary relief of nasal congestion due to colds, sinusitis, hay fever, other upper respiratory allergies (allergic rhinitis) and for headache, tubal block, and serous otitis media associated with nasal congestion.

Congestion, sinus (treatment)—Nasal xylometazoline is used for the relief of sinus congestion.

PHENYLEPHRINE PRODUCTS	
Brand Name	**Dosage Form**
Neo-Synephrine (Bayer)	**Solution:** 0.50% 1% **Spray:** 0.25%, 0.50%, 1%
Nostril (Novartis)	**Spray:** 0.25% 0.50%
Vicks Sinex (Procter & Gamble)	**Spray:** 0.50%

PSEUDOEPHEDRINE PRODUCTS	
Brand Name	**Dosage Form**
Chlor-Trimeton Nasal Decongestant (Schering)	**Tablet:** 60mg
Dimetapp Decongestant (Wyeth)	**Capsule:** 30mg
Simply Stuffy (McNeil)	**Liquid:** 15mg/5mL
Sudafed (Pfizer)	**Tablet:** 30mg
Sudafed 12 Hour (Pfizer)	**Tablet:** 120mg
Sudafed 24 Hour (Pfizer)	**Solution:** 240mg
Sudafed Children's (Pfizer)	**Solution:** 15mg/5mL **Tablet:** 15mg

DOSING INFORMATION FOR ALLERGIC RHINITIS PRODUCTS

The following table provides a quick comparison of the ingredients and dosages of common brand-name OTC drugs. Products are listed alphabetically by drug category and brand name.

BRAND NAME	INGREDIENT/STRENGTH	DOSE
ANTIHISTAMINE		
Alavert 24-Hour Allergy tablets (*Wyeth Consumer Healthcare*)	Loratadine 10mg	**Adults & Peds** ≥**6 yo:** 1 tab qd. **Max:** 1 tab q24h.
Benadryl Allergy capsules (*Pfizer Consumer Healthcare*)	Diphenhydramine HCl 25mg	**Adults** ≥**12 yo:** 1-2 caps q4-6h. **Peds 6-12 yo:** 1 cap q4-6h. **Max:** 6 doses q24h.
Benadryl Allergy chewable tablets (*Pfizer Consumer Healthcare*)	Diphenhydramine HCl 12.5mg	**Adults** ≥**12 yo:** 2-4 tabs q4-6h. **Peds 6-12 yo:** 1-2 tabs q4-6h. **Max:** 6 doses q24h.
Benadryl Allergy liquid (*Pfizer Consumer Healthcare*	Diphenhydramine HCl 12.5mg/5mL	**Adults** ≥**12 yo:** 2-4 tsps (10-20mL) q4-6h. **Peds 6-12 yo:** 1-2 tsp (5-10mL) q4-6h. **Max:** 6 doses q24h.
Benadryl Allergy Ultratab (*Pfizer Consumer Healthcare*)	Diphenhydramine HCl 25mg	**Adults** ≥**12 yo:** 1-2 tabs q4-6h. **Peds 6-12 yo:** 1 tab q4-6h. **Max:** 6 doses q24h.
Benadryl Children's Allergy fastmelt tablets (*Pfizer Consumer Healthcare*)	Diphenhydramine Citrate HCl 19mg	**Adults** ≥**12 yo:** 2-4 tabs q4-6h. **Peds 6-12 yo:** 1-2 tabs q4-6h. **Max:** 6 doses q24h.
Chlor-Trimeton 4-Hour Allergy tablets (*Schering-Plough*)	Chlorpheniramine Maleate 4mg	**Adults** ≥**12 yo:** 1 tab q4-6h. **Max:** 6 tabs q24h. **Peds 6-12 yo:** 1/2 tab q4-6h. **Max:** 3 tabs q24h.
Claritin 24 Hour Allergy tablets (*Schering-Plough*)	Loratadine 10mg	**Adults & Peds** ≥**6 yo:** 1 tab qd. **Max:** 1 tab q24h.
Claritin Children's syrup (*Schering-Plough*)	Loratadine 5mg/5mL	**Adults** ≥**6 yo:** 2 tsp qd. **Max:** 2 tsp q24h. **Peds 2-6 yo:** 1 tsp qd. **Max:** 1 tsp q24h.
Claritin RediTabs (*Schering-Plough*)	Loratadine 10mg	**Adults & Peds** ≥**6 yo:** 1 tab qd. **Max:** 1 tab q24h.
Dimetapp ND Children's Allergy liquid (*Wyeth Consumer Healthcare*)	Loratadine 5mg/5mL	**Adults** ≥**6 yo:** 2 tsp qd. **Max:** 2 tsp q24h. **Peds 2-6 yo:** 1 tsp qd. **Max:** 1 tsp q24h.
Dimetapp ND Children's Allergy tablets (*Wyeth Consumer Healthcare*)	Loratadine 10mg	**Adults** ≥**6 yo:** 1 tab qd. **Max:** 1 tab q24h.
Tavist Allergy tablets (*Novartis Consumer Health*)	Clemastine Fumarate 1.34mg	**Adults & Peds** ≥**12 yo:** 1 tab q12h. **Max:** 2 tabs q24h.
Tavist ND 24-Hour Allergy tablets (*Novartis Consumer Health*)	Loratadine 10mg	**Adults & Peds** ≥**6 yo:** 1 tab qd. **Max:** 1 tab q24h.
Triaminic Allerchews (*Novartis Consumer Health*)	Loratadine 10mg	**Adults & Peds** ≥**6 yo:** 1 tab qd. **Max:** 1 tab q24h.
ANTIHISTAMINE COMBINATION		
Advil Allergy Sinus caplets (*Wyeth Consumer Healthcare*)	Chlorpheniramine Maleate/Ibuprofen/Pseudoephedrine HCl 2mg-200mg-30mg	**Adults & Peds** ≥**12 yo:** 1 tab q4-6h. **Max:** 6 tabs q24h.
Alavert D-12 Hour Allergy tablets (*Wyeth Consumer Healthcare*)	Loratadine/Pseudoephedrine Sulfate 5mg-120mg	**Adults & Peds** ≥**12 yo:** 1 tab q12h. **Max:** 2 tabs q24h.
Benadryl Allergy & Sinus Headache gelcaps (*Pfizer Consumer Healthcare*)	Diphenhydramine HCl/Acetaminophen/Pseudoephedrine HCl 12.5mg-500mg-30mg	**Adults & Peds** ≥**12 yo:** 2 caps q6h. **Max:** 8 caps q24h.
Benadryl Severe Allergy & Sinus Headache caplets (*Pfizer Consumer Healthcare*)	Diphenhydramine HCl/Acetaminophen/Pseudoephedrine HCl 25mg-500mg-30mg	**Adults & Peds** ≥**12 yo:** 2 tabs q6h. **Max:** 8 tabs q24h.
Benadryl-D Allergy & Sinus fastmelt tablets (*Pfizer Consumer Healthcare*)	Diphenhydramine Citrate/Pseudoephedrine HCl 19mg-30mg	**Adults & Peds** ≥**12 yo:** 2 tabs q4-6h. **Max:** 8 tabs q24h.
Benadryl-D Allergy & Sinus liquid (*Pfizer Consumer Healthcare*)	Diphenhydramine HCl/Pseudoephedrine HCl 12.5mg-30mg/5mL	**Adults** ≥**12 yo:** 2 tsp q4-6h. **Peds 6-12 yo:** 1 tsp q4-6h. **Max:** 4 doses q24h.
Benadryl-D Allergy & Sinus tablets (*Pfizer Consumer Healthcare*)	Diphenhydramine HCl/Pseudoephedrine HCl 25mg-60mg	**Adults & Peds** ≥**12 yo:** 1 tab q4-6h. **Max:** 4 tabs q24h.
Chlor-Trimeton 4-Hour Allergy-D tablets (*Schering-Plough*)	Chlorpheniramine Maleate/Pseudoephedrine HCl 4mg-60mg	**Adults** ≥**12 yo:** 1 tab q4-6h. **Max:** 4 tabs q24h. **Peds 6-12 yo:** 1/2 tab q4-6h. **Max:** 2 tabs q24h.
Claritin-D 12 Hour Allergy & Congestion tablets (*Schering-Plough*)	Loratadine/Pseudoephedrine Sulfate 5mg-120mg	**Adults & Peds** ≥**12 yo:** 1 tab q12h. **Max:** 2 tabs q24h.
Claritin-D 24 Hour Allergy & Congestion tablets (*Schering-Plough*)	Loratadine/Pseudoephedrine Sulfate 10mg-240mg	**Adults & Peds** ≥**12 yo:** 1 tab qd. **Max:** 1 tab q24h.

DOSING INFORMATION FOR ALLERGIC RHINITIS PRODUCTS (cont.)

Brand Name	Ingredient/Strength	Dose
Contac Day & Night Allergy/Sinus Relief caplets (GlaxoSmithKline Consumer Healthcare)	Diphenhydramine HCl/Acetaminophen/ Pseudoephedrine HCl 50mg-650mg-60mg (Night) Acetaminophen/Pseudoephedrine HCl 650mg-60mg (Day)	**Adults & Peds ≥12 yo:** 1 tab q6h. **Max:** 4 tabs q24h.
Drixoral Allergy Sinus sustained-action tablets (Schering-Plough)	Dexbrompheniramine Maleate/ Acetaminophen/Pseudoephedrine HCl 3mg-500mg-60mg	**Adults & Peds ≥12 yo:** 2 tabs q12h. **Max:** 4 tabs q24h.
Sinutab Maximum Strength Sinus Allergy caplets (Pfizer Consumer Healthcare)	Chlorpheniramine Maleate/Acetaminophen/ Pseudoephedrine HCl 2mg-500mg-30mg	**Adults & Peds ≥12 yo:** 2 tabs q6h. **Max:** 8 tabs q24h.
Sudafed Sinus & Allergy tablets (Pfizer Consumer Healthcare)	Chlorpheniramine Maleate/Pseudoephedrine HCl 4mg-60mg	**Adults ≥12 yo:** 1 tab q4-6h. **Peds 6-12 yo:** 1/2 tab q4-6h. **Max:** 4 doses q24h.
Tavist Allergy/Sinus/Headache caplets (Novartis Consumer Health)	Clemastine Fumarate/Acetaminophen/ Pseudoephedrine HCl 0.335mg-500mg-30mg	**Adults & Peds ≥12 yo:** 2 tab q6h. **Max:** 8 tabs q24h.
Tavist Sinus caplets (Novartis Consumer Health)	Acetaminophen/Pseudoephedrine HCl 500mg-30mg	**Adults & Peds ≥12 yo:** 2 tab q6h. **Max:** 8 tabs q24h.
Tylenol Allergy Complete Multi-Symptom Cool Burst caplets (McNeil Consumer)	Chlorpheniramine Maleate/Acetaminophen/ Pseudoephedrine HCl 2mg-500mg-30mg	**Adults & Peds ≥12 yo:** 2 tabs q6h. **Max:** 8 tabs q24h.
Tylenol Allergy Complete Nighttime Cool Burst caplets (McNeil Consumer)	Diphenhydramine HCl/Acetaminophen/ Pseudoephedrine HCl 25mg-500mg-30mg	**Adults & Peds ≥12 yo:** 2 tabs q4-6h. **Max:** 8 tabs q24h.
Tylenol Allergy Sinus Day Time caplets (McNeil Consumer)	Chlorpheniramine Maleate/Acetaminophen/ Pseudoephedrine HCl 2mg-500mg-30mg	**Adults & Peds ≥12 yo:** 2 tabs q4-6h. **Max:** 8 tabs q24h.
Tylenol Allergy Sinus Night Time caplets (McNeil Consumer)	Diphenhydramine HCl/Acetaminophen/ Pseudoephedrine HCl 25mg-500mg-30mg	**Adults & Peds ≥12 yo:** 2 tabs q4-6h. **Max:** 8 tabs q24h.
Tylenol Severe Allergy caplets (McNeil Consumer)	Diphenhydramine HCl/Acetaminophen 12.5mg-500mg	**Adults & Peds ≥12 yo:** 2 tabs q4-6h. **Max:** 8 tabs q24h.

TOPICAL NASAL DECONGESTANTS

Brand Name	Ingredient/Strength	Dose
4-Way Fast Acting Nasal Decongestant Spray (Bristol-Myers Squibb)	Phenylephrine Hydrochloride 1%	**Adults & Peds ≥12 yo:** Instill 2-3 spray per nostril q4h.
4-Way Nasal Decongestant Spray, 12 Hour (Bristol-Myers Squibb)	Phenylephrine Hydrochloride 1%	**Adults & Peds ≥12 yo:** Instill 2-3 spray per nostril q4h.
4-Way No Drip Nasal Decongestant Spray (Bristol-Myers Squibb)	Phenylephrine Hydrochloride 1%	**Adults & Peds ≥12 yo:** Instill 2-3 spray per nostril q4h.
Afrin Extra Moisturizing Nasal Spray (Schering-Plough)	Oxymetazoline Hydrochloride 0.05%	**Adults & Peds ≥6 yo:** Instill 2-3 spray per nostril q10-12h.
Afrin No Drip Nasal Spray (Schering-Plough)	Oxymetazoline Hydrochloride 0.05%	**Adults & Peds ≥6 yo:** Instill 2-3 spray per nostril q10-12h.
Afrin No Drip Sinus Nasal Spray (Schering-Plough)	Oxymetazoline Hydrochloride 0.05%	**Adults & Peds ≥6 yo:** Instill 2-3 spray per nostril q10-12h.
Afrin Original Nasal Spray (Schering-Plough)	Oxymetazoline Hydrochloride 0.05%	**Adults & Peds ≥6 yo:** Instill 2-3 spray per nostril q10-12h.
Afrin Original Pumpmist Nasal Spray (Schering-Plough)	Oxymetazoline Hydrochloride 0.05%	**Adults & Peds ≥6 yo:** Instill 2-3 spray per nostril q10-12h.
Afrin Severe Congestion Nasal Spray (Schering-Plough)	Oxymetazoline Hydrochloride 0.05%	**Adults & Peds ≥6 yo:** Instill 2-3 spray per nostril q10-12h.
Afrin Sinus Nasal Spray (Schering-Plough)	Oxymetazoline Hydrochloride 0.05%	**Adults & Peds ≥6 yo:** Instill 2-3 spray per nostril q10-12h.
Benzedrex Inhaler (B.F. Ascher)	Propylhexedrine 250 mg	**Adults & Peds ≥6 yo:** Inhale 2 spray per nostril q2h.
Neo-Synephrine 12 Hour Extra Moisturizing Nasal Spray (Bayer Healthcare)	Oxymetazoline HCl 0.05%	**Adults & Peds ≥6 yo:** Instill 2-3 spray per nostril q10-12h.
Neo-Synephrine 12 Hour Nasal Decongestant Spray (Bayer Healthcare)	Oxymetazoline HCl 0.05%	**Adults & Peds ≥6 yo:** Instill 2-3 spray per nostril q10-12h.
Neo-Synephrine Extra Strength Nasal Decongestant Drops (Bayer Healthcare)	Phenylephrine Hydrochloride 1%	**Adults & Peds ≥12 yo:** Instill 2-3 drops per nostril q4h.
Neo-Synephrine Extra Strength Nasal Spray (Bayer Healthcare)	Phenylephrine Hydrochloride 1%	**Adults & Peds ≥6 yo:** Instill 2-3 spray per nostril q4h.

DOSING INFORMATION FOR ALLERGIC RHINITIS PRODUCTS (cont.)

Brand Name	Ingredient/Strength	Dose
Neo-Synephrine Mild Formula Nasal Spray (Bayer Healthcare)	Phenylephrine Hydrochloride 0.25%	**Adults & Peds ≥6 yo:** Instill 2-3 spray per nostril q4h.
Neo-Synephrine Regular Strength Nasal Decongestant Spray (Bayer Healthcare)	Phenylephrine Hydrochloride 0.5%	**Adults & Peds ≥12 yo:** Instill 2-3 spray per nostril q4h.
Nostrilla 12 Hour Nasal Decongestant spray (Bayer Healthcare)	Oxymetazoline Hydrochloride 0.05%	**Adults & Peds ≥6 yo:** Instill 2-3 spray per nostril q10-12h.
Vicks Sinex 12 Hour Ultra Fine Mist For Sinus Relief (Procter & Gamble)	Oxymetazoline Hydrochloride 0.05%	**Adults & Peds ≥12 yo:** Instill 2-3 spray per nostril q10-12h.
Vicks Sinex Long Acting Nasal Spray For Sinus Relief (Procter & Gamble)	Oxymetazoline HCl 0.05%	**Adults & Peds ≥12 yo:** Instill 2-3 spray per nostril q10-12h.
Vicks Sinex Nasal Spray For Sinus Relief (Procter & Gamble)	Phenylephrine Hydrochloride 0.5%	**Adults & Peds ≥12 yo:** Instill 2-3 spray per nostril q4h.
TOPICAL NASAL MOISTURIZERS		
4-Way Saline Moisturizing Mist (Bristol-Myers Squibb Co)	Water, Boric Acid, Glycerin, Sodium Chloride, Sodium Borate, Eucalyptol, Menthol, Polysorbate 80, Benzalkonium Chloride	**Adults & Peds ≥2 yo:** Instill 2-3 spray per nostril prn.
Ayr Baby's Saline Nose Spray, Drops (B.F. Ascher)	Sodium Chloride 0.65%	**Peds:** Instill 2 to 6 drops to each nostril.
Ayr Saline Nasal Gel (B.F. Ascher)	Aloe Vera Gel, Carbomer, Diazolidinyl Urea, Dimethicone Copolyol, FD&C Blue 1, Geranium Oil, Glycerin, Glyceryl Polymethacrylate, Methyl Gluceth 10, Methylparaben, Poloxamer 184, Propylene Glycol, Propylparaben, Sodium Chloride, Tocopherol Acetate, Triethanolamine, Xanthan Gum, Water	**Adults & Peds ≥12 yo:** Apply to nostril prn.
Ayr Saline Nasal Gel, No-Drip Sinus Spray (B.F. Ascher)	Water, Sodium Carbomethyl Starch, Propylene Glycol, Glycerin, Aloe Barbadensis Leaf Juice (Aloe Vera Gel), Sodium Chloride, Cetyl Pyridinium Chloride, Citric Acid, Disodium EDTA, Glycine Soja (Soybean Oil), Tocopheryl Acetate, Benzyl Alcohol, Benzalkonium Chloride, Geranium Maculatum Oil	**Adults & Peds ≥12 yo:** Use prn as directed.
Ayr Saline Nasal Mist (B.F. Ascher)	Sodium Chloride 0.65%	**Adults & Peds ≥12 yo:** Instill 2 spray per nostril prn.
Breathe Right Saline Nasal Spray (CNS)	Sodium Chloride 0.65%	**Adults & Peds ≥12 yo:** Use prn as directed.
ENTSOL Mist, Buffered Hypertonic Nasal Irrigation Mist (Bradley Pharmaceuticals)	Purified Water, Sodium Chloride, Sodium Phosphate Dibasic, Edetate Disodium, Potassium Phosphate Monobasic, Benzalkonium Chloride	**Adults & Peds ≥12 yo:** Instill 1-2 spray per nostril prn.
ENTSOL Single Use, Pre-Filled Nasal Wash Squeeze Bottle (Bradley Pharmaceuticals)	Purified Water, Sodium Chloride, Sodium Phosphate Dibasic, Potassium Phosphate Monobasic	**Adults & Peds ≥12 yo:** Use as directed
ENTSOL Spray, Buffered Hypertonic Saline Nasal Spray (Bradley Pharmaceuticals)	Purified Water, Sodium Chloride, Sodium Phosphate Dibasic, Potassium Phosphate Monobasic	**Adults & Peds ≥12 yo:** Instill 1 spray per nostril bid, 6 times daily
Little Noses Moisturizing Saline Gel with Aloe Vera & Vitamin E (Vetco)	Purified Water, Propylene Glycol, Glycerine, Glyceryl Stearate and PEG-100 Stearate, Hydroxyethylcellulose, Aloe Vera Gel, Methyl Gluceth 10, Dimethicone Copolyol, Sodium Chloride, Allantoin, Diazolidinyl Urea, Methylparaben, Vitamin E, Olive Oil, Geranium Oil, Propyl Paraben	**Peds:** Use as directed.
Little Noses Saline Spray/Drops, Non-Medicated (Vetco)	Sodium Chloride 0.65%	**Peds:** Use as directed.
Ocean Premium Saline Nasal Spray (Fleming)	Sodium Chloride (0.65%), Phenylcarbinol, Benzalkonium Chloride, Chloride	**Adults & Peds ≥6 yo:** Instill 2 spray per nostril prn.

DOSING INFORMATION FOR ALLERGIC RHINITIS PRODUCTS (cont.)

BRAND NAME	INGREDIENT/STRENGTH	DOSE
Simply Saline Sterile Saline Nasal Mist (Blairex)	Sodium Chloride 0.9%	**Adults & Peds ≥12 yo:** Use prn as directed.
SinoFresh Moisturizing Nasal & Sinus Spray (SinoFresh HealthCare)	Cetylpyridinium Cloride 0.05%	**Adults & Peds ≥12 yo:** Instill 1-3 spray per nostril qd.
Zicam Nasal Moisturizer (Zicam)	Purified Water, Sodium Phosphate, Hydroxethylcellulose, Disodium Phosphate, Glycerin, Alkoxylated Diester, Aloe Barbadensis Gel, Hydrolyzed Algin, Chlorella Vulgaris Extract, Sea Water, Benzalkonium Chloride, Benzyl Alcohol, Disodium EDTA, Hydroxylated Lecithin, Tocopherol, Polysorbate 80	**Adults & Peds ≥12 yo:** Use as directed.
MISCELLANEOUS		
NasalCrom Allergy Prevention Nasal Spray (Pfizer Consumer Healthcare)	Cromolyn Sodium 5.2 mg	**Adults & Peds ≥6 yo:** Instill 1 spray per nostril q4-6h.
NasalCrom Nasal Allergy Symptom Controller, Nasal Spray (Pfizer Consumer Healthcare)	Cromolyn Sodium 5.2 mg	**Adults & Peds ≥2 yo:** Instill 1 spray per nostril q4-6h.
Similasan Hay Fever Relief, Non-Drowsy Formula, Nasal Spray (Similasan)	Cardiospermum HPUS 6X, Galphimia Glauca HPUS 6X, Luffa Operculata HPUS 6X, Sabadilla HPUS 6x	**Adults & Peds ≥12 yo:** Use as directed.
Zicam Allergy Relief, Homeopathic Nasal Solution, Pump (Zicam)	Luffa Operculata 4x, 12x, 30x, Galphimia Glauca 12x, 30x, Histaminum Hydrochloricum 12x, 30x, 200x, Sulphur 12x, 30x, 200x	**Adults & Peds ≥6 yo:** Instill 2-3 spray per nostril q4h.

Asthma

Asthma is a chronic lower airway disease typically involving airway obstruction, airway inflammation, and increased airway responsiveness to a variety of stimuli. Asthma affects about 5% of the general population and is responsible for approximately 500,000 hospital admissions yearly in the United States. Hospitalization is largely preventable when a patient receives appropriate primary care.

Asthma is characterized by bronchial hyperreactivity, mucous production, bronchial edema, and eosinophilic and lymphocytic inflammation; it is at least partially reversible (either spontaneously or with treatment). The airway inflammatory response may be divided into three phases: *acute, late (chronic)*, and *remodeling*. The acute phase is triggered by immunologic or nonimmunologic stimuli including allergens, respiratory virus infection, exercise, irritants, and medications (e.g., aspirin). In the acute phase, activated airway mast cells release chemical mediators including histamine, leukotrienes, prostaglandins, platelet activating factor, and thromboxanes. These chemical mediators result in smooth muscle contraction, bronchial hyperresponsiveness, and airway wall edema and lead to recruitment of other inflammatory cells and mediators. The late (chronic) phase of the asthmatic response is marked by airway infiltration of mast cells, eosinophils, lymphocytes, and macrophages. The subsequent release of cytokines, chemokines, cationic proteins, and enzymes by these cells causes the marked inflammatory response that is typical in asthmatic airways. These primary and secondary mediators result in bronchial hyperresponsiveness, airway wall edema, and mucous production, which collectively compromise airflow. The remodeling phase is characterized by an aberrant restorative process that results in airway remodeling. Histologically, this phase is marked by basement membrane thickening and fibrosis, mucous gland hypertrophy and hypersecretion, smooth muscle hypertrophy, inflammatory cell infiltration, angiogenesis, and epithelial damage. If the inflammatory component of asthma is not adequately treated, it can be followed by this phase, which is eventually associated with an irreversible loss of lung function.

Asthma is a condition that normally requires the use of prescription medications to control it. However, there are a few OTC products that have been used to treat minor symptoms of asthma, most of which contain ephinephrine or ephedrine.

EPHEDRINE

PHARMACOLOGY

Ephedrine is a CNS stimulant that acts directly on both alpha- and beta-adrenergic receptors. It also acts indirectly by stimulating release of endogenous norepinephrine from sympathetic neurons, resulting in increased blood pressure and cardiac output.

INDICATIONS

Unaccepted indications: Ephedrine has been used as a bronchodilator, a nasal decongestant, and to treat urinary incontinence; however, it has been generally replaced by safer and more effective medications.

CONTRAINDICATIONS

Except under special circumstances, this medication should not be used when the following medical problems exist:

- Brain damage, organic.
- Cerebral arteriosclerosis.
- Glaucoma, narrow-angle.
- Prostatic hypertrophy.

WARNINGS/PRECAUTIONS

Pregnancy: FDA Category C.

Breastfeeding: It is not known whether ephedrine is distributed into human breast milk. Irritability, excessive crying, and disturbed sleeping patterns were reported in the breast-fed infant of a mother taking a long-acting preparation containing d-isoephedrine and dexbrompheniramine. The symptoms resolved when breastfeeding was discontinued.

DRUG INTERACTIONS

Urinary acidifiers or alkalizers, guanadrel, guanethidine.

ADVERSE REACTIONS

Those indicating need for medical attention: Incidence less frequent or rare

Palpitations and tachycardia.

ADMINISTRATION AND DOSING

For asthma:

Adults/Pediatrics: Use has been generally replaced by safer and more effective agents.

EPINEPHRINE

PHARMACOLOGY

Epinephrine is a direct-acting, potent stimulant of both alpha- and beta-adrenergic receptors.

EPHEDRINE SULFATE/GUAIFENESIN PRODUCTS	
Brand Name	**Dosage Form**
Bronkaid (Bayer)	**Tablets:** 25mg-400mg
Primatene Bronchial Asthma Relief (Whitehall Labs)	**Tablets:** 12.5mg-200mg
EPINEPHRINE PRODUCTS	
Brand Name	**Dosage Form**
Primatene Mist (Whitehall Labs)	**Inhaler:** 0.22mg

INDICATIONS

Unaccepted indications: Epinephrine has been used as a bronchodilator in the treatment of asthma; however, it has been generally replaced by safer and more effective medications.

CONTRAINDICATIONS

Except under special circumstances, this medication should not be used when the following medical problems exist:

- Cardiac disease.
- Cerebral arteriosclerosis.
- Organic brain damage.
- Glaucoma, narrow angle.
- Parkinson's disease.
- Psychoneurotic disorders.
- Nonasthmatic shock.

WARNINGS/PRECAUTIONS

Pregnancy: FDA Category C.

Breastfeeding: Epinephrine is distributed into human breast milk. Risk-benefit should be considered because of potential adverse effects in the nursing infant.

DRUG INTERACTIONS

Insulin, oral antidiabetic agents, cocaine.

ADVERSE REACTIONS

Those indicating need for medical attention:

Hypertension and anxiety (more common), tachycardia and palpitations, psychoneurotic disorders (rare).

ADMINISTRATION AND DOSAGE

For asthma:

Adults/Pediatrics: Use has been generally replaced by safer and more effective agents.

DOSING INFORMATION FOR EPHEDRINE/EPINEPHRINE PRODUCTS

The following table provides a quick comparison of the ingredients and dosages of common brand-name OTC drugs.

BRAND NAME	INGREDIENT/STRENGTH	DOSE
Bronkaid Dual Action Bronchial Relief Caplets *(Bayer Corporation)*	Ephedrine Sulfate/Guaifenesin 25mg-400mg	**Adults & Peds** ≥**12 yo:** Take 1 tab q4h. **Max:** 6 tab q24h.
Primatene Bronchial Asthma Relief, Tablets *(Whitehall Labs)*	Ephedrine HCl/Guaifenesin 12.5mg-200mg	**Adults & Peds** ≥**12 yo:** Take 2 tab q4h. **Max:** 12 tab q24h.
Primatene Mist Inhaler *(Whitehall Labs)*	Epinephrine 0.22 mg	**Adults & Peds** ≥**4 yo:** Inhale 1 puff q3h.

Cough, Cold, and Flu

The diagnosis of a typical viral upper-respiratory infection (VURI) in a healthy individual is usually relatively uncomplicated. Determining which specific virus has caused the VURI, however, is difficult. Although clinical manifestations and epidemiologic factors may suggest a specific respiratory virus infection (e.g., influenza virus in an nonimmunized, febrile adult with a painful bronchial cough during an influenza epidemic, or RSV [respiratory syncytial virus] in a minimally febrile infant with "wheeze bronchitis" in the spring), each of these can cause such a variety of clinical manifestations that attempting to identify the specific virus that is causing the respiratory infection results in an educated guess at best.

The general symptoms of VURI include general malaise, laryngitis, injection of conjunctiva, decrease in appetite, headache, fever (≥100.3° F for 1-3 days), and nasal discharge. The three most frequent symptoms of a cold are runny nose, nasal congestion, and sneezing. Adults and children with colds generally have minimal or no fever; young children often run a fever around 100° to 102° F. Other symptoms of a cold include sore throat, cough, muscle aches, headache, postnasal drip, and decreased appetite.

An estimated two thirds to three fourths of acute respiratory illnesses are caused by viruses. The incidence of acute respiratory disease in the United States ranges from 3 to 5.6 cases per person per year. The rate is 6.1 to 8.3 cases per year in children younger than 12 months and remains high until 6 years of age. The frequency of viral respiratory infections is highest in children up to 4 years of age, gradually decreases in the teenage years, rises again in parents exposed to infected children, and is lowest in the elderly. This age-related cycle suggests gradual acquisition of immunity to some agents. In general, the major reservoir for most respiratory viruses is schoolchildren, who acquire the infection in the classroom and introduce it into their homes. Moreover, a number of respiratory viruses have been shown to cause outbreaks in hospitals, day-care centers, and nursing homes. Seasonality and transmission patterns of the viruses vary from one virus to another. Survival of the virus is aided by the presence of a lipid-containing envelope. For example, in temperate areas enveloped viruses (influenza and coronaviruses) are found in midwinter, whereas nonenveloped viruses are found most often in the spring and fall, when indoor relative humidity is high.

Alleviation of VURI symptoms using OTC medications and supportive measures is the primary strategy for managing the condition. Symptoms peak in 3 to 5 days and resolve in 7 to 14 days. There are numerous OTC medications available to treat the symptoms of cold, including nasal decongestants (pseudoephedrine, phenylephrine, naphazoline, oxymetazoline, xylometazoline), antihistamines (diphenhydramine, loratadine, chlorpheniramine, brompheniramine), antitussives (dextromethorphan), expectorants (guaifenesin), and analgesics (acetaminophen, ibuprofen, naproxen).

ACETAMINOPHEN

Analgesic—The mechanism of analgesic action has not been fully determined. Acetaminophen may act predominantly by inhibiting prostaglandin synthesis in the central nervous system and, to a lesser extent, through a peripheral action by blocking pain-impulse generation. The peripheral action may also be due to inhibition of prostaglandin synthesis or to inhibition of the synthesis or actions of other substances that sensitize pain receptors to mechanical or chemical stimulation.

Antipyretic—Acetaminophen probably produces antipyresis by acting centrally on the hypothalamic heat-regulating center to produce peripheral vasodilation, resulting in increased blood flow to the skin, sweating, and heat loss. The central action probably involves inhibition of prostaglandin synthesis in the hypothalamus.

Acetaminophen is often used in many multi-ingredient products for the treatment of symptoms of cough, cold, and flu.

For more information, refer to the complete monograph for acetaminophen in "Aches and Pains" under Musculoskeletal Systems.

ANTIHISTAMINES

Antihistaminic (H_1-receptor)—Antihistamines used in the treatment of allergy act by competing with histamine for H_1-receptor sites on effector cells. They thereby prevent, but do not reverse, responses mediated by histamine alone. Antihistamines antagonize, in varying degrees, most of the pharmacological effects of histamine, including urticaria and pruritus. Also, the anticholinergic actions of most antihistamines provide a drying effect on the nasal mucosa.

Antitussive—Diphenhydramine suppresses the cough reflex by a direct effect on the cough center in the medulla of the brain.

Antihistamines are often used in many multi-ingredient products for the treatment of symptoms of cough, cold, and flu.

For more information, refer to the complete monograph for antihistamines in "Allergic Rhinitis" under Respiratory System.

DEXTROMETHORPHAN

PHARMACOLOGY

Dextromethorphan suppresses the cough reflex by a direct action on the cough center in the medulla of the brain.

INDICATIONS

Cough (treatment)—Dextromethorphan is indicated for the temporary symptomatic relief of nonproductive cough due to minor throat and bronchial irritation occurring with colds or inhaled irritants.

CONTRAINDICATIONS

Risk-benefit should be considered when the following medical problems exist:

- Asthma (dextromethorphan may impair expectoration and thus increase airway resistance.

- Bronchitis, chronic.

- Cough, productive.

- Emphysema or (inhibition of cough reflex by dextromethorphan may lead to retention of secretions).

- Diabetes (some dextromethorphan products contain sugar and may impair blood glucose control).

- Hepatic function impairment (metabolism of dextromethorphan may be impaired).
- Respiratory depression (dextromethorphan may make this condition worse).
- Sensitivity to dextromethorphan, other ingredients, such as procaine, butacaine, benzocaine, or other "caine" anesthetics, or other inactive ingredients (may result in adverse effects such as insomnia, dizziness, weakness, tremors, and arrhythmias).

WARNINGS/PRECAUTIONS

Pregnancy: Adequate and well-controlled studies in humans have not been done.

Breastfeeding: Problems in humans have not been documented.

ADVERSE REACTIONS

Those indicating need for medical attention only if they continue or are bothersome: Incidence less frequent or rare

Confusion, constipation, headache, mild dizziness, mild drowsiness, nausea or vomiting, stomach pain.

ADMINISTRATION AND DOSAGE

Lozenges

Adults/Pediatrics ≥12 years of age: 5 to 15mg every 2 to 4 hours as needed. Max: 90mg/day.

Pediatrics 6 to 12 years of age: 5 to 15mg every 2 to 6 hours as needed. Max: 60mg/day.

Pediatrics 2 to 6 years of age: 5mg every 4 hours as needed. Max: 30mg/day.

Syrup

Adults/Pediatrics ≥12 years of age: 30mg every 6 to hours as needed. Max: 120mg/day.

Pediatrics 6 to 12 years of age: 7mg every four hours or 15mg every six to eight hours as needed. Max: 60mg/day.

Pediatrics 2 to 6 years of age: 3.5mg every 4 hours or 7.5mg every 6 to 8 hours as needed. Max: 30mg/day.

Suspension, extended-release

Adults/Pediatrics ≥12 years of age: 60mg every 12 hours as needed. Max: 120mg/day.

Pediatrics 6 to 12 years of age: 5 to 30mg every 12 hours as needed. Max: 60mg/day.

Pediatrics 2 to 6 years of age: 15mg every 12 hours as needed. Max: 30mg/day.

Drug Interactions for Dextromethorphan

Precipitant Drug	Object Drug	Effect On Object Drug	Description
◆ Amiodarone ◆ Fluoxetine ◆ Quinidine	Dextromethorphan	↑	Inhibition of the CYP-450 2D6 enzyme system by these drugs may cause a decrease in the hepatic metabolism of dextromethorphan, which may result in increased dextromethorphan serum concentrations; higher concentrations of dextromethorphan have been associated with an increased incidence of side effects.
Dextromethorphan	◆ CNS Depressants	↑	Concurrent use may potentiate the CNS depressant effects of these medications or dextromethorphan.
◆ MAOIs (furazolidone, phenelzine, procarbazine, selegiline, tranylcypromine)	Dextromethorphan	↔	Concurrent use with dextromethorphan, and also use of MAOIs within 2 to 3 weeks of dextromethorphan, may cause adrenergic crisis, collapse, coma, dizziness, excitation, hypertension, hyperpyrexia, intracerebral bleeding, lethargy, nausea, psychotic behavior, spasms, and tremors.

◆ = Major clinical significance. MAOI = monoamine oxidase inhibitor.

DEXTROMETHORPHAN PRODUCTS

Brand Name	Dosage Form
Benylin Pediatric Formula (Pfizer)	**Syrup:** 15mg/5mL
Delsym (Celltech)	**Suspension:** 30mg/5mL
Pediacare Long-Acting Cough (Pfizer)	**Solution:** 7.5mg/0.8mL
Pediacare Medicated Freezer Pops (Pfizer)	**Solution:** 7.5mg/25mL
Robitussin Cough Calmers (Wyeth)	**Lozenge:** 5mg
Robitussin Maximum Strength (Wyeth)	**Syrup:** 15mg/5mL
Robitussin Pediatric Cough (Wyeth)	**Syrup:** 7.5mg/5mL
Simply Cough (McNeil)	**Liquid:** 5mg/5mL
Vicks 44 Cough Relief (Procter & Gamble)	**Liquid:** 10mg/5mL

GUAIFENESIN

PHARMACOLOGY

Guaifenesin is thought to act as an expectorant by increasing the volume and reducing the viscosity of secretions in the trachea and bronchi. Thus, it may increase the efficiency of the cough reflex and facilitate removal of the secretions; however, objective evidence for this is limited and conflicting.

INDICATIONS

Cough (treatment)—Guaifenesin is indicated as an expectorant in the temporary symptomatic management of cough due to minor upper respiratory infections and related conditions, such as sinusitis, pharyngitis, and bronchitis, when these conditions are complicated by viscous mucus and congestion. However, because supporting data are very limited, there is some controversy about its effectiveness.

CONTRAINDICATIONS

Risk-benefit should be considered when the following medical problems exist:

- Sensitivity to guaifenesin.

WARNINGS/PRECAUTIONS

Pregnancy: FDA Category C.

Breastfeeding: Problems in humans have not been documented.

ADVERSE REACTIONS

Those indicating need for medical attention only if they continue or are bothersome: Incidence less frequent or rare

Diarrhea, dizziness, headache, nausea or vomiting, skin rash, stomach pain, urticaria.

ADMINISTRATION AND DOSAGE

Capsules/Solution/Syrup/Tablets

Adults/Pediatrics ≥12 years of age: 200 to 400mg every 4 hours. Max: 2400mg/day.

Pediatrics 2 to 6 years of age: 50 to 100mg every 4 hours. Max: 600mg/day.

Pediatrics 6 to 12 years of age: 100 to 200mg every 4 hours. Max: 1200mg/day.

Capsules, extended-release/Tablets, extended-release

Adults/Pediatrics ≥12 years of age: 600 to 1200mg every 12 hours. Max: 2400mg/day.

Pediatrics 2 to 6 years of age: 300mg every 12 hours. Max: 600mg/day.

Pediatrics 6 to 12 years of age: 600mg every 12 hours. Max: 1200mg/day.

NONSTEROIDAL ANTI-INFLAMMATORY DRUGS (NSAIDs)

Analgesic—NSAIDs may block pain-impulse generation via a peripheral action that may involve reduction of the activity of prostaglandins, and possibly inhibition of the synthesis or actions of other substances that sensitize pain receptors to mechanical or chemical stimulation.

Antipyretic—NSAIDs Probably produce antipyresis by acting centrally on the hypothalamic heat-regulating center to produce peripheral vasodilation, resulting in increased blood flow to the skin, sweating, and heat loss. The central action probably involves reduction of prostaglandin activity in the hypothalamus.

NSAIDs are often used in many multi-ingredient products for the treatment of symptoms of cough, cold, and flu.

For more information, as well as a list of products and dosages, refer to the complete monograph for NSAIDs in "Aches and Pains" under Musculoskeletal System.

PSEUDOEPHEDRINE

Pseudoephedrine acts on alpha-adrenergic receptors in the mucosa of the respiratory tract, producing vasoconstriction. The medication shrinks swollen nasal mucous membranes; reduces tissue hyperemia, edema, and nasal congestion; and increases nasal airway patency. Also, drainage of sinus secretions may be increased and obstructed eustachian ostia may be opened.

Pseudoephedrine is often used in many multi-ingredient products for the treatment of symptoms of cough, cold, and flu.

For more information, refer to the complete monograph for pseudoephedrine in "Nasal Congestion" under Respiratory System.

GUAIFENESIN PRODUCTS	
Brand Name	**Dosage Form**
Mucinex (Adams)	**Tablet:** 600mg
Robitussin (Wyeth)	**Syrup:** 100mg/5mL

DOSING INFORMATION FOR COUGH, COLD, AND FLU PRODUCTS

The following table provides a quick comparison of the ingredients and dosages of common brand-name OTC drugs. Products are listed alphabetically by drug category and brand name.

ANTIHISTAMINE & DECONGESTANT

Brand Name	Analgesic	Antihistamine	Decongestant	Cough Suppressant	Expectorant	Dose
Actifed Cold & Allergy caplets (*Pfizer Consumer Healthcare*)		Triprolidine Hydrochloride 2.5mg	Pseudoephedrine HCl 60mg			**Adults ≥12 yo:** 1 tabs q4-6h. **Max:** 4 tabs q24h. **Peds 3-12 yo:** 1/2 tab q4-6h. **Max:** 2 tabs q24h.
Alka-Seltzer Ready Relief Multi-Symptom Cold Relief (*Bayer Healthcare*)		Chlorpheniramine Maleate 2mg	Pseudoephedrine HCl 30mg			**Adults ≥12 yo:** 2 tab q4-6h. **Max:** 8 tab q24h. **Peds 6-12 yo:** 1 tab q4-6h. **Max:** 4 tab q24h.
Benadryl Children's Allergy & Cold Fastmelt tablets (*Pfizer Consumer Healthcare*)		Diphenhydramine 19mg	Pseudoephedrine HCl 30mg			**Adults ≥12 yo:** 2 tabs q4h. **Max:** 8 tabs q24h. **Peds 6-12 yo:** 1 tab q4h. **Max:** 4 tabs q24h.
Benadryl-D Allergy & Sinus Fastmelt Tablets (*Pfizer Consumer Healthcare*)		Diphenhydramine Citrate 19mg	Pseudoephedrine HCl 30mg			**Adults & Peds ≥12 yo:** 2 tabs q4-6h. **Max:** 8 tabs q24h.
Benadryl-D Allergy/Sinus Tablets (*Pfizer Consumer Healthcare*)		Diphenhydramine HCl 25mg	Pseudoephedrine HCl 30mg			**Adults & Peds ≥12 yo:** 1 tab q4-6h. **Max:** 4 tab q24h.
Children's Benadryl-D Allergy & Sinus Liquid (*Pfizer Consumer Healthcare*)		Diphenhydramine HCl 12.5mg/5mL	Pseudoephedrine HCl 30mg/5mL			**Adults >12 yo:** 2 tsp (10mL) q4-6h. **Peds 6-12 yo:** 1 tsp (5mL) q4-6h. **Max:** 4 doses q24h.
Dimetapp Children's Cold & Allergy elixir (*Wyeth Consumer Healthcare*)		Brompheniramine Maleate 1mg/5mL	Pseudoephedrine HCl 15mg/5mL			**Adults ≥12 yo:** 4 tsp (20mL) q4h. **Peds 6-12 yo:** 2 tsp (10mL) q4h. **Max:** 4 doses q24h.
PediaCare Children's Cold & Allergy liquid (*Pharmacia Consumer Healthcare*)		Chlorpheniramine Maleate 1mg/5mL	Pseudoephedrine HCl 15mg/5mL			**Peds 6-12 yo:** 2 tsp (10ml) q4-6h. **Max:** 4 doses q24.
Sudafed Sinus Nighttime tablets (*Pfizer Consumer Healthcare*)		Triprolidine Hydrochloride 2.5mg	Pseudoephedrine HCl 60mg			**Adults ≥12 yo:** 1 tabs q4-6h. **Peds 6-12 yo:** 1/2 tab q4-6h. **Max:** 4 doses q24h.
Triaminic Cold & Allergy liquid (*Novartis Consumer Health*)		Chlorpheniramine Maleate 1mg/5mL	Pseudoephedrine HCl 15mg/5mL			**Peds 6-12 yo:** 2 tsp (10mL) q4-6h. **Max:** 8 tsp (40mL) q24h.

DOSING INFORMATION FOR COUGH, COLD, AND FLU PRODUCTS (cont.)

Brand Name	Analgesic	Antihistamine	Decongestant	Cough Suppressant	Expectorant	Dose
Triaminic Softchews Cold & Allergy (*Novartis Consumer Health*)		Chlorpheniramine Maleate 1mg	Pseudoephedrine HCl 15mg			**Peds 6-12 yo:** 2 tabs q4-6h. **Max:** 4 doses q24.
ANTIHISTAMINE & DECONGESTANT & ANALGESIC						
Actifed Cold & Sinus caplets (*Pfizer Consumer Healthcare*)	Acetaminophen 500mg	Chlorpheniramine Maleate 2mg	Pseudoephedrine HCl 30mg			**Adults & Peds ≥12 yo:** 2 tabs q6h. **Max:** 8 tabs q24h.
Advil Multi-Symptom Cold caplets (*Wyeth Consumer Healthcare*)	Ibuprofen 200mg	Chlorpheniramine Maleate 2mg	Pseudoephedrine HCl 30mg			**Adults & Peds ≥12 yo:** 1 tab q4-6h. **Max:** 6 tabs q24h.
Alka-Seltzer Plus Cold effervescent tablets (*Bayer Healthcare*)	Acetaminophen 250mg	Chlorpheniramine Maleate 2mg	Phenylephrine HCl 5mg			**Adults & Peds ≥12 yo:** 2 tabs q4h. **Max:** 8 tabs q24h.
Alka-Seltzer Plus Cold liqui-gels (*Bayer Healthcare*)	Acetaminophen 325mg	Chlorpheniramine Maleate 2mg	Pseudoephedrine HCl 30mg			**Adults ≥12 yo:** 2 caps q4h. **Peds 6-12 yo:** 1 cap q4h. **Max:** 4 doses q24h.
Benadryl Allergy & Cold caplets (*Pfizer Consumer Healthcare*)	Acetaminophen 500mg	Diphenhydramine HCl 25mg	Pseudoephedrine HCl 60mg			**Adults & Peds ≥12 yo:** 2 cap q6h. **Max:** 8 q24h.
Benadryl Children's Allergy & Cold caplets (*Pfizer Consumer Healthcare*)	Acetaminophen 500mg	Diphenhydramine 12.5mg	Pseudoephedrine HCl 30mg			**Adults & Peds ≥12 yo:** 2 tabs q6h. **Max:** 8 tabs q24h.
Benadryl Severe Allergy & Sinus Headache caplets (*Pfizer Consumer Healthcare*)	Acetaminophen 500mg	Diphenhydramine HCl 25mg	Pseudoephedrine HCl 30mg			**Adults & Peds ≥12 yo:** 2 tab q6h. **Max:** 8 tab q24h.
Comtrex Acute Head Cold caplets (*Bristol-Myers Squibb*)	Acetaminophen 500mg	Brompheniramine Maleate 2mg	Pseudoephedrine HCl 30mg			**Adults & Peds ≥12 yo:** 2 tabs q6h. **Max:** 8 tabs q24h.
Comtrex Flu Therapy Maximum Strength liquid (*Bristol-Myers Squibb*)	Acetaminophen 1000mg/30mL	Chlorpheniramine Maleate 4mg/30mL	Pseudoephedrine HCl 60mg/30mL			**Adults & Peds ≥12 yo: Max:** 2 tbl (30mL) q6h. **Max:** 8 tbl (240mL) q24h.
Comtrex Nighttime Acute Head Cold liquid (*Bristol-Myers Squibb*)	Acetaminophen 1000mg/30mL	Brompheniramine Maleate 4mg/30mL	Pseudoephedrine HCl 60mg/30mL			**Adults & Peds ≥12 yo: Max:** 2 tbl (30mL) q6h. **Max:** 8 tbl (240mL) q24h.
Coricidin D Cold, Flu & Sinus tablets (*Schering-Plough*)	Acetaminophen 325mg	Chlorpheniramine Maleate 2mg	Pseudoephedrine Sulfate 30mg			**Adults ≥12 yo:** 2 tabs q4-6h. **Max:** 8 tabs q24h. **Peds 6-12 yo:** 1 tab q4h. **Max:** 4 tabs q24h.

DOSING INFORMATION FOR COUGH, COLD, AND FLU PRODUCTS (cont.)

Brand Name	Analgesic	Antihistamine	Decongestant	Cough Suppressant	Expectorant	Dose
Dristan Cold Multi-Symptom tablets (*Wyeth Consumer Healthcare*)	Acetaminophen 325mg	Chlorpheniramine Maleate 2mg	Phenylephrine HCl 5mg			**Adults & Peds ≥12 yo:** 2 tabs q4h. **Max:** 12 caps q24h.
Sudafed Sinus Nighttime Plus Pain Relief caplets (*Pfizer Consumer Healthcare*)	Acetaminophen 500mg	Diphenhydramine HCl 25mg	Pseudoephedrine HCl 30mg			**Adults & Peds ≥12 yo:** 2 tabs q6h. **Max:** 8 tabs q24h.
Theraflu Flu & Sore Throat packets (*Novartis Consumer Health*)	Acetaminophen 1000mg/packet	Chlorpheniramine Maleate 4mg/packet	Pseudoephedrine HCl 60mg/packet			**Adults & Peds ≥12 yo:** 1 packet q6h. **Max:** 4 packets q24h.
Tylenol Children's Plus Cold & Allergy liquid (*McNeil Consumer*)	Acetaminophen 160mg/5mL	Diphenhydramine HCl 12.5mg/5mL	Pseudoephedrine HCl 15mg/5mL			**Peds 6-12 yo (48-95 lbs):** 2 tsp 10mL) q4-6h. **Max:** 8 tsp 40mL) q24h.
Tylenol Children's Plus Cold Nighttime suspension (*McNeil Consumer*)	Acetaminophen 160mg/5mL	Chlorpheniramine Maleate 1mg/5mL	Pseudoephedrine HCl 15mg/5mL			**Peds 6-12 yo (48-95 lbs):** 2 tsp (10mL) q4-6h. **Max:** 8 tsp (40mL) q24h.
Tylenol Flu Nighttime gelcaps (*McNeil Consumer*)	Acetaminophen 500mg	Diphenhydramine HCl 25mg	Pseudoephedrine HCl 30mg			**Adults & Peds ≥12 yo:** 2 caps q6h. **Max:** 8 caps q24h.
Tylenol Sinus Nighttime caplets (*McNeil Consumer*)	Acetaminophen 500mg	Doxylamine Succinate 6.25mg	Pseudoephedrine HCl 30mg			**Adults & Peds ≥12 yo:** 2 tabs q4-6h. **Max:** 8 tabs q24h.
COUGH SUPPRESSANT						
Benylin Adult Formula liquid (*Pfizer Consumer Healthcare*)				Dextromethorphan HBr 15mg/5mL		**Adults & Peds ≥12 yo:** 2 tsp (10mL) q6-8h. **Peds 6-12 yo:** 1 tsp (5mL) q6-8h. **2-6 yo:** 1/2 tsp 2.5mL) q6-8h. **Max:** 4 doses q24h.
Benylin Pediatric liquid (*Pfizer Consumer Healthcare*)				Dextromethorphan HBr 7.5mg/5mL		**Adults & Peds ≥12 yo:** 4 tsp (20mL) q6-8h. **Peds 6-12 yo:** 2 tsp (10mL) q6-8h. **2-6 yo:** 1 tsp (5mL) q6-8h. **Max:** 4 doses q24h.
Delsym 12 Hour Cough Relief liquid (*Celltech Pharmaceuticals*)				Dextromethorphan Polistrex 30mg/5mL		**Adults ≥12 yo:** 2 tsp (10mL) q12h. **Peds 6-12 yo:** 1 tsp (5mL) q12h. **2-6 yo:** 1/2 tsp (2.5mL) q12h. **Max:** 4 doses q24h.

DOSING INFORMATION FOR COUGH, COLD, AND FLU PRODUCTS (cont.)

Brand Name	Analgesic	Antihistamine	Decongestant	Cough Suppressant	Expectorant	Dose
PediaCare Long-Acting Cough freezer pops (*Pharmacia Consumer Healthcare*)				Dextromethorphan HBr 7.5mg/pop		**Peds 6-12 yo:** 2 pops q6-8h. **2-6 yo:** 1 pop (5mL) q6-8h. **Max:** 4 doses q24h.
Robitussin Cough Maximum Strength liquid (*Wyeth Consumer Healthcare*)				Dextromethorphan HBr 15mg/5mL		**Adults & Peds ≥12 yo:** 2 tsp (10mL) q6-8h. **Max:** 8 tsp (40mL) q24h.
Robitussin CoughGels liqui-gels (*Wyeth Consumer Healthcare*)				Dextromethorphan HBr 15mg		**Adults & Peds ≥12 yo:** 2 caps q6-8h. **Max:** 8 caps q24h.
Robitussin Honey Cough syrup (*Wyeth Consumer Healthcare*)				Dextromethorphan HBr 10mg/5mL		**Adults ≥12 yo:** 3 tsp (15mL) q6-8h. **Peds 6-12 yo:** 1.5 tsp (7.5mL) q6-8h. **Max:** 4 doses q24h.
Robitussin Pediatric Cough liquid (*Wyeth Consumer Healthcare*)				Dextromethorphan HBr 7.5mg		**Adults ≥12 yo (≥96 lbs):** 4 tsp (20mL) q6-8h. **Peds 6-12 yo (48-95 lbs):** 2 tsp (10mL) q6-8h. **2-6 yo:** 1 tsp (5mL) q6-8h. **Max:** 4 doses q24h.
Simply Cough liquid (*McNeil Consumer*)				Dextromethorphan HBr 5mg/5mL		**Peds 6-12 yo (48-95 lbs):** 2 tsp (10mL) q4h. **2-6 yo (24-47 lbs):** 1 tsp (5mL) q4h. **Max:** 4 doses q24h.
Theraflu Long Acting Cough thin strips (*Novartis Consumer Health*)				Dextromethorphan 11mg/strip		**Adults & Peds ≥12 yo:** 2 strips q6-8h. **Max:** 8 strips q24h.
Triaminic Long Acting Cough thin strips (*Novartis Consumer Health*)				Dextromethorphan 5.5mg/strip		**Peds 6-12 yo:** 2 strips q6-8h. **Max:** 8 strips q24h.
Triaminic Vapor Patch Cough (*Novartis Consumer Health*)				Camphor 4.7% Menthol 2.6%		**Peds 2-12 yo:** 1 patch q8h.
Vicks 44 liquid (*Procter & Gamble*)				Dextromethorphan HBr 30mg/15mL		**Adults & Peds ≥12 yo:** 1 tbl (15mL) q6-8h. **Peds 6-12 yo:** 1.5 tsp (7.5mL) q6-8h. **Max:** 4 doses q24h.

DOSING INFORMATION FOR COUGH, COLD, AND FLU PRODUCTS (cont.)

Brand Name	Analgesic	Antihistamine	Decongestant	Cough Suppressant	Expectorant	Dose
Vicks BabyRub (*Procter & Gamble*)				Eucalyptus		Peds ≥3 mth: Apply q8h.
Vicks Cough Drops Cherry Flavor (*Procter & Gamble*)				Menthol 1.7mg		Adults & Peds ≥5 yo: 3 drops q1-2h.
Vicks Cough Drops Original Flavor (*Procter & Gamble*)				Menthol 3.3mg		Adults & Peds ≥5 yo: 2 drops q1-2h.
Vicks VapoRub (*Procter & Gamble*)				Camphor 5.2% Menthol 2.8% Eucalyptus1.2%		Adults & Peds ≥2 yo: Apply q8h.
Vicks VapoRub Cream (*Procter & Gamble*)				Camphor 4.8% Menthol 2.6% Eucalyptus 1.2%		Adults & Peds ≥2 yo: Apply q8h.
Vicks VapoSteam (*Procter & Gamble*)				Camphor 6.2%		Adults & Peds ≥2 yo: 1 tbl/quart q8h.
COUGH SUPPRESSANT & ANTIHISTAMINE						
Coricidin HBP Cough & Cold tablets (*Schering-Plough*)		Chlorpheniramine Maleate 4mg		Dextromethorphan HBr 30mg		Adults & Peds ≥12 yo: 1 tabs q6h. Max: 4 tabs q24h.
Vicks NyQuil Cough liquid (*Procter & Gamble*)		Doxylamine Succinate 6.25mg/15mL		Dextromethorphan HBr 15mg/15mL		Adults & Peds ≥12 yo: 2 tbl (30mL) q6h. Max: 8 tbl (120mL) q24h.
COUGH SUPPRESSANT & ANTIHISTAMINE & ANALGESIC						
Alka-Seltzer Plus Flu effervescent tablets (*Bayer Healthcare*)	Aspirin 500mg	Chlorpheniramine Maleate 2mg		Dextromethorphan HBr 15mg		Adults & Peds ≥12 yo: 2 tabs q6h. Max: 8 tabs q24h.
Coricidin HBP Maximum Strength Flu tablets (*Schering-Plough*)	Acetaminophen 500mg	Chlorpheniramine Maleate 2mg		Dextromethorphan HBr 15mg		Adults & Peds ≥12 yo: 2 tabs q6h. Max: 8 tabs q24h.
Tylenol Nighttime Cough & Sore Throat Cool Burst liquid (*McNeil Consumer*)	Acetaminophen 1000mg/30mL	Doxylamine 12.5mg/30mL		Dextromethorphan HBr 30mg/30mL		Adults & Peds ≥12 yo: 2 tbl (30mL) q6h. Max: 8 tbl (120mL) q24h.
COUGH SUPPRESSANT & ANTIHISTAMINE & ANALGESIC & DECONGESTANT						
Alka-Seltzer Plus Cold & Cough liqui-gels (*Bayer Healthcare*)	Acetaminophen 325mg	Chlorpheniramine Maleate 2mg	Pseudoephedrine HCl 30mg	Dextromethorphan HBr 10mg		Adults ≥12 yo: 2 caps q4h. **Peds 6-12 yo:** 1 cap q4h. **Max:** 4 doses q24h.
Alka-Seltzer Plus Night-Time liqui-gels (*Bayer Healthcare*)	Acetaminophen 325mg	Doxylamine 6.25mg	Pseudoephedrine HCl 30mg	Dextromethorphan HBr 10mg		Adults & Peds ≥12 yo: 2 caps q6h. **Max:** 8 caps q24h.

DOSING INFORMATION FOR COUGH, COLD, AND FLU PRODUCTS (cont.)

Brand Name	Analgesic	Antihistamine	Decongestant	Cough Suppressant	Expectorant	Dose
Alka-Seltzer Plus Nose & Throat effervescent tablets (Bayer Healthcare)	Acetaminophen 250mg	Chlorpheniramine Maleate 2mg	Phenylephrine HCl 5mg	Dextromethorphan HBr 10mg		**Adults & Peds ≥12 yo:** 2 tabs q4h. **Max:** 8 tabs q24h.
Comtrex Cold & Cough Nighttime caplets (Bristol-Myers Squibb)	Acetaminophen 500mg	Chlorpheniramine Maleate 2mg	Pseudoephedrine HCl 30mg	Dextromethorphan HBr 15mg		**Adults & Peds ≥12 yo:** 2 tabs q6h. **Max:** 8 tabs q24h.
Comtrex Nighttime Cold & Cough liquid (Bristol-Myers Squibb)	Acetaminophen 1000mg/ 30mL	Chlorpheniramine Maleate 4mg/30mL	Pseudoephedrine HCl 60mg/30mL	Dextromethorphan HBr 30mg/30mL		**Adults & Peds ≥12 yo:** 2 tbl (30mL) q6h. **Max:** 8 tbl (240mL) q24h.
Contac Cold & Flu Maxium Strength caplets (GlaxoSmithKline Consumer Healthcare)	Acetaminophen 500mg	Chlorpheniramine Maleate 2mg	Pseudoephedrine HCl 30mg	Dextromethorphan HBr 15mg		**Adults & Peds ≥12 yo:** 2 tabs q6h. **Max:** 8 tabs q24h.
Dimetapp Children's Nigttime Flu liquid (Wyeth Consumer Healthcare)	Acetaminophen 160mg/ 5mL	Brompheniramine Maleate 1mg/5mL	Pseudoephedrine HCl 15mg/5mL	Dextromethorphan HBr 5mg/5mL		**Adults ≥12 yo:** 4 tsp (20mL) q4h. **Peds 6-12 yo:** 2 tsp (10mL) q4h. **Max:** 4 doses q24h.
Robitussin Flu liquid (Wyeth Consumer Healthcare)	Acetaminophen 160mg/ 5mL	Chlorpheniramine Maleate 1mg/5mL	Psuedoephedrine HCl 15mg/5mL	Dextromethorphan HBr 5mg/5mL		**Adults ≥12 yo:** 4 tsp (20mL) q4h. **Peds 6-12 yo:** 2 tsp (10mL) q4h. **Max:** 4 doses q24h.
Robitussin Night Relief liquid (Wyeth Consumer Healthcare)	Acetaminophen 650mg/ 30mL	Pyrilamine maleate 50mg/30mL	Pseudoephedrine HCl 60mg/30mL	Dextromethorphan HBr 30mg/30mL		**Adults & Peds ≥12 yo:** 2 tbl (30mL) q6h. **Max:** 8 tbl (240mL) q24h.
Theraflu Cold & Cough packets (Novartis Consumer Health)	Acetaminophen 650mg/ packet	Chlorpheniramine Maleate 4mg/packet	Pseudoephedrine HCl 60mg/packet	Dextromethorphan HBr 20mg/packet		**Adults & Peds ≥12 yo:** 1 packet q4-6h. **Max:** 4 packets q24h.
Theraflu Severe Cold & Cough packets (Novartis Consumer Health)	Acetaminophen 1000mg/ packet	Chlorpheniramine Maleate 4mg/packet	Pseudoephedrine HCl 60mg/packet	Dextromethorphan HBr 30mg/packet		**Adults & Peds ≥12 yo:** 1 packet q6h. **Max:** 4 packets q24h.
Theraflu Severe Cold caplets (Novartis Consumer Health)	Acetaminophen 500mg	Chlorpheniramine Maleate 2mg	Pseudoephedrine HCl 30mg	Dextromethorphan HBr 15mg		**Adults & Peds ≥12 yo:** 2 tabs q6h. **Max:** 8 tabs q24h.
Theraflu Severe Cold packets (Novartis Consumer Health)	Acetaminophen 1000mg/ packet	Chlorpheniramine Maleate 4mg/packet	Pseudoephedrine HCl 60mg/packet	Dextromethorphan HBr 30mg/packet		**Adults & Peds ≥12 yo:** 1 packet q6h. **Max:** of 4 packets q24h.
Triaminic Flu, Cough, & Fever liquid (Novartis Consumer Health)	Acetaminophen 160mg/ 5mL	Chlorpheniramine Maleate 1mg/5mL	Pseudoephedrine HCl 15mg/5mL	Dextromethorphan HBr 7.5mg/5mL		**Peds 6-12 yo:** 2 tsp (10mL) q6h. **Max:** 8 tsp (40mL) q24h.

DOSING INFORMATION FOR COUGH, COLD, AND FLU PRODUCTS (cont.)

Brand Name	Analgesic	Antihistamine	Decongestant	Cough Suppressant	Expectorant	Dose
Tylenol Children's Cold Plus Cough liquid (McNeil Consumer)	Acetaminophen 160mg/5mL	Chlorpheniramine Maleate 1mg/5mL	Pseudoephedrine HCl 15mg/5mL	Dextromethorphan HBr 5mg/5mL		**Peds 6-12 yo (48-95 lbs):** 2 tsp (10mL) q4-6h. **Max:** 8 tsp (40mL) q24h.
Tylenol Children's Flu liquid (McNeil Consumer)	Acetaminophen 160mg/5mL	Chlorpheniramine Maleate 1mg/5mL	Pseudoephedrine HCl 15mg/5mL	Dextromethorphan HBr 7.5mg/5mL		**Peds 6-12 yo (48-95 lbs):** 2 tsp (10mL) q6-8h. **Max:** 8 tsp (40mL) q24h.
Tylenol Cold & Flu Severe Nighttime Cool Burst liquid (McNeil Consumer)	Acetaminophen 1000mg/30mL	Doxylamine 12.5mg/30mL	Pseudoephedrine HCl 60mg/30mL	Dextromethorphan HBr 30mg/30mL		**Adults & Peds ≥12 yo:** 2 tbl (30mL) q6h. **Max:** 8 tbl (120mL) q24h.
Tylenol Cold Nighttime Cool Burst caplets (McNeil Consumer)	Acetaminophen 325mg	Chlorpheniramine Maleate 2mg	Pseudoephedrine HCl 30mg	Dextromethorphan HBr 15mg		**Adults & Peds ≥12 yo:** 2 tabs q6h. **Max:** 8 tabs q24h.
Vicks 44M liquid (Procter & Gamble)	Acetaminophen 162.5mg/5mL	Chlorpheniramine Maleate 1mg/5mL	Pseudoephedrine HCl 15mg/5mL	Dextromethorphan HBr 7.5mg/5mL		**Adults & Peds ≥12 yo:** 4 tsp (20mL) q6h. **Max:** 16 tsp (80mL) q24h.
Vicks NyQuil liquicaps (Procter & Gamble)	Acetaminophen 325mg	Doxylamine Succinate 6.25mg	Pseudoephedrine HCl 30mg	Dextromethorphan HBr 15mg		**Adults & Peds ≥12 yo:** 2 caps q6h. **Max:** 8 caps q24h.
Vicks NyQuil liquid (Procter & Gamble)	Acetaminophen 500mg/15mL	Doxylamine Succinate 6.25mg/15mL	Pseudoephedrine HCl 30mg/15mL	Dextromethorphan HBr 15mg/15mL		**Adults & Peds ≥12 yo:** 2 tbl (30mL) q6h. **Max:** 8 tbl (120mL) q24h.
COUGH SUPPRESSANT & ANTIHISTAMINE & DECONGESTANT						
Alka-Seltzer Plus Cold & Cough effervescent tablets (Bayer Healthcare)		Chlorpheniramine Maleate 2mg	Phenylephrine HCl 5mg	Dextromethorphan HBr 10mg		**Adults & Peds ≥12 yo:** 2 tabs q4h. **Max:** 8 tabs q24h.
Alka-Seltzer Plus Night-Time effervescent tablets (Bayer Healthcare)		Doxylamine 6.25mg	Phenylephrine HCl 5mg	Dextromethorphan HBr 10mg		**Adults & Peds ≥12 yo:** 2 tabs q4h. **Max:** 8 caps q24h.
Dimetapp DM Children's Cold & Cough elixir (Wyeth Consumer Healthcare)		Brompheniramine Maleate 1mg/5mL	Pseudoephedrine HCl 15mg/5mL	Dextromethorphan HBr 5mg/5mL		**Adults ≥12 yo:** 4 tsp (20mL) q4h. **Peds 6-12 yo:** 2 tsp (10mL) q4h. **Max:** 4 doses q24h.
PediaCare Multi-Symptom chewable tablets (Pharmacia Consumer Healthcare)		Chlorpheniramine Maleate 1mg	Pseudoephedrine HCl 15mg	Dextromethorphan HBr 5mg		**Peds 6-12 yo:** 2 tabs q4-6h. **Max:** 8 tabs q24h.

DOSING INFORMATION FOR COUGH, COLD, AND FLU PRODUCTS (cont.)

Brand Name	Analgesic	Antihistamine	Decongestant	Cough Suppressant	Expectorant	Dose
PediaCare Multi-Symptom liquid (*Pharmacia Consumer Healthcare*)		Chlorpheniramine Maleate 1mg/5mL	Pseudoephedrine HCl 15mg/5mL	Dextromethorphan HBr 5mg/5mL		**Peds 6-12 yo:** 2 tsp (10mL) q4-6h. **Max:** 8 tsp (40mL) q24h.
PediaCare Night Rest Cough & Cold liquid (*Pharmacia Consumer Healthcare*)		Chlorpheniramine Maleate 1mg/5mL	Pseudoephedrine HCl 15mg/5mL	Dextromethorphan HBr 7.5mg/5mL		**Peds 6-12 yo:** 2 tsp (10mL) q6-8h. **Max:** 8 tsp (40mL) q24h.
Robitussin Allergy & Cough liquid (*Wyeth Consumer Healthcare*)		Brompheniramine Maleate 2mg/5mL	Pseudoephedrine HCl 30mg/5mL	Dextromethorphan HBr 10mg/5ml		**Adults ≥12 yo:** 2 tsp (10mL) q4h. **Peds 6-12 yo:** 1 tsp (5mL) q4h. **Max:** 4 doses q24h.
Robitussin Pediatric Night Relief liquid (*Wyeth Consumer Healthcare*)		Chlorpheniramine Maleate 1mg/5mL	Pseudoephedrine HCl 15mg/5mL	Dextromethorphan HBr 7.5mg/5mL		**Adults & Peds ≥12 yo (≥96 lbs):** 4 tsp (20mL) q6h. **Peds 6-12 yo (48-95 lbs):** 2 tsp (10mL) q6h.
Robitussin PM liquid (*Wyeth Consumer Healthcare*)		Chlorpheniramine Maleate 1mg/5mL	Pseudoephedrine HCl 15mg/5mL	Dextromethorphan HBr 7.5mg/5mL		**Adults ≥12 yo:** 4 tsp (20mL) q6h. **Peds 6-12 yo:** 2 tsp (10mL) q6h. **Max:** 4 doses q24h.
Triaminic Cold & Cough liquid (*Novartis Consumer Health*)		Chlorpheniramine Maleate 1mg/5mL	Pseudoephedrine HCl 15mg/5mL	Dextromethorphan HBr 5mg/5mL		**Peds 6-12 yo:** 2 tsp (10mL) q4-6h. **Max:** 8 tsp (40mL) q24h.
Triaminic Cold & Cough softchews (*Novartis Consumer Health*)		Chlorpheniramine Maleate 1mg	Pseudoephedrine HCl 15mg	Dextromethorphan HBr 5mg		**Peds 6-12 yo:** 2 tabs q4-6h. **Max:** 8 tabs q24h.
Triaminic Night Time Cough & Cold liquid (*Novartis Consumer Health*)		Chlorpheniramine Maleate 1mg/5mL	Pseudoephedrine HCl 15mg/5mL	Dextromethorphan HBr 7.5mg/5mL		**Peds 6-12 yo:** 2 tsp (10mL) q6h. **Max:** 8 tsp (40mL) q24h.
Vicks Children's NyQuil liquid (*Procter & Gamble*)		Chlorpheniramine Maleate 2mg/15ml	Pseudoephedrine HCl 30mg/15ml	Dextromethorphan HBr 15mg/15ml		**Adults & Peds ≥12 yo:** 2 tbl (30ml) q6h. **Peds 6-12 yo:** 1 tbl (15ml) q6h. **Max:** 4 doses q24h.
Vicks Pediatric 44M liquid (*Procter & Gamble*)		Chlorpheniramine Maleate 2mg/15ml	Pseudoephedrine HCl 30mg/15ml	Dextromethorphan HBr 15mg/15ml		**Adults ≥12 yo:** 2 tbl (30ml) q6h. **Peds 6-12 yo:** 1 tbl (15ml) q6h. **Max:** 4 doses q24h.
COUGH SUPPRESSANT & DECONGESTANT						
Dimetapp Children's Decongestant Infant Plus Cough drops (*Wyeth Consumer Healthcare*)			Pseudoephedrine HCl 7.5mg/0.8mL	Dextromethorphan HBr 2.5mg/0.8mL		**Peds 2-3 yo:** 1.6mL q4-6h. **Max:** 6.4mL q24h.

DOSING INFORMATION FOR COUGH, COLD, AND FLU PRODUCTS (cont.)

Brand Name	Analgesic	Antihistamine	Decongestant	Cough Suppressant	Expectorant	Dose
Dimetapp Children's Long Acting Cough Plus Cold elixir (Wyeth Consumer Healthcare)			Pseudoephedrine HCl 15mg/5mL	Dextromethorphan HBr 7.5mg/5mL		**Adults ≥12 yo:** 4 tsp (20mL) q6h. **Peds 6-12 yo:** 2 tsp (10mL) q6h. **2-6 yo:** 1 tsp q6h. **Max:** 4 doses q24h.
PediaCare Decongestant & Cough Infants' drops (Pharmacia Consumer Healthcare)			Pseudoephedrine HCl 7.5mg/0.8mL	Dextromethorphan HBr 2.5mg/0.8mL		**Peds 2-3 yo:** 1.6mL q4-6h. **Max:** 6.4mL q24h.
PediaCare Long-Acting Cough Plus Cold liquid (Pharmacia Consumer Healthcare)			Pseudoephedrine HCl 15mg/5mL	Dextromethorphan HBr 7.5mg/5mL		**Peds 6-12 yo:** 2 tsp (10mL) q6-8h. **2-6 yo:** 1 tsp (5mL) q6-8h. **Max:** 4 doses q24h.
Robitussin Honey Cold liquid (Wyeth Consumer Healthcare)			Psuedoephedrine HCl 20mg/5mL	Dextromethorphan HBr 10mg/5mL		**Adults & Peds ≥12 yo:** 3 tsp (15mL) q6h. **Max:** 12 tsp (180mL) q24h.
Robitussin Maximum Strength Cough & Cold liquid (Wyeth Consumer Healthcare)			Pseudoephedrine HCl 30mg/5mL	Dextromethorphan HBr 15mg/5mL		**Adults & Peds ≥12 yo:** 2 tsp (10mL) q4h. **Max:** 12 tsp (120mL) q24h.
Robitussin Pediatric Cough & Cold liquid (Wyeth Consumer Healthcare)			Pseudoephedrine HCl 15mg/5mL	Dextromethorphan HBr 7.5mg/5mL		**Adults ≥12 yo (≥96 lbs):** 4 tsp (20mL) q6h. **Peds 6-12 yo (48-95 lbs):** 2 tsp (10mL) q6h. **2-6 yo (24-47 lbs):** 1 tsp (2.5-5mL) q6h. **Max:** 4 doses q24h.
Sudafed Children's Cold & Cough liquid (Pfizer Consumer Healthcare)			Pseudoephedrine HCl 15mg/5mL	Dextromethorphan HBr 5mg/5mL		**Adults ≥12 yo:** 4 tsp (20mL) q4h. **Peds 6-12 yo:** 2 tsp (10mL) q4h. **2-6 yo:** 1 tsp (5mL) q4h. **Max:** 4 doses q24h.
Triaminic Cough & Nasal Congestion liquid (Novartis Consumer Health)			Pseudoephedrine HCl 15mg/5mL	Dextromethorphan HBr 7.5mg/5mL		**Peds 6-12 yo:** 2 tsp (10mL) q6h. **2-6 yo:** 1 tsp (5mL) q6h. **Max:** 4 doses q24h.
Triaminic Cough liquid (Novartis Consumer Health)			Pseudoephedrine HCl 15mg/5mL	Dextromethorphan HBr 5mg/5mL		**Peds 6-12 yo:** 2 tsp (10mL) q4-6h. **2-6 yo:** 1 tsp (5mL) q4-6h. **Max:** 4 doses q24h.
Vicks 44D liquid (Procter & Gamble)			Pseudoephedrine HCl 60mg/15mL	Dextromethorphan HBr 30mg/15mL		**Adults ≥12 yo:** 1 tbl (15mL) q6h. **Peds 6-12 yo:** 1.5 tsp (7.5mL) q6h. **Max:** 4 doses q24h.

DOSING INFORMATION FOR COUGH, COLD, AND FLU PRODUCTS (cont.)

COUGH SUPPRESSANT & DECONGESTANT & ANALGESIC

Brand Name	Analgesic	Antihistamine	Decongestant	Cough Suppressant	Expectorant	Dose
Alka-Seltzer Plus Cold Non-Drowsy effervescent tablets (*Bayer Healthcare*)	Acetaminophen 250mg		Phenylephrine HCl 5mg	Dextromethorphan HBr 10mg		**Adults & Peds ≥12 yo:** 2 tabs q4h. **Max:** 8 tabs q24h.
Alka-Seltzer Plus Non-Drowsy Cold Effervescent tablets (*Bayer Healthcare*)	Acetaminophen 250mg		Phenylepherine HCl 5mg	Dextromethorphan HBr 10mg		**Adults & Peds ≥12 yo:** 2 tab q4h. **Max:** 8 tab q24h.
Alka-Seltzer Plus Non-Drowsy Cold Medicine liqui-gels (*Bayer Healthcare*)	Acetaminophen 325mg		Pseudoephedrine HCl 30mg	Dextromethorphan HBr 30mg		**Adults ≥12 yo:** 2 caps q4h. **Max:** 8 cap q24h. **Peds 6-12 yo:** 1 cap q4h. **Max:** 4 tab q24h.
Comtrex Cold & Cough caplets (*Bristol-Myers Squibb*)	Acetaminophen 500mg		Pseudoephedrine HCl 30mg	Dextromethorphan HBr 15mg		**Adults & Peds ≥12 yo:** 2 tabs q6h. **Max:** 8 tabs q24h.
Contac Cold & Flu caplets (*GlaxoSmithKline Consumer Healthcare*)	Acetaminophen 325mg		Pseudoephedrine HCl 30mg	Dextromethorphan HBr 15mg		**Adults & Peds ≥12 yo:** 2 tabs q6h. **Max:** 8 tabs q24h.
Sudafed Severe Cold caplets (*Pfizer Consumer Healthcare*)	Acetaminophen 500mg		Pseudoephedrine HCl 30mg	Dextromethorphan HBr 15mg		**Adults & Peds ≥12 yo:** 2 tabs q6h. **Max:** 8 tabs q24h.
Theraflu Severe Cold Non-Drowsy caplets (*Novartis Consumer Health*)	Acetaminophen 500mg		Pseudoephedrine HCl 30mg	Dextromethorphan HBr 15mg		**Adults & Peds ≥12 yo:** 2 tabs q6h. **Max:** 8 tabs q24h.
Theraflu Severe Cold Non-Drowsy packets (*Novartis Consumer Health*)	Acetaminophen 1000mg/packet		Pseudoephedrine HCl 60mg/packet	Dextromethorphan HBr 30mg/packet		**Adults & Peds ≥12 yo:** 1 packet q6h. **Max:** 4 packets q24h.
Triaminic Cough & Sore Throat liquid (*Novartis Consumer Health*)	Acetaminophen 160mg/5mL		Pseudoephedrine HCl 15mg/5mL	Dextromethorphan HBr 7.5mg/5mL		**Peds 6-12 yo:** 2 tsp (10mL) q6h. **2-6 yo:** 1 tsp (5mL) q6h. **Max:** 4 doses q24h.
Triaminic Softchews Cough & Sore Throat tablets (*Novartis Consumer Health*)	Acetaminophen 160mg		Pseudoephedrine HCl 15mg	Dextromethorphan HBr 5mg		**Peds 6-12 yo:** 2 tabs q4-6h. **2-6 yo:** 1tab q4-6h. **Max:** 4 doses q24h.
Tylenol Cold & Flu Severe Daytime Cool Burst liquid (*McNeil Consumer*)	Acetaminophen 1000mg/30mL		Pseudoephedrine HCl 60mg/30mL	Dextromethorphan HBr 30mg/30mL		**Adults & Peds ≥12 yo:** 2 tbl (30mL) q6h. **Max:** 8 tbl (120mL) q24h.

DOSING INFORMATION FOR COUGH, COLD, AND FLU PRODUCTS (cont.)

Brand Name	Analgesic	Antihistamine	Decongestant	Cough Suppressant	Expectorant	Dose
Tylenol Cold Daytime Cool Burst caplets (McNeil Consumer)	Acetaminophen 325mg		Pseudoephedrine HCl 30mg	Dextromethorphan HBr 15mg		**Adults & Peds ≥12 yo:** 2 tabs q6h. **Max:** 8 tabs q24h.
Tylenol Cold Daytime gelcaps (McNeil Consumer)	Acetaminophen 325mg		Pseudoephedrine HCl 30mg	Dextromethorphan HBr 15mg		**Adults & Peds ≥12 yo:** 2 caps q6h. **Max:** 8 caps q24h.
Tylenol Cold Plus Cough Infants' drops (McNeil Consumer)	Acetaminophen 80mg/ 0.8mL		Pseudoephedrine HCl 7.5mg/0.8mL	Dextromethorphan HBr 5mg/0.8mL		**Peds 2-3 yo (24-35 lbs):** 1.6mL q4-6h. **Max:** 6.4mL q24h.
Tylenol Flu Daytime gelcaps (McNeil Consumer)	Acetaminophen 500mg		Pseudoephedrine HCl 30mg	Dextromethorphan HBr 15mg		**Adults & Peds ≥12 yo:** 2 caps q6h. **Max:** 8 caps q24h.
Vicks DayQuil liquicaps (Procter & Gamble)	Acetaminophen 325mg		Pseudoephedrine HCl 30mg	Dextromethorphan HBr 15mg		**Adults & Peds ≥12 yo:** 2 caps q6. **Max:** 8 caps q24h.
Vicks DayQuil liquid (Procter & Gamble)	Acetaminophen 325mg/ 15mL		Pseudoephedrine HCl 30mg/15mL	Dextromethorphan HBr 15mg/15mL		**Adults & Peds ≥12 yo:** 2 tbl (30mL) q6h. **Max:** 8 tbl (120mL) q24h.
COUGH SUPPRESSANT & DECONGESTANT & EXPECTORANT						
Robitussin CF liquid (Wyeth Consumer Healthcare)			Pseudoephedrine HCl 30mg/5mL	Dextromethorphan HBr 10mg/5mL	Guaifenesin 100mg/5mL	**Adults ≥12 yo:** 2 tsp (10mL) q4h. **Peds 6-12 yo:** 1 tsp (5mL) q4h. **2-6 yo:** 1/2 tsp (2.5mL) q4h. **Max:** 4 doses q24h.
Robitussin Pediatric Cough & Cold Infant Drops (Wyeth Consumer Healthcare)			Pseudoephedrine HCl 15mg/2.5mL	Dextromethorphan HBr 5mg/2.5mL	Guaifenesin 100mg/ 2.5mL	**Peds 2-6 yo (24-47 lbs):** 2.5ml q4h. **Max:** 4 doses q24h.
COUGH SUPPRESSANT & DECONGESTANT & EXPECTORANT & ANALGESIC						
Comtrex Chest Cold capsules (Bristol-Myers Squibb)	Acetaminophen 250mg		Pseudoephedrine HCl 30mg	Dextromethorphan HBr 10mg	Guaifenesin 100mg	**Adults & Peds ≥12 yo:** 2 caps q4h. **Max:** 12 caps q24h.
Robitussin Multi-Sympton Cold & Flu liqui-gels (Wyeth Consumer Healthcare)	Acetaminophen 250mg		Pseudoephedrine HCl 30mg	Dextromethorphan HBr 10mg	Guaifenesin 100mg	**Adults & Peds ≥12 yo:** 2 caps q4h. **Max:** 8 caps q24h.
Sudafed Cold & Cough liquid caps (Pfizer Consumer Healthcare)	Acetaminophen 250mg		Pseudoephedrine HCl 30mg	Dextromethorphan HBr 10mg	Guaifenesin 100mg	**Adults & Peds ≥12 yo:** 2 caps q4h. **Max:** 8 caps q24h.

DOSING INFORMATION FOR COUGH, COLD, AND FLU PRODUCTS (cont.)

Brand Name	Analgesic	Antihistamine	Decongestant	Cough Suppressant	Expectorant	Dose
Theraflu Flu & Chest Congestion packets (*Novartis Consumer Health*)	Acetaminophen 1000mg/ packet		Pseudoephedrine HCl 60mg/packet	Dextromethorphan HBr 30mg/packet	Guaifenesin 400mg/ packet	**Adults & Peds ≥12 yo:** 1 packet q6h. **Max:** 4 packets q24h.
Tylenol Cold Severe Congestion Non-Drowsy caplets (*McNeil Consumer*)	Acetaminophen 325mg		Pseudoephedrine HCl 30mg	Dextromethorphan HBr 15mg	Guaifenesin 200mg	**Adults & Peds ≥12 yo:** 2 tabs q6h. **Max:** 8 tabs q24h.
COUGH SUPPRESSANT & EXPECTORANT						
Benylin liquid (*Pfizer Consumer Healthcare*)				Dextromethorphan HBr 5mg/5mL	Guaifenesin 100mg/5mL	**Adults ≥12 yo:** 4 tsp (20mL) q4h. **Peds 6-12 yo:** 2 tsp (10mL) q4h. **2-6 yo:** 1 tsp (5mL) q4h. **Max:** 6 doses q24h.
Coricidin HBP Chest Congestion & Cough softgels (*Schering-Plough*)				Dextromethorphan HBr 10mg	Guaifenesin 200mg	**Adults & Peds ≥12 yo:** 1-2 caps q4h. **Max:** 12 caps q24h.
Mucinex DM extended-release tablets (*Adams Respiratoy Therapeutics*)				Dextromethorphan HBr 30mg	Guaifenesin 600mg	**Adults & Peds ≥12 yo:** 1-2 tabs q12h. **Max:** 4 tabs q24h.
Robitussin Cough & Congestion liquid (*Wyeth Consumer Healthcare*)				Dextromethorphan HBr 10mg/5mL	Guaifenesin 200mg/5mL	**Adults ≥12 yo:** 2 tsp (10mL) q4h. **Peds 6-12 yo:** 1 tsp (5mL) q4h. **2-6 yo:** 1/2 tsp (2.5mL) q4h. **Max:** 6 doses q24h.
Robitussin DM Infant Drops (*Wyeth Consumer Healthcare*)				Dextromethorphan HBr 5mg/2.5mL	Guaifenesin 100mg/ 2.5mL	**Peds 2-6 yo (24-47lbs):** 2.5ml q4h. **Max:** 6 doses q24h.
Robitussin DM liquid (*Wyeth Consumer Healthcare*)				Dextromethorphan HBr 10mg/5mL	Guaifenesin 100mg/5mL	**Adults ≥12 yo:** 2 tsp (10mL) q4h. **Peds 6-12 yo:** 1 tsp (5mL) q4h. **2-6 yo:** 1/2 tsp (2.5mL) q4h. **Max:** 6 doses q24h.
Robitussin Sugar Free Cough liquid (*Wyeth Consumer Healthcare*)				Dextromethorphan HBr 10mg/5mL	Guaifenesin 200mg/5mL	**Adults ≥12 yo:** 2 tsp (10ml) q4h. **Peds 6-12 yo:** 1 tsp (5ml) q4h. **2-6 yo:** 1/2 tsp (2.5ml). **Max:** 4 doses q24h.

DOSING INFORMATION FOR COUGH, COLD, AND FLU PRODUCTS (cont.)

Brand Name	Analgesic	Antihistamine	Decongestant	Cough Suppressant	Expectorant	Dose
Vicks 44E liquid *(Procter & Gamble)*				Dextromethorphan HBr 20mg/15mL	Guaifenesin 200mg/15mL	**Adults ≥12 yo:** 1 tbl (15mL) q4h. **Peds 6-12 yo:** 1.5 tsp (7.5mL) q4h. **Max:** of 6 doses q24h.
Vicks 44E Pediatric liquid *(Procter & Gamble)*				Dextromethorphan HBr 10mg/15mL	Guaifenesin 100mg/15mL	**Adults ≥12 yo:** 2 tbl (30mL) q4h. **Peds 6-12 yo:** 1 tbl (15mL) q4h. **2-5 yo:** 0.5 tbl (7.5mL) q4h. **Max:** 6 doses q24h.
DECONGESTANT						
Contac Cold timed-release caplets *(GlaxoSmithKline Consumer Healthcare)*			Pseudoephedrine HCl 120mg			**Adults & Peds ≥12 yo:** 1 tabs q12h. **Max:** 2 tabs q24h.
Dimetapp Children's Decongestant Infant Drops *(Wyeth Consumer Healthcare)*			Pseudoephedrine HCl 7.5mg/0.8mL			**Peds 2-3 yo:** 1.6mL q4-6h. **Max:** 6.4mL q24h.
Dimetapp Extentabs caplets *(Wyeth Consumer Healthcare)*			Pseudoephedrine HCl 120mg			**Adults & Peds ≥12 yo:** 1 tab q12h. **Max:** 2 tabs q24h.
PediaCare Decongestan Infants' drops *(Pharmacia Consumer Healthcare)*			Pseudoephedrine HCl 7.5mg/0.8mL			**Peds 2-3 yo:** 1.6mL q4-6h. **Max:** 6.4mL q24h.
Simply Stuffy liquid *(McNeil Consumer)*			Pseudoephedrine HCl 15mg/5mL			**Peds 6-12 yo (48-95 lbs):** 2 tsp (10mL) q4-6h. **2-6 yo (24-47 lbs):** 1 tsp (5mL) q4-6h. **Max:** 4 doses q24h.
Sudafed 12 Hour tablets *(Pfizer Consumer Healthcare)*			Pseudoephedrine HCl 120mg			**Adults & Peds ≥12 yo:** 1 tab q12h. **Max:** 2 tabs q24h.
Sudafed 24 Hour tablets *(Pfizer Consumer Healthcare)*			Pseudoephedrine HCl 240mg			**Adults & Peds ≥12 yo:** 1 tab q24h. **Max:** 1 tab q24h.
Sudafed Children's chewable tablets *(Pfizer Consumer Healthcare)*			Pseudoephedrine HCl 15mg			**Peds 6-12 yo:** 2 tabs q4-6h. **Max:** 8 tabs q24h.

DOSING INFORMATION FOR COUGH, COLD, AND FLU PRODUCTS (cont.)

Brand Name	Analgesic	Antihistamine	Decongestant	Cough Suppressant	Expectorant	Dose
Sudafed Children's liquid (*Pfizer Consumer Healthcare*)			Pseudoephedrine HCl 15mg/5mL			**Adults ≥12 yo:** 4 tsp (20mL) q4-6h. **Peds 6-12 yo:** 2 tsp (10mL) q4-6h. **2-6 yo:** 1 tsp (5mL) q4-6h. **Max:** 4 doses q24h.
Sudafed PE tablets (*Pfizer Consumer Healthcare*)			Phenylephrine HCl 10mg			**Adults & Peds ≥12 yo:** 1 tab q4h. **Max:** 6 tabs q24h.
Sudafed tablets (*Pfizer Consumer Healthcare*)			Pseudoephedrine HCl 30mg			**Adults ≥12 yo:** 2 tabs q4-6h. **Peds 6-12 yo:** 1 tab q4-6h. **Max:** 4 doses q24h.
Vicks Sinex 12-hour nasal spray (*Procter & Gamble*)			Oxymetazoline HCl 0.05%			**Adults & Peds ≥6 yo:** 2-3 sprays q10-12h. **Max:** 2 doses q24h.
Vicks Sinex Nasal Spray (*Procter & Gamble*)			Phenylephrine HCl 0.5%			**Adults & Peds ≥12 yo:** 2-3 sprays q4h. **Max:** 18 sprays q24h.
Vicks Sinex UltraFine Mist (*Procter & Gamble*)			Phenylephrine HCl 0.5%			**Adults & Peds ≥12 yo:** 2-3 sprays q4h. **Max:**18 sprays q24h.
Vicks Sinex UltraFine Mist (*Procter & Gamble*)			Oxymetazoline HCl 0.05%			**Adults & Peds ≥6 yo:** 2-3 sprays q10-12h. **Max:** 2 doses q24h
Vicks Vapor Inhaler (*Procter & Gamble*)			Levmetamfetamine 50mg			**Adults ≥12 yo:** 2 inhalations q2h. **Max:** 24 inhalations q24h **Peds 6-12 yo:** 1 inhalation q2h. **Max:** 12 inhalations q24h.
DECONGESTANT & ANALGESIC						
Advil Children's Cold liquid (*Wyeth Consumer Healthcare*)	Ibuprofen 100mg		Pseudoephedrine HCl 15mg			**Peds 6-12 yo (49-95 lbs):** 2 tsp (10ml) q 6h. **2-6 yo (24-47 lbs):** 1 tsp (5ml) q6h. **Max:** 4 doses q24h
Advil Children's Cold suspension (*Wyeth Consumer Healthcare*)	Ibuprofen 100mg/5mL		Pseudoephedrine HCl 15mg/5mL			**Peds 6-12 yo (48-95 lbs):** 2 tsp (10mL) q6h. **2-6 yo (24-47 lbs):** 1 tsp (5mL) q6h. **Max:** 4 doses q24h.

DOSING INFORMATION FOR COUGH, COLD, AND FLU PRODUCTS (cont.)

Brand Name	Analgesic	Antihistamine	Decongestant	Cough Suppressant	Expectorant	Dose
Advil Cold & Sinus caplets/liqui-gels (*Wyeth Consumer Healthcare*)	Ibuprofen 200mg		Pseudoephedrine HCl 30mg			**Adults & Peds ≥12 yo:** 1-2 caps q4-6h. **Max:** 6 caps q24h.
Advil Flu & Body Ache caplets (*Wyeth Consumer Healthcare*)	Ibuprofen 200mg		Pseudoephedrine HCl 30mg			**Adults & Peds ≥12 yo:** 1-2 tabs q4-6h. **Max:** 6 tabs q24h.
Alka-Seltzer Plus Cold & Sinus tablets (*Bayer Healthcare*)	Acetaminophen 250mg		Phenylephrine HCl 5mg			**Adults & Peds ≥12 yo:** 2 tabs q4h. **Max:** 8 tab q24h.
Dimetapp Children's Cold & Fever liquid (*Wyeth Consumer Healthcare*)	Ibuprofen 100mg		Pseudoephedrine HCl 15mg			**Peds 6-12 yo (49-95 lbs):** 2 tsp (10ml) q 6h. **2-6 yo (24-47 lbs):** 1 tsp (5ml) q6h. **Max:** 4 doses q24h.
Dimetapp Children's Cold and Fever liquid (*Wyeth Consumer Healthcare*)	Ibuprofen 100mg/5mL		Pseudoephedrine HCl 15mg/5mL			**Peds 6-12 yo (48-95 lbs):** 2 tsp (10mL) q6h. **2-6 yo (24-47 lbs):** 1 tsp (5mL) q6h. **Max:** 4 doses q24h.
Dristan Cold capsules (*Wyeth Consumer Healthcare*)	Acetaminophen 500mg		Pseudoephedrine HCl 30mg			**Adults & Peds ≥12 yo:** 2 caps q6h. **Max:** 8 caps q24h.
Motrin Children's Cold suspension (*McNeil Consumer*)	Ibuprofen 100mg/5mL		Pseudoephedrine HCl 15mg/5mL			**Peds 6-12 yo (48-95 lbs):** 2 tsp (10mL) q6h. **2-6 yo (24-47 lbs):** 1 tsp (5mL) q6h. **Max:** 4 doses q24h.
Motrin Cold & Sinus caplets (*McNeil Consumer*)	Ibuprofen 200mg		Pseudoephedrine HCl 30mg			**Adults & Peds ≥12 yo:** 1-2 tabs q4-6h. **Max:** 6 caps q24h.
Sinutab Sinus tablets (*Pfizer Consumer Healthcare*)	Acetaminophen 500mg		Pseudoephedrine HCl 30mg			**Adults & Peds ≥12 yo:** 2 tabs q6h. **Max:** 8 tabs q24h.
Sudafed Sinus and Cold liquid caps (*Pfizer Consumer Healthcare*)	Acetaminophen 325mg		Pseudoephedrine HCl 30mg			**Adults & Peds ≥12 yo:** 2 caps q4-6h. **Max:** 8 caps q24h.
Tylenol Children's Plus Cold Daytime liquid (*McNeil Consumer*)	Acetaminophen 160mg/5mL		Pseudoephedrine HCl 15mg/5mL			**Peds 6-12 yo (48-95 lbs):** 2 tsp (10mL) q4-6h. **2-6 yo (24-47 lbs):** 1 tsp (5mL) q4-6h. **Max:** 4 doses q24h.

DOSING INFORMATION FOR COUGH, COLD, AND FLU PRODUCTS (cont.)

Brand Name	Analgesic	Antihistamine	Decongestant	Cough Suppressant	Expectorant	Dose
Tylenol Cold Infants' Drops (McNeil Consumer)	Acetaminophen 80mg/0.8mL		Pseudoephedrine HCl 7.5mg/0.8mL			**Peds 2-3 yo (24-25 lbs):** 1.6mL q4-6h. **Max:** 6.4mL q24h.
Tylenol Sinus Maximum Strength gelcaps (McNeil Consumer)	Acetaminophen 500mg		Pseudoephedrine HCl 30mg			**Adults & Peds ≥12 yo:** 2 caps q4-6h. **Max:** 8 caps q24h.
Vicks DayQuil Sinus liquicaps (Procter & Gamble)	Acetaminophen 325mg		Pseudoephedrine HCl 30mg			**Adults & Peds ≥12 yo:** 2 caps q6h. **Max:** 8 caps q24h.
DECONGESTANT & EXPECTORANT						
Robitussin PE liquid (Wyeth Consumer Healthcare)			Pseudoephedrine HCl 30mg/5mL		Guaifenesin 100mg/5mL	**Adults ≥12 yo:** 2 tsp (10mL) q4h. **Peds 6-12 yo:** 1 tsp (5mL) q4h. **2-6 yo:** 1/2 tsp (2.5mL) q4h. **Max:** 4 doses q24h.
Robitussin Severe Congestion liqui-gels (Wyeth Consumer Healthcare)			Pseudoephedrine HCl 30mg		Guaifenesin 200mg	**Adults ≥12 yo:** 2 caps q4h. **Peds 6-12 yo:** 1 cap q4h. **Max:** 4 doses q24h.
Sinutab Non-Drying Liquid Caps (Pfizer Consumer Healthcare)			Pseudoephedrine HCl 30mg		Guaifenesin 200mg	**Adults & Peds ≥12 yo:** 2 cap q4h. **Max:** 8 q24h
Sudafed Non-Drying Sinus liquid caps (Pfizer Consumer Healthcare)			Pseudoephedrine HCl 30mg		Guaifenesin 200mg	**Adults & Peds ≥12 yo:** 2 caps q4h. **Max:** 8 caps q24h.
Triaminic Chest & Nasal Congestion liquid (Novartis Consumer Health)			Pseudoephedrine HCl 15mg/5mL		Guaifenesin 50mg/5mL	**Peds 6-12 yo:** 2 tsp (10mL) q4-6h. **2-6 yo:** 1 tsp (5mL) q4-6h. **Max:** 4 doses q24h.
DECONGESTANT & EXPECTORANT & ANALGESIC						
Tylenol Sinus Severe Congestion Daytime caplets (McNeil Consumer)	Acetaminophen 325 mg		Pseudoephedrine HCl 30mg		Guaifenesin 200mg	**Adults & Peds ≥12 yo:** 2 tab q6h. **Max:** 8 tab q24h.
EXPECTORANT						
Mucinex extended-release tablets (Adams Respiratoy Therapeutics)					Guaifenesin 600mg	**Adults & Peds ≥12 yo:** 1-2 tabs q12h. **Max:** 4 tabs q24h.
Robitussin liquid (Wyeth Consumer Healthcare)					Guaifenesin 100mg/5mL	**Adults ≥12 yo:** 2-4 tsp (10-20mL) q4h. **Peds 6-12 yo:** 1-2 tsp (5-10mL) q4h. **2-6 yo:** 1/2-1 tsp (2.5-5mL) q4h. **Max:** 6 doses q24h.

Nasal Congestion

Nasal congestion occurs when the membranes lining the nose become swollen from inflamed blood vessels. It is often caused by the same conditions that cause a runny nose (e.g., colds, allergies, and the flu). The most common culprits are viruses, hay fever, and sinus infection. Overuse of some nasal sprays or drops can also lead to nasal congestion. Clogged nasal passages can affect the ears, the sense of hearing, and speech development. Significant congestion can also disrupt sleep and cause snoring and sometimes sleep apnea. Typically, nasal congestion resolves spontaneously within a week. There are several OTC products available to treat the symptoms of nasal congestion, including nasal decongestants (pseudoephedrine, phenylephrine, naphazoline, oxymetazoline, xylometazoline), antihistamines (diphenhydramine, loratadine, chlorpheniramine), and saline nasal products.

OXYMETAZOLINE (nasal)

PHARMACOLOGY

Oxymetazoline is a direct-acting sympathomimetic amine. It acts on alpha-adrenergic receptors in the arterioles of the nasal mucosa to produce constriction, resulting in decreased blood flow and decreased nasal congestion, for up to 12 hours.

INDICATIONS

Congestion, nasal (treatment)—Oxymetazoline is indicated for temporary relief of nasal congestion, up to 12 hours, due to the common cold, sinusitis, hay fever, or other upper respiratory allergies (allergic rhinitis).

Congestion, sinus (treatment)—Nasal oxymetazoline is used for the relief of sinus congestion.

CONTRAINDICATIONS

Risk-benefit should be considered when the following medical problems exist:

- Coronary artery disease; heart disease, including angina; hypertension (condition may be exacerbated due to drug-induced cardiovascular effects).

- Enlarged prostate (difficulty of urination due to enlarged prostate may be exacerbated because of vasoconstrictive effects).

- Diabetes mellitus.

- Glaucoma, narrow-angle.

- Hyperthyroidism.

- Rhinitis, sicca (may exacerbate already dry mucous membranes).

- Sensitivity to oxymetazoline or other nasal decongestants (may exacerbate side effects such as sleepiness, dizziness, lightheadedness, weakness, tremulousness, and cardiac arrhythmia).

WARNINGS/PRECAUTIONS

Patients sensitive to other nasal decongestants may be sensitive to this medication also.

Pregnancy: Oxymetazoline may be systemically absorbed. However, adequate and well-controlled studies in humans have not been done.

Breastfeeding: Oxymetazoline may be systemically absorbed. However, problems in humans have not been documented.

Pediatrics: Children may be especially prone to systemic absorption of oxymetazoline with resulting side/adverse effects.

DRUG INTERACTIONS

Antidepressants, tricylic; maprotiline; monoamine oxidase inhibitors: If significant systemic absorption of nasal oxymetazoline occurs, concurrent use may potentiate the pressor effect of oxymetazoline.

ADVERSE REACTIONS

Those indicating need for medical attention:

Rebound congestion (increase in runny or stuffy nose).

Symptoms of systemic absorption:

Blurred vision; fast, irregular, or pounding heartbeat; headache, dizziness, drowsiness, or lightheadedness; high blood pressure; nervousness; trembling; trouble in sleeping; weakness.

Those indicating need for medical attention only if they continue or are bothersome:

Burning, dryness, or stinging of nasal mucosa; increase in nasal discharge; sneezing.

OXYMETAZOLINE PRODUCTS	
Brand Name	**Dosage Form**
4-Way Long Lasting (BMS)	**Spray:** 0.05%
Afrin (Schering)	**Spray:** 0.05% **Solution:** 0.05%
Afrin Extra Moisturizing (Schering)	**Spray:** 0.05%
Afrin w/menthol (Schering)	**Spray:** 0.05%
Afrin Sinus (Schering)	**Spray:** 0.05%
Duration (Schering)	**Spray:** 0.05%
Neo-Synephrine 12 Hour (Bayer)	**Spray:** 0.05%
Sinarest Nasal (Novartis)	**Spray:** 0.05%
Vicks Sinex 12 Hour Procter & Gamble)	**Spray:** 0.05%

ADMINISTRATION AND DOSAGE

General Dosing Information

Prolonged or excessive use of this medication will cause rebound congestion with chronic swelling of nasal mucosa.

Adults/Pediatrics >6 years of age: 2 or 3 drops or sprays of a 0.05% solution into each nostril every 10 to 12 hours. Maximum of 2 doses in 24 hours.

PHENYLEPHRINE (nasal)

PHARMACOLOGY

Phenylephrine is primarily a direct-acting sympathomimetic amine. It acts on alpha-adrenergic receptors in the arterioles of the nasal mucosa to produce constriction, resulting in decreased nasal congestion.

INDICATIONS

Congestion, nasal (treatment)—Nasal phenylephrine is indicated for the symptomatic relief of nasal congestion due to the common cold, hay fever, sinusitis, or other upper respiratory allergies.

Congestion, sinus (treatment)—Nasal phenylephrine is used for relief of sinus congestion.

Congestion, eustachian tube (treatment)—Nasal phenylephrine may be useful in the adjunctive therapy of middle ear infections by decreasing congestion around the eustachian ostia.

CONTRAINDICATIONS

Risk-benefit should be considered when the following medical problems exist:

- Coronary artery disease; heart disease, including angina; hypertension (condition may be exacerbated because of drug-induced cardiovascular effects).
- Diabetes mellitus.
- Hyperthyroidism.
- Sensitivity to phenylephrine or other nasal decongestants.

PRECAUTIONS TO CONSIDER

Patients sensitive to other nasal decongestants may be sensitive to this medication also.

Drug Interactions: See chart on page 316.

Pregnancy: Problems in humans have not been documented; however, nasal phenylephrine may be systemically absorbed.

Breastfeeding: Problems in humans have not been documented; however, nasal phenylephrine may be systemically absorbed.

Pediatrics: Children may be especially prone to systemic absorption of nasal phenylephrine and resulting side/adverse effects.

ADVERSE REACTIONS

Those indicating need for medical attention:

Rebound congestion (increase in runny or stuffy nose).

Symptoms of systemic absorption:

Fast, irregular, or pounding heartbeat; headache or dizziness; increased sweating; nervousness; paleness; trembling; trouble in sleeping.

Those indicating need for medical attention only if they continue or are bothersome:

Burning, dryness, or stinging of nasal mucosa.

ADMINISTRATION AND DOSAGE

General Dosing Information

Prolonged or excessive use of this medication will cause rebound congestion with chronic swelling of nasal mucosa. To reduce the chance of rebound congestion and systemic side effects, the weakest strength that is effective should be used.

Nasal jelly

Adults: Place a small amount of 0.5% jelly into each nostril and sniff well back into the nasal passages every 3 or 4 hours as needed.

Solution

Adults/Pediatrics ≥12 years of age: 2 or 3 drops or sprays of a 0.25% to 0.5% solution into each nostril every 4 hours as needed.

Pediatrics 2 to 6 years of age: 2 or 3 drops or sprays of a 0.125% to 0.16% solution into each nostril every 4 hours as needed.

Pediatrics 6 to 12 years of age: 2 or 3 drops or sprays of a 0.25% solution into each nostril every 4 hours as needed.

PSEUDOEPHEDRINE

PHARMACOLOGY

Pseudoephedrine acts on alpha-adrenergic receptors in the mucosa of the respiratory tract, producing vasoconstriction. The medication shrinks swollen nasal mucous membranes; reduces tissue hyperemia, edema, and nasal congestion; and increases nasal airway patency. Also, drainage of sinus secretions may be increased, and obstructed eustachian ostia may be opened.

INDICATIONS

Congestion, nasal (treatment); *congestion, sinus* (treatment); *congestion, eustachian tube* (treatment)—Pseudoephedrine is indicated for temporary relief of congestion associated with acute coryza, acute eustachian salpingitis, serous otitis media with eustachian tube congestion, vasomotor rhinitis, and aerotitis (barotitis) media. Pseudoephedrine may also be indicated as an adjunct to analgesics, antihistamines, antibiotics, antitussives, or expectorants for optimum results in allergic rhinitis, croup, acute and subacute sinusitis, acute otitis media, and acute tracheobronchitis.

CONTRAINDICATIONS

Risk-benefit should be considered when the following medical problems exist:

- Cardiovascular disease, including ischemic heart disease; hypertension, mild to moderate (condition may be exacerbated due to drug-induced cardiovascular effects).

PHENYLEPHRINE PRODUCTS	
Brand Name	**Dosage Form**
Neo-Synephrine (Bayer)	**Solution:** 0.50%, 1% **Spray:** 0.25%, 0.50%, 1%
Nostril (Novartis)	**Spray:** 0.25%, 0.50%
Vicks Sinex (Procter & Gamble)	**Spray:** 0.50%

Drug Interactions for Phenylephrine (nasal)

Precipitant Drug	Object Drug	Effect On Object Drug	Description
Guanadrel Guanethidine	Phenylephrine	↑	If significant systemic absorption of nasal phenylephrine occurs, concurrent use of guanadrel or guanethidine may potentiate the pressor effect of phenylephrine, possibly resulting in hypertension and/or cardiac arrhythmias.
MAOIs (furazolidone, procarbazine, selegiline) Maprotiline Tricyclic antidepressants	Phenylephrine	↑	If significant systemic absorption of nasal phenylephrine occurs, concurrent use of these medications may potentiate the pressor effect of phenylephrine; nasal phenylephrine should not be administered within 14 days following the administration of MAOIs.

- Coronary artery disease, severe; hypertension, severe —*major clinical significance* (condition may be exacerbated due to drug-induced cardiovascular effects).
- Diabetes mellitus (may lead to increased blood glucose concentrations).
- Glaucoma, predisposition to (condition may be aggravated).
- Hyperthyroidism (symptoms may be exacerbated).
- Prostatic hypertrophy (urinary retention may be precipitated).
- Sensitivity to pseudoephedrine or other sympathomimetics.

WARNINGS/PRECAUTIONS

Patients sensitive to other sympathomimetics (eg, albuterol, amphetamines, ephedrine, epinephrine, isoproterenol, metaproterenol, norepinephrine, phenylephrine, phenylpropanolamine, terbutaline) may be sensitive to this medication also.

Pregnancy: FDA Category B. Studies in humans have not been done.

Breastfeeding: Pseudoephedrine is distributed into breast milk; use by nursing mothers is not recommended because of the higher than usual risk to infants, especially newborn and premature infants, of side effects from sympathomimetic amines.

Pediatrics: Pseudoephedrine should be used with caution in infants, especially newborn and premature infants, because of the higher than usual risk of side/adverse effects.

ADVERSE REACTIONS

Those indicating need for medical attention: Incidence rare

Convulsions; hallucinations; irregular or slow heartbeat; shortness of breath or troubled breathing.

Those indicating need for medical attention only if they continue or are bothersome:

Incidence more frequent

Nervousness; restlessness; trouble in sleeping.

Incidence less frequent:

Difficult or painful urination; dizziness or lightheadedness; fast or pounding heartbeat; headache; increased sweating; nausea or vomiting; trembling; unusual paleness; weakness.

ADMINISTRATION AND DOSAGE

General Dosing Information

To minimize the possibility of insomnia, the last dose of pseudoephedrine for each day should be administered a few hours before bedtime. For patients who have difficulty in swallowing the extended-release capsule, the contents of the capsule may be mixed with jam or jelly and taken without chewing.

Capsules/Tablets

Adults/Pediatrics ≥*12 years of age*: 60mg every 4 to 6 hours, not to exceed 240mg in 24 hours.

Capsules, extended-release/Tablets, extended-release:

Adults/Pediatrics ≥*12 years of age*: 120mg every 12 hours, not to exceed 240mg in 24 hours.

Solution/Syrup

Adults/Pediatrics ≥*12 years of age*: 60mg every 4 to 6 hours, not to exceed 240mg in 24 hours.

Pediatrics 4 to 12 months of age (5.4-7.7kg): 7.5mg every 4 to 6 hours, not to exceed 4 doses (30mg) in 24 hours.

Pediatrics 12 to 23 months of age (8.2-10.4kg): 11.25mg every 4 to 6 hours, not to exceed 4 doses (45mg) in 24 hours.

Pediatrics 2 to 6 years of age: 15mg every 4 to 6 hours, not to exceed 60mg in 24 hours.

Pediatrics 6 to 12 years of age: 30mg every 4 to 6 hours, not to exceed 120mg in 24 hours.

Drug Interactions for Pseudoephedrine

Precipitant Drug	Object Drug	Effect On Object Drug	Description
Anesthetics, hydrocarbon inhalation (e.g., chloroform, cyclopropane, enflurane, halothane, isoflurane, methoxyflurane, trichloroethylene)	Pseudoephedrine	↑	Administration of pseudoephedrine prior to or shortly after anesthesia may increase the risk of severe ventricular arrhythmias, especially in patients with preexisting heart disease, because these anesthetics greatly sensitize the myocardium to the effects of sympathomimetics.

Drug Interactions for Pseudoephedrine (cont.)

Precipitant Drug	Object Drug	Effect On Object Drug	Description
Citrates	Pseudoephedrine	↑	Concurrent use may inhibit urinary excretion and prolong the duration of action of pseudoephedrine.
Levodopa	Pseudoephedrine	↑	Concurrent use may increase the possibility of cardiac arrhythmias; dosage reduction of the sympathomimetic is recommended.
♦ MAOIs (furazolidone, procarbazine, selegiline)	Pseudoephedrine	↑	Concurrent use may prolong and intensify the cardiac stimulant and vasopressor effects of pseudoephedrine because of release of catecholamines, which accumulate in intraneuronal storage sites during MAOI therapy, resulting in headache, cardiac arrhythmias, vomiting, or sudden and severe hypertensive and/or hyperpyretic crises; pseudoephedrine should not be administered during or within 14 days following administration of MAOIs.
Pseudoephedrine	Antihypertensives Diuretics used as antihypertensives	↓	Antihypertensive effects may be reduced when these medications are used concurrently with pseudoephedrine; the patient should be monitored carefully to confirm that the desired effect is being obtained.
♦ Pseudoephedrine	Beta-blockers	↓	Concurrent use with pseudoephedrine may inhibit the therapeutic effect of these medications; B-blockade may result in unopposed a-adrenergic activity of pseudoephedrine, with a risk of hypertension and excessive bradycardia and possible heart block.
Pseudoephedrine	CNS stimulants, other	↑	Concurrent use with pseudoephedrine may result in additive CNS stimulation to excessive levels, which may cause unwanted effects such as nervousness, irritability, insomnia, or possibly convulsions or cardiac arrhythmias; close observation is recommended.
♦ Pseudoephedrine	Cocaine	↑	In addition to increasing CNS stimulation, concurrent use with pseudoephedrine may increase the cardiovascular effects of either or both medications and the risk of adverse effects.
Pseudoephedrine	Digitalis glycosides	↑	Concurrent use may increase the risk of cardiac arrhythmias; caution and ECG monitoring are very important if concurrent use is necessary.
Pseudoephedrine	Nitrates	↓	Concurrent use with pseudoephedrine may reduce the antianginal effects of these medications.
Pseudoephedrine	Sympathomimetics, other	↑	In addition to possibly increasing CNS stimulation, concurrent use may increase the cardiovascular effects of either the other sympathomimetics or pseudoephedrine and the potential for side effects.
Pseudoephedrine	Thyroid hormones	↑	Concurrent use may increase the effects of either these medications or pseudoephedrine; thyroid hormones enhance risk of coronary insufficiency when sympathomimetic agents are administered to patients with coronary artery disease; dosage adjustment is recommended, although problem is reduced in euthyroid patients.

♦ = Major clinical significance. CNS = central nervous system; ECG = electrocardiogram; MAOI = monoamine oxidase inhibitor.

PSEUDOEPHEDRINE PRODUCTS	
Brand Name	**Dosage Form**
Chlor-Trimeton Nasal Decongestant (Schering)	**Tablet:** 60mg
Dimetapp Decongestant (Wyeth)	**Capsule:** 30mg
Simply Stuffy (McNeil)	**Liquid:** 15mg/ 5mL
Sudafed (Pfizer)	**Tablet:** 30mg
Sudafed 12 Hour (Pfizer)	**Tablet:** 120mg
Sudafed 24 Hour (Pfizer)	**Tablet:** 240mg
Sudafed Children's (Pfizer)	**Solution:** 15mg/ 5mL **Tablet:** 15mg

XYLOMETAZOLINE

PHARMACOLOGY

A direct-acting sympathomimetic amine, xylometazoline acts on alpha-adrenergic receptors in the nasal mucosa to produce vasoconstriction, resulting in decreased blood flow and decreased nasal congestion.

INDICATIONS

Congestion, nasal (treatment)—Xylometazoline is indicated for the temporary relief of nasal congestion due to colds, sinusitis, hay fever, and other upper respiratory allergies (allergic rhinitis) and for headache, tubal block, and otitis media associated with nasal congestion.

Congestion, sinus (treatment)—Nasal xylometazoline is used for the relief of sinus congestion.

CONTRAINDICATIONS

Risk-benefit should be considered when the following medical problems exist:

- Coronary artery disease; heart disease, including angina; hypertension (condition may be exacerbated due to drug-induced cardiovascular effects).

- Enlarged prostate (urination difficulty may worsen due to drug-induced cardiovascular effects).

- Diabetes mellitus (vasoconstriction may be exacerbated due to drug-induced cardiovascular effects).

- Glaucoma, narrow-angle, predisposition to—*major clinical significance* (vasoconstriction may be exacerbated due to drug-induced cardiovascular effects).

- Hyperthyroidism.

- Sensitivity to xylometazoline or other nasal decongestants.

WARNINGS/PRECAUTIONS

Patients sensitive to other nasal decongestants may be sensitive to this medication also.

Pregnancy: FDA Category C. Adequate and well-controlled studies in humans have not been done.

Breastfeeding: It is not known whether xylometazoline is distributed into breast milk. However, problems in humans have not been documented.

Pediatrics: Children may be especially prone to systemic absorption of xylometazoline with resulting side effects, especially sedation.

Drug Interactions

Antidepressants, tricyclic; maprotiline; monoamine oxidase inhibitors (MAOIs): If significant systemic absorption of xylometazoline occurs, concurrent use of tricyclic antidepressants, maprotiline, or MAOIs may potentiate the pressor effect of xylometazoline.

ADVERSE REACTIONS

Those indicating need for medical attention:

Rebound congestion (increase in runny or stuffy nose).

Symptoms of systemic absorption:

Allergic reaction or hypersensitivity (hives; rash; shortness of breath; swelling of eyelids, face, or lips; troubled breathing; wheezing).

Blurred vision.

Dizziness.

Headache or lightheadedness.

Nausea.

Nervousness.

Pounding, irregular, or fast heartbeat.

Trouble in sleeping.

Those indicating need for medical attention only if they continue or are bothersome:

Burning, dryness, or stinging of nasal mucosa; increase in nasal discharge; sneezing.

ADMINISTRATION AND DOSAGE

General Dosing Information

Prolonged or excessive use of this medication, ie, for more than 3 days, will cause rebound congestion with chronic swelling of nasal mucosa. Medication is more effective if 3 to 5 minutes are allowed to elapse between each spray per nostril, and nose is blown thoroughly before next spray is administered. Continue until complete dose is used.

Adults/Pediatrics ≥12 years of age: 1 to 3 drops or sprays of a 0.1% solution into each nostril every 8 to 10 hours as needed. Maximum of 3 doses per day.

Pediatrics 2 to 12 years of age: 2 or 3 drops or sprays of a 0.05% solution into each nostril every 8 to 10 hours as needed. Maximum of 3 doses per day.

XYLOMETAZOLINE PRODUCTS	
Brand Name	**Dosage Form**
Otrivin (Novartis)	**Solution:** 0.1% **Spray:** 0.1%
Otrivin Pediatric (Novartis)	**Solution:** 0.05%

DOSING INFORMATION FOR NASAL DECONGESTANT/MOISTURIZING PRODUCTS

The following table provides a quick comparison of the ingredients and dosages of common brand-name OTC drugs. Products are listed alphabetically by drug category and brand name.

BRAND NAME	INGREDIENT/STRENGTH	DOSE
PSEUDOEPHEDRINE		
Dimetapp 12-Hour tablets (*Wyeth Consumer Healthcare*)	Pseudoephedrine Hydrochloride 120mg	**Adults & Peds** ≥**12 yo:** 1 tab q12h. **Max:** 2 tabs/day.
Dimetapp Decongestant Infant drops (*Wyeth Consumer Healthcare*)	Pseudoephedrine Hydrochloride 7.5mg/ 0.8mL	**Peds 2-3 yo:** 1.6mL q4-6h. **Max:** 4 doses/ day.
Simply Stuffy liquid (*McNeil Consumer*)	Pseudoephedrine Hydrochloride 15mg/5mL	**Peds 6-11 yo (48-95 lbs):** 2 tsp q4-6h. **2-5 yo (24-47 lbs):** 1 tsp q4-6h. **Max:** 4 doses/ day.
Sudafed 12 Hour tablets (*Pfizer Consumer Healthcare*)	Pseudoephedrine Hydrochloride 120mg	**Adults & Peds** ≥**12 yo:** 1 tab q12h. **Max:** 2 tabs/day.
Sudafed 24 Hour tablets (*Pfizer Consumer Healthcare*)	Pseudoephedrine Hydrochloride 240mg	**Adults & Peds** ≥**12 yo:** 1 tab q24h. **Max:** 1 tab/day.
Sudafed Children's Nasal Decongestant chewable tablets (*Pfizer Consumer Healthcare*)	Pseudoephedrine Hydrochloride 15mg	**Peds 6-12 yo:** 2 tabs q4-6h. **Max:** 4 doses/ day.
Sudafed Children's Nasal Decongestant liquid (*Pfizer Consumer Healthcare*)	Pseudoephedrine Hydrochloride 15mg/5mL	**Adults** ≥**12 yo:** 4 tsp q4-6h. **Peds 6-12 yo:** 2 tsp q4-6h. **2-6 yo:** 1 tsp q4-6h. **Max:** 4 doses/day.
Sudafed Nasal Decongestant tablets (*Pfizer Consumer Healthcare*)	Pseudoephedrine Hydrochloride 30mg	**Adults** ≥**12 yo:** 2 tabs q4-6h. **Peds 6-12 yo:** 1 tab q4-6h. **Max:** 4 doses/day.
Sudafed PE tablets (*Pfizer Consumer Healthcare*)	Pseudoephedrine Hydrochloride 10mg	**Adults & Peds** ≥**12 yo:** 1 tab q4h. **Max:** 6 tabs/day.
TOPICAL NASAL DECONGESTANTS		
4-Way Fast Acting Nasal Decongestant Spray (*Bristol-Myers Squibb*)	Phenylephrine Hydrochloride 1%	**Adults & Peds** ≥**12 yo:** Instill 2-3 spray per nostril q4h.
4-Way Nasal Decongestant Spray, 12 Hour (*Bristol-Myers Squibb*)	Phenylephrine Hydrochloride 1%	**Adults & Peds** ≥**12 yo:** Instill 2-3 spray per nostril q4h.
4-Way No Drip Nasal Decongestant Spray (*Bristol-Myers Squibb*)	Phenylephrine Hydrochloride 1%	**Adults & Peds** ≥**12 yo:** Instill 2-3 spray per nostril q4h.
Afrin Extra Moisturizing Nasal Spray (*Schering-Plough*)	Oxymetazoline Hydrochloride 0.05%	**Adults & Peds** ≥**6 yo:** Instill 2-3 spray per nostril q10-12h.
Afrin No Drip Nasal Spray (*Schering-Plough*)	Oxymetazoline Hydrochloride 0.05%	**Adults & Peds** ≥**6 yo:** Instill 2-3 spray per nostril q10-12h.
Afrin No Drip Sinus Nasal Spray (*Schering-Plough*)	Oxymetazoline Hydrochloride 0.05%	**Adults & Peds** ≥**6 yo:** Instill 2-3 spray per nostril q10-12h.
Afrin Original Nasal Spray (*Schering-Plough*)	Oxymetazoline Hydrochloride 0.05%	**Adults & Peds** ≥**6 yo:** Instill 2-3 spray per nostril q10-12h.
Afrin Original Pumpmist Nasal Spray (*Schering-Plough*)	Oxymetazoline Hydrochloride 0.05%	**Adults & Peds** ≥**6 yo:** Instill 2-3 spray per nostril q10-12h.
Afrin Severe Congestion Nasal Spray (*Schering-Plough*)	Oxymetazoline Hydrochloride 0.05%	**Adults & Peds** ≥**6 yo:** Instill 2-3 spray per nostril q10-12h.
Afrin Sinus Nasal Spray (*Schering-Plough*)	Oxymetazoline Hydrochloride 0.05%	**Adults & Peds** ≥**6 yo:** Instill 2-3 spray per nostril q10-12h.
Benzedrex Inhaler (*B.F. Ascher*)	Propylhexedrine 250 mg	**Adults & Peds** ≥**6 yo:** Inhale 2 spray per nostril q2h.
Neo-Synephrine 12 Hour Extra Moisturizing Nasal Spray (*Bayer Healthcare*)	Oxymetazoline HCl 0.05%	**Adults & Peds** ≥**6 yo:** Instill 2-3 spray per nostril q10-12h.
Neo-Synephrine 12 Hour Nasal Decongestant Spray (*Bayer Healthcare*)	Oxymetazoline HCl 0.05%	**Adults & Peds** ≥**6 yo:** Instill 2-3 spray per nostril q10-12h.
Neo-Synephrine Extra Strength Nasal Decongestant Drops (*Bayer Healthcare*)	Phenylephrine Hydrochloride 1%	**Adults & Peds** ≥**12 yo:** Instill 2-3 drops per nostril q4h.
Neo-Synephrine Extra Strength Nasal Spray (*Bayer Healthcare*)	Phenylephrine Hydrochloride 1%	**Adults & Peds** ≥**6 yo:** Instill 2-3 spray per nostril q4h.
Neo-Synephrine Mild Formula Nasal Spray (*Bayer Healthcare*)	Phenylephrine Hydrochloride 0.25%	**Adults & Peds** ≥**6 yo:** Instill 2-3 spray per nostril q4h.

DOSING INFORMATION FOR NASAL DECONGESTANT/MOISTURIZING PRODUCTS (cont.)

Brand Name	Ingredient/Strength	Dose
Neo-Synephrine Regular Strength Nasal Decongestant Spray (Bayer Healthcare)	Phenylephrine Hydrochloride 0.5%	**Adults & Peds ≥12 yo:** Instill 2-3 spray per nostril q4h.
Nostrilla 12 Hour Nasal Decongestant (Bayer Healthcare)	Oxymetazoline Hydrochloride 0.05%	**Adults & Peds ≥6 yo:** Instill 2-3 spray per nostril q10-12h.
Vicks Sinex 12 Hour Ultra Fine Mist For Sinus Relief (Procter & Gamble)	Oxymetazoline Hydrochloride 0.05%	**Adults & Peds ≥12 yo:** Instill 2-3 spray per nostril q10-12h.
Vicks Sinex Long Acting Nasal Spray For Sinus Relief (Procter & Gamble)	Oxymetazoline HCl 0.05%	**Adults & Peds ≥12 yo:** Instill 2-3 spray per nostril q10-12h.
Vicks Sinex Nasal Spray For Sinus Relief (Procter & Gamble)	Phenylephrine Hydrochloride 0.5%	**Adults & Peds ≥12 yo:** Instill 2-3 spray per nostril q4h.
TOPICAL NASAL MOISTURIZERS		
4-Way Saline Moisturizing Mist (Bristol-Myers Squibb)	Water, Boric Acid, Glycerin, Sodium Chloride, Sodium Borate, Eucalyptol, Menthol, Polysorbate 80, Benzalkonium Chloride	**Adults & Peds ≥2 yo:** Instill 2-3 spray per nostril prn.
Ayr Baby's Saline Nose Spray, Drops (B.F. Ascher)	Sodium Chloride 0.65%	**Peds:** Instill 2 to 6 drops to each nostril.
Ayr Saline Nasal Gel (B.F. Ascher)	Aloe Vera Gel, Carbomer, Diazolidinyl Urea, Dimethicone Copolyol, FD&C Blue 1, Geranium Oil, Glycerin, Glyceryl Polymethacrylate, Methyl Gluceth 10, Methylparaben, Poloxamer 184, Propylene Glycol, Propylparaben, Sodium Chloride, Tocopherol Acetate, Triethanolamine, Xanthan Gum, Water	**Adults & Peds ≥12 yo:** Apply to nostril prn.
Ayr Saline Nasal Gel, No-Drip Sinus Spray (B.F. Ascher)	Water, Sodium Carbomethyl Starch, Propylene Glycol, Glycerin, Aloe Barbadensis Leaf Juice (Aloe Vera Gel), Sodium Chloride, Cetyl Pyridinium Chloride, Citric Acid, Disodium EDTA, Glycine Soja (Soybean Oil), Tocopheryl Acetate, Benzyl Alcohol, Benzalkonium Chloride, Geranium Maculatum Oil	**Adults & Peds ≥12 yo:** Use prn as directed.
Ayr Saline Nasal Mist (B.F. Ascher)	Sodium Chloride 0.65%	**Adults & Peds ≥12 yo:** Instill 2 spray per nostril prn.
Breathe Right Saline Nasal Spray (CNS)	Sodium Chloride 0.65%	**Adults & Peds ≥12 yo:** Use prn as directed.
ENTSOL Mist, Buffered Hypertonic Nasal Irrigation Mist (Bradley Pharmaceuticals)	Purified Water, Sodium Chloride, Sodium Phosphate Dibasic, Edetate Disodium, Potassium Phosphate Monobasic, Benzalkonium Chloride	**Adults & Peds ≥12 yo:** Instill 1-2 spray per nostril prn.
ENTSOL Single Use, Pre-Filled Nasal Wash Squeeze Bottle (Bradley Pharmaceuticals)	Purified Water, Sodium Chloride, Sodium Phosphate Dibasic, Potassium Phosphate Monobasic	**Adults & Peds ≥12 yo:** Use as directed
ENTSOL Spray, Buffered Hypertonic Saline Nasal Spray (Bradley Pharmaceuticals)	Purified Water, Sodium Chloride, Sodium Phosphate Dibasic, Potassium Phosphate Monobasic	**Adults & Peds ≥12 yo:** Instill 1 spray per nostril bid, 6 times daily
Little Noses Moisturizing Saline Gel with Aloe Vera & Vitamin E (Vetco)	Purified Water, Propylene Glycol, Glycerine, Glyceryl Stearate and PEG-100 Stearate, Hydroxyethylcellulose, Aloe Vera Gel, Methyl Gluceth 10, Dimethicone Copolyol, Sodium Chloride, Allantoin, Diazolidinyl Urea, Methylparaben, Vitamin E, Olive Oil, Geranium Oil, Propyl Paraben	**Peds:** Use as directed.
Little Noses Saline Spray/Drops, Non-Medicated (Vetco)	Sodium Chloride 0.65%	**Peds:** Use as directed.
Ocean Premium Saline Nasal Spray (Fleming)	Sodium Chloride (0.65%), Phenylcarbinol, Benzalkonium Chloride, Chloride	**Adults & Peds ≥6 yo:** Instill 2 spray per nostril prn.
Simply Saline Sterile Saline Nasal Mist (Blairex)	Sodium Chloride 0.9%	**Adults & Peds ≥12 yo:** Use prn as directed.

DOSING INFORMATION FOR NASAL DECONGESTANT/MOISTURIZING PRODUCTS (cont.)

Brand Name	Ingredient/Strength	Dose
SinoFresh Moisturizing Nasal & Sinus Spray *(SinoFresh HealthCare)*	Cetylpyridinium Cloride 0.05%	**Adults & Peds ≥12 yo:** Instill 1-3 spray per nostril qd.
Zicam Nasal Moisturizer *(Zicam)*	Purified Water, Sodium Phosphate, Hydroxethylcellulose, Disodium Phosphate, Glycerin, Alkoxylated Diester, Aloe Barbadensis Gel, Hydrolyzed Algin, Chlorella Vulgaris Extract, Sea Water, Benzalkonium Chloride, Benzyl Alcohol, Disodium EDTA, Hydroxylated Lecithin, Tocopherol, Polysorbate 80	**Adults & Peds ≥12 yo:** Use as directed.

Sinusitis

Sinusitis is an infectious or inflammatory condition of the paranasal sinuses typically associated with rhinitis (rhinosinusitis). Although the term *sinusitis* traditionally indicates a presumed bacterial infection of the sinuses, sinus infection or inflammation may also be due to various viral, fungal, or noninfectious causes. About 90% of patients with viral colds have rhinosinusitis as part of their illness, and 0.2% to 2% of these patients develop a secondary acute bacterial infection of the sinuses.

The paranasal sinuses comprise four symmetrical systems of air-filled sacs surrounding the nasal cavity: the maxillary, ethmoidal, frontal, and sphenoid sinuses. The sinuses are lined by pseudostratified, ciliated, columnar epithelium covered with a mucous blanket, and they each drain through a narrow opening (ostium) into the nasal cavity. The sweep of cilia drives mucus naturally toward the ostium. The ostia are the focal point for sinus infections. Regardless of cause, mucosal swelling narrows the ostia and impedes sinus drainage, leading to retention of secretions and decreased sinus ventilation. Fluid accumulation, decreased pH, and lowered oxygen tension create an ideal environment for bacterial growth. In addition, sniffing, sneezing, and nose blowing may facilitate the displacement of bacteria from the posterior nasal chamber, which is heavily colonized, into the normally sterile sinus cavities. The ostiomeatal complex, which drains the frontal, ethmoidal, and maxillary sinuses, is a key structure in the development of sinusitis. Mucosal layers approximate near the ostiomeatal complex, making the area especially vulnerable to inflammatory changes that limit sinus drainage.

Factors contributing to impaired sinus drainage and the development of sinusitis include systemic disorders and local insults that result in mucosal swelling, and mechanical obstructions. A viral upper respiratory infection (URI) is the most common precipitating cause of acute bacterial sinusitis. On average, adults develop 2 to 3 colds per year and children 6 to 8 colds per year; at most, 2% of colds are complicated by acute bacterial infection of the sinuses. Other major causes of impaired sinus drainage and sinusitis include iatrogenic factors (e.g., mechanical ventilation, nasogastric tubes), dental procedures, pregnancy, puberty-related hormonal changes, and anatomic variations (e.g., a deviated nasal septum). The nasal passages and nasopharynx are commonly colonized with the same bacterial species that cause acute bacterial sinusitis (ABS) or otitis media, and the bacteria in these areas probably serve as the reservoir for such infections. The organisms most frequently cultured in acute sinusitis are *Streptococcus pneumoniae* and *Haemophilus influenzae*, which together account for approximately 70% of cases of sinusitis. *Staphylococcus aureus*, other streptococcal species, *Moraxella (Branhamella) catarrhalis*, and anaerobic bacteria each account for a small percentage of ABS cases in adults. In children, *M catarrhalis* causes up to 20% of ABS cases, whereas anaerobic infections are uncommon. The presence of anaerobic bacteria usually suggests a dental infection as the source of ABS, unless the patient is immunocompromised or hospitalized. The microbiology of chronic sinusitis is typically polymicrobial, and *S aureus* (approximately 10%) and anaerobic organisms (48%-88%) are isolated more frequently. Fungal sinusitis is rare and typically occurs in immunocompromised or debilitated persons (e.g., with poorly controlled diabetes or metabolic acidosis-associated conditions such as chronic renal failure or diarrhea).

Aspergillus is often isolated in immunosuppressed patients, whereas *Mucor* predominates in patients with diabetes. *Candida* species are also occasionally pathogens.

Sinusitis is one of the most common conditions treated by primary care physicians (PCPs). Approximately 15% of the population is affected annually by presumed (self-reported) sinusitis, with rates relatively higher for women than for men. Children younger than 15 years and adults aged 25 to 64 years are most frequently affected. Despite the self-reported high incidence of ABS—13.5% of US adults annually—the amount of high-quality evidence pertaining to ABS is still remarkably limited. However, relatively clear major guidelines for the diagnosis and treatment of ABS are available. Most symptoms of ABS are nonspecific and are difficult to differentiate from symptoms of URI or allergic rhinitis, and none of the available diagnostic tools are cost-effective for routine use in differentiating bacterial sinusitis from colds and allergic rhinitis. Current management guidelines emphasize that uncomplicated ABS is generally a clinical diagnosis based on the history and physical examination. The mainstays of treatment are antibiotics combined with adjunctive symptomatic therapy, but the overuse of antibiotics to treat ill-defined URIs is contributing to the rapidly increasing antibiotic resistance of bacterial pathogens and is becoming a major public health concern. Epidemiologic evidence suggests that approximately 15% of people with URI symptoms seek medical care. If about 1% of people with a URI develop ABS, approximately 15% of all URI patients seek medical care, and all ABS patients seek medical care, then about 7% of patients presenting for medical care with URI symptoms have ABS. However, about 50% of patients presenting to PCPs with URI symptoms are diagnosed as having sinusitis, and 85% to 98% of patients diagnosed as having sinusitis are prescribed antibiotics.

If PCPs (who treat most cases of presumed ABS in the United States) could more accurately diagnose bacterial sinusitis and prescribe antibiotics only for patients who are likely to benefit, the inappropriate use of antibiotics would be markedly reduced. Recent guidelines endorsed by the Centers for Disease Control and Prevention, the American Academy of Family Physicians, the American College of Physicians-American Society of Internal Medicine, and the Infectious Diseases Society of America recommend that clinical diagnosis of acute bacterial rhinosinusitis be reserved for patients who experience symptoms that do not improve after 7 or more days and have maxillary pain or tenderness in the face or teeth (especially if unilateral) and purulent nasal secretions. An exception is the rare patient who presents with dramatic symptoms of severe unilateral maxillary pain, swelling, and fever. Recent pediatric guidelines recommend that the clinical diagnosis of ABS be applicable to children who present with URI symptoms that are persistent (do not improve after 10-14 days or more) or severe (3-4 days or more of concurrent purulent nasal discharge, fever of 39°C [102°F] or greater, and ill appearance).

Even though prescription antibiotic therapy is the mainstay of sinusitis therapy, there are a number of OTC products available to treat the symptoms of sinusitis, most of which contain a nasal decongestant (pseudoephedrine, phenylephrine, naphazoline, oxymetazoline, xylometazoline).

OXYMETAZOLINE

Oxymetazoline is a direct-acting sympathomimetic amine. It acts on alpha-adrenergic receptors in the arterioles of the nasal mucosa to produce constriction, resulting in decreased blood flow and decreased nasal congestion for up to 12 hours.

Congestion, nasal (treatment)—Oxymetazoline is indicated for temporary relief of nasal congestion, up to 12 hours, due to the common cold, sinusitis, hay fever, or other upper respiratory allergies (allergic rhinitis).

Congestion, sinus (treatment)—Nasal oxymetazoline is used for the relief of sinus congestion.

Topical solution

Adults/Pediatrics ≥6 years of age: 2 or 3 drops or sprays of a 0.05% solution into each nostril every 10 to 12 hours. Maximum of 2 doses in 24 hours.

For more information, refer to the complete monograph for oxymetazoline in "Allergic and Conjuctivitis" under Ophthalmologic System.

PHENYLEPHRINE

Phenylephrine is primarily a direct-acting sympathomimetic amine. It acts on alpha-adrenergic receptors in the arterioles of the nasal mucosa to produce constriction, resulting in decreased nasal congestion.

Congestion, nasal (treatment)—Nasal phenylephrine is indicated for the symptomatic relief of nasal congestion due to the common cold or hay fever, sinusitis, or other upper respiratory allergies.

Congestion, sinus (treatment)—Nasal phenylephrine is used for relief of sinus congestion.

Topical solution

Adults/Pediatrics ≥12 years of age: 2 or 3 drops or sprays of a 0.25% to 0.5% solution into each nostril every 4 hours as needed.

Pediatrics 2 to 6 years of age: 2 or 3 drops or sprays of a 0.125% to 0.16% solution into each nostril every 4 hours as needed.

Pediatrics 6 to 12 years of age: 2 or 3 drops or sprays of a 0.25% solution into each nostril every 4 hours as needed.

For more information, refer to the complete monograph for phenylephrine in "Nasal Congestion" under Respiratory System.

PSEUODEPHEDRINE

Pseudoephedrine acts on alpha-adrenergic receptors in the mucosa of the respiratory tract, producing vasoconstriction. The medication shrinks swollen nasal mucous membranes; reduces tissue hyperemia, edema, and nasal congestion; and increases nasal airway patency. Also, drainage of sinus secretions may be increased and obstructed eustachian ostia may be opened.

Congestion, nasal (treatment); *congestion, sinus* (treatment); *congestion, eustachian tube* (treatment)—Pseudoephedrine is indicated for temporary relief of congestion associated with acute coryza, acute eustachian salpingitis, serous otitis media with eustachian tube congestion, vasomotor rhinitis, and aerotitis (barotitis) media. Pseudoephedrine also may be indicated as an adjunct to analgesics, antihistamines, antibiotics, antitussives, or expectorants for optimum results in allergic rhinitis, croup, acute and subacute sinusitis, acute otitis media, and acute tracheobronchitis.

Capsules/Tablets

Adults/Pediatrics ≥12 years of age: 60mg every 4 to 6 hours. Max of 240mg/day.

Capsules, extended-release/Tablets, extended-release

Adults/Pediatrics ≥12 years of age: 120mg every 12 hours. Max of 240mg/day.

Solution/Syrup

Adults/Pediatrics ≥12 years of age: 60mg every 4 to 6 hours. Max of 240mg/day.

Pediatrics 4 to 12 months of age (5.4 to 7.7kg): 7.5mg every 4 to 6 hours, not to exceed 4 doses (30mg) in 24 hours.

Pediatrics 12 to 23 months of age (8.2 to 10.4kg): 11.25mg every 4 to 6 hours, not to exceed 4 doses (45mg) in 24 hours.

Pediatrics 2 to 6 years of age: 15mg every 4 to 6 hours, not to exceed 60mg in 24 hours.

OXYMETAZOLINE PRODUCTS	
Brand Name	**Dosage Form**
4-Way Long Lasting (BMS)	**Spray:** 0.05%
Afrin (Schering)	**Solution:** 0.05% **Spray:** 0.05%
Afrin Extra Moisturizing (Schering)	**Spray:** 0.05%
Afrin w/menthol (Schering)	**Spray:** 0.05%
Afrin Sinus (Schering)	**Spray:** 0.05%
Duration (Schering)	**Spray:** 0.05%
Neo-Synephrine 12 Hour (Bayer)	**Spray:** 0.05%
Sinarest Nasal (Novartis)	**Spray:** 0.05%
Vicks Sinex 12 Hour (Procter & Gamble)	**Spray:** 0.05%

PHENYLEPHRINE PRODUCTS	
Brand Name	**Dosage Form**
Neo-Synephrine (Bayer)	**Solution:** 0.50%, 1%
	Spray: 0.25%, 0.50%, 1%
Nostril (Novartis)	**Spray:** 0.25%, 0.50%
Vicks Sinex (Procter & Gamble)	**Spray:** 0.50%

Pediatrics 6 to 12 years of age: 30mg every 4 to 6 hours, not to exceed 120mg in 24 hours.

For more information, refer to the complete monograph for pseudoephedrine in "Nasal Congestion" under Respiratory System.

XYLOMETAZOLINE

Xylometazoline is a direct-acting sympathomimetic amine. It acts on alpha-adrenergic receptors in the nasal mucosa to produce vasoconstriction, resulting in decreased blood flow and decreased nasal congestion.

Congestion, nasal (treatment)—Xylometazoline is indicated for the temporary relief of nasal congestion due to colds, sinusitis, hay fever, and other upper respiratory allergies (allergic rhinitis); and for headache, tubal block, and serious otitis media associated with nasal congestion.

Congestion, sinus (treatment)—Nasal xylometazoline is used for the relief of sinus congestion.

Adults/Pediatrics ≥12 years of age: 1 to 3 drops or sprays of a 0.1% solution into each nostril every 8 to 10 hours as needed. Maximum of 3 doses per day.

Pediatrics 2 to 12 years of age: 2 or 3 drops or sprays of a 0.05% solution into each nostril every 8 to 10 hours as needed. Maximum of 3 doses per day.

PSEUDOEPHEDRINE PRODUCTS

Brand Name	Dosage Form
Chlor-Trimeton Nasal Decongestant (Schering)	**Tablet:** 60mg
Dimetapp Decongestant (Wyeth)	**Capsule:** 30mg
Simply Stuffy (McNeil)	**Liquid:** 15mg/5mL
Sudafed (Pfizer)	**Tablet:** 30mg
Sudafed 12 Hour (Pfizer)	**Tablet:** 120mg
Sudafed 24 Hour (Pfizer)	**Tablet:** 240mg
Sudafed Children's (Pfizer)	**Solution:** 15mg/5mL
	Tablet: 15mg

XYLOMETAZOLINE PRODUCTS

Brand Name	Dosage Form
Otrivin (Novartis)	**Solution:** 0.1% **Spray:** 0.1%
Otrivin Pediatric (Novartis)	**Solution:** 0.05%

DOSING INFORMATION FOR NASAL DECONGESTANT/MOISTURIZING PRODUCTS

The following table provides a quick comparison of the ingredients and dosages of common brand-name OTC drugs. Products are listed alphabetically by drug category and brand name.

BRAND NAME	INGREDIENT/STRENGTH	DOSE
PSEUDOEPHEDRINE		
Dimetapp 12-Hour tablets *(Wyeth Consumer Healthcare)*	Pseudoephedrine Hydrochloride 120mg	**Adults & Peds ≥12 yo:** 1 tab q12h. **Max:** 2 tabs/day.
Dimetapp Decongestant Infant drops *(Wyeth Consumer Healthcare)*	Pseudoephedrine Hydrochloride 7.5mg/0.8mL	**Peds 2-3 yo:** 1.6mL q4-6h. **Max:** 4 doses/day.
Simply Stuffy liquid *(McNeil Consumer)*	Pseudoephedrine Hydrochloride 15mg/5mL	**Peds 6-11 yo (48-95 lbs):** 2 tsp q4-6h. **2-5 yo (24-47 lbs):** 1 tsp q4-6h. **Max:** 4 doses/day.
Sudafed 12 Hour tablets *(Pfizer Consumer Healthcare)*	Pseudoephedrine Hydrochloride 120mg	**Adults & Peds ≥12 yo:** 1 tab q12h. **Max:** 2 tabs/day.
Sudafed 24 Hour tablets *(Pfizer Consumer Healthcare)*	Pseudoephedrine Hydrochloride 240mg	**Adults & Peds ≥12 yo:** 1 tab q24h. **Max:** 1 tab/day.
Sudafed Children's Nasal Decongestant chewable tablets *(Pfizer Consumer Healthcare)*	Pseudoephedrine Hydrochloride 15mg	**Peds 6-12 yo:** 2 tabs q4-6h. **Max:** 4 doses/day.
Sudafed Children's Nasal Decongestant liquid *(Pfizer Consumer Healthcare)*	Pseudoephedrine Hydrochloride 15mg/5mL	**Adults ≥12 yo:** 4 tsp q4-6h. **Peds 6-12 yo:** 2 tsp q4-6h. **2-6 yo:** 1 tsp q4-6h. **Max:** 4 doses/day.
Sudafed Nasal Decongestant tablets *(Pfizer Consumer Healthcare)*	Pseudoephedrine Hydrochloride 30mg	**Adults ≥12 yo:** 2 tabs q4-6h. **Peds 6-12 yo:** 1 tab q4-6h. **Max:** 4 doses/day.
Sudafed PE tablets *(Pfizer Consumer Healthcare)*	Pseudoephedrine Hydrochloride 10mg	**Adults & Peds ≥12 yo:** 1 tab q4h. **Max:** 6 tabs/day.

DOSING INFORMATION FOR NASAL DECONGESTANT/MOISTURIZING PRODUCTS (cont.)

BRAND NAME	INGREDIENT/STRENGTH	DOSE
TOPICAL NASAL DECONGESTANTS		
4-Way Fast Acting Nasal Decongestant Spray (Bristol-Myers Squibb)	Phenylephrine Hydrochloride 1%	**Adults & Peds ≥12 yo:** Instill 2-3 spray per nostril q4h.
4-Way Nasal Decongestant Spray, 12 Hour (Bristol-Myers Squibb)	Phenylephrine Hydrochloride 1%	**Adults & Peds ≥12 yo:** Instill 2-3 spray per nostril q4h.
4-Way No Drip Nasal Decongestant Spray (Bristol-Myers Squibb)	Phenylephrine Hydrochloride 1%	**Adults & Peds ≥12 yo:** Instill 2-3 spray per nostril q4h.
Afrin Extra Moisturizing Nasal Spray (Schering-Plough)	Oxymetazoline Hydrochloride 0.05%	**Adults & Peds ≥6 yo:** Instill 2-3 spray per nostril q10-12h.
Afrin No Drip Nasal Spray (Schering-Plough)	Oxymetazoline Hydrochloride 0.05%	**Adults & Peds ≥6 yo:** Instill 2-3 spray per nostril q10-12h.
Afrin No Drip Sinus Nasal Spray (Schering-Plough)	Oxymetazoline Hydrochloride 0.05%	**Adults & Peds ≥6 yo:** Instill 2-3 spray per nostril q10-12h.
Afrin Original Nasal Spray (Schering-Plough)	Oxymetazoline Hydrochloride 0.05%	**Adults & Peds ≥6 yo:** Instill 2-3 spray per nostril q10-12h.
Afrin Original Pumpmist Nasal Spray (Schering-Plough)	Oxymetazoline Hydrochloride 0.05%	**Adults & Peds ≥6 yo:** Instill 2-3 spray per nostril q10-12h.
Afrin Severe Congestion Nasal Spray (Schering-Plough)	Oxymetazoline Hydrochloride 0.05%	**Adults & Peds ≥6 yo:** Instill 2-3 spray per nostril q10-12h.
Afrin Sinus Nasal Spray (Schering-Plough)	Oxymetazoline Hydrochloride 0.05%	**Adults & Peds ≥6 yo:** Instill 2-3 spray per nostril q10-12h.
Benzedrex Inhaler (B.F. Ascher)	Propylhexedrine 250 mg	**Adults & Peds ≥6 yo:** Inhale 2 spray per nostril q2h.
Neo-Synephrine 12 Hour Extra Moisturizing Nasal Spray (Bayer Healthcare)	Oxymetazoline HCl 0.05%	**Adults & Peds ≥6 yo:** Instill 2-3 spray per nostril q10-12h.
Neo-Synephrine 12 Hour Nasal Decongestant Spray (Bayer Healthcare)	Oxymetazoline HCl 0.05%	**Adults & Peds ≥6 yo:** Instill 2-3 spray per nostril q10-12h.
Neo-Synephrine Extra Strength Nasal Decongestant Drops (Bayer Healthcare)	Phenylephrine Hydrochloride 1%	**Adults & Peds ≥12 yo:** Instill 2-3 drops per nostril q4h.
Neo-Synephrine Extra Strength Nasal Spray (Bayer Healthcare)	Phenylephrine Hydrochloride 1%	**Adults & Peds ≥6 yo:** Instill 2-3 spray per nostril q4h.
Neo-Synephrine Mild Formula Nasal Spray (Bayer Healthcare)	Phenylephrine Hydrochloride 0.25%	**Adults & Peds ≥6 yo:** Instill 2-3 spray per nostril q4h.
Neo-Synephrine Regular Strength Nasal Decongestant Spray (Bayer Healthcare)	Phenylephrine Hydrochloride 0.5%	**Adults & Peds ≥12 yo:** Instill 2-3 spray per nostril q4h.
Nostrilla 12 Hour Nasal Decongestant spray (Bayer Healthcare)	Oxymetazoline Hydrochloride 0.05%	**Adults & Peds ≥6 yo:** Instill 2-3 spray per nostril q10-12h.
Vicks Sinex 12 Hour Ultra Fine Mist For Sinus Relief (Procter & Gamble)	Oxymetazoline Hydrochloride 0.05%	**Adults & Peds ≥12 yo:** Instill 2-3 spray per nostril q10-12h.
Vicks Sinex Long Acting Nasal Spray For Sinus Relief (Procter & Gamble)	Oxymetazoline HCl 0.05%	**Adults & Peds ≥12 yo:** Instill 2-3 spray per nostril q10-12h.
Vicks Sinex Nasal Spray For Sinus Relief (Procter & Gamble)	Phenylephrine Hydrochloride 0.5%	**Adults & Peds ≥12 yo:** Instill 2-3 spray per nostril q4h.
TOPICAL NASAL MOISTURIZERS		
4-Way Saline Moisturizing Mist (Bristol-Myers Squibb)	Water, Boric Acid, Glycerin, Sodium Chloride, Sodium Borate, Eucalyptol, Menthol, Polysorbate 80, Benzalkonium Chloride	**Adults & Peds ≥2 yo:** Instill 2-3 spray per nostril prn.
Ayr Baby's Saline Nose Spray, Drops (B.F. Ascher)	Sodium Chloride 0.65%	**Peds:** Instill 2 to 6 drops to each nostril.
Ayr Saline Nasal Gel (B.F. Ascher)	Aloe Vera Gel, Carbomer, Diazolidinyl Urea, Dimethicone Copolyol, FD&C Blue 1, Geranium Oil, Glycerin, Glyceryl Polymethacrylate, Methyl Gluceth 10, Methylparaben, Poloxamer 184, Propylene Glycol, Propylparaben, Sodium Chloride, Tocopherol Acetate, Triethanolamine, Xanthan Gum, Water	**Adults & Peds ≥12 yo:** Apply to nostril prn.

DOSING INFORMATION FOR NASAL DECONGESTANT/MOISTURIZING PRODUCTS (cont.)

BRAND NAME	INGREDIENT/STRENGTH	DOSE
Ayr Saline Nasal Gel, No-Drip Sinus Spray *(B.F. Ascher)*	Water, Sodium Carbomethyl Starch, Propylene Glycol, Glycerin, Aloe Barbadensis Leaf Juice (Aloe Vera Gel), Sodium Chloride, Cetyl Pyridinium Chloride, Citric Acid, Disodium EDTA, Glycine Soja (Soybean Oil), Tocopheryl Acetate, Benzyl Alcohol, Benzalkonium Chloride, Geranium Maculatum Oil	**Adults & Peds ≥12 yo:** Use prn as directed.
Ayr Saline Nasal Mist *(B.F. Ascher)*	Sodium Chloride 0.65%	**Adults & Peds ≥12 yo:** Instill 2 spray per nostril prn.
Breathe Right Saline Nasal Spray *(CNS)*	Sodium Chloride 0.65%	**Adults & Peds ≥12 yo:** Use prn as directed.
ENTSOL Mist, Buffered Hypertonic Nasal Irrigation Mist *(Bradley Pharmaceuticals)*	Purified Water, Sodium Chloride, Sodium Phosphate Dibasic, Edetate Disodium, Potassium Phosphate Monobasic, Benzalkonium Chloride	**Adults & Peds ≥12 yo:** Instill 1-2 spray per nostril prn.
ENTSOL Single Use, Pre-Filled Nasal Wash Squeeze Bottle *(Bradley Pharmaceuticals)*	Purified Water, Sodium Chloride, Sodium Phosphate Dibasic, Potassium Phosphate Monobasic	**Adults & Peds ≥12 yo:** Use as directed
ENTSOL Spray, Buffered Hypertonic Saline Nasal Spray *(Bradley Pharmaceuticals)*	Purified Water, Sodium Chloride, Sodium Phosphate Dibasic, Potassium Phosphate Monobasic	**Adults & Peds ≥12 yo:** Instill 1 spray per nostril bid, 6 times daily
Little Noses Moisturizing Saline Gel with Aloe Vera & Vitamin E *(Vetco)*	Purified Water, Propylene Glycol, Glycerine, Glyceryl Stearate and PEG-100 Stearate, Hydroxyethylcellulose, Aloe Vera Gel, Methyl Gluceth 10, Dimethicone Copolyol, Sodium Chloride, Allantoin, Diazolidinyl Urea, Methylparaben, Vitamin E, Olive Oil, Geranium Oil, Propyl Paraben	**Peds:** Use as directed.
Little Noses Saline Spray/Drops, Non-Medicated *(Vetco)*	Sodium Chloride 0.65%	**Peds:** Use as directed.
Ocean Premium Saline Nasal Spray *(Fleming)*	Sodium Chloride (0.65%), Phenylcarbinol, Benzalkonium Chloride, Chloride	**Adults & Peds ≥6 yo:** Instill 2 spray per nostril prn.
Simply Saline Sterile Saline Nasal Mist *(Blairex)*	Sodium Chloride 0.9%	**Adults & Peds ≥12 yo:** Use prn as directed.
SinoFresh Moisturizing Nasal & Sinus Spray *(SinoFresh HealthCare)*	Cetylpyridinium Cloride 0.05%	**Adults & Peds ≥12 yo:** Instill 1-3 spray per nostril qd.
Zicam Nasal Moisturizer *(Zicam)*	Purified Water, Sodium Phosphate, Hydroxethylcellulose, Disodium Phosphate, Glycerin, Alkoxylated Diester, Aloe Barbadensis Gel, Hydrolyzed Algin, Chlorella Vulgaris Extract, Sea Water, Benzalkonium Chloride, Benzyl Alcohol, Disodium EDTA, Hydroxylated Lecithin, Tocopherol, Polysorbate 80	**Adults & Peds ≥12 yo:** Use as directed.

Sore Throat

A sore throat is defined as discomfort, pain, or scratchiness in the throat. The soreness often makes it painful to swallow. The symptoms are usually worse in the morning and improve throughout the day. Like colds, the vast majority of sore throats are caused by viral infections. The common causes of sore throat include breathing through the mouth, which can result in drying and irritation; the common cold; viral pharyngitis; influenza; streptococcal bacteria (strep throat); infectious mononucleosis; endotracheal intubation; and tonsillectomy or adenoidectomy.

Pharyngitis is one of the most common reasons for visits to doctors' offices and is a significant cause of absence from work. Acute pharyngitis and tonsillitis typically present with throat pain that sometimes radiates to the ears, and occasionally with dysphagia. Most cases of pharyngitis and tonsillitis are viral in origin: 90% of pharyngitis in adults and 60% to 75% in children are caused by viruses including influenza virus, adenoviruses, and Epstein-Barr virus, many of which are associated with the common cold. About 15% of cases are caused by group A ß-hemolytic streptococcus (*Streptococcus pyogenes*) infection. Fever is more commonly associated with the bacterial than the viral form of pharyngitis. Viral thyroiditis may also present as a sore throat.

Noninfectious causes of sore throat include mouth breathing secondary to nasal obstruction, which may result from an upper respiratory infection. Carotidynia, which is characterized by tenderness over the carotid artery, painful swallowing, and pain radiating to the ears, may also present as a sore throat. Even with elaborate culture techniques, no microbiological etiology can be detected in approximately one third of patients with pharyngitis or tonsillitis. . Furthermore, nonpathogenic resident flora frequently contaminate the microbiological specimen, rendering the results of laboratory culture of doubtful clinical value. Human rhinoviruses (at least 90 to 100 species) are the most common cause of common colds, responsible for 30% to 50%; peak incidence is in the early fall. In a study of 364 adults with colds during the fall, viruses were detected in 83% of patients. In the same study, sore throat was the most common first symptom among patients who tested positive by culture with human rhinovirus (40%); stuffy nose was the most common first symptom among those who tested negative for human rhinovirus (27%). Colds lasted 9.5 to 11.5 days (median), and there were no significant differences in the clinical course between groups who tested positive or negative for viral infection (using multiple laboratory techniques).

There are many products available OTC to relieve sore throat, including oral analgesics (acetaminophen, ibuprofen, naproxen) and topical anesthetic lozenges and sprays.

TOPICAL ANESTHETICS

Local anesthetics block both the initiation and conduction of nerve impulses by decreasing the neuronal membrane's permeability to sodium ions. This reversibly stabilizes the membrane and inhibits depolarization, resulting in the failure of a propagated action potential and subsequent conduction blockade.

Pain, pharyngeal (treatment)—Benzocaine (lozenges); benzocaine and menthol (lozenges); dyclonine (lozenges); and lidocaine hydrochloride (oral topical solution).

Benzocaine

Lozenges

Adults: One 10-mg lozenge every 2 hours as needed.

Pediatrics >2 years of age: One 5-mg lozenge every 2 hours as needed. Max: 12 lozenges/day.

Benzocaine/Menthol

Lozenges

Adults/Pediatrics >2 years of age: One lozenge every 2 hours as needed.

Dyclonine

Lozenges

Adults: One 2-mg or 3-mg lozenge every 2 hours as needed.

Pediatrics >2 years of age: One 1.2-mg lozenge every 2 hours as needed.

For product and dosing information, refer to the complete monograph for topical anesthetics (mucosal) in "Canker and Cold Sores" under Oral Cavity.

DOSING INFORMATION FOR SORE THROAT PRODUCTS

The following table provides a quick comparison of the ingredients and dosages of common brand-name OTC drugs. Products are listed alphabetically by brand name.

Brand Name	Ingredient/Strength	Dose
Alka-Seltzer Plus Nose & Throat effervescent tablets *(Bayer Healthcare)*	Acetaminophen/Chlorpheniramine Maleate/ Phenylephrine HCl/Dextromethorphan 250mg-2mg-5mg-10mg	**Adults & Peds ≥12 yo:** 2 tabs q4h. **Max:** 8 tabs q24h.
Cepacol Extra Strength Sore Throat Lozenges Cherry *(Combe)*	Benzocaine/Menthol 10mg-3.6mg	**Adults & Peds ≥5 yo:** 1 loz q2h.
Cepacol Extra Strength Sore Throat Lozenges Citrus *(Combe)*	Benzocaine/Menthol 10mg-2.1mg	**Adults & Peds ≥5 yo:** 1 loz q2h.
Cepacol Extra Strength Sore Throat Lozenges Sugar Free Cherry *(Combe)*	Benzocaine/Menthol 10mg-4.5mg	**Adults & Peds ≥5 yo:** 1 loz q2h.
Cepacol Maximum Strength Sore Throat Spray *(Combe)*	Dyclonine Hydrochloride/Glycerin 0.1%-33.0%	**Adults ≥12 yo:** 1-4 sprays qid. **Peds 3-12 yo:** 1-3 sprays qid.
Cepacol Sore Throat from Post Nasal Drip Lozenges *(Combe)*	Menthol 3.6mg	**Adults & Peds ≥2 yo:** 1 loz q2h.
Cepacol Sore Throat Lozenges Vapor Formula *(Combe)*	Menthol 5.4mg	**Adults & Peds ≥5 yo:** 1 loz q2h.
Cepastat Extra-Strength Lozenges *(Heritage)*	Phenol 29mg	**Adults ≥12 yo:** 1 loz q2h. **Max:** 18 loz/day. **Peds 6-12 yo:** 1 loz q2h. **Max:** 10 loz/day.
Cepastat Lozenges *(Heritage)*	Phenol 14.5mg	**Adults ≥12 yo:** 1 loz q2h. **Max:** 18 loz/day. **Peds 6-12 yo:** 1 loz q2h. **Max:** 10 loz/day.
Cepastat Sugar Free Lozenges *(Heritage)*	Anitfoam Emulsion, Caramel, Eucalyptus Oil, Gum Crystal, Menthol, Sorbitol	**Adults ≥12 yo:** 1-2 loz q2h. **Peds 6-12 yo:** 1 loz q2h. **Max:** 10 loz/day.
Chloraseptic Sore Throat Gargle *(Prestige Brands)*	Phenol 1.4%	**Adults ≥12 yo:** Swish/spit q2h.
Chloraseptic Sore Throat Lozenges *(Prestige Brand)*	Benzocaine/Menthol 6mg-10mg	**Adults & Peds ≥5 yo:** 1 loz q2h.
Chloraseptic Sore Throat Relief Spray *(Prestige Brands)*	Phenol 1.4%	**Adults ≥12 yo:** 5 sprays q2h. **Peds 2-12 yo:** 3 sprays q2h.
Chloraseptic Sore Throat Relief Strips *(Prestige Brands)*	Benzocaine/Menthol 3mg-3mg	**Adults & Peds ≥5 yo:** 2 strips q2h.
Chloraseptic Sore Throat Relief Strips for Kids *(Prestige Brands)*	Benzocaine/Menthol 2mg-2mg	**Adults & Peds ≥5 yo:** 2 strips q2h.
Chloraseptic Sore Throat Spray For Kids *(Prestige Brands)*	Phenol 0.5%	**Peds 2-11 yo:** 5 sprays q2h.
Comtrex Maximum Strength Sore Throat Relief *(Bristol-Myer Squibb)*	Acetaminophen 1000mg	**Adults & Peds ≥12 yo:** 2 tbsp q6h. **Max:** 4 doses q24h
Fisherman's Friend Cough Suppressant/Oral Anesthetic Lozenges *(Pez Candy)*	Menthol 10mg	**Adults & Peds ≥5 yo:** 1 loz q2h.
Halls Cherry Cough Drops *(Cadbury Adams)*	Menthol 7mg	**Adults & Peds ≥5 yo:** 1 loz q2h.
Halls Fruit Breezers *(Cadbury Adams)*	Pectin 7mg	**Adults & Peds ≥5 yo:** 1-2 lozs prn.
Halls Honey Lemon Cough Drops *(Cadbury Adams)*	Menthol 8mg	**Adults & Peds ≥5 yo:** 1 loz q2h.
Halls Ice Blue Peppermint Cough Drops *(Cadbury Adams)*	Menthol 10mg	**Adults & Peds ≥5 yo:** 1 loz q2h.
Halls Max Sore Throat Relief Lozenges *(Cadbury Adams)*	Benzocaine/Menthol 6mg-10mg	**Adults & Peds ≥5 yo:** 1-2 loz q2h.
Halls Mentho-Lyptus Cough Drops *(Cadbury Adams)*	Menthol 6.5mg	**Adults & Peds ≥5 yo:** 1 loz q2h.
Halls Plus Cough Drops *(Cadbury Adams)*	Menthol 10mg	**Adults & Peds ≥5 yo:** 1 loz q2h.
Halls Spearmint Cough Drops *(Cadbury Adams)*	Menthol 5.6mg	**Adults & Peds ≥5 yo:** 1 loz q2h.
Halls Strawberry Cough Drops *(Cadbury Adams)*	Menthol 3.1mg	**Adults & Peds ≥5 yo:** 2 loz q2h.
Halls Sugar Free Black Cherry Cough Drops *(Cadbury Adams)*	Menthol 5mg	**Adults & Peds ≥5 yo:** 1 loz q2h.

DOSING INFORMATION FOR SORE THROAT PRODUCTS (cont.)

BRAND NAME	INGREDIENT/STRENGTH	DOSE
Halls Sugar Free Citrus Blend Cough Drops *(Cadbury Adams)*	Menthol 5mg	**Adults & Peds ≥5 yo:** 1 loz q2h.
Halls Sugar Free Honey-Lemon Cough Drops *(Cadbury Adams)*	Menthol 7.6mg	**Adults & Peds ≥5 yo:** 1 loz q2h.
Halls Sugar Free Mountain Menthol Cough Drops *(Cadbury Adams)*	Menthol 5mg	**Adults & Peds ≥5 yo:** 1 loz q2h.
Halls Sugar Free Squares Black Cherry Cough Drops *(Cadbury Adams)*	Menthol 5.9mg	**Adults & Peds ≥5 yo:** 1 loz q2h.
Halls Sugar Free Squares Mountain Menthol Cough Drops *(Cadbury Adams)*	Menthol 6.8mg	**Adults & Peds ≥5 yo:** 1 loz q2h.
Halls Tropical Fruit Cough Drops *(Cadbury Adams)*	Menthol 3.1mg	**Adults & Peds ≥5 yo:** 2 loz q2h.
Little Colds Sore Throat Saf-T-Pops *(Vetco)*	Pectin 19mg	**Adults & Peds ≥2 yo:** Use prn. **Max 2-3 yo:** 3 pops/day. **4-8 yo:** 5 pops/day. **9-13 yo:** 8 pops/day.
N'ICE Sugar Free Cough Suppressant/Oral Anesthetic Drops *(Insight Pharmaceutical)*	Menthol 5mg	**Adults & Peds ≥12 yo:** 1 loz q2h. **Max:** 10 loz/day.
Nuprin Cold Relief Sore Throat Liquid *(Bristol-Myers Squibb)*	Phenol 1.4%	**Adults ≥12 yo:** 5 sprays q2h. **Peds 2-12 yo:** 3 sprays q2h.
Ricola Herb Throat Drops Lemon Mint *(Ricola)*	Menthol 1.1mg	**Adults & Peds ≥6 yo:** 2 loz q2h.
Robitussin Almond with Natural Honey Center Cough Drops *(Wyeth Consumer Healthcare)*	Menthol 2.5mg	**Adults & Peds ≥4 yo:** 2 loz q2h.
Robitussin Cherry Cough Drops *(Wyeth Consumer Healthcare)*	Menthol 5mg	**Adults & Peds ≥4 yo:** 1 loz q2h.
Robitussin Honey Citrus Cough Drops *(Wyeth Consumer Healthcare)*	Menthol 2.5mg	**Adults & Peds ≥4 yo:** 2 loz q2h.
Robitussin Honey-Lemon Cough Drops *(Wyeth Consumer Healthcare)*	Menthol 5mg	**Adults & Peds ≥4 yo:** 1 loz q2h.
Robitussin Honey-Lemon Tea Cough Drops *(Wyeth Consumer Healthcare)*	Menthol 5mg	**Adults & Peds ≥4 yo:** 1 loz q2h.
Robitussin Menthol Eucalyptus Cough Drops *(Wyeth Consumer Healthcare)*	Menthol 10mg	**Adults & Peds ≥4 yo:** 1 loz q2h.
Robitussin Natural Honey Center Cough Drops *(Wyeth Consumer Healthcare)*	Menthol 5mg	**Adults & Peds ≥4 yo:** 1 loz q2h.
Robitussin Sugar Free Throat Drops *(Wyeth Consumer Healthcare)*	Menthol 2.5mg	**Adults & Peds ≥4 yo:** 2 loz q2h. **Max:** 9 loz/day.
Sucret Children's Lozenges *(Heritage)*	Dyclonine Hydrochloride 1.2mg	**Peds ≥2 yo:** 1 loz q2h.
Sucret Maximum Strength Lozenges *(Heritage)*	Dyclonine Hydrochloride 3mg	**Adults & Peds ≥2 yo:** 1 loz q2h. **Max:** 10 loz/day.
Sucret Regular Strength Lozenges *(Heritage)*	Dyclonine Hydrochloride 2mg	**Adults & Peds ≥2 yo:** 1 loz q2h. **Max:** 10 loz/day.
Theraflu Flu & Sore Throat packets *(Novartis Consumer Health)*	Acetaminophen/Chlorpheniramine Maleate/Pseudoephedrine HCl 1000mg-4mg-60mg/packet	**Adults & Peds ≥12 yo:** 1 packet q6h. **Max:** 4 packets q24h.
Triaminic Cough & Sore Throat liquid *(Novartis Consumer Health)*	Acetaminophen/Pseudoephedrine HCl/Dextromethorphan 160mg-15mg-7.5mg/5mL	**Peds 6-12 yo:** 2 tsp (10mL) q6h. **2-6 yo:** 1 tsp (5mL) q6h. **Max:** 4 doses q24h.
Triaminic Softchews Cough & Sore Throat tablets *(Novartis Consumer Health)*	Acetaminophen/Pseudoephedrine HCl/Dextromethorphan 160mg-15mg-5mg	**Peds 6-12 yo:** 2 tabs q4-6h. **2-6 yo:** 1 tab q4-6h. **Max:** 4 doses q24h.
Tylenol Daytime Cough & Sore Throat Cool Burst liquid *(McNeil Consumer)*	Acetaminophen/Dextromethorphan 1000mg-30mg/30mL	**Adults & Peds ≥12 yo:** 2 tbl (30mL) q6h. **Max:** 8 tbl (120mL) q24h.
Tylenol Nighttime Cough & Sore Throat Cool Burst liquid *(McNeil Consumer)*	Acetaminophen/Doxylamine/Dextromethorphan 1000mg-12.5-30mg/30mL	**Adults & Peds ≥12 yo:** 2 tbl (30mL) q6h. **Max:** 8 tbl (120mL) q24h.
Tylenol Sore Throat Liquid *(McNeil Consumer)*	Acetaminophen 1000mg/30mL	**Adults & Peds ≥12 yo:** 2 tbsp q4-6h. **Max:** 8 tbl/day.

Atrophic Vaginitis

Atrophic vaginitis is an inflammation of the vagina caused by thinning and shrinking of tissues and decreased lubrication of the vaginal walls. It is due to decreased levels of circulating estrogen resulting from menopause or other events that produce long-term estrogen loss. Thinned endometrium and increased vaginal pH levels induced by estrogen deficiency predispose the vagina and urinary tract to infection and mechanical weakness. Reduction in lactic acid production and an increase in vaginal pH (>5.0) encourage overgrowth of nonacidophilic coliforms and the disappearance of lactobacillus.

Predisposing factors for atrophic vaginitis include menopause, decreased ovarian functioning (eg, from radiation therapy orchemotherapy), immunologic disorders, oophorectomy, post-partum loss of placental estrogen, elevated prolactin levels during lactation, antiestrogenic medications (eg, tamoxifen, danazol, medroxyprogesterone, leuprolide, nafarelin), cigarette smoking, vaginal multiparity, nonfluctuating estrogen levels, and cessation of coital activity. Most women with mild-to-moderate atrophy are asymptomatic. Symptoms and signs of advanced atrophy include decreased vaginal lubrication, vaginal soreness, postcoital burning, dyspareunia, occasional spotting, thin vaginal mucosa with diffuse redness, occasional petechiae, or ecchymoses, and few or no vaginal folds. Prescription topical estrogen and estrogen replacement therapy are often used for treatment for atrophic vaginits. There are also OTC vaginal lubricants available to alleviate symptoms of atrophic vaginitis.

DOSING INFORMATION FOR VAGINAL LUBRICANT PRODUCTS

The following table provides a quick comparison of the ingredients and dosages of common brand-name OTC products. Entries are listed alphabetically by brand name.

BRAND NAME	INGREDIENT/STRENGTH	DOSE
Astroglide Personal Lubricant (Biofilm)	Purified Water; Glycerin; Propylene Glycol; Polyquaternium 15; Methylparaben; Propylparaben	**Adults:** Use prn.
Astroglide Personal Lubricant Gel (Biofilm)	Purified Water; Glycerin; Hydroxyethylcellulose; Chorhexidine Gluconate; Methylparaben; Glucono Delta Lactone; Sodium Hydroxide	**Adults:** Use prn.
Astroglide Warming Liquid (Biofilm)	Propylene Glycol; Glycerin; Purified Water; Acacia Honey; Methylparaben; Polyquaternium 15	**Adults:** Use prn.
Gynecort Maximum Strength Anti-Itch Creme (Combe)	Hydrocortisone Acetate 1.0%	**Adults & Peds ≥2 yo:** Apply to affected area bid-tid.
Hyland's Vaginitis Natural Relief Tablets (Hyland)	Natrum Muriaticum 12X, HPUS, Candida Albicans 30X HPUS, Kreosotum 12X, HPUS, Carbolicum Acidum 12X, HPUS in a Base of Lactose, USP	**Adults:** 2-3 tabs q4h.
K-Y Jelly (McNeil Consumer)	Chlorhexidine Gluconate; Glucono Delta Lactone; Glycerin; Hydroxyethylcellulose; Methylparaben; Purified Water; Sodium Hydroxide	**Adults:** Use prn.
K-Y Liquid (McNeil Consumer)	Purified Water; Glycerin; Sorbitol; Propylene Glycol; Natrosol 250H; Benzoic Acid; Methylparaben; Sodium Hydroxide	**Adults:** Use prn.
K-Y Silk-E Vaginal Moisturizer (McNeil Consumer)	Purified Water; Propylene Glycol; Sorbitol; Polysorbate 60; Natrosol 250H; Benzoic Acid; Methylparaben; Vitamin E; Aloe Vera	**Adults:** Use prn.
K-Y Silk-E Vaginal Moisturizer Pre-Filled Applicators (McNeil Consumer)	Purified Water; Propylene Glycol; Sorbitol; Polysorbate 60; Natrosol 250H; Benzoic Acid; Methylparaben; Vitamin E; Aloe Vera	**Adults:** Use one application every 2 to 3 days.
K-Y Ultra Gel (McNeil Consumer)	Purified Water; Propylene Glycol; Sorbitol; Polysorbate 60; Natrosol 250H; Benzoic Acid; Methylparaben; Vitamin E	**Adults:** Use prn.
K-Y Warming Jelly (McNeil Consumer)	Propylene Glycol; Polyethylene Glycol; Hydroxypropylcellulose; Lactic Acid	**Adults:** Use prn.
K-Y Warming Liquid (McNeil Consumer)	Propylene Glycol; Glycerin; Acacia Honey Type O; Methylparaben	**Adults:** Use prn.

DOSING INFORMATION FOR VAGINAL LUBRICANT PRODUCTS (cont.)

Brand Name	Ingredient/Strength	Dose
K-Y Warming Ultra Gel *(McNeil Consumer)*	Propylene Glycol; Polyethylene Glycol; Hydroxypropylcellulose; Lactic Acid	**Adults:** Use prn.
Monistat Soothing Care Chafing Relief Powder-Gel *(McNeil Consumer)*	Dimethicone	**Adults & Peds ≥12 yo:** Apply as needed.
Monistat Soothing Care Itch Relief Cream *(McNeil Consumer)*	Hydrocortisone 1%	**Adults & Peds ≥2 yo:** Apply to affected area bid-tid.
Monistat Soothing Care Itch Relief Spray *(McNeil Consumer)*	Pramoxine HCl 1%	**Adults & Peds ≥2 yo:** Apply to affected area bid-tid.
Monistat Soothing Care Medicated Powder *(McNeil Consumer)*	Zinc Oxide 10%	**Adults & Peds ≥12 yo:** Apply as needed.
Replens Vaginal Moisturizer Pre-Filled Applicators *(Lil Drug Store)*	Purified Water; Glycerin; Mineral Oil; Polycarbophil; Carbopol 974P; Hydrogenated Palm Oil Glyceride; Sorbic Acid; Methylparaben; Sodium Hydroxide	**Adults:** Use one application every 2 to 3 days.
Vagi-Gard Medicated Cream, Advanced Sensitive Formula *(Lake Consumer Products)*	Benzocaine/Benzalkonium Chloride 5%-0.13%	**Adults & Peds ≥2 yo:** Apply to affected area tid-qid.
Vagi-Gard Medicated Cream, Maximum Strength *(Lake Consumer Products)*	Benzocaine/Benzalkonium Chloride 20%-0.13%	**Adults & Peds ≥2 yo:** Apply to affected area tid-qid.
Vagisil Anti-Itch Creme, Maximum Strength *(Combe)*	Benzocaine/Resorcinol 20%-3%	**Adults & Peds ≥12 yo:** Apply to affected area tid-qid.
Vagisil Anti-Itch Creme, Original Formula *(Combe)*	Benzocaine/Resorcinol 5%-2%	**Adults & Peds ≥2 yo:** Apply to affected area tid-qid.

Dysmenorrhea

Dysmenorrhea is defined as painful menses and is characterized as the menstrual period accompanied by either sharp, intermittent pain or dull, aching pain, usually in the pelvis or lower abdomen. The pain may begin several days before or just at the start of the menstrual period and usually subsides as menstrual bleeding tapers off. Painful menstruation is the leading cause of lost time and work among women in their teens and 20s. There are two general types of dysmenorrhea, primary and secondary.

Primary dysmenorrhea refers to menstrual pain that occurs in an otherwise healthy woman. *Secondary dysmenorrhea* is menstrual pain attributed to some underlying disease process or structural abnormality within or outside the uterus. Abnormal conditions associated with secondary dysmenorrhea include endometriosis, pelvic inflammatory disease, vaginal agenesis, and ovarian cysts. Primary dysmenorrhea in adolescents usually begins 2 to 3 years following the onset of menses and consists of crampy lower abdominal pain that generally starts several hours prior to the onset of a menstrual period. Pain may be mild to severe and may be associated with nausea and vomiting and constipation or diarrhea. Primary dysmenorrhea is caused by prostaglandin-induced uterine contractions. OTC nonsteroidal anti-inflammatory drugs such as ibuprofen and naproxen can be used to treat dysmenorrhea.

NONSTEROIDAL ANTI-INFLAMMATORY DRUGS (NSAIDs)

Antidysmenorrheal—By inhibiting the synthesis and activity of intrauterine prostaglandins (which are thought to be responsible for the pain and other symptoms of primary dysmenorrhea), NSAIDs decrease uterine contractility and uterine pressure, increase uterine perfusion, and relieve ischemic as well as spasmodic pain. The antibradykinin activity of NSAIDs may also be involved in relief of dysmenorrhea, since bradykinin has been shown to induce uterine contractions and act together with prostaglandins to cause pain. In addition, NSAIDs may, to some extent, relieve extrauterine symptoms (such as headache, nausea, and vomiting) that are associated with excessive prostaglandin production.

Dysmenorrhea (treatment)—Ibuprofen, ketoprofen, and naproxen are indicated for relief of the pain and other symptoms of primary dysmenorrhea.

Ibuprofen

Adults: 200 to 400mg every 4 to 6 hours as needed.

Ketoprofen

Adults: 25 to 50mg every 6 to 8 hours as needed.

Naproxen

Adults: 500mg initially, then 250mg every 6 to 8 hours as needed.

IBUPROFEN PRODUCTS	
Brand Name	**Dosage Form**
Advil (Wyeth)	**Capsule:** 200mg **Tablet:** 200mg
Advil Children's (Wyeth)	**Tablet:** 50mg
Advil Junior (Wyeth)	**Tablet:** 100mg
Midol Cramp Formula (Bayer)	**Tablet:** 200mg
Motrin IB (McNeil)	**Tablet:** 200mg
Motrin Children's (McNeil)	**Suspension:** 100mg/5mL
Motrin Infants' (McNeil)	**Suspension:** 50mg/1.25mL
Motrin Junior (McNeil)	**Tablet:** 100mg
Motrin Migraine Pain (McNeil)	**Tablet:** 200mg
KETOPROFEN PRODUCTS	
Brand Name	**Dosage Form**
Orudis KT (Wyeth)	**Tablet:** 12.5mg
NAPROXEN PRODUCTS	
Brand Name	**Dosage Form**
Aleve (Bayer)	**Capsule:** 220mg **Tablet:** 220mg
Aleve Arthritis (Bayer)	**Tablet:** 220mg
Midol Extended Relief (Bayer)	**Tablet:** 220mg

DOSING INFORMATION FOR ANALGESIC PRODUCTS

The following table provides a quick comparison of the ingredients and dosages of common brand-name OTC drugs. Products are listed alphabetically by brand name.

BRAND NAME	INGREDIENT/STRENGTH	DOSE
NSAIDs		
Advil caplets *(Wyeth Consumer Healthcare)*	Ibuprofen 200mg	**Adults & Peds ≥12 yo:** 1-2 tabs q4-6h. **Max:** 6 tabs q24h.
Advil gelcaps *(Wyeth Consumer Healthcare)*	Ibuprofen 200mg	**Adults & Peds ≥12 yo:** 1-2 caps q4-6h. **Max:** 6 caps q24h.
Advil liqui-gels *(Wyeth Consumer Healthcare)*	Ibuprofen 200mg	**Adults & Peds ≥12 yo:** 1-2 caps q4-6h. **Max:** 6 caps q24h.
Advil tablets *(Wyeth Consumer Healthcare)*	Ibuprofen 200mg	**Adults & Peds ≥12 yo:** 1-2 tabs q4-6h. **Max:** 6 tabs q24h.
Aleve caplets *(Bayer Healthcare)*	Naproxen Sodium 220mg	**Adults ≥65 yo:** 1 tab q12h. **Max:** 2 tabs q24h. **Adults & Peds ≥12 yo:** 1 tab q8-12h. **Max:** 3 tabs q24h.
Aleve gelcaps *(Bayer Healthcare)*	Naproxen Sodium 220mg	**Adults ≥65 yo:** 1 cap q12h. **Max:** 2 caps q24h. **Adults & Peds ≥12 yo:** 1 cap q8-12h. **Max:** 3 caps q24h.
Aleve tablets *(Bayer Healthcare)*	Naproxen Sodium 220mg	**Adults ≥65 yo:** 1 tab q12h. **Max:** 2 tabs q24h. **Adults & Peds ≥12 yo:** 1 tab q8-12h. **Max:** 3 tabs q24h.
Midol Cramps and Body Aches tablets *(Bayer Healthcare)*	Ibuprofen 200mg	**Adults & Peds ≥12 yo:** 1-2 tabs q4-6h. **Max:** 6 tabs q24h.
Midol Extended Relief caplets *(Bayer Healthcare)*	Naproxen Sodium 220mg	**Adults & Peds ≥12 yo:** 1 tabs q8-12h. **Max:** 3 tabs q24h.
Motrin IB caplets *(McNeil Consumer)*	Ibuprofen 200mg	**Adults & Peds ≥12 yo:** 1-2 tabs q4-6h. **Max:** 6 tabs q24h.
Motrin IB gelcaps *(McNeil Consumer)*	Ibuprofen 200mg	**Adults & Peds ≥12 yo:** 1-2 tabs q4-6h. **Max:** 6 tabs q24h.
Motrin IB tablets *(McNeil Consumer)*	Ibuprofen 200mg	**Adults & Peds ≥12 yo:** 1-2 tabs q4-6h. **Max:** 6 tabs q24h.
Nuprin caplets *(Bristol-Myers Squibb)*	Ibuprofen 200mg	**Adults & Peds ≥12 yo:** 1-2 tabs q4-6h. **Max:** 6 tabs q24h.
Nuprin tablets *(Bristol-Myers Squibb)*	Ibuprofen 200mg	**Adults & Peds ≥12 yo:** 1-2 tabs q4-6h. **Max:** 6 tabs q24h.
Orudis KT tablets *(Wyeth Consumer Healthcare)*	Ketoprofen Magnesium 12.5mg	**Adults:** 1-2 tabs q4-6h. **Max:** 6 tabs q24h.

Premenstrual Syndrome

There is no clear consensus on a definition of premenstrual syndrome (PMS), which may be associated with more than 150 different symptoms. PMS is generally understood to refer to a cluster of mood, behavioral, and/or physical symptoms that (1) reccur during the luteal phase (second half, premenstrual phase) of consecutive menstrual cycles, (2) are of sufficient severity to interfere with some aspect of life, and (3) largely disappear within a few hours or days of menses onset. The most common symptoms include headache, backache, abdominal pain, abdominal heaviness, abdominal cramps, abdominal fullness, muscle spasms, breast tenderness, weight gain, recurrent cold sores, acne flare-ups, nausea, bloating, constipation, diarrhea, decreased coordination, food craving, painful menstruation, and swelling of the ankles, feet, and hands. Other symptoms include anxiety or panic, confusion, difficulty concentrating, forgetfulness, poor judgment, depression, increased guilt feelings, fatigue, lethargic movement, decreased self-image, sex drive changes, paranoia or increased fears, low self-esteem, and irritability, hostility, or aggressive behavior.

If the symptoms are primarily affective (emotional), markedly impair work, school, social activities, and/or interpersonal relationships, and satisfy stringent temporal and operational criteria of the American Psychiatric Association's *Diagnostic and Statistical Manual of Mental Disorders, Fourth Edition, Text Revision (DSM-IV-TR)*, the patient is classified as having premenstrual dysphoric disorder (PMDD). Although PMDD is a credible diagnosis, its classification criteria are primarily designed to standardize research populations and may be too narrow for general clinical use, given the various symptoms of anxiety often present in women with PMS or PMDD. In contrast, the diagnosis of PMS according to the *Tenth Revision of the International Classification of Disease (ICD-10)* requires that only a single physical or mood symptom recur in a cyclic fashion; prospective recording and functional impairment are not required. Thus, according to the broader *ICD-10* criteria, about 20% to 30% of reproductive-age women in the general population have PMS, whereas only about 5% of otherwise similar women have PMDD according to the *Diagnostic and Statistical Manual of Mental Disorders, Fourth Edition (DSM-IV)* criteria.

Regardless of classification (ie, either severe PMS or PMDD), 5 key symptom patterns appear to predominate: anger/irritability, depressed mood, anxiety/tension, decreased energy/interest (with physical symptoms), and appetite changes. Moreover, clinical studies have failed to demonstrate any significant differences in treatment response between women who meet the *DSM-IV* criteria for PMDD and women who are strictly classified as having severe PMS. Regardless of the individual symptoms, the most important diagnostic key is the timing of symptoms in relation to the menstrual cycle. Significant symptomatology that continues well into the follicular (postmenstrual) phase automatically rules out PMS or PMDD according to standard criteria.

The diagnosis of PMS is frequently confounded by other chronic disorders that are exacerbated premenstrually. Importantly, premenstrual disturbances often coexist with psychiatric disorders. For example, more than 50% of women with a history of major depression experience premenstrual depression or exacerbation of symptoms. There is some controversy regarding the percentage of women with a current premenstrual syndrome who

have had a prior episode of major depression; several studies have found a rate of lifetime major depression among women with confirmed PMDD of about 40%. Furthermore, several studies suggest that PMS is a stable diagnosis over time, indicating that the higher risk attendant to the history of major depression in women with PMS existed at baseline. In summary, some women with major depression may develop PMDD and some women with PMDD develop major depression, but more study is necessary to determine the specific nature and predictors of the relationship between the two disorders. Diagnostic criteria require that exacerbation of coexisting psychiatric disorders be ruled out prior to diagnosis of PMDD.

Although the underlying etiology of PMS is uncertain, the pathophysiology appears to be multifactorial. PMS does not depend on menses (it can occur in a woman who has undergone a hysterectomy without bilateral oophorectomy— the "ovarian cycle syndrome"), but PMS does not occur if there is no ovarian function (eg, before menarche or after the menopause). However, women with PMDD do not differ from controls with respect to serum ovarian steroid levels. Rather, the serotonergic systems of women with PMDD may be more vulnerable to interactions with the ovarian steroids, as well as other endocrine factors, neurotransmitters, and biological systems (eg, calcium regulation). Several studies support the serotonin theory, which postulates that altered serotoninergic system sensitivity in response to essentially normal phasic fluctuations in female gonadal hormone(s) causes PMS or PMDD. Moreover, the effectiveness of selective serotonin reuptake inhibitors (SSRIs) administered only during the luteal phase emphasizes a significant difference between PMS and typical depressive disorders. Acute SSRI treatment, which increases synaptic serotonin, relieves many PMS symptoms within 1 to 2 days, whereas chronic SSRI treatment, which down-regulates serotonin receptors, requires 3 to 6 weeks to relieve major depressive symptoms.

A National Institutes of Health (NIH) study that used metergoline (a serotonin receptor antagonist) provided additional support for the hypothesis that altered serotonergic transmission accounts for the efficacy of SSRIs in PMS or PMDD. In the NIH study, women with PMDD (whose symptoms had remitted on fluoxetine) and control women received metergoline. Within 24 hours, the symptoms of the women who had received fluoxetine returned, whereas women with PMDD who received the placebo and women without PMDD had no changes in mood. Some women with PMS have no depressive or mood symptoms, and some do not respond to SSRIs. Thus, the pathophysiology of PMS is likely to be multifactorial, and mechanisms other than those primarily related to serotonin may be involved. Genetic factors are also involved in PMS. Seventy percent of women whose mothers have had PMS have PMS themselves, whereas 37% of women whose mothers have not had PMS have PMS themselves. Monozygotic twins have a 93% concordance rate, whereas dizygotic twins have a 44% concordance rate for PMS.

There are several OTC products available to treat many of the symptoms of PMS, most of which contain an analgesic such as acetaminophen, ibuprofen, or naproxen.

ACETAMINOPHEN

Analgesic—The mechanism of analgesic action has not been fully determined. Acetaminophen may act predominantly by inhibiting prostaglandin synthesis in the central nervous system and, to a lesser extent, through a peripheral action by blocking pain-impulse generation. The peripheral action may also be due to inhibition of prostaglandin synthesis or to inhibition of the synthesis or actions of other substances that sensitize pain receptors to mechanical or chemical stimulation.

Acetaminophen is used in several combination products to treat symptoms of PMS.

For more information, refer to the complete monograph for acetaminophen in "Aches and Pains" under Musculoskeletal System.

NONSTEROIDAL ANTI-INFLAMMATORY DRUGS (NSAIDs)

Antidysmenorrheal—By inhibiting the synthesis and activity of intrauterine prostaglandins (which are thought to be responsible for the pain and other symptoms of primary dysmenorrhea), NSAIDs decrease uterine contractility and uterine pressure, increase uterine perfusion, and relieve ischemic as well as spas-modic pain. The antibradykinin activity of NSAIDs may also be involved in relief of dysmenorrhea, since bradykinin has been shown to induce uterine contractions and to act together with prostaglandins to cause pain. In addition, NSAIDs may, to some extent, relieve extrauterine symptoms (such as headache, nausea, and vomiting) that are associated with excessive prostaglandin production.

Dysmenorrhea (treatment)—Ibuprofen, ketoprofen, and naproxen are indicated for relief of the pain and other symptoms of primary dysmenorrhea.

Ibuprofen

Adults: 200 to 400mg every 4 to 6 hours as needed.

Ketoprofen

Adults: 25 to 50mg every 6 to 8 hours as needed.

Naproxen

Adults: 500mg initially, then 250mg every 6 to 8 hours as needed.

For more information, refer to the complete monograph for NSAIDs in "Aches and Pains" under Musculoskeletal System.

IBUPROFEN PRODUCTS	
Brand Name	**Dosage Form**
Advil (Wyeth)	**Capsule:** 200mg **Tablet:** 200mg
Advil Children's (Wyeth)	**Tablet:** 50mg
Advil Junior (Wyeth)	**Tablet:** 100mg
Midol Cramp Formula (Bayer)	**Tablet:** 200mg
Motrin IB (McNeil)	**Tablet:** 200mg
Motrin Children's (McNeil)	**Suspension:** 100mg/5mL
Motrin Infants' (McNeil)	**Suspension:** 50mg/1.25mL
Motrin Junior (McNeil)	**Tablet:** 100mg
Motrin Migraine Pain (McNeil)	**Tablet:** 200mg
KETOPROFEN PRODUCTS	
Brand Name	**Dosage Form**
Orudis KT (Wyeth)	**Tablet:** 12.5mg
NAPROXEN PRODUCTS	
Brand Name	**Dosage Form**
Aleve (Bayer)	**Capsule:** 220mg **Tablet:** 220mg
Aleve Arthritis (Bayer)	**Tablet:** 220mg
Midol Extended Relief (Bayer)	**Tablet:** 220mg

DOSING INFORMATION FOR PREMENSTRUAL SYNDROME PRODUCTS

The following table provides a quick comparison of the ingredients and dosages of common brand-name OTC drugs. Products are listed alphabetically by drug category and brand name.

BRAND NAME	INGREDIENT/STRENGTH	DOSE
ACETAMINOPHEN COMBINATION		
Midol Menstrual Complete caplets (Bayer Healthcare)	Acetaminophen/Caffeine/Pyrilamine Maleate 500mg-60mg-15mg	**Adults & Peds ≥12 yo:** 2 tabs q6h. **Max:** 8 tabs q24h.
Midol Menstrual Complete caplets (Bayer Healthcare)	Acetaminophen/Caffeine/Pyrilamine Maleate 500mg-60mg-15mg	**Adults & Peds ≥12 yo:** 2 tabs q6h. **Max:** 8 tabs q24h.
Midol PMS caplets (Bayer Healthcare)	Acetaminophen/Pamabrom/Pyrilamine 500mg-25mg-15mg	**Adults & Peds ≥12 yo:** 2 tabs q6h. **Max:** 8 tabs q24h.
Midol Teen caplets (Bayer Healtcare)	Acetaminophen/Pamabrom 500mg-25mg	**Adults & Peds ≥12 yo:** 2 tabs q6h. **Max:** 8 tabs q24h.
Pamprin Multi-Symptom caplets (Chattem Consumer Products)	Acetaminophen/Pamabrom/Pyrilamine 500mg-25mg-15mg	**Adults & Peds ≥12 yo:** 2 tabs q4-6h. **Max:** 8 tabs q24h.
Premsyn PMS caplets (Chattem Consumer Products)	Acetaminophen/Pamabrom/Pyrilamine 500mg-25mg-15mg	**Adults & Peds ≥12 yo:** 2 tabs q4-6h. **Max:** 8 tabs q24h.
Tylenol Women's caplets (McNeil Consumer)	Acetaminophen/Pamabrom 500mg-25mg	**Adults & Peds ≥12 yo:** 2 tabs q4-6h. **Max:** 8 tabs q24h.
NSAIDs		
Advil caplets (Wyeth Consumer Health)	Ibuprofen 200mg	**Adults & Peds ≥12 yo:** 1-2 tabs q4-6h. **Max:** 6 tabs q24h.
Advil gelcaps (Wyeth Consumer Healthcare)	Ibuprofen 200mg	**Adults & Peds ≥12 yo:** 1-2 caps q4-6h. **Max:** 6 caps q24h.
Advil liqui-gels (Wyeth Consumer Healthcare)	Ibuprofen 200mg	**Adults & Peds ≥12 yo:** 1-2 caps q4-6h. **Max:** 6 caps q24h.
Advil tablets (Wyeth Consumer Healthcare)	Ibuprofen 200mg	**Adults & Peds ≥12 yo:** 1-2 tabs q4-6h. **Max:** 6 tabs q24h.
Aleve caplets (Bayer Healthcare)	Naproxen Sodium 220mg	**Adults ≥65 yo:** 1 tab q12h. **Max:** 2 tabs q24h. **Adults & Peds ≥12 yo:** 1 tab q8-12h. **Max:** 3 tabs q24h.
Aleve gelcaps (Bayer Healthcare)	Naproxen Sodium 220mg	**Adults ≥65 yo:** 1 cap q12h. **Max:** 2 caps q24h. **Adults & Peds ≥12 yo:** 1 cap q8-12h. **Max:** 3 caps q24h.
Aleve tablets (Bayer Healthcare)	Naproxen Sodium 220mg	**Adults ≥65 yo:** 1 tab q12h. **Max:** 2 tabs q24h. **Adults & Peds ≥12 yo:** 1 tab q8-12h. **Max:** 3 tabs q24h.
Midol Cramps and Body Aches tablets (Bayer Healthcare)	Ibuprofen 200mg	**Adults & Peds ≥12 yo:** 1-2 tabs q4-6h. **Max:** 6 tabs q24h.
Midol Extended Relief caplets (Bayer Healthcare)	Naproxen Sodium 220mg	**Adults & Peds ≥12 yo:** 1 tabs q8-12h. **Max:** 3 tabs q24h.
Motrin IB caplets (McNeil Consumer)	Ibuprofen 200mg	**Adults & Peds ≥12 yo:** 1-2 tabs q4-6h. **Max:** 6 tabs q24h.
Motrin IB gelcaps (McNeil Consumer)	Ibuprofen 200mg	**Adults & Peds ≥12 yo:** 1-2 tabs q4-6h. **Max:** 6 tabs q24h.
Motrin IB tablets (McNeil Consumer)	Ibuprofen 200mg	**Adults & Peds ≥12 yo:** 1-2 tabs q4-6h. **Max:** 6 tabs q24h.
Nuprin caplets (Bristol-Myers Squibb)	Ibuprofen 200mg	**Adults & Peds ≥12 yo:** 1-2 tabs q4-6h. **Max:** 6 tabs q24h.
Nuprin tablets (Bristol-Myers Squibb)	Ibuprofen 200mg	**Adults & Peds ≥12 yo:** 1-2 tabs q4-6h. **Max:** 6 tabs q24h.
Orudis KT tablets (Wyeth Consumer Healthcare)	Ketoprofen Magnesium 12.5mg	**Adults:** 1-2 tabs q4-6h. **Max:** 6 tabs q24h.

Vaginal Candidiasis

Vaginal candidiasis is a vaginal infection caused most commonly by the fungal organism *Candida albicans*. Vaginal candidiasis is the second most common cause of vaginitis. An estimated 75% of women will experience at least one episode during their lifetime, and 40% to 45% will experience two or more episodes; a small percentage of women (probably <5%) experience recurrent infection. *Candida albicans* causes most cases of clinical vaginal "yeast infections." Approximately 10% of infections are caused by *Candida* (formerly *Torulopsis*) *glabrata*. Nonalbicans candidiasis is increasing in incidence and is associated with relapsing candidiasis.

Vaginal candidiasis is usually not sexually acquired or transmitted. However, sexual activity may be more contributory to the production of clinical disease (causing mild abrasions) than simple transmission of the organism. A higher incidence of candidiasis is noted in the summer months. Candidiasis is thought to be a hormonally dependent disease supported by its frequent occurrence in women between menarche and menopause. Vaginal candidiasis usually begins with the adherence of candidal cells to the vaginal epithelium and changes to the mycelial form. This can be enhanced in the presence of estrogen. This is believed to be followed by a release of a cellular toxin or a protease enzyme leading to extensive damage of normal cells and resulting in the symptoms of vaginal candidiasis.

Vaginal candidiasis is classified on the basis of clinical presentation, microbiology, and host factors. Uncomplicated vulvovaginal candidiasis is characterized as sporadic, infrequent, or mild to moderate; is likely to be caused by *C albicans*; and appears in nonimmunocompromised women. Diagnosis is suggested clinically by pruritus and erythema in the vulvovaginal area; a white discharge may be present. Diagnosis can be made with clinical signs and symptoms and either (1) a wet prep (saline, 10% KOH) or Gram's stain of vaginal discharge that demonstrates yeasts or pseudohyphae or (2) a culture or other test that yields a positive result for a yeast species.

Complicated vulvovaginal candidiasis (CVC) is classified as recurrent or severe and is generally not caused by *C albicans*. It often appears in women who are pregnant, debilitated, immunocompromised, or have uncontrolled diabetes. Recurrent CVC is defined as 4 or more symptomatic episodes a year. It occurs in less than 5% of women. Pathogenesis is poorly understood, and some women with recurrent CVC do not have apparent predisposing or underlying conditions. Vaginal cultures should be obtained from patients with recurrent episodes to confirm the clinical diagnosis and to identify unusual species, including nonalbicans species. Severe CVC (e.g., extensive vulvar erythema, edema, excoriation, or fissure formation) has lower clinical response rates in patients treated with short courses of topical or oral therapy.

The predisposing factors for recurrent candidiasis include high-dose oral contraceptives; IUD use; broad-spectrum antibiotic therapy; diabetes mellitus; estrogen therapy in postmenopausal women; pregnancy; young age at first intercourse; intercourse more than 4 times per month; receptive oral sex; localized allergic reactions from semen or douching with commercially available solutions; and immunosuppression. Intravaginal trauma (e.g., microscopic abrasions) associated with sexual activity may also be a risk factor for recurrent candidiasis, as well as HIV infection. Premenstrual onset is typical; postmenopausal disease should prompt a search for predisposing factors such as diabetes mellitus.

The hallmark symptom of vaginal candidiasis is pruritus; as the disease progresses, burning, soreness, and pain upon urination or wiping occurs. Vaginal discharge is a frequent but not universal complaint, and dyspareunia or dysuria may be reported. Erythema, excoriation (from scratching), and small, red satellite lesions may be present. Vaginal secretions may range from a scanty discharge to a thick, white, and curdy one (often called "cottage-cheese" discharge, which occurs only in a minority of patients).

There are a several OTC vaginal antifungal agents available to treat vaginal candidiasis; many contain clotrimazole, miconazole, tioconazole, or butoconazole.

AZOLE ANTIFUNGALS (VAGINAL)

PHARMACOLOGY

These drugs are fungistatic and may be fungicidal, depending on concentration. Their exact mechanism of action is unknown. Azoles inhibit biosynthesis of ergosterol or other sterols, damaging the fungal cell membrane and altering its permeability. As a result, loss of essential intracellular elements may occur.

Azoles also inhibit biosynthesis of triglycerides and phospholipids by fungi. In addition, azoles inhibit oxidative and peroxidative enzyme activity, resulting in intracellular buildup of toxic concentrations of hydrogen peroxide, which may contribute to deterioration of subcellular organelles and cellular necrosis. In *Candida albicans,* azoles inhibit transformation of blastospores into invasive mycelial form.

INDICATIONS

Candidiasis, vulvovaginal (treatment)—Vaginal azoles are indicated in the local treatment of vulvovaginal candidiasis caused by *Candida albicans* and other species of Candida in pregnant (second and third trimesters only) and nonpregnant women. Nonpregnant women should self-medicate with nonprescription antifungal vaginal medications only if they have been diagnosed previously with vulvovaginal candidiasis and have the same symptoms. If symptoms recur within 2 months, women should seek professional medical care. Pregnant women treating vulvovaginal candidiasis with antifungal vaginal agents should use at least a 7-day treatment regimen and seek their physician's advice before using medication in the first trimester.

CONTRAINDICATIONS

Risk-benefit should be considered when the following medical problems exist:

• Allergy to azoles

WARNINGS/PRECAUTIONS

Pregnancy: Pregnant women treating vulvovaginal candidiasis with antifungal vaginal agents should use at least a 7-day treatment regimen. A decision to use antifungal vaginal agents during the first trimester should be based on risk-benefit status and on advice of the physician.

Butoconazole: FDA Pregnancy Category C.

Clotrimazole: FDA Pregnancy Category B.

Miconazole: FDA Pregnancy Category B.

Terconazole: FDA Pregnancy Category C.

Tioconazole: FDA Pregnancy Category C.

Breastfeeding: It is not known whether vaginal azoles are distributed into breast milk. However, problems in humans have not been documented.

Pediatrics: Safety and efficacy have not been established in children up to 12 years of age.

Drug Interactions

• Warfarin (concurrent use may cause bleeding and/or bruising).

ADVERSE REACTIONS

Those indicating need for medical attention: Incidence less frequent

Vaginal burning, itching, discharge, or other irritation not present before therapy.

Incidence rare:

Hypersensitivity skin rash or hives.

Those indicating need for medical attention only if they continue or are bothersome:

Incidence less frequent or rare:

Abdominal or stomach cramps or pain; burning or irritation of penis of sexual partner; headache.

ADMINISTRATION AND DOSAGE

General Dosing Information

Physicians should diagnose vulvovaginal candidiasis and prescribe vaginal azole antifungal agents for first-time users. Patients should consult a physician if symptoms return within 2 months or if exposure to HIV occurs. Recurring yeast infections may be a sign of other conditions, such as diabetes or impaired immune function. Recurring conditions or severe local vaginal infections may benefit from vaginal treatments of longer duration, such as 10 to 14 days, or from the use of appropriate oral medications instead.

If there is no response to therapy, the course of therapy may be repeated after other pathogens have been ruled out by potassium hydroxide (KOH) smears and cultures. If sensitization or irritation occurs, treatment with vaginal azoles should be discontinued. It is recommended that the patient wait 3 days after treatment with azole antifungal agents to resume using latex barrier devices such as condoms or diaphragms. The vehicles for

some vaginal azole products contain lipid-based components. It is likely that many of these products affect the performance of latex contraceptive devices, such as cervical caps, condoms, or diaphragms. Unmedicated tampons may absorb vaginal creams, ointments, or suppositories and are not recommended for use concurrently with vaginal azole antifungal agents.

Butoconazole Nitrate

Cream

Adults/Pediatrics ≥12 years of age: Nonpregnant: 100mg (1 applicatorful of a 2% cream) intravaginally once a day at bedtime for three days. May be repeated for an additional 3 days if needed. *Pregnant (second and third trimesters)*: 100mg (1 applicatorful of a 2% cream) intravaginally once a day at bedtime for 6 days.

Clotrimazole

Cream

Adults/Pediatrics ≥12 years of age: 50mg (1 applicatorful of a 1% cream) intravaginally once a day at bedtime for 6 to 14 days; or 100mg (1 applicatorful of a 2% cream) intravaginally once a day at bedtime for 3 days.

Tablets, Vaginal

Adults/Pediatrics ≥12 years of age: Nonpregnant: 200mg intravaginally once a day at bedtime for 3 days; or 100mg intravaginally once a day at bedtime for 6 or 7 days.

Miconazole Nitrate

Cream

Adults/Pediatrics ≥12 years of age: 1 applicatorful of a 2% cream intravaginally once a day at bedtime for 7 days. May repeat if needed.

Suppositories

Adults/Pediatrics ≥12 years of age: 100mg intravaginally once a day at bedtime for 7 days; or 200mg to 400mg intravaginally once a day at bedtime for 3 days; or 1200mg as a single dose at bedtime.

Tioconazole

Ointment

Adults/Pediatrics ≥12 years of age: 300mg (1 applicatorful of a 6.5% ointment) intravaginally as single dose at bedtime.

Suppositories

Adults/Pediatrics ≥12 years of age: 300mg intravaginally as a single dose at bedtime.

CLOTRIMAZOLE PRODUCTS	
Brand Name	**Dosage Form**
Gyne-Lotrimin 3-Day (Schering)	**Cream:** 2% (100mg)
Gyne-Lotrimin 7 (Schering)	**Cream:** 1% (50mg)
MICONAZOLE PRODUCTS	
Brand Name	**Dosage Form**
Monistat 1 (McNeil)	**Suppository:** 1200mg
Monistat 3 (McNeil)	**Cream:** 4% (200mg)
Monistat 7 (McNeil)	**Cream:** 2% (100mg)
TIOCONAZOLE PRODUCTS	
Brand Name	**Dosage Form**
Monistat 1 (McNeil)	**Ointment:** 6.5% (300mg)
Vagistat-1 (Bristol-Myers Squibb)	**Ointment:** 6.5% (300mg)

DOSING INFORMATION FOR ANTIFUNGAL PRODUCTS

The following table provides a quick comparison of the ingredients and dosages of common brand-name OTC drugs. Products are listed alphabetically by brand name.

BRAND NAME	INGREDIENT/STRENGTH	DOSE
Gyne-Lotrimin 3-Day Treatment Applicators *(Schering-Plough)*	Clotrimazole 2% (100mg)	**Adults & Peds ≥12 yo:** 1 applicatorful qhs x 3d.
Gyne-Lotrimin 7 Vaginal Cream *(Schering-Plough)*	Clotrimazole 1% (50mg)	**Adults & Peds ≥12 yo:** 1 applicatorful qhs x 7d.
Monistat 1 Combination Pack *(McNeil Consumer)*	Cream: Miconazole Nitrate 2%; Vaginal Inset: 1200mg	**Adults & Peds ≥12 yo:** 1 vaginal insert hs x 1d. Apply cream externally bid for up to 7 days.
Monistat 1 Combination Pack With Coolwipes *(McNeil Consumer)*	Cream: Miconazole Nitrate 2%; Vaginal Inset: 1200mg	**Adults & Peds ≥12 yo:** 1 vaginal insert hs x 1d. Apply cream externally bid for up to 7 days.
Monistat 1 Prefilled Applicator *(McNeil Consumer)*	Tioconazole 6.5% (300mg)	**Adults & Peds ≥12 yo:** 1 applicatorful hs x 1d.
Monistat 3 Combination Pack *(McNeil Consumer)*	Cream: Miconazole Nitrate 4%; Suppositories: Miconazole Nitrate 200mg	**Adults & Peds ≥12 yo:** 1 suppository qhs x 3d. Apply cream externally bid for up to 7 days.
Monistat 3 Combination Pack With Coolwipes *(McNeil Consumer)*	Applicator: Miconazole Nitrate 4% (200mg); Cream: Miconazole Nitrate 2%;	**Adults & Peds ≥12 yo:** 1 applicatorful qhs x 3d. Apply cream externally bid for up to 7 days.
Monistat 3 Cream Prefilled Appplicators *(McNeil Consumer)*	Miconazole Nitrate 4% (200mg)	**Adults & Peds ≥12 yo:** 1 applicatorful qhs x 3d.
Monistat 7 Combination Pack *(McNeil Consumer)*	Cream: Miconazole Nitrate 2%; Applicator: Miconazole Nitrate 2%	**Adults & Peds ≥12 yo:** 1 applicatorful qhs x 7d. Apply cream externally bid for up to 7 days.
Vagistat-1 Ointment *(Bristol-Myers Squibb)*	Tioconazole 6.5% (300mg)	**Adults & Peds ≥12 yo:** 1 applicatorful hs x 1d.

DIETARY SUPPLEMENT
PROFILES

Dietary Supplements

Alpha Lipoic Acid

EFFECTS

ALA is an important coenzyme with antioxidant and antidiabetic properties. It is an endogenous substance that acts as a cofactor in the pyruvate-dehydrogenase complex, the alpha-ketoglutarate-dehydrogenase complex, and the amino acid-hydrogenase complex. Reduced levels of ALA have been found in patients with liver cirrhosis, diabetes mellitus, atherosclerosis, and polyneuritis. During metabolism, ALA may be transformed from its oxidized form (with the disulfide bridge in the molecule) to its reduced dihydroform with two free sulfide groups. Both forms have strong antioxidant effects. They protect the cell from free radicals that result from intermediate metabolites, from the degradation of exogenous molecules, and from heavy metals.

ALA is available in oral and parenteral formulations. The scope of this monograph is limited to the oral formulations. Information on the parenteral use of ALA can be found in *PDR for Herbal Medicines*

COMMON USAGE

Unproven uses: Studies of the efficacy of ALA for treating complications of diabetes mellitus are conflicting. ALA may be beneficial for alleviating pain and paresthesia caused by diabetic neuropathy. It is probably ineffective for the treatment of alcohol-related liver disease, Amanita ("death cap" mushroom) poisoning, and HIV-associated cognitive impairment. More placebo-controlled trials are needed.

CONTRAINDICATIONS

There are no known contraindications to the oral formulation of ALA.

WARNINGS/PRECAUTIONS

Hypoglycemia: Patients with diabetes may need additional blood-sugar monitoring.

Paresthesia: Symptoms may temporarily worsen at the beginning of therapy; some research shows that antidepressants or neuroleptics may be used concurrently to treat the pain.

Pregnancy and breastfeeding: Scientific evidence for the safe use of ALA during pregnancy is not available; it is not recommended during lactation.

DRUG INTERACTIONS

Antidiabetic agents: Additive hypoglycemic effects may occur with concurrent use of antidiabetic agents. Close monitoring of blood-sugar control is recommended when initiating therapy with ALA.

Cisplatin: ALA antagonizes the action of cisplatin.

FOOD INTERACTIONS

The bioavailability of ALA is decreased with food.

ADVERSE REACTIONS

Nausea has been reported.

ADMINISTRATION AND DOSAGE

Adults

Diabetic neuropathy: Initiate treatment at 600mg daily in two or three divided doses. Maintenance doses range from 200mg to 600mg daily in single or divided doses.

Bromelain

EFFECTS

Bromelain is a concentrated mixture of proteolytic enzymes derived from the pineapple plant. It has anti-inflammatory, anti-tumor, and digestive properties.

Commercial bromelain is not a chemically homogeneous substance because if the enzyme is highly purified it loses its stability and most of its physiological activity. The main ingredient is a proteolytic enzyme (a glycoprotein), but it also contains small amounts of an acid phosphatase, a peroxidase, several protease inhibitors, and organically bound calcium.

COMMON USAGE

Accepted uses: Bromelain is approved by the German Commission E as an anti-edematous agent.

Unproven uses: Bromelain may be of therapeutic value in modulating inflammation, tumor growth, blood coagulation, and debridement of third-degree burns. It could possibly enhance absorption of some drugs, including antibiotics.

CONTRAINDICATIONS

Bromelain is contraindicated in patients who have severe liver or kidney impairment or who need dialysis. The supplement should also be avoided by patients who have a coagulation disorder such as hemophilia or who have demonstrated hypersensitivity to bromelain, pineapple, or the inactive ingredients of enzyme preparations.

WARNINGS/PRECAUTIONS

Allergic reactions/hypersensitivity: Bromelain is capable of inducing IgE-mediated respiratory and gastrointestinal reactions. Cross-sensitivity reactions between bromelain and papain can occur.

Pregnancy and breastfeeding: Scientific evidence for the safe use of bromelain during pregnancy and lactation in not available.

Tachycardia: Bromelain may increase heart rate at higher doses. It should be used cautiously (doses <500mg per day) in patients with heart palpitations or tachycardia.

DRUG INTERACTIONS

Anticoagulants, low molecular weight heparins, or thrombolytic agents: Theoretically, there is an increased risk of bleeding if bromelain is used with these medications. Avoid concomitant use.

ADVERSE REACTIONS

Mild hypersensitivity reactions such as erythema and pruritus occur infrequently. Gastrointestinal side effects are infrequent but may include stomach ache and/or diarrhea.

ADMINISTRATION AND DOSAGE

Bromelain is administered orally and topically. Available preparations of bromelain tablets vary widely in their concentrations, and caution must be exercised in determining dosage regimens.

Take one hour before or after food.

Adults

General use: 500mg to 2,000mg daily in divided doses.

Carpal tunnel syndrome: 1000mg (with a potency of at least 3,000 microunits/gram) given 3 times a day, between meals.

Debridement: Administer a 35% topical suspension in a liquid base.

Inflammation: 500mg to 2,000mg per day. A European manufacturer recommends 450mg to 1,500 Federation Internationale Pharmaceutique (FIP) units divided into 3 daily doses and administered over 8 to 10 days.

Platelet aggregation inhibition: 160mg to 1400mg daily.

Pediatrics

150FIP to 300FIP units daily, divided into 3 doses.

Calcium

EFFECTS

Calcium is an electrolyte, a nutrient, and a mineral that demonstrates anti-osteoporotic, antihypertensive, antihyperlipidemic, and possible anticarcinogenic properties. Calcium functions as a regulator in the release and storage of neurotransmitters and hormones, in the uptake and binding of amino acids, and in vitamin B^{12} absorption and gastrin secretion. Calcium is required to maintain the function of the nervous, muscular, and skeletal systems and cell membrane and capillary permeability. It is an activator in many enzyme reactions and is essential in the transmission of nerve impulses; contraction of cardiac, smooth, and skeletal muscles; respiration; blood coagulation; and renal function.

The scope of this monograph will be limited to the oral salt formulations, including carbonate, citrate, glubionate, gluconate, lactate, phosphate, and other calcium salts.

COMMON USAGE

Accepted uses: Calcium salts are FDA-approved for the prophylaxis of calcium deficiency and osteoporosis. Calcium acetate is approved for the treatment of hyperphosphatemia related to renal failure and hemodialysis. Calcium carbonate is used alone or in combination products as an antacid to relieve symptoms of heartburn, acid indigestion, and stomach upset.

Unproven uses: Calcium supplementation may reduce premenstrual pain, total and LDL cholesterol levels, hypertension, and the occurrence of colorectal polyps. Studies show it may also reverse fluorosis in children (when combined with vitamins C and D), control age-related increases in parathyroid hormone, and reduce plasma bilirubin in patients with Crigler-Najjar syndrome (calcium phosphate only). Weaker evidence shows calcium supplementation may be helpful for leg cramps, pre-eclampsia, and prophylaxis of urinary crystallization of calcium oxalate in patients with nephrolithiasis (calcium citrate only).

CONTRAINDICATIONS

Calcium supplements are contraindicated in patients with hypercalcemia.

WARNINGS/PRECAUTIONS

Arrhythmia: Calcium enhances the effect of cardiac glycosides on the heart and may precipitate arrhythmia.

Hypercalcemia: Oral calcium—including antacids containing calcium carbonate or other absorbable calcium salts—can cause hypercalcemia, which may result in nephrolithiasis, anorexia, nausea, vomiting, and ocular toxicity.

Milk-alkali syndrome: Doses higher than 4g daily can result in milk-alkali syndrome. Symptoms include hypercalcemia, uremia, calcinosis, nausea, vomiting, headache, weakness, azotemia, and alterations in taste.

Pregnancy and breastfeeding: Calcium is safe in normal dietary amounts. It is FDA-rated as Pregnancy Category C.

Prostate cancer: A high intake of calcium, whether from food alone or including supplements, was associated in an epidemiological study with an increased incidence of prostate cancer, possibly due to calcium's inhibitory effect on vitamin D conversion.

DRUG INTERACTIONS

Aspirin: Concurrent use may result in decreased effectiveness of aspirin due to increased urinary pH and subsequent increased renal elimination of salicylates. Monitor for reduced aspirin effectiveness upon initiation of calcium-containing products or for possible aspirin toxicity upon withdrawal of calcium-containing products. Adjust the dose accordingly. Using buffered aspirin may limit the degree to which the urine is alkalinized.

Atenolol: Concomitant use may decrease the bioavailability of atenolol; administer atenolol 2 hours before or 6 hours after calcium-containing products.

Bismuth subcitrate: Concomitant use may result in decreased effectiveness of bismuth subcitrate. Administer at least 30 minutes apart.

Bisphosphonates: Concurrent use may interfere with the absorption of bisphosphonates such as alendronate, etidronate, tiludronate, and risedronate. Administer bisphosphonates 2 hours before or 3 to 4 hours after a dose of calcium.

Calcium channel blockers: Concomitant use can result in decreased effectiveness of calcium channel blockers. Monitor the patient and adjust dose accordingly.

Cefpodoxime: Concomitant use may result in decreased effectiveness of cefpodoxime. Concurrent administration of cefpodoxime and calcium-containing products is not recommended. If concurrent use cannot be avoided, cefpodoxime should be taken at least 2 to 3 hours before the administration of calcium. Because staggered administration may not be completely reliable, aggressively monitor patients for continued antibiotic efficacy. Alternative antibiotic therapy may need to be considered.

Diuretics: Thiazide and thiazide-like diuretics may cause hypercalcemia by decreasing renal calcium excretion. Concomitant ingestion of calcium salts and thiazide diuretics may predispose patients to developing the milk-alkali syndrome. Instruct patients to avoid excessive ingestion of calcium in any form (e.g., antacids, dairy products) during thiazide diuretic therapy. Consider monitoring the patient's serum calcium level and/or parathyroid function if calcium replacement therapy is clinically necessary.

Fluoroquinolones: Concomitant use may result in decreased effectiveness of fluoroquinolones such as ciprofloxacin and enoxacin. Concurrent administration of fluoroquinolones with calcium—including calcium-fortified foods and drinks such as orange juice—should be avoided. Fluoroquinolones may be taken 2 hours before or 6 hours after taking calcium-containing products.

Hyoscyamine: Concomitant use may result in decreased absorption of hyoscyamine. Hyoscyamine should be taken prior to meals and calcium-containing products should be taken after meals.

Itraconazole: Concomitant use may result in decreased effectiveness of itraconazole. Calcium-containing products should be taken at least 1 hour before or 2 hours after itraconazole.

Ketoconazole: Concomitant use may result in decreased effectiveness of ketoconazole. Concurrent administration of ketoconazole and calcium-containing products is not recommended. If concurrent use cannot be avoided, ketoconazole should be taken at least 2 hours before calcium-containing products. Because staggered administration may not be completely reliable, aggressively monitor patients for continued antifungal efficacy.

Levothyroxine: Concurrent use with calcium carbonate may result in decreased absorption of levothyroxine. Separate the administration of levothyroxine and calcium carbonate by at least 4 hours.

Methscopolamine: Concomitant use may result in decreased absorption of methscopolamine, although the effect is minor. Monitor the patient for drug effectiveness.

Polystyrene sulfonate: Concomitant administration of calcium-containing antacids and sodium polystyrene sulfonate resin therapy has resulted in the elevation of serum carbon dioxide content levels, associated with varying degrees of metabolic alkalosis. Separate the oral administration of sodium polystyrene sulfonate and calcium-containing products by as much time as possible. Another alternative is to administer the sodium polystyrene sulfonate rectally. If concurrent oral administration cannot be avoided, monitor the patient for evidence of alkalosis.

Sucralfate: Concurrent use may result in decreased effectiveness of sucralfate. Calcium-containing products should not be taken 30 minutes before or after sucralfate administration.

Sulfasalazine: Concomitant sulfasalazine and calcium gluconate therapy has been reported to result in delayed absorption of sulfasalazine.

Tetracyclines: Concurrent use may result in decreased effectiveness of tetracyclines and is not recommended. If concurrent use cannot be avoided, tetracyclines should be taken at least 1 to 3 hours before calcium-containing products. Because staggered administration may not be completely reliable, aggressively monitor patients for continued antibiotic efficacy.

Ticlopidine: Concurrent use may result in decreased effectiveness of ticlopidine. Concurrent administration of ticlopidine and calcium-containing products is not recommended. If concurrent use cannot be avoided, ticlopidine should be taken at least 1 to 2 hours before the administration of calcium.

Zalcitabine: Concurrent use may result in decreased effectiveness of zalcitabine. Separate the administration of zalcitabine and calcium-containing products as far apart as possible.

ADVERSE REACTIONS

Constipation: Oral calcium supplementation can cause constipation.

ADMINISTRATION AND DOSAGE

Because calcium salts are bound with other molecules such as oxygen and carbon, supplements often list the percentage of elemental calcium in each tablet along with the total salt weight, usually in milligrams. The table below lists common examples.

Elemental calcium/1,000 mg of salt (percentage and weight)		
Carbonate	40%	(400mg)
Citrate	21%	(210mg)
Lactate	13%	(130mg)
Gluconate	9%	(90mg)

Daily Dosage: The National Institute of Medicine recommends the following Adequate Intakes (AIs) for males and females:

Adults 19 to 50 years: 1,000mg daily; *51+ years*: 1,200mg daily.

Infants and children 0 to 6 months: 210mg daily; *7 to 12 months*: 270mg daily; *1 to 3 years*: 500mg daily; *4 to 8 years*: 800mg daily; *9 to 18 years*: 1,300mg daily.

The same AIs apply to pregnant or lactating women.

Adults

Deficiency: Calcium carbonate—1g to 2g three times daily with meals; calcium citrate—950mg to 1.9g given 3 or 4 times a day after meals; calcium gluconate—15g daily in divided doses; calcium lactate—7.7g daily in divided doses with meals; calcium glubionate—15g daily in divided doses; dibasic calcium phosphate—4.4g daily in divided doses with or after meals; tribasic calcium phosphate—1.6g twice daily with or after meals.

Colorectal cancer prevention: 1,200mg to 2,000mg daily.

Crigler-Najjar syndrome: 4,000mg daily

Dysmenorrhea: 1,000mg to 1,300mg daily

Hypercholesterolemia: 250mg to 400mg daily with meals

Hyperphosphatemia: 1,334mg of calcium acetate with each meal initially. Most patients will require 2,001mg to 2,668mg with each meal. The dosage may be increased as necessary to obtain serum phosphate levels below 6mg/dL as long as hypercalcemia does not occur or, alternatively, 1g to 17g calcium carbonate daily in divided doses.

Hyperphosphatemia of renal failure and hemodialysis: 4,000mg to 8,000mg daily of calcium acetate or 2,500mg to 8,500mg daily of calcium carbonate

Hypertension, idiopathic: 1,000mg to 2,000mg per day

Hypertension, pregnancy-related: 1,000 to 2,000mg per day

Nephrolithiasis, prevention: 200mg to 300mg with meals or as the citrate salt between meals

Osteoporosis, glucocorticoid-induced, prevention of bone loss: 1,000mg daily

Osteoporosis, idiopathic, prevention of bone loss and fractures: 500mg to 2,400mg daily

Pre-eclampsia, prevention: 1,000mg to 2,000mg daily

Premenstrual syndrome: 1,000mg to 1,200mg daily

Pediatrics

Bone mass accretion (adolescents): 500mg daily

Fluorosis: 250mg daily

Hypertension, prevention: 600mg daily

Hypocalcemia: calcium chloride—200mg/kg/d in divided doses every 4 to 6 hours; calcium glubionate—infants up to 1 year old should receive 1.8g calcium glubionate five times a day before meals, children 1 to 4 years old should receive 3.6g three times a day before meals; children over age 4 should receive 15g per day in divided doses; calcium gluconate—200mg to 800mg/kg/d in divided doses; calcium lactate—500mg/kg/24 hours given orally in divided doses; calcium levulinate—500mg/kg/24 hours (12g/square meter/24 hours) given orally in divided doses;

dibasic calcium phosphate—200mg to 280mg/kg of body weight a day, in divided doses with or after meals.

Chondroitin Sulfate

EFFECTS

Chondroitin sulfate is a mucopolysaccharide found in most mammalian cartilaginous tissues. It has a molecular configuration similar to sodium hyaluronate, although chondroitin has a considerably shorter chain length. Chondroitin sulfate has protective effects on cartilage as well as viscoelastic effects. Preliminary evidence suggests it may also have antilipidemic, anticoagulant, and antithrombogenic properties.

Ophthalmic preparations of chondroitin are FDA-approved used for ophthalmic procedures. The scope of this monograph, however, is limited to the oral preparations.

COMMON USAGE

Unproven uses: Chondroitin sulfate is used to reduce pain, improve functional capacity, and reduce the use of pain medications in patients with osteoarthritis and rheumatic disease. Oral chondroitin is sometimes used to treat the following: TMJ disorder, coronary heart disease, hypercholesterolemia, and nephrolithiasis. It is also used to prevent or treat disorders of connective tissue structures such as the aorta, vascular tissues, and soft tissues involved in musculoskeletal trauma.

CONTRAINDICATIONS

Patients with asthma may be at risk for symptom exacerbation.

WARNINGS/PRECAUTIONS

Pregnancy and breastfeeding: Information is not available regarding the safe use of chondroitin during pregnancy and lactation.

DRUG INTERACTIONS

Antiplatelet and anticoagulant agents: Theoretically, concurrent use with chondroitin may increase the risk of bleeding.

ADVERSE REACTIONS

Adverse reactions have not been reported with oral chondroitin.

ADMINISTRATION AND DOSAGE

Adults

Osteoarthritis: 800mg to 1200mg orally in single or divided doses

Pediatrics

Information on pediatric dosing is not available.

Chromium

EFFECTS

Chromium is an essential trace mineral that plays a role in glucose metabolism. It is believed to potentiate the action of insulin at the cellular level. Chromium may also play a role in lipoprotein metabolism. Chromium deficiency may lead to glucose intolerance and neuropathies.

Chromium is available in oral and intravenous formulations. The scope of this monograph is limited to the oral formulation.

COMMON USAGE

Accepted uses: Prevention and treatment of chromium deficiency.

Unproven Uses: Chromium supplementation may aid in glycemic control in a subset of patients with type 2 diabetes and gestational diabetes. The use of chromium for glucose regulation in both hypoglycemia and diabetes has been longstanding but without uniform positive results.

Chromium is not widely used in diabetics and is not endorsed by the American Diabetes Association. The optimal dose for glycemic control is not known and may exceed the estimated safe and adequate daily dietary intake of 10mcg to 200mcg, and the available studies, while of high quality, need to be expanded. Preliminary data from the diabetes studies also suggest that chromium may positively affect serum lipids. There is some interest in chromium's use in reactive hypoglycemia mostly from small clinical studies and case reports. A recent study reported that chromium supplementation (1000mcg daily) shortened the QT interval in patients with type 2 diabetes.

Popular literature touts chromium as a weight loss and body-building supplement, but there is little evidence to support chromium use for these indications.

CONTRAINDICATIONS

Do not use in patients who have exhibited hypersensitivity to chromium.

WARNINGS/PRECAUTIONS

Diabetes: Improved glucose tolerance my affect blood glucose levels. Close monitoring of blood glucose levels is recommended.

Pregnancy and breastfeeding: Scientific evidence for the safe use of chromium in doses exceeding the recommended adequate intake is not available.

DRUG INTERACTIONS

Insulin: There is an increased risk of hypoglycemia.

ADVERSE REACTIONS

Insomnia and irritability have been reported.

ADMINISTRATION AND DOSAGE

Daily Dosage (Adequate Intakes [AI]):

Males—9 to 13 years: 25mcg/day; *14 to 50 years*: 35mcg/day; *50+ years*: 30mcg/day. *Females—9 to 13 years*: 21mcg/day; *14 to 18 years*: 24mcg/day; *19 to 50*: 25mcg/day; *50+ years*: 20mcg/day.

During pregnancy—up to 18 years: 29mcg/day; *19 years and older*: 30mcg/day.

During lactation—up to 18 years: 44mcg/day; *19 years and older*: 45mcg/day.

Infants and children—up to 6 months: 0.2mcg/day; *7 to 12 months*: 5.5mcg/day; *1-3 years*: 11mcg/day; *4 to 8 years*: 15mcg/day.

Adults

Deficiency: Treatment is individualized by the prescriber based on the severity of the deficiency.

Non-insulin dependent diabetes: 200mcg to 1000mcg daily

Coenzyme Q10

EFFECTS

Coenzyme Q10 is a fat-soluble quinone that is synthesized intracellularly and participates in a variety of important cellular processes. It has vitamin-like characteristics and is structurally similar to vitamin K. Coenzyme Q10 is a vital component of the inner mitochondrial membrane.

Coenzyme Q10 is an antioxidant and cardiotonic. Some evidence suggests it may also have cytoprotective and neuroprotective qualities. An endogenous deficiency of coenzyme Q10 has been suggested in a variety of disorders, including cancer, congestive heart failure, hypertension, chronic hemodialysis, mitochondrial disease, and periodontal disease.

Coenzyme Q10 is available for oral and parenteral administration. The scope of this monograph is limited to the oral formulation; information on the parenteral form can be found in *PDR for Herbal Medicines*.

COMMON USAGE

Accepted uses: FDA-approved for use as an orphan product in the treatment of Huntington's disease and mitochondrial cytopathies.

Unproven uses: Coenzyme Q10 is used mainly for the treatment of various heart conditions, including congestive heart failure, cardiomyopathy, ischemic heart disease, and angina. Studies have shown it may benefit patients having cardiovascular surgery such as cardiac valve replacement, coronary artery bypass grafting, and repair of abdominal aortic aneurysms. Coenzyme Q10 has also been used for asthenozoospermia, central nervous system problems, and muscle disorders. Athletes sometimes take it to improve performance, but current evidence does not justify this use.

CONTRAINDICATIONS

Hypersensitivity to coenzyme Q10 or its excipients.

WARNINGS/PRECAUTIONS

Hepatic failure is a precaution for use, since the primary site of metabolism is the liver. However, coenzyme Q10 has a very low toxicity profile, and higher plasma levels seem to be well-tolerated. There have been no reports of overt hepatotoxicity with coenzyme Q10.

DRUG INTERACTIONS

HMG-CoA reductase inhibitors: Use of these drugs may inhibit the natural synthesis of coenzyme Q10. Patients who have reduced levels of coenzyme Q10 may be at risk for side effects of HMG-CoA reductase inhibitors, particularly myopathy.

Oral hypoglycemic agents and insulin: Dosage adjustment may be necessary, since coenzyme Q10 could reduce insulin requirements.

Warfarin: Concurrent use could reduce anticoagulant effectiveness; monitor the INR as necessary.

ADVERSE REACTIONS

Gastrointestinal disturbances, including nausea, epigastric discomfort, diarrhea, heartburn, and appetite suppression, are the most common adverse effects, occurring in less than 1% in large studies. Rare side effects may include skin rash, pruritus, photophobia, irritability, agitation, headache, and dizziness. Transient minor abnormalities of urinary sediment (protein, granular, and hyaline casts) were reported in patients with Parkinson's disease given doses of 400 to 800mg of coenzyme Q10 daily for 1 month. Problems resolved following discontinuation of therapy. Fatigue and increased involuntary movements were reported in patients with Huntington's chorea taking high doses.

ADMINISTRATION AND DOSAGE

For best absorption, coenzyme Q10 should be taken with food.

Adults

Angina: 150 to 600mg daily in divided doses.

Cardiac Surgery: 100mg daily for 14 days before surgery, followed by 100mg daily for 30 days postoperatively.

Congestive Heart Failure: 50 to 150mg daily in two or three divided doses

Migraine Prevention: 150mg daily.

Neurological Disease: (associated with mitochondrial ATP producing deficiency): 150mg or more daily.

Parkinson's Disease/Huntington's Disease: 800 to 1,200mg daily.

Periodontal Disease: 25mg twice daily; or topical solution consisting of 85mg/mL in soybean oil applied twice daily.

Pediatrics

General Use: 2.4 to 3.8mg/kg daily.

Pediatric Mitochondrial Encephalomyopathy: 30mg daily.

Folic Acid

EFFECTS

Folic acid is a water-soluble B vitamin that has antidepressant, antiproliferative, antiteratogenic, antihomocysteinemic, and gingival anti-inflammatory effects. The coenzymes formed from folic acid are instrumental in the following intracellular metabolisms: conversion of homocysteine to methionine, conversion of serine to glycine, synthesis of thymidylate, histidine metabolism, synthesis of purines, and utilization or generation of formate.

COMMON USAGE

Accepted uses: Prevention of neural tube defects in pregnancy; treatment of megaloblastic anemias caused by folic acid deficiency; and treatment of folic acid deficiency caused by oral contraceptive or anticonvulsant therapy.

Unproven uses: Strong evidence shows that folic acid therapy can reduce high levels of homocysteine, which has been linked to coronary heart disease. Other studies have suggested that folic acid supplementation may be helpful for atherosclerosis, colon cancer prevention, coronary heart disease, depression, gingival hyperplasia, hyperhomocysteinemia, iron deficiency or sickle-cell anemia, lung cancer prevention, methotrexate toxicity, prevention of restenosis following coronary angiography, ulcerative colitis, and vitiligo.

Weaker evidence suggests that folic acid may be of some benefit for cervical cancer prevention, aphthous ulcers, geriatric memory deficit, and the prevention of fragile x syndrome in children.

CONTRAINDICATIONS

Do not use in the presence of pernicious anemia and megaloblastic anemia caused by vitamin B_{12} deficiency.

WARNINGS/PRECAUTIONS

Folic acid doses above 0.1mg/day may obscure pernicious anemia.

Pregnancy and breastfeeding: FDA-rated as Pregnancy Category A (relatively safe) at doses below 0.8mg/day; doses higher than this are rated as Pregnancy Category C (effects unknown). It is safe to use during lactation.

DRUG INTERACTIONS

Barbiturates: May interfere with folate utilization, resulting in the need for folate supplementation.

Metformin: May interfere with the utilization of folate, resulting in increased need for folate supplementation.

Methotrexate: Interferes with the utilization of folate.

Pancreatic enzymes: Concurrent use may interfere with the absorption of folic acid. Patients taking pancreatin may require folic acid supplementation.

Phenytoin and fosphenytoin: Concurrent use may decrease phenytoin or fosphenytoin levels and increase seizure frequency. If folic acid is added to phenytoin therapy, monitor patients for decreased seizure control.

Pyrimethamine: Concurrent use may reduce the effectiveness of pyrimethamine. Folic acid should not be used as a folate supplement during pyrimethamine therapy as it is ineffective in preventing megaloblastic anemia. Leucovorin (folinic acid) may be added to pyrimethamine therapy to prevent hematologic toxicity without affecting pyrimethamine efficacy. However, the use of leucovorin may worsen leukemia.

Sulfasalazine: Concurrent use may decrease the absorption of folic acid; monitor patients for signs of deficiency.

Triamterine: Concurrent use may cause decreased utilization of dietary folate; monitor patient for signs of deficiency.

ADVERSE REACTIONS

Side effects of folic acid therapy include erythema, pruritus, urticaria, irritability, excitability, nausea, bloating, and flatulence.

A variety of central nervous system effects have been reported following 5mg of folic acid three times a day, including altered sleep patterns, vivid dreaming, irritability, excitability, and overactivity. Discontinuation of the drug usually results in rapid improvement but in some cases may require 3 weeks to resolve.

High-dose folic acid has been associated with zinc depletion. Evidence suggests that up to 5mg to 15mg daily of folic acid does not have significant adverse effects on zinc status in healthy, nonpregnant individuals.

ADMINISTRATION AND DOSAGE

Daily Dosage: Recommended dietary allowance (RDA): *Adults and adolescents 14 years and older*: 400mcg daily.

During pregnancy: 600mcg daily.

During lactation: 500mcg daily.

Infants and children 0 to 6 months: 65mcg daily, *7 to 12 months*: 80mcg daily; *1 to 3 years*: 150mcg daily; *4 to 8 years*: 200mcg daily; *9 to 13 years*: 300mcg daily.

Adults

Deficiency: Up to 1mg daily until clinical symptoms of deficiency have resolved and blood levels have returned to normal.

Anticonvulsant-induced folate deficiency: 15mg daily.

Aphthous ulcers (canker sores): treat folic acid deficiency.

Hyperhomocysteinemia: 500mcg to 5,000mcg daily.

Methotrexate toxicity: 5mg orally per week.

Oral contraceptive-induced folate deficiency: 2mg daily.

Periodontal disease: 2mg twice daily, or 5mL of 0.1% topical mouth rinse twice daily.

Prevention of birth defects: 400mcg to 4,000mcg orally daily beginning 1 month before conception.

Prevention of cerebrovascular disease: treat folic acid deficiency or hyperhomocysteinemia.

Prevention of cervical cancer: 800mcg to 1,000mcg daily.

Prevention of colorectal cancer: 1mg to 5mg daily.

Prevention of lung cancer: 10mg daily.

Prevention of neural tube defects: 0.4mg of folic acid daily. Doses from 0.5mg to 1mg daily are often administered during pregnancy. Patients with a previous history of neural tube defects during pregnancy should receive 4mg daily starting 1 month before pregnancy and throughout the first 3 months of pregnancy.

Prevention of restenosis following coronary angiography: 1mg in combination with 400mcg vitamin B_{12} and 10mg vitamin B_6 daily.

Sickle cell anemia: 1mg daily.

Ulcerative colitis: 15mg daily.

Vitiligo: 2,000mcg to 10,000mcg daily.

Pediatrics

Anticonvulsant-induced folate deficiency: 5mg daily

Folic acid deficiency: Up to 1mg daily until clinical symptoms of deficiency have resolved and blood levels have returned to normal

Gingival hyperplasia: 5mg daily

Hyperhomocysteinemia: 500mcg to 5,000mcg daily.

Glucosamine

EFFECTS

Glucosamine is an endogenous aminomonosaccharide synthesized from glucose and utilized for biosynthesis of two larger compounds—glycoproteins and glycosaminoglycans. These compounds are necessary for the construction and maintenance of virtually all connective tissues and lubricating fluids in the body. The sulfate salt of glucosamine forms half of the disaccharide subunit of keratan sulfate, which is decreased in osteoarthritis, and of hyaluronic acid, which is found in both articular cartilage and synovial fluid.

Supplemental glucosamine is generally used to reduce pain and immobility associated with osteoarthritis, especially in the knee joint. The supplements are usually derived from crab shells, although a corn source is also available. Most studies of osteoarthritis have used the sulfate form of glucosamine. Other forms include glucosamine hydrochloride and N-acetyl glucosamine.

Glucosamine is available in oral and parenteral formulations. The scope of this monograph is limited to the oral formulations. Information on the parenteral use of glucosamine can be found in *PDR for Herbal Medicine*.

COMMON USAGE

Unproven uses: Glucosamine, especially the sulfate form, is a popular treatment for pain and immobility associated with osteoarthritis. Glucosamine is classified by the European League Against Rheumatism (EULAR) as a "symptomatic slow-acting drug in osteoarthritis." This drug group is characterized by slow-onset improvement in osteoarthritis with persistent benefits after discontinuation. Whether long-term use of glucosamine can reverse the course of osteoarthritis is a theory that has yet to be investigated. Supplemental glucosamine has also been used for articular injury repair, TMJ, and cutaneous aging (wrinkles).

CONTRAINDICATIONS

Do not use in patients who have experienced hypersensitivity reactions to glucosamine.

WARNINGS/PRECAUTIONS

Allergic reactions: Glucosamine should be used with caution in patients with an allergy to shellfish and shellfish products.

Asthma: Patients with asthma may be at risk for symptom exacerbation.

Diabetes: Patients with diabetes should be cautious, since glucosamine may affect insulin sensitivity or glucose tolerance.

Pregnancy and breastfeeding: Scientific evidence for the safe use of glucosamine during pregnancy and lactation is not available.

DRUG INTERACTIONS

Antidiabetic Drugs: Glucosamine may reduce their effectiveness. Glucosamine is likely safe for patients with diabetes that is well controlled with diet only or with one or two oral antidiabetic agents (HbA$_{1c}$ less than 6.5%). In patients with higher HbA$_{1c}$ concentrations or for those requiring insulin, closely monitor blood glucose concentrations.

Doxorubicin, etoposide, and teniposide: Glucosamine may reduce their effectiveness; avoid concomitant use.

ADVERSE REACTIONS

The most commonly reported adverse effects are gastrointestinal disturbances, including nausea, dyspepsia, heartburn, vomiting, constipation, diarrhea, anorexia, and epigastric pain. Less than 1% of patients have reported edema, tachycardia, drowsiness, insomnia, headache, erythema, and pruritus.

ADMINISTRATION AND DOSAGE

Adults

Osteoarthritis: 1,500mg in single or three divided doses daily.

Pediatrics

Information on pediatric dosing is not available.

Glutamine

EFFECTS

Glutamine is a nonessential amino acid; it is the most abundant amino acid in the body. Glutamine stimulates anabolism of protein and inhibits catabolism of protein. Glutamine is essential for maintaining intestinal function, the immune response, and amino acid homeostasis. Glutamine serves as a metabolic fuel for rapidly proliferating cell lines such as enterocytes, colonocytes, fibroblasts, lymphocytes, and macrophages. The body is depleted of glutamine stores during trauma, hypercatabolism, immunodeficiency, malnutrition, or extreme stress and in these states it may be considered an essential amino acid.

Human and animal studies have shown that glutamine has antioxidant, antitumor, chemoprotective, and immunostimulatory effects.

Glutamine is available in oral, enteral, and parenteral formulations. The scope of this monograph is limited to the oral formulations. Information on the enteral and parenteral use of glutamine is available in the *PDR for Herbal Medicines*.

COMMON USAGE

Unproven uses: Glutamine is used for a wide variety of digestive disorders such as ulcers, food allergies, leaky gut syndrome, reflux disease, and symptoms of malabsorption, including diarrhea and drug-induced diarrhea. Glutamine is being used to treat environmental and multiple-chemical sensitivity and for its reported benefit in supporting Phase II liver detoxification pathways. In the practice of lifestyle and longevity medicine, glutamine is widely used to promote the release of growth hormone. Glutamine is accepted as a biomarker in determining and treating diseases of aging. In "wasting" diseases, such as cancer and AIDS, glutamine is used to support T-cell function in the immune system, to augment lean muscle mass, and to decrease cachexia. More recently, the athletic community has embraced glutamine as a muscle enhancer and recovery aid. In children

with sickle cell disease, it is being used to decrease resting energy expenditure and improve nutritional status.

CONTRAINDICATIONS

Patients with liver disease should not use glutamine. This supplement is also contraindicated for patients with any condition that puts them at risk for accumulation of nitrogenous wastes in the blood—such as Reye's syndrome or cirrhosis—since it can lead to ammonia-induced encephalopathy and coma.

Patients who have had a previous hypersensitivity reaction to glutamine should not use it.

WARNINGS/PRECAUTIONS

Pregnancy and breastfeeding: Scientific evidence for the safe use of glutamine during pregnancy and lactation is not available.

DRUG INTERACTIONS

No drug interaction data is available.

ADVERSE REACTIONS

Patients who are taking glutamine and have chronic renal failure should have their kidney function monitored. Extreme caution is also advised when adding glutamine to the total parenteral nutrition of cancer patients, since glutamine serves as the main substrate for many tumors. The most common side effects of supplemental glutamine are constipation, gastrointestinal upset, and bloating.

ADMINISTRATION AND DOSAGE

Adults

Cancer: 30g daily, usually taken in 3 divided doses

Chemoprotective: 10g daily taken in 3 divided doses, or 0.5g/kg/day

Intestinal permeability: 7g to 21g daily in single or divided doses

Short-bowel syndrome: 0.4g/kg/day to 0.63g/kg/day

Stomatitis (oral solution): 2g twice daily used as a mouthwash and then swallowed

Pediatrics

Stomatitis (oral solution): 2g twice daily used as a mouthwash and then swallowed

Sickle cell disease: 600mg/kg/day

Iron

EFFECTS

Iron is an essential trace mineral involved in the process of respiration, including oxygen and electron transport. The function and synthesis of hemoglobin, which carries most of the oxygen in the blood, is dependent on iron. Iron is also involved in the production of cytochrome oxidase, myoglobin, L-carnitine, and aconitase, all of which are involved in energy production in the body. In addition to its fundamental roles in energy production, iron is involved in DNA synthesis and may also play roles in normal brain development and immune function. Iron is involved in the synthesis of collagen and the neurotransmitters serotonin, dopamine, and norepinephrine. Iron has putative immune-enhancing, anticarcinogenic, and cognition-enhancing activities.

Iron also has oxidative effects. Iron is able to catalyze reactions that produce free radical metabolites, which may damage cell membranes, cause chromosomal mutations, or oxidize low-density lipoproteins (LDL) into more atherogenic particles. Animal studies have confirmed that atherosclerotic plaques contain a high concentration of iron, and rats given large amounts of iron have increased LDL lipid peroxidation, In human studies, atherosclerosis has been associated with increased iron levels.

Supplemental iron is administered orally or by intramuscular injection. The scope of this monograph is limited to oral iron preparations. Information on parenteral forms of iron is available in *PDR for Herbal Medicines*.

COMMON USAGE

Accepted uses: Prophylaxis and treatment of iron-deficiency anemia.

Unproven uses: Limited research suggests that supplemental iron could be helpful for reducing the frequency of breath-holding spells in children. It may also enhance cognition in children and adolescents who have a documented iron deficiency. Likewise, iron may have some favorable effects on immunity and exercise performance—but again, these benefits are most likely limited to those with acute or borderline iron deficiency. Iron supplementation has also been used for the following: Plummer-Vinson syndrome, malaria, herpes simplex outbreaks, pediatric diarrhea, intestinal helminth infection, microcephaly prophylaxis, and decreased thyroid function in individuals consuming very-low-calorie diets.

CONTRAINDICATIONS

Iron supplementation is contraindicated in patients with hemochromatosis and hemosiderosis. It is also contraindicated for treating anemias not caused by iron deficiency, such as hemolytic anemia or thalassemia, due to the risk of excess iron storage. Sustained-release dosage forms should be avoided in patients who have conditions associated with intestinal strictures.

WARNINGS/PRECAUTIONS

Toxicity: Treatment of iron-deficiency anemia must only be done under medical supervision. Iron supplements should be used with extreme caution in those with chronic liver failure, alcoholic cirrhosis, chronic alcoholism, and pancreatic insufficiency. Iron supplements can be highly toxic or lethal to small children. Those who take iron supplements should use childproof bottles and store them away from children.

Gastrointestinal irritation: Iron should be used cautiously in those with a history of gastritis, peptic ulcer disease, and gastrointestinal bleeding.

Elevated ferritin levels: Patients with elevated serum ferritin levels should generally avoid iron supplements.

Infection: Individuals with an active or suspected infection should generally avoid iron supplements.

Ischemic heart disease and cancer: A moderate increase in iron stores has been associated with an increased risk of ischemic heart disease and cancer.

Pregnancy and breastfeeding: FDA-rated as Pregnancy Category C. Pregnant and lactating women should not exceed the RDA unless their physician recommends it.

DRUG INTERACTIONS

Antacids: Concomitant use of aluminum- or magnesium-containing antacids may decrease the absorption of iron.

Bisphosphonates (e.g., alendronate, etidronate, risedronate): Concomitant use with ferrous (II) iron supplements may decrease the absorption of bisphosphonates.

H_2 blockers (e.g., cimetidine, famotidine, nizatidine, ranitidine): Concomitant use may suppress the absorption of carbonyl iron.

Levodopa: Concomitant use with iron may reduce the absorption of levodopa.

Levothyroxine: Concomitant use with iron may decrease the absorption of levothyroxine.

Penicillamine: Concomitant use with iron may decrease the absorption of penicillamine.

Proton pump inhibitors (e.g., lansoprazole, omeprazole, pantoprazole, rabeprazole): Concomitant use may suppress the absorption of carbonyl iron.

Quinolones (e.g., ciprofloxacin, gatifloxacin, levofloxacin, lomefloxacin, moxifloxacin, norfloxacin, ofloxacin, sparfloxacin, trovafloxacin): Concomitant use may decrease the absorption of both the quinolone and iron supplement.

Tetracyclines (e.g., doxycycline, minocycline, tetracycline): Concomitant use may decrease the absorption of both the tetracycline and iron supplement.

SUPPLEMENT INTERACTIONS

Beta-carotene: Concomitant use may enhance the absorption of iron.

Calcium carbonate: Concomitant use may decrease the absorption of iron.

Copper: Concomitant use with iron supplements may decrease the copper status of tissues.

Inositol hexaphosphate: Concomitant use may decrease the absorption of iron.

L-cysteine: Concomitant use may increase the absorption of iron.

Magnesium: Concomitant use may decrease the absorption of iron.

N-Acetyl-L-Cysteine: Concomitant use may increase the absorption of iron.

Tocotrienols: Concomitant use of iron and tocotrienols, which are typically used in their nonesterified forms, may cause oxidation of tocotrienols.

Vanadium: Concomitant use may decrease the absorption of iron.

Vitamin C: Concomitant use may enhance the absorption of iron.

Vitamin E (e.g., alpha-tocopherol, gamma-tocopherol, mixed tocopherols): Concomitant use of nonesterified tocopherols and iron may cause oxidation of the tocopherols.

Zinc: Concomitant use may decrease the absorption of iron.

FOOD INTERACTIONS

Caffeine (e.g., coffee): Concomitant use may decrease the absorption of iron.

Cysteine-containing proteins (e.g., meat): Concomitant use may increase the absorption of iron.

Dairy foods and eggs: Concomitant use may decrease the absorption of iron.

Oxalic Acid (e.g., spinach, sweet potatoes, rhubarb, beans): Concomitant use may decrease the absorption of iron.

Phytic acid (e.g., unleavened bread, raw beans, seeds, nuts and grains, soy isolates): Concomitant use may decrease the absorption of iron.

Teas and tannin-containing herbs: Concomitant use may cause decrease the absorption of iron.

ADVERSE REACTIONS

The most common side effects of iron supplements are gastrointestinal problems, including nausea, vomiting, bloating, abdominal discomfort, black stools, diarrhea, constipation, and anorexia.

Enteric-coated iron preparations may prevent some of the gastro-intestinal complaints associated with iron therapy. Temporary staining of teeth may occur from iron-containing liquids.

ADMINISTRATION AND DOSAGE

Daily Dosage: Recommended Dietary Allowance (RDA):

Adult males: *14 to 18 years*: 11mg daily; *19 years and older*: 8mg daily

Adult females: *14 to 18 years*: 15mg daily; *19 to 50 years*: 18mg daily; *51 years and older*: 8mg daily.

During pregnancy (all ages): 27mg daily.

During lactation: *14 to 18 years*: 10mg daily; *19 to 50 years*: 9mg daily.

Infants and children: *0 to 6 months*: 0.27mg daily; *7 to 12months*: 11mg daily; *1 to 3 years*: 7mg daily; *4 to 8 years*: 10mg daily; *9 to 13 years*: 8mg daily.

The following lists the elemental iron content of various forms:

Iron Salt	% Iron
Ferrous fumarate	33
Ferrous gluconate	11.6
Ferrous sulfate	20
Ferrous sulfate, anhydrous	30

Adults

Deficiency: immediate-release dosage forms: 2mg/kg to 3 mg/kg daily in 3 divided doses; sustained-release dosage forms: 50mg to 100mg daily.

Iron deficiency in pregnancy: 60mg to 100mg daily; *prevention of*: 40mg to 100mg daily

Decreased thyroid function during very-low-calorie diets: 9mg/d or more to bring total iron intake to 1.5 times the RDA.

Impaired athletic performance: Treat only confirmed iron deficiency.

Inflammatory bowel disease: Treat only confirmed iron deficiency.

Plummer-Vinson Syndrome: 2mg/kg to 3mg/kg daily.

Pediatrics

Adolescent girls with low ferritin: 105mg to 260mg daily.

Breath-holding syndrome (ferrous sulfate solution): 5mg/kg daily.

Cognitive function: 105mg to 260mg daily.

Iron-deficiency anemia: *Premature infants*: 2mg to 4mg/kg/d in 2 to 4 divided doses, up to a maximum of 15mg/d; *Children*: 3mg to 6mg/kg/d in 1 to 3 divided doses.

Lutein

EFFECTS

Lutein is an antioxidant that has immunostimulant and photoprotectant properties. It is a naturally occurring carotenoid used to improve eye health, especially in people with age-related macular degeneration (AMD) and cataracts. Studies show that the retina selectively accumulates two carotenoids, lutein and its chemical cousin zeaxanthin. Within the central macula, zeaxanthin is the dominant component (up to 75%), whereas in the peripheral retina, lutein predominates (greater than 67%). The macular concentration of lutein and zeaxanthin is so high that they are visible as a dark yellow spot called the macular pigment. Because these carotenoids are powerful antioxidants and absorb blue light, researchers have hypothesized that they protect the retina. While both are abundant in green and yellow fruits and vegetables, lutein is the carotenoid most often used as a supplement.

Dietary intake of lutein and zeaxanthin is estimated at 1mg to 3mg daily. Sources include spinach, collard greens, corn, kiwifruit, zucchini, pumpkin, squash, peas, cucumbers, green peppers, and egg yolks.

COMMON USAGE

Unproven uses: Increased consumption of lutein may prevent, delay, or modify the course of age-related macular degeneration, although conclusive evidence is not available. Lutein has also been used to help prevent or treat various cancers, including breast, ovarian, endometrial, lung, and prostate. Some advocates have promoted lutein as a general anti-aging supplement.

CONTRAINDICATIONS

No data available.

WARNINGS/PRECAUTIONS

No data available.

DRUG INTERACTIONS

No data available.

ADVERSE REACTIONS

No data available.

ADMINISTRATION AND DOSAGE

Adults

Cancer Prevention: ≥5921mcg daily from dietary sources

Macular degeneration prevention: 10mg daily

Lysine

EFFECTS

Lysine is an essential amino acid involved in many biological processes, including receptor affinity, protease-cleavage points, retention of endoplasmic reticulum, nuclear structure and function, muscle elasticity, and chelation of heavy metals. Like other amino acids, the metabolism of free lysine follows two principal paths: protein synthesis and oxidative catabolism. It is required for biosynthesis of such substances as carnitine, collagen, and elastin. Lysine appears to have antiviral, anti-osteoporotic, cardiovascular, and lipid-lowering effects, although more controlled human studies are needed.

The terms L-lysine and lysine are used interchangeably. The D-stereoisomer (D-lysine) is not biologically active.

COMMON USAGE

Unproven uses: The most common use of supplemental lysine is for preventing and treating episodes of herpes simplex virus. Lysine has been used in conjunction with calcium to prevent and treat osteoporosis. It has also been used for treating pain, aphthous ulcers, migraine attacks, rheumatoid arthritis, and opiate withdrawal. Many "body-building" formulations contain lysine to aid in muscle repair.

CONTRAINDICATIONS

Patients who have kidney or liver disease should not use lysine.

WARNINGS/PRECAUTIONS

Hypercholesterolemia: Patients with hypercholesterolemia should be aware that supplemental lysine has been linked to increased cholesterol levels in animal studies. However, other studies have shown lysine can also decrease cholesterol levels.

DRUG INTERACTIONS

Aminoglycoside antibiotics (eg, gentamicin, neomycin, streptomycin): Concurrent use may increase the risk of nephrotoxicity.

ADVERSE REACTIONS

Renal dysfunction, including Fanconi's syndrome and renal failure, has been reported.

ADMINISTRATION AND DOSAGE

Adults

Herpes simplex virus: 1g to 3g daily, divided and taken with meals.

Migraine headache: Oral sachet of lysine acetylsalicylate 1620mg plus metoclopramide 10mg

Osteoporosis prophylaxis: 400mg to 800mg daily. Take with calcium.

Pediatrics

Hyperargininemia: 250mg/kg/day. Take with ornithine 100mg/kg/day.

Magnesium

EFFECTS

Magnesium is an essential mineral said to have anti-osteoporotic, anti-arrhythmic, antihypertensive, glucose regulatory, and bronchodilating effects. It is an electrolyte, a nutrient, and a mineral. Magnesium is important as a cofactor in many enzymatic reactions in the body. There are at least 300 enzymes that are dependent upon magnesium for normal functioning. Its effects on lipoprotein lipase play an important role in reducing serum cholesterol. Magnesium is necessary for maintaining serum potassium and calcium levels due to its effect on the renal tubule. In the heart, magnesium acts as a calcium channel blocker. It also activates sodium-potassium ATPase in the cell membrane to promote resting.

Magnesium is available for oral, parenteral, and topical administration. The scope of this discussion will be limited to the oral and topical formulations.

COMMON USAGE

Accepted uses: Magnesium sulfate (Epsom salt) is approved as a laxative for the temporary relief of constipation. Magnesium sulfate is used for replacement therapy for hypomagnesemia.

Unproven uses: Magnesium is used in pregnant women to treat leg cramps and to control and prevent seizures in pre-eclampsia. Magnesium is used for migraine, bone resorption, diabetes, hypertension, arrhythmias, PMS, nephrolithiasis, and spasms. Magnesium may also be effective in treating certain cardiac arrhythmias, in asthma that is unresponsive to other treatments, during alcohol withdrawal, and for ischemic heart disease. Magnesium therapy has inconsistent effects on hypertension, but should be considered in those at risk of deficiency, including patients taking magnesium-depleting medications.

CONTRAINDICATIONS

Magnesium is not to be used in the presence of heart block, severe renal disease, or toxemia in the 2 hours preceding delivery.

WARNINGS/PRECAUTIONS

Administration of magnesium, especially in patients with renal impairment, may lead to loss of deep tendon reflexes, hypoten-sion, confusion, respiratory paralysis, cardiac arrhythmias, or cardiac arrest. Increased bleeding time has been reported. Monitor to avoid magnesium toxicity.

Pregnancy and breastfeeding: Rickets in the newborn may result from prolonged magnesium sulfate administration in the second trimester of pregnancy. It is safe to use while breastfeeding.

DRUG INTERACTIONS

Aminoglycosides: Concomitant use with magnesium may precipitate neuromuscular weakness and possibly paralysis.

Calcium channel blockers: Concurrent use may enhance hypotensive effects.

Fluoroquinolones: Concomitant use with magnesium may decrease absorption and effectiveness. Fluoroquinolones should be administered at least 4 hours before magnesium or any product containing magnesium.

Labetalol: Concomitant use with magnesium may cause bradycardia and reduced cardiac output.

Levomethadyl: Concomitant use with magnesium may precipitate QT prolongation.

Neuromuscular blockers: Concomitant use with magnesium may enhance neuromuscular blocking effects.

Tetracycline: Magnesium decreases the absorption of tetracycline.

ADVERSE REACTIONS

Side effects include blurred vision, photophobia, diarrhea, hypermagnesemia, hypotension, increased bleeding times, neuromuscular blockade (in higher doses), and vasodilation.

ADMINISTRATION AND DOSAGE

Daily Dosage: Recommended Dietary Allowance:

Males—14 to 18 years: 410mg/day; *19 to 30 years*: 400mg/day; *31+ years*: 420mg/day. *Females—14 to 18 years*: 360mg/day; *19 to 30 years*: 310mg/day; *31+ years*: 320mg/day

During pregnancy—14 to 18 years: 400mg/day; *19 to 30 years*: 350mg/day; *31 years and over*: 360mg/day

During lactation: 14 to 18 years: 360mg/day; *19 to 30 years*: 310mg/day; *31+ years*: 320mg/day.

Children—1 to 3 years: 80mg/day; *4 to 8 years*: 130mg/day; *9-13 years*: 240mg/day

There is insufficient data to establish a RDA for infants. The adequate intake (AI) for infants is 30mg/day for infants 0 to 6 months and 75mg/day for infants 7 to 12 months.

Adults

Abdominal and perineal incision wound healing: (magnesium hydroxide ointment, topical) Apply twice daily along with zinc chloride spray for 7 days

Congestive heart failure: (enteric-coated magnesium chloride) 3,204mg/d in divided doses (equal to 15.8mmol elemental Mg)

Detrusor instability: (magnesium hydroxide) 350mg for 4 weeks; double after 2 weeks if there is an unsatisfactory response

Diabetes mellitus type 2: 15.8mmol/d to 41.4mmol/d

Dietary supplementation: 54mg to 483mg daily in divided doses

Dyslipidemia: (enteric-coated magnesium chloride) Studies have used a mean dose of 17.92mmol for a mean duration of 118 days; (magnesium oxide) 15mmol/d for 3 months.

Hypertension: 360mg/d to 600mg/d

Migraine prophylaxis: 360mg/d to 600mg/d

Mitral valve prolapse: (magnesium carbonate capsules) During the first week of treatment, 21 mmol/d is used; then 14mmol/d is used during Weeks 2 to 5.

Nephrolithiasis prophylaxis: (magnesium hydroxide) 400mg/d to 500mg/d.

Osteoporosis: 250mg taken at bedtime on an empty stomach, increased to 250mg three times daily for 6 months, followed by 250mg daily for 18 months.

Premenstrual syndrome: 200mg/dto 360mg/d.

Pediatrics

Deficiency: The oral dose of magnesium sulfate to treat hypomagnesemia in children is 100mg/d to 200mg/kg four times daily.

Dietary supplementation: 3mg/kg to 6mg/kg body weight per day in divided doses three to four times daily, up to a maximum of 400mg daily.

Laxative: The recommended dose of magnesium citrate for children 2 to 5 years of age is 2.7g to 6.25g daily as a single dose or as divided doses. For children 6 to 11 years of age, the dose is 5.5g to 12.5g daily in a single dose or as divided doses.

Melatonin

EFFECTS

Melatonin (N-acetyl-5-methoxytryptamine) is a neurohormone produced by pinealocytes in the pineal gland during the dark hours of the day-night cycle. Serum levels of melatonin are very low during most of the day, and it has been labeled the "hormone of darkness." The hormone serves as a messenger to the neuroendocrine system regarding environmental conditions (especially the photoperiod). Putative functions of endogenous melatonin in this regard include regulation of sleep cycles, hormonal rhythms, and body temperature. Melatonin is involved in the induction of sleep, may play a role in the internal synchronization of the mammalian circadian system, and may serve as a marker of the "biologic clock." In addition, melatonin is thought to have antioxidant and immunomodulator effects.

Melatonin is administered by the oral, transdermal, transmucosal, and parenteral route. The scope of this discussion is limited the oral formulation.

COMMON USAGE

Accepted uses: Melatonin is FDA-approved as an orphan drug for the treatment of sleep disorders in blind individuals with no light perception.

Unproven uses: Melatonin is commonly used as a sleep aid. Evidence suggests that it is effective for the short-term treatment of delayed sleep phase syndrome. However, available data indicate that it is not effective for treating most primary or secondary sleep disorders. There is no evidence to support the claims that melatonin is effective for alleviating the sleep disturbance aspect of jet lag or shift-work disorder.

Melatonin has been used in the treatment of a variety of solid tumors (in combination with interleukin-2), and to improve thrombocytopenia and other toxicities induced by cancer chemotherapy and from other conditions. In addition, melatonin is used for the treatment of cluster headaches and tinnitus.

CONTRAINDICATIONS

Hypersensitivity to melatonin or its excipients.

WARNINGS/PRECAUTIONS

Depressive symptoms: Melatonin can exacerbate dysphoria in depressed patients and cause mood swings. It can cause depressive symptoms when used with interleukin-2 in cancer therapy.

Liver disease: Increased risk of liver dysfunction.

History of neurological disorders: Increased risk of CNS effects.

Seizures: Increased risk of seizures.

DRUG INTERACTIONS

Fluvoxamine: Increased risk of CNS depression with concomitant use. Patients should be monitored for signs of CNS depression and appropriate dosage adjustments should be made.

Nifedipine: Melatonin may reduce the effectiveness of nifedipine. Close monitoring of blood pressure is advised.

Warfarin: Increased risk of bleeding with concomitant use. If both agents are taken together, monitor prothrombin time, INR, and signs and symptoms of excessive bleeding.

ADVERSE REACTIONS

Adverse effects of commercially available melatonin have generally been minimal. Drowsiness, fatigue, headache, confusion, gastrointestinal complaints, and reduced body temperature have been reported. Rarely, tachycardia, seizures, acute psychotic reactions, autoimmune hepatitis, and pruritus have been reported.

ADMINISTRATION AND DOSAGE

Adults

Cancer as combination therapy: 40mg or 50mg oral tablets given once daily at night, initiated 7 days prior to interleukin-2 and continued throughout the cycle.

Chronic insomnia: 1mg to 10mg orally daily

Delayed sleep phase syndrome: 5mg orally daily

Jet lag: 5mg orally daily for 3 days prior to departure, then 5mg for 4 additional days

Sleep disorders: 5mg at the usual bedtime

Pediatrics

Congenital sleep disorder: 2.5mg oral tablet

Neurological disability: 0.5mg to 10mg oral tablet at bedtime

Sleep-wake cycle disorder: An average dose of 5.7mg, administered as a controlled-release tablet, was used in children ages 4 to 21 years, with neurodevelopmental disabilities. Doses ranged from 2mg to 12mg.

Omega-3 Fatty Acids

EFFECTS

Eicosapentaenic acid (EPA) and docosahexaenoic acid (DHA) are nonessential omega-3 fatty acids that are synthesized in the body. The omega-3 fatty acids have anticoagulant and anti-inflammatory effects. They also lower cholesterol and triglyceride levels, and reduce blood pressure.

Omega-3 fatty acids are abundant in oily fish such as salmon, tuna, and mackerel. For this reason, they are sometimes referred to as "omega-3 fish oils" or simply "fish oil". Linoleic acid is a plant-derived omega-3 fatty acid. The proven health benefits of the omega-3 fish oils have not been demonstrated in studies of linoleic acid. For the purposes of this discussion, the term "omega-3 fatty acids" refers to the omega-3 fish oils, EPA and DHA.

COMMON USAGE

Accepted uses: The FDA has acknowledged the cardiovascular benefits of omega-3 fatty acids by granting a "qualified health claim" for foods and supplements containing fish oil. The claim states, "Supportive but not conclusive research shows that consumption of EPA and DHA omega-3 fatty acids may reduce the risk of coronary heart disease."

Unproven uses: A review of available data on omega-3 fatty acids concluded that they have mixed effects on people with inflammatory bowel disease, kidney disease, and osteoporosis and no effect on people with arthritis. Data are inconclusive regarding the effect of omega-3 fatty acids on adults and children who have asthma.

In addition, omega-3 fatty acids have also been used in the following conditions: aggression, Alzheimer's disease, atopic dermatitis, cachexia, cancer, cyclosporine protectant, dementia, dermatitis, gestation prolongation, gingivitis, pediatric growth and development, hyperlipidemia, hypertension, inflammation, lupus erythematosus, osteoporosis, persistent antiphospholipid syndrome, platelet aggregation inhibition, psoriasis, respiratory illness, rheumatoid arthritis, and stroke.

CONTRAINDICATIONS

Hypersensitivity to EPA, DHA, or fish oils.

WARNINGS/PRECAUTIONS

Bleeding disorders: There is an increased risk of bleeding with high doses.

Diabetics: Omega-3 fatty acids may increase blood glucose levels, decrease glucose tolerance, and decrease plasma insulin levels.

Pregnancy and breastfeeding: EPA and DHA are safe at normal doses during pregnancy and are safe for maternal use during lactation.

DRUG INTERACTIONS

Anticoagulants: Increased risk of bleeding.

ADVERSE REACTIONS

Side effects include abdominal pain, bloating, diarrhea, fatigue, gas, increased renal clearance, nausea, oxidative damage in large doses, skin irritation, somnolence, thrombocytopenia, and vitamin toxicity.

ADMINISTRATION AND DOSAGE

The FDA recommends that daily consumption of fish oils be limited to 2g per day from dietary supplements and 3g per day from food sources.

DHA

Adults

Cancer: 4.1g/day of EPA and 3.6g/day of DHA

Coronary artery restenosis: 4.5g EPA and DHA daily, or 3g to 7g fish oils daily

Dementia: 0.72g DHA daily

Hyperlipidemia: 2.2g daily combined with EPA

Hypertension: 1.8 to 2.8g daily combined with EPA

Inflammatory bowel disease: 1.8g to 2.6g daily combined with EPA

Platelet aggregation inhibition: 2790mg EPA plus 1698mg DHA daily

Rheumatoid arthritis: 1.8g DHA daily

Pediatrics

Deficiency: 200 to 300mg daily

EPA

Adults

Cancer: 4.1g/day of EPA and 3.6g/day of DHA

Colitis: 2.7g to 3.2g daily

Coronary artery restenosis: 2g to 11g daily

Hyperlipidemia: 1.8g to 18g daily

Hypertension: 1g to 16g daily

Platelet aggregation inhibition: 2g to 18g daily

Psoriasis: 9g to 18g daily; or 25mL to 80mL of fish oils daily

Rheumatoid arthritis: 2.7g daily

Pediatrics

Hypertriglyceridemia: 3g to 8g fish oils daily

Potassium

EFFECTS

Potassium is an electrolyte that plays a role in numerous cellular, neurologic, and metabolic processes. It maintains intracellular and extracellular fluid volume. It also blunts the hypertensive response to excess sodium intake. Potassium plays a role in cardiac, skeletal, and smooth muscle contraction; energy production; nerve impulse transmission; and nucleic acid synthesis. Potassium may have a protective effect against cardiovascular disease, hypertension, strokes and possibly other degenerative diseases as well.

Potassium is available for oral and intravenous administration. The intravenous use of potassium is beyond the scope of this discussion.

COMMON USAGE

Accepted uses: Potassium is FDA-approved for the prevention and treatment of hypokalemia.

Unproven uses: Arrhythmias, arthritis, bone turnover, hypercalciuria, fasting hyperinsulinemia, hypertension, malnutrition, myocardial infarction, nephrolithiasis, premenstrual syndrome, stroke, cardiac surgery

CONTRAINDICATIONS

Potassium supplementation is contraindicated in patients who are experiencing acute dehydration or heat cramps. It should not be used in patients who have adynamia episodica hereditaria. Patients who have hyperkalemia, severe renal impairment, or untreated Addison's disease should not receive potassium supplementation.

WARNINGS/PRECAUTIONS

Pregnancy and breastfeeding: Pregnant women and nursing mothers should avoid potassium supplements unless they are prescribed by their physicians.

Renal disease, diabetes: Patients with chronic renal insufficiency and diabetes are at increased risk of hyperkalemia.

DRUG INTERACTIONS

Angiotensin converting enzyme (ACE) inhibitors (e.g., benazepril, captopril, enalapril, fosinopril, lisinopril, moexipril, perindopril, quinapril, ramipril, trandolapril): Increased risk of hyperkalemia.

Angiotensin receptor blockers: Increased risk of hyperkalemia.

Potassium-sparing diuretics (amiloride, triamterene, spironolactone): Increased risk of hyperkalemia.

Indomethacin: Potential for hyperkalemia, especially if the patient has underlying renal dysfunction.

HERBAL INTERACTIONS

Dandelion: Concurrent use may result in hyperkalemia due to the high potassium content of dandelion leaves and roots. Monitor serum potassium levels if the two agents are used together.

Gossypol: Gossypol may cause hypokalemia unresponsive to potassium supplementation. Monitoring of serum potassium levels is recommended if the two agents are used together.

Licorice: Hypokalemia and paralysis may result. Avoid concurrent use of licorice and potassium supplements.

ADVERSE REACTIONS

The most common adverse reactions of potassium supplements are gastrointestinal and include abdominal discomfort, diarrhea, flatulence, nausea, and vomiting. Rashes are occasionally reported. ECG changes may occur.

ADMINISTRATION AND DOSAGE

Potassium supplements are available as potassium aspartate, potassium bicarbonate, potassium chloride, potassium citrate, potassium gluconate, and potassium orotate. One milliequivalent (mEq) or millimole (mmol) of potassium is equal to 39.09 milligrams (mg).

Daily Dosage:

Because of the risks associated with hyperkalemia, potassium supplementation should be done under medical supervision. The recommended adequate intake (AI) of potassium from dietary sources is as follows:

Adults (19 years and older): 4.7g/day; *during pregnancy*: 4.7g/day; *during lactation*: 5.1g/day

Children 0 to 6 months: 0.4g/day; *7 to 12 months*: 0.7g/day; *1 to 3 years*: 3.0g/day; *4 to 8 years*: 3.8g/day; *9 to 13 years*: 4.5g/day.

Adults

Deficiency: Doses are individualized and typically begin with 40mEq to 100mEq/day, with serum level monitoring

Pediatrics

Deficiency: Doses are individualized and begin with 3mEq to 5mEq/kg/day, in divided doses, with serum level monitoring

Probiotics

EFFECTS

Lactobacillus products are often called probiotics, translated as "for life," a popular term used to refer to bacteria in the intestine considered beneficial to health. At least 400 different species of microflora colonize the human gastrointestinal tract. The most important commercially available lactobacillus species are *L acidophilus* and *L casei* GG. Other lactobaccilli inhabiting the human gastrointestinal (GI) tract include *L brevis*, *L cellobiosus*, *L fermentum*, *L leichmannii*, *L plantarum*, and *L salivaroes*. As the intestinal flora is intimately involved in the host's nutritional status and affects immune system function, cholesterol metabolism, carcinogenesis, toxin load, and aging, lactobacillus supplementation is often used to promote overall good health.

Possible mechanisms for the effective action of lactobacilli in the treatment of various GI tract pathologies include replacement of pathogenic organisms in the GI tract by lactobacilli, elicitation of an immune response, lowering of fecal pH, and interfering with the ability of pathogenic bacteria to adhere to intestinal mucosal cells.

Commercially available lactobacillus products are designed to be taken orally with the intent to colonize the intestine and establish a balanced ecosystem. It has been proposed that lactobacilli must possess properties including adhesion, competitive exclusion, and inhibitor production to colonize a mucosal surface.

COMMON USAGE

Unproven uses: Lactobacilli are used primarily for diarrhea. Other uses include treatment of irritable bowel syndrome, urinary tract infection, vaginal candidiasis, and bacterial vaginosis.

CONTRAINDICATIONS

Lactobacillus is contraindicated in patients who have a hypersensitivity to lactose or milk.

WARNINGS/PRECAUTIONS

Infants and small children: Over-the-counter commercial preparations are not to be used in children under the age of 3 unless directed by a physician.

Liver disease: Stupor with EEG-slowing has been reported with high oral doses in patients with hepatic encephalopathy.

DRUG INTERACTIONS

Data are not available.

ADVERSE REACTIONS

Burping, diarrhea, flatulence, hiccups, increased phlegm production, rash, and vomiting have been reported infrequently with oral administration. Disagreeable sensation and burning is possible with vaginal formulations.

ADMINISTRATION AND DOSAGE

Adults

Radiation-induced diarrhea: Lactobacillus rhamnosus (Antibiophilus®) 1.5×10^9 colony-forming units three times daily for up to one week.

Uncomplicated diarrhea: 1 to 2 billion viable cells of *L acidophilus* or other Lactobacillus species daily.

Pediatrics

Diarrhea in undernourished children: Lactobacillus rhamnosus: GG 37 billion organisms daily six days per week up to 15 months.

Infantile diarrhea: Lactobacillus reuteri: 10^{10} CFU daily for up to 5 days or Lactobacillus strain GG 5×10^9 CFU daily for up to 5 days, under doctor's supervision.

Quercetin

EFFECTS

Quercetin is a bioflavinoid abundant in fruits and vegetables. It may have antioxidant, antineoplastic, anti-inflammatory, and antiviral activity. As an anticancer agent, quercetin interrupts cell cycles, ATPase activity, signal transduction, and phosphorylation. Some activity had been found against viral reverse transcriptases.

Quercetin has been shown to inhibit platelet aggregation and thrombus formation. It has also been shown to stabilize the membranes of mast cells and basophils, thereby inhibiting histamine release. It has also demonstrated activity as a leukotriene inhibitor.

Quercetin is available for oral and intravenous administration. The scope of this discussion will be limited to the oral formulations.

COMMON USAGE

Unproven uses: Quercetin may protect against the development of cardiovascular disease and alleviate the symptoms of prostatitis. It is used for the treatment of acute and chronic asthma symptoms, inflammation, and cancer.

CONTRAINDICATIONS

Hypersensitivity to quercetin.

WARNINGS/PRECAUTIONS

Nephrotoxicity has been a dose-limiting side effect of quercetin administration in humans.

DRUG INTERACTIONS

Cyclosporine: Concomitant use may reduce cyclosporine effectiveness; monitor cyclosporine levels.

Digoxin: Concomitant use may increase the risk of digoxin toxicity.

Fluoroquinolones: Concomitant use may reduce the effectiveness of this antibiotic class.

ADVERSE REACTIONS

Oral quercetin is well tolerated. Pain, flushing, dyspnea, and emesis have been reported after intravenous injection.

ADMINISTRATION AND DOSAGE

Daily dosage: 400mg to 500mg orally three times daily is recommended by practitioners of natural medicine. If the water-soluble quercetin chalcone is used, the dose is reduced to about 250mg three times daily.

Adults

Acute allergic symptoms: 2g every two hours for a maximum of two days.

Chronic allergies: 2g daily

Prostatitis: 500mg twice daily

SAMe

EFFECTS

S-Adenosylmethionine (SAMe) is a naturally occurring substance present in virtually all body tissues and fluids. SAMe is produced in the body from the amino acid methionine and adenosine triphosphate. It serves as a source of methyl groups in numerous biochemical reactions involving the synthesis, activation, and metabolism of hormones, proteins, catecholamines, nucleic acids, and phospholipids. Release of methyl groups also promotes the formation of glutathione, the chief cellular antioxidant, thereby favoring detoxification processes. SAMe is closely linked with the metabolism of folate and vitamin B12, which accounts for its ability to lower excessive homocysteine serum concentrations resulting from a deficiency of one or both of these nutrients. SAMe is postulated to increase the turnover of the neurotransmitters dopamine and serotonin in the central nervous system. It has been shown to increase the levels of the serotonin metabolite 5-hydroxyindoleacetic acid in the cerebrospinal fluid.

SAMe has antidepressant action. SAMe promotes bile flow and may relieve cholestasis. It is claimed that SAMe may increase the detoxification and elimination of pharmaceuticals from the body. There is also evidence that SAMe may lessen the severity of chronic liver disease and, in animal studies, prevent liver cancer.

COMMON USAGE

Unproven uses: The clinical application of SAMe centers on the treatment of depression, pain disorders such as osteoarthritis, and liver conditions such as cholestasis.

CONTRAINDICATIONS

Hypersensitivity to SAMe.

WARNINGS/PRECAUTIONS

Bipolar disorder: Strict medical supervision is warranted when SAMe is used in individuals with bipolar disorder.

Pregnancy and breastfeeding: Data are not available.

DRUG INTERACTIONS

Tricyclic antidepressants (e.g., amitriptyline, amoxapine, clomipramine, desipramine, doxepin, imipramine, nortriptyline): Concurrent use of SAMe and tricyclic antidepressants may result in an increased risk of serotonin syndrome. If SAMe and a tricyclic antidepressant are used together, use low doses of each and titrate upward slowly, while monitoring closely for early signs of serotonin syndrome such as increasing anxiety, confusion, and disorientation.

ADVERSE REACTIONS

Reported side effects are rare and include anxiety, headache, urinary frequency, pruritus, nausea, and diarrhea.

ADMINISTRATION AND DOSAGE

Tablets containing 768mg of sulfo-adenosyl-L-methionine (SAMe) sulfate-p-toluene sulfonate are equivalent to 400mg of SAMe.

Adults

Arthritis: 600mg to 800mg daily. Dosage may be reduced to 400mg, depending on response.

Depression: 200mg to 1600mg orally daily in the form of enteric-coated tablets; dosage often is graduated in increments of 200mg.

Fibromyalgia: 600mg or 800mg daily. Dosage may be reduced to 400mg daily depending on response.

Liver toxicity, estrogen-related: In one study, women treated for estrogen-related liver toxicity received 800mg of SAMe daily by the oral route. In general, the minimum recommended daily dose by mouth is 1600mg but no dose-finding studies have been done in patients with liver disease. Patients with less well-compensated disease may require larger doses.

Mood disorders, mild: Standard dosing regimens are not available. However, an open-label study (n = 192) demonstrated improved mild mood disorders in subjects treated with ademetionine (SAMe) 100mg orally two times a day for two months.

Selenium

EFFECTS

Selenium is a trace mineral with antioxidant properties. Selenium is a component of the cytosolic enzyme Se-dependent glutathione peroxidase (SeGSHpx), which reduces hydrogen peroxide and thereby prevents initiation of lipid peroxidation. In platelets, SeGSHpx is required for the conversion of HPETE (L-12-hydroperoxy-5,8,14-eicosatetraenoic acid) to prostacyclin. Low SeGSHpx results in an imbalance of prostacyclin and thromboxanes, which, in cell and tissue cultures, leads to platelet aggregation and vasoconstriction. Selenium supplementation in humans has led to increased bleeding times.

COMMON USAGE

Accepted uses: Trace mineral.

Unproven uses: Selenium is often used in combination with other antioxidants as a tool in the prevention of degenerative diseases, such as cancer and cardiovascular disease. No coronary disease risk intervention studies with selenium have been done, though certain cardiomyopathies appear to be related to selenium deficiency and preliminary evidence exists of post-myocardial infarction protection.

Antioxidant therapy is also considered in other chronic inflammatory or degenerative diseases, such as arthritis. Only rheumatoid arthritis has been studied, with mixed results, suggesting only milder, early disease responds to selenium supplementation.

Studies concluded beneficial effects of selenium supplementation in intrinsic asthma, bronchopneumonia prevention in burn patients, erysipelas prevention in mastectomy patients, male infertility, and possibly myocardial infarction. Uncontrolled reports of success using selenium to prevent Kaschin-Beck osteoarthropathy and viral hepatitis in Chinese populations have been documented.

CONTRAINDICATIONS

Selenium hypersensitivity

WARNINGS/PRECAUTIONS

Pregnancy and breastfeeding: Selenium is safe to use during pregnancy and lactation.

Toxicity: High blood levels of selenium can lead to selenosis. Symptoms include fatigue, garlic breath odor, gastrointestinal upset, hair loss, irritability, mild nerve damage, and white blotchy nails.

DRUG INTERACTIONS

Data are not available.

ADVERSE REACTIONS

Side effects include abdominal pain and cramps, diarrhea, fatigue, garlicky breath, irritability, nail and hair changes, nausea, and vomiting

ADMINISTRATION AND DOSAGE

Many forms of selenium are available and include: selenium selenite, selenomethionine, and selenium-enriched yeast. Organically bound forms may have a slight advantage.

Daily dosage: Recommended Dietary Allowance:

Adults 19 years and over: 55mcg daily; *during pregnancy:* 60 mcg daily; *during lactation:* 70mcg daily.

Children: 1 to 3 years: 20mcg daily; *4 to 8 years:* 30mcg daily; *9 to 13 years:* 40mcg daily; *14 to 18 years:* 55mcg daily.

Daily dosage: Adequate intake (AI): *Infants: 0 to 6 months:* 15mcg daily; *7 to 12 months:* 20mcg daily.

Adults

Asthma: 100mcg daily

Cancer prevention: 200mcg daily

Erysipelas infection: 300mg to 1000mg daily as selenium selenite

HIV: 80mcg daily

Male infertility: 100mcg daily

Myocardial infarction: 100mcg daily

Rheumatoid arthritis: 200mcg daily

Vitamin A

EFFECTS

Vitamin A is a fat-soluble vitamin required for growth and bone development, vision, reproduction, and for differentiation and maintenance of epithelial tissue. The biologically active forms of vitamin A are retinol, retinal, and retinoic acid. Retinyl esters, or fatty acid esters of retinol, are the storage form of vitamin A in the body. Beta-carotene is a precursor to vitamin A.

Retinol is required as a cofactor in the glycosylation of glycoproteins. Vitamin A may enhance the function of the immune system, and some evidence indicates that it affords protection against cancer. Vitamin A may also affect membrane systems such as the mitochondria and lysosomes; however, further research is necessary to confirm this finding.

Retinol is the parent compound of vitamin A, and the form that is transported within the body. Retinol is released from the liver and is bound to a serum retinol binding protein (RBP), which facilitates absorption, transport and mediation of the biological activity. Retinal is the active form required for formation of the visual pigment rhodopsin in the rods and cones of the retina.

Retinoic acid may be the active form for processes involving growth and differentiation. Although the exact mechanism of action is unknown, retinoic acid may act directly at the level of genetic transcription via a nuclear receptor to promote the synthesis of some proteins and inhibit the synthesis of others.

Vitamin A is involved in vision after conversion in the body to 11-*cis*-retinal. The latter interacts with opsin, a protein, to form rhodopsin, which is the light-sensitive pigment in the rods and cones of the retina. The exact mechanism of action of retinoids is not understood at the molecular level, except for their role in vision.

COMMON USAGE

Accepted uses: Treatment of vitamin A deficiency.

Unproven uses: Topical ophthalmic solutions of vitamin A have been successful in treating dry-eye syndromes. Large doses of vitamin A have shown some success in the treatment of acne with retinol therapy and in Kyrle's disease. Vitamin A in combination with vitamin E is beneficial in the treatment of abetalipoproteinemia and in Darier's disease cutaneous lesions. Studies evaluating the benefit of vitamin A therapy in conditions of cancer, Crohn's disease, and growth promotion produced controversial results. Other studies concluded that vitamin A had no overall effect in the treatment of coronary heart disease, HIV prophylaxis, and respiratory syncytial viral infections.

CONTRAINDICATIONS

Doses above 5000 U are contraindicated in pregnancy.

Do not use in persons who have exhibited hypersensitivity to vitamin A.

Do not administer to persons with hypervitaminosis A.

Oral preparations should not be used for treating vitamin A deficiency in persons with malabsorption syndromes.

WARNINGS/PRECAUTIONS

Hepatotoxicity: Chronic consumption may cause liver damage.

Pregnancy and breastfeeding: Doses exceeding 5000 U are contraindicated during pregnancy. Retinoids, chemically synthesized analogs of vitamin A, are known to cause severe birth defects in humans. Vitamin A is excreted in human breast milk. The dangers to the nursing infant are unknown.

Toxicity: High doses can cause: blurred vision, depression, dizziness, drowsiness, headache, insomnia, irritability, lack of muscle coordination, nausea, osteoporosis, osteosclerosis, seizures, somnolence, and vomiting.

DRUG INTERACTIONS

Anticoagulants: Increased risk of bleeding.

Cholestyramine: Decreased absorption of vitamin A; separate administration times.

Colestipol: Decreased absorption of vitamin A; separate administration times.

Minocycline: Increased risk of pseudotumor cerebri.

Retinoids (e.g., acitretin, bexarotene, etretinate, isotretinoin, tretinoin:): Increased risk of vitamin A toxicity.

FOOD INTERACTIONS

Carob: Caution is advised for patients who ingest large amounts of carob foods and take vitamin A supplements, due to increased bioavailability of vitamin A.

ADVERSE REACTIONS

Dermatitis and photosensitivity reactions may occur.

ADMINISTRATION AND DOSAGE

The RDAs for vitamin A are listed as Retinol Activity Equivalents (RAE) to account for the different activities of retinol and provitamin A carotenoids. 1 RAE in mcg = 3.3 IU.

Daily Dosage: Recommended Dietary Allowance:

Males 14 years and over: 900mcg or 3000IU daily

Females 14 years and over: 700mcg or 2330IU

Pregnancy—14 to 18 years: 750mcg or 2500 IU; *19 years and over*: 700mcg or 2330IU.

Lactation: 14 to 18 years: 1200mcg or 4000 IU; *19 years and over*: 1300mcg or 4335 IU.

Children—1 to 3 years: 300mcg or 1000IU; *4 to 8 years*: 400mcg or 1333IU; *9 to 13 years*: 600mcg or 2000IU.

Infants—0 to 6 months (Adequate Intake [AI]): 400mcg or 1330IU; *7 to 12 months*: 500mcg or 1665IU.

Adults

Deficiency: 100,000 U daily for 3 days, followed by 50,000 U daily for 2 weeks.

Maintenance doses of 10,000 to 20,000 U daily for 2 months are recommended.

Topical use: Apply daily as needed

Xerophthalmia: 110mg vitamin A palmitate or 66mg vitamin A acetate, repeat the following day and one to two weeks later.

Vitamin C

EFFECTS

Vitamin C, also known as ascorbic acid, has atherogenic, anticarcinogenic, antihypertensive, antiviral, antihistamine, immunomodulatory, ophthalmoprotective, airway-protective, and heavy-metal detoxifying properties. Antioxidant effects have been demonstrated as increased resistance of red blood cells to free radical attack in elderly persons and reduced activated oxygen species in patients receiving chemotherapy and radiation. Antioxidant mechanisms have been shown in the reduction of LDL oxidation as well, though studies on the prevention of heart disease and stroke are conflicting.

COMMON USAGE

Accepted uses: FDA-approved prophylaxis of vitamin C deficiency and to increase iron absorption.

Unproven uses: Vitamin C has been used in the prevention of heart disease, pneumonia, sunburn, hyperlipidemia, cancer prevention, muscle soreness, asthma, common cold, erythema (after CO2 laser skin resurfacing), and for fluorosis, wound healing after severe trauma, and as an antioxidant.

CONTRAINDICATIONS

Hypersensitivity to vitamin C.

WARNINGS/PRECAUTIONS

Medical conditions: Use cautiously in patients with preexisting kidney stone disease, erythrocyte G6PD deficiency, hemochromatosis, thalassemia, or sideroblastic anemia.

Laboratory tests: Vitamin C interferes with the results of the following laboratory tests: acetaminophen, AST (SGOT), bilirubin, carbamazepine, creatinine, glucose, LDH, stool guiac, theophylline, and uric acid.

Pregnancy and breastfeeding: Vitamin C is safe at the Recommended Dietary Allowance doses.

DRUG INTERACTIONS

Antacids: Increased risk of aluminum toxicity with concomitant use. Concurrent administration is not recommended, especially in patients with renal insufficiency. If concurrent use cannot be avoided, monitor patients for possible acute aluminum toxicity (eg, encephalopathy, seizures, or coma) and adjust the doses accordingly.

Aspirin: Increased ascorbic requirements with concomitant use. Increased dietary or supplemental vitamin C intake (100mg to 200mg daily) should be considered for patients on chronic high-dose aspirin.

Cyanocobalmin: Reduced the absorption and bioavailability of cyanocobalmin with concomitant use. Vitamin C should be administered 2 or more hours after a meal.

ADVERSE REACTIONS

Adverse effects of oral vitamin C include diarrhea, esophagitis (rare), and intestinal obstruction (rare).

ADMINISTRATION AND DOSAGE

Daily Dosage: Recommended Dietary Allowance:

Males—14 to 18 years: 75mg daily; *19+ years*: 90mg daily.

Females—14 to 18 years: 65mg daily; *19+ years*: 75mg daily

During pregnancy—less than 18 years: 80mg daily; *19 to 50 years*: 85mg daily.

Lactation—18 years and younger: 115mg daily; *19 to 50 years*: 120mg daily.

Infants and children— 0 to 6 months: 40mg daily; *7 to 12 months*: 50mg daily; *1 to 3 years*: 15mg daily; *4 to 8 years*: 25mg daily; *9 to 13 years*: 45mg daily.

Individuals who smoke require an additional 35mg/day of vitamin C over the established RDA.

Adults

Antioxidant effects: 120mg/day to 450mg/day

Asthma: 500mg/day to 2000mg/day or prior to exercise

Atherosclerosis prevention: 45mg/day to 1000mg/day

Delayed-onset muscle soreness: 3000mg/day

Gastric cancer: 50mg/day

Histamine detoxification: 2000mg/day

Hypercholesterolemia: 300mg/day to 3000mg/day

Respiratory infection: 1000mg/day to 2000mg/day

Scurvy: The recommended dose for the treatment of scurvy is 1g to 2g administered for the first 2 days, then 500mg daily for a week. Alternately, the AMA recommends 100mg 3 times a day for 1 week then 100mg daily for several weeks until tissue saturation is normal.

Skin erythema: Apply a topical 10% aqueous solution once daily.

Sunburn prevention: 2000mg/day

Urine acidification: 3g/day to 12g/day titrated to desired effect and given as divided doses every 4 hours

Wound healing: 1000mg/day to 1500mg/day

Pediatrics

Daily Dosage: The recommended prophylactic dose for infants on formula feedings is 35mg/day orally or intramuscularly for the first few weeks of life. If the formula contains 2 to 3 times the amount of protein in human milk, the dose should be 50mg/day.

Infants and children require 30 to 60mg of crystalline ascorbic acid daily. This may be taken as oral tablets or as part of the normal diet (i.e., 2 to 4 oz. of orange juice)

Fluorosis: 500mg/day

Scurvy: 100mg 3 times a day for 1 week, then 100mg daily for several weeks until tissue saturation is normal.

Vitamin D

EFFECTS

Vitamin D is both a vitamin and a steroid hormone. The vitamin can be consumed from dietary sources and the hormone synthesized in the skin with exposure to sunlight. The active metabolite operates via both nuclear receptors and nongenomic systems. However, vitamin D must first undergo a two-step metabolic process en route to the biologically active form of the drug. The first metabolic step occurs in the microsomal fraction of the liver in which vitamin D is hydroxylated at the C25 position. The compound 25-hydroxyvitamin D is the major circulating and storage form of vitamin D. Its level reflects sunlight exposure and dietary intake, and it is generally used as a clinical indicator of vitamin D stores. Next, 25-hydroxyvitamin D is bound to the same carrier protein as the parent compound and carried in the bloodstream to the kidney where it is hydroxylated at the "1" position to produce 1,25-dihydroxyvitamin D_3 (1,25D or calcitriol), the biologically active product. This final step in the production of vitamin D is dependent on the complex interaction of calcium, phosphorus, and parathyroid hormone.

Vitamin D is critical to normal bone mineralization and insufficient mineralization produces rickets in children and osteomalacia in children and adults. In addition to its effects on bone, in vitro vitamin D enhances cell differentiation and inhibits cell proliferation, actions that oppose those of cancer.

Vitamin D is available for oral, topical and parenteral administration. The scope of this discussion will be limited to the oral and topical formulations.

COMMON USAGE

Accepted uses: Vitamin D is FDA-approved for the prevention and treatment of vitamin D deficiency, and for the treatment of familial hypophosphatemia, hypoparathyroidism, malabsorption syndromes, and vitamin D-resistant rickets.

Unproven uses: Vitamin D supplementation is used to prevent and treat rickets in children and osteomalacia in adults. Vitamin D prevents and treats osteopenia and osteoporosis. Patients with secondary hyperparathyroidism who are vitamin D deficient may benefit from vitamin D supplementation.

Sick sinus syndrome and chronic atrial fibrillation respond successfully to vitamin D supplementation. Supplementation with vitamin D appears to decrease symptoms associated with asthma, perhaps because of its influence on calcium metabolism. It also improves expiratory volume and decreases airway resistance. Ingestion and topical application of vitamin D, alone or in combination with ultraviolet light, is used to treat plaque psoriasis. Localized and systemic scleroderma can be treated with oral or topical vitamin D. Supplementation with vitamin D is helpful in Crohn's disease-related osteomalacia. Supplementation with vitamin D and calcium may improve hearing. Vitamin D alleviates migraine headaches and headaches associated with menses.

CONTRAINDICATIONS

Do not use in patient with hypercalcemia.

Do not use in individuals who have exhibited hypersensitivity to vitamin D.

Vitamin D is contraindicated in patients who have systemic lupus erythematosus.

WARNINGS/PRECAUTIONS

Pregnancy and breastfeeding: Vitamin D is safe during pregnancy and lactation.

DRUG INTERACTIONS

Orlistat: Treatment with Orlistat has been shown to reduce serum levels of vitamin D (cholecalciferol).

ADVERSE REACTIONS

Potential adverse reactions include constipation, cardiac arrhythmia, hypercalcemia, nausea, nocturia, polydipsia, polyuria, and vomiting.

ADMINISTRATION AND DOSAGE

Note that 1mcg calciferol is equivalent to 40IU vitamin D. "Ergocalciferol" is vitamin D_2; "cholecalciferol" is vitamin D_3.

Daily Dosage: Recommended Dietary Allowance:

Adults—19 to 50 years: 5mcg daily; *50 to 70 years*: 10mcg daily; *Over 70 years*: 15mcg daily.

During pregnancy: 5mcg daily

During lactation: 5mcg daily

Children 1 to 18 years: 5mcg daily.

Infants 0 to 12 months: 5mcg daily.

These values are based on the absence of adequate exposure to sunlight.

Adults

Epilepsy: Initial dose of Vitamin D_2 4000IU daily for 105 days, followed by 150 days of 1000IU daily

Familial hypophosphatemia: Vitamin D_2 50,000IU to 75,000IU and phosphorus 2g daily.

Hepatic osteodystrophy: Vitamin D_2 100,000IU monthly

Hyperparathyroidism: 50,000IU vitamin D_2 daily, increased to 200,000IU daily

Hypoparathyroidism: 2.5mg to 6.25mg vitamin D_2 daily

Osteomalacia: 36,000IU vitamin D_2 daily in addition to calcium supplementation

Osteoporosis prophylaxis: Vitamin D 400IU to 800IU daily

Pregnancy supplementation: Vitamin D_2 given in two large doses of 600,000IU during the 7th and 8th months of pregnancy

Pseudohypoparathyroidism: 2.5mg to 6.25mg vitamin D_2 daily

Psoriasis: 1mcg vitamin D_3 daily for 6 months

Psoriasis: Topical formulation consisting of 0.5mcg vitamin D_3 per gram base. Apply daily for 8 weeks.

Renal oseodystrophy: 15,000 to 20,000 IU vitamin D_2 daily

Systemic scleroderma: 1.75mcg vitamin D_3 for 6 months to 3 years

Vitamin D-resistant rickets: 50,000IU to 300,000IU vitamin D_2 daily

Pediatrics

Anticonvlsant osteomalacia: 15,000IU in daily doses to 600,000IU in a single dose vitamin D_2

Hypoparathyroidism: 200mcg/kg of body weight (8000IU/kg) vitamin D_2 daily for 1 to 2 weeks

Pseudohypoparathyroidism: 200mcg/kg of body weight (8000IU/kg) vitamin D_2 daily for 1 to 2 weeks

Renal osteodystrophy: Ergocalciferol 25mcg/kg to 100mcg/kg daily

Vitamin E

EFFECTS

Vitamin E is a powerful antioxidant that plays a role in immune function, DNA repair, and cell-membrane stabilization. Research suggests it may also have the following effects: antiplatelet, antiatherogenic, antithrombotic, anti-inflammatory, and anticarcinogenic. Vitamin E appears to have neuroprotective actions as well.

Keep in mind that vitamin E is divided chemically into two groups, tocopherols and tocotrienols. The most biologically active—and the most studied—form is alpha-tocopherol. However, limited research indicates possible benefits of the other forms of vitamin E as well.

COMMON USAGE

Accepted uses: Prevention and treatment of vitamin E deficiency due to intestinal malabsorption caused by premature birth or disorders such as Crohn's disease, cystic fibrosis, and rare genetic disorders (e.g., abetalipoproteinemia).

Unproven uses: Some evidence suggests supplemental vitamin E may be helpful as adjunctive treatment for type 1 diabetes, anemia in hemodialysis patients, intermittent claudication, some types of male infertility, tardive dyskinesia, osteoarthritis, rheumatoid arthritis, premenstrual syndrome, and enhanced immune function in the elderly. It may also be helpful for decreasing platelet adhesion and improving the effectiveness of antiplatelet therapy with aspirin.

Studies have reported conflicting results when vitamin E was used for preventing or treating Alzheimer's disease, heart disease, stroke, certain cancers (eg, breast, colon, prostate, and bladder), seizures, cataracts, fibrocystic breast problems, and exercise-induced tissue damage. A few small preliminary studies suggest vitamin E may be useful for sunburn protection and nitrate tolerance, but more research is needed.

Currently, clinical trials have demonstrated no benefit when vitamin E was used for Huntington's chorea, ischemia reperfusion in heart surgery, lung cancer, muscular dystrophy, myotonic dystrophy, Parkinson's disease, or decreasing the rate of chronic hemolysis.

CONTRAINDICATIONS

Because of potential blood-thinning effects, supplemental vitamin E is contraindicated in patients with coagulation disorders and during anticoagulation therapy. Topical use of vitamin E is contraindicated after a recent chemical peel or dermabrasion.

WARNINGS/PRECAUTIONS

Blood-clotting disorders: Supplementation is not advised. Monitor bleeding time in patients who decide to use vitamin E.

High doses: Research suggests a slight dose-response increase in all-cause mortality as vitamin E dosages exceed 400 IU/day, although conflicting evidence indicates that dosages are unsafe only when they exceed 1600 IU. Another study reported a higher risk of hospitalization and heart failure in older patients ($\geq$55 years) with vascular disease or diabetes who took 400 IU/day.

Pregnancy and breastfeeding: Vitamin E is safe at RDA levels but avoid higher doses.

Thrombophlebitis: This problem has been reported in patients at risk of small-vessel disease who were taking $\geq$400 IU/day.

DRUG INTERACTIONS

Anticoagulants: Avoid concomitant use. Vitamin E could potentiate their effects.

Colestipol: Concomitant use may reduce vitamin E absorption. Allow as much time as possible between doses.

Orlistat: Concomitant use may reduce vitamin E absorption. Allow at least 2 hours between doses.

ADVERSE REACTIONS

No side effects have been reported at recommended doses. Occasionally, doses greater than 400 IU/day have been associated with diarrhea, nausea, headache, blurred vision, dizziness, and fatigue. Doses greater than 800 IU/day may increase the risk of bleeding, especially in patients deficient in vitamin K.

ADMINISTRATION AND DOSAGE

Because vitamin E is fat soluble, supplements should be taken with a meal that contains fat to enhance absorption.

Daily Dosage: 1mg of alpha-tocopherol is approximately equal to 1.5 International Units (IU). Recommended Dietary Allowance (RDA)—*Adults and adolescents 14 years and older*: 15mg (22.5 IU) daily. *During pregnancy*: 15mg (22.5 IU) daily. *During lactation*: 19mg (28.5 IU) daily. *Infants and children—0 to 6 months*: 4mg (6 IU) daily; *7 to 12 months*: 5mg (7.5 IU) daily; *1 to 3 years*: 6mg (9 IU) daily; *4 to 8 years*: 7mg (10.5 IU) daily; *9 to 13 years*: 11mg (16.5 IU) daily.

Adults

Deficiency: 32-50mg/day. The usual oral dose for vitamin E deficiency is 4 to 5 times the RDA. Doses as high as 300mg may be necessary.

Alzheimer's disease: 2000 IU/day

Anemia in hemodialysis patients: 500mg/day

Angina pectoris: 50-300mg/day

Antioxidant effects: 100-800mg/day

Antiplatelet effects: 200-400 IU/day

Cerebrovascular disease: 400 IU/day with aspirin 325mg/day

Colorectal cancer prevention: 50mg/day

Coronary heart disease prevention: 100-800 IU/day

Cystic fibrosis: 50mg/day for correction of anemia

Diabetes: 100-900 IU/day for improving glucose tolerance and reducing protein glycation in insulin-dependent (and some non-insulin-dependent) patients.

Enhanced exercise performance at high altitude: 400mg/day

Epilepsy: 400 IU/day

Exercise-induced tissue damage (prevention): 500-1200 IU/day

Immune system support in geriatric patients: 200mg/day

Intermittent claudication: 600-1600mg/day

Infertility (male): 200-300mg/day

Nitrate tolerance: 600mg/day

Oral leukoplakia and oropharyngeal cancer prevention: 800 IU/day

Osteoarthritis: 400-1200 IU/day

Premenstrual symptoms: 150-600 IU/day

Prostate cancer prevention: 50mg/day

Rheumatoid arthritis: 800-1200 IU/day

Sunburn protection: 1000 IU of vitamin E combined with 2000mg of vitamin C daily

Tardive dyskinesia: 1200-1600 IU/day

Pediatrics

Children with malabsorption syndrome: 1 unit/kg/day of water-miscible vitamin E is given to raise plasma tocopherol to within the normal range within 2 months and for maintenance of normal plasma concentrations (1 unit = 1mg alpha-tocopherol acetate).

Premature or low-birth-weight neonates: 25-50 units/day results in normal plasma tocopherol levels in 1 week (1 unit = 1mg alpha-tocopherol acetate).

Zinc

EFFECTS

Zinc is an essential trace element thought to have antimicrobial, anti-sickling, cell-protective, copper-absorbing, enzyme-regulating, and growth-stimulating effects.

COMMON USAGE

Accepted uses: Zinc is approved by the FDA for the treatment of zinc deficiency.

Unproven uses: Zinc supplements are used for numerous conditions, including the following: acne vulgaris, acrodermatitis enteropathica, Alzheimer's disease, common cold, dental hygiene, diabetes mellitus, diarrhea, eczema, eye irritation, growth, Hansen's disease, herpes simplex infection, hypertension, hypogeusia (decreased sense of taste), immunodeficiency, impotence, infertility, leg ulcers, lipid peroxidation, macular degeneration, necrolytic migratory erythema, parasites, peptic ulcer disease, psoriasis, scalp dermatoses, schistosomiasis, sepsis, sickle cell anemia, stomatitis, thalassemia major, trichomoniasis, Wilson's disease, and wound healing.

CONTRAINDICATIONS

Do not use in patients who have exhibited hypersensitivity reactions to zinc-containing products.

WARNINGS/PRECAUTIONS

Ophthalmic use: Zinc ophthalmic solution should be used cautiously in patients with glaucoma. Do not use zinc ophthalmic solutions that have changed color.

Pregnancy and breastfeeding: Zinc is safe at RDA doses. Zinc should not be used in doses greater than the RDA during lactation.

DRUG INTERACTIONS

Copper or iron: Concurrent administration with zinc inhibits the absorption of copper and iron. Administer zinc and copper or iron as far apart as possible.

Penicillamine: Concurrent administration with zinc reduces zinc absorption.

Quinolones: Zinc decreases absorption of quinolone antibiotics (eg, ciprofloxacin, gatifloxacin, ofloxacin). Zinc salts or vitamins containing zinc should be given 2 hours after or 6 hours before antibiotics.

Tetracycline: Concurrent administration results in decreased tetracycline effectiveness. Administer tetracycline at least 2 hours before or 3 hours after zinc.

DRUG-FOOD INTERACTIONS

Concurrent administration of caffeine with zinc reduces zinc absorption. Foods containing high amounts of phosphorus, calcium (dairy), or phytates (eg, bran, brown bread) may reduce absorption.

ADVERSE REACTIONS

Side effects include gastrointestinal discomfort, nausea, vomiting, headaches, drowsiness, and metallic taste.

ADMINISTRATION AND DOSAGE

Daily Dosage: Recommended Dietary Allowance:

Males 14 and older: 11mg daily

Females—14 to 18 years: 9 mg daily; *19+ years*: 8mg daily

During pregnancy—younger than 18 years: 12mg daily; *19+ years*: 11mg daily

During lactation—younger than 18 years: 13mg daily; *19+ years*: 12mg daily

Infants and children—7 months to 3 years: 3 mg daily; *4 to 8 years*: 5mg daily; *9 to 13 years*: 8mg daily.

Adults

Dietary supplement: Daily oral doses range from 9mg to 25mg.

Acne and dermatitis: A topical preparation (cream or gel) of 10mg zinc sulfate per gram or 27mg to 30mg zinc oxide per gram used several times daily.

Acne: 90mg to 135mg orally daily

Zinc deficiency/acrodermatitis: maximum doses up to 40mg orally daily

Wilson's disease: 300mg to 1200mg orally daily in divided doses

Pediatrics

Acne: 135mg orally daily.

Zinc deficiency: Daily doses range from 1.5mg to 12mg, depending on age.

HERBAL MEDICINE PROFILES

Herbal Medicines

Aloe Vera

EFFECTS

Aloe gel, from the pulp of the *Aloe vera* leaf, has soothing and healing effects. A juice is made from the gel as well as from the whole leaf. A component with very different effects is taken from specialized cells of the leaf's inner lining as a liquid then dried into a yellow powder. Called aloe vera latex, this powder has powerful laxative properties.

COMMON USAGE

Accepted uses: Commission E approves of the use of aloe vera latex for constipation (the anthraquinone laxative portion of aloe is primarily used for short-term treatment of this condition) and to clear out the colon for rectal and bowel examination.

Unproven uses: Aloe vera gel is used topically to hasten healing in mild first-degree burns (such as sun burns), wounds, and other skin infections and conditions. Its ability to treat varying degrees of more serious burns, frostbite, herpes simplex, and psoriasis remains unclear. Aloe juice and derivatives are taken for heartburn and other digestive complaints, but the effectiveness remains uncertain. Likewise unproven is its ability to help with AIDS, arthritis, asthma, cancer, diabetes, and ulcers.

CONTRAINDICATIONS

Aloe products should not be taken by mouth by people with kidney or heart disease, or with electrolyte abnormalities. In addition to hypersensitivity, contraindications to the use of aloe latex include pregnancy and breastfeeding, nausea, vomiting, symptoms of appendicitis, undiagnosed abdominal pain, and temporary paralysis of the bowel (ileus) such as bowel obstruction, fecal impaction, and acute surgical abdomen. The use of aloe latex is not recommended for children under age 12.

WARNINGS/PRECAUTIONS

Overuse as laxative: Exercise caution in taking oral aloe formulations. More than seven consecutive days of use may cause dependency or worsening of constipation once aloe latex is stopped. Possible risk of colorectal cancer with more than 12 months of use.

Diabetes or kidney disease: Exercise caution in using aloe orally as a laxative, as electrolyte imbalances such as low potassium levels can occur, potentially causing complications such as muscle weakness or abnormal heart rhythms.

Wound healing: There have been cases of slowed healing and skin irritation and redness following application of aloe juice. Avoid applying prior to sun exposure. Do not apply the gel following cesarean delivery.

Pregnancy and breastfeeding: While topical use of the gel likely poses no risk, oral use of aloe forms is contraindicated during pregnancy or breastfeeding. Compounds in aloe could, theoretically, stimulate uterine contractions. Breastfeeding women should not consume the dried juice of aloe leaves. It remains unclear whether active aloe ingredients appear in breast milk.

DRUG INTERACTIONS

Antidiabetic agents: Avoid concomitant use of oral aloe forms due to increased risk of hypoglycemia.

Digoxin: Avoid concomitant use with oral aloe forms given the theoretical risk of hypokalemia resulting in digoxin toxicity.

ADVERSE REACTIONS

Using aloe or aloe latex orally for laxative effects can cause excessive bowel activity (bloody diarrhea, nausea), cramping, and diarrhea. Oral use may lower blood sugar levels (according to a small number of human studies). In overdose, electrolyte imbalances such as low potassium levels, as well as kidney damage, are a risk. Doses of 1g/day for several days may be fatal.

Usually safe when used topically, although cases of delayed wound healing and skin irritation have been reported following application of juice to skin. Avoid applying prior to sun exposure.

Administration by injection is dangerous and linked to fatalities; more research is needed.

ADMINISTRATION AND DOSAGE

The dosing of aloe vera products is highly dependent on such varied factors as plant part used, growing and harvesting condition, and extraction methods employed.

Adults

Daily dosage: As an oral laxative, the usual (and maximum) single daily oral dose at bedtime of dried aloe extract or powdered aloe: 0.05-0.2g. Do not exceed commonly recommended dosage.

Topical use: Some sources recommend that commercial aloe gel solutions contain at least a 70% concentration of aloe to positively influence inflammation and healing. Follow directions on commercial creams and ointments for wounds or burns.

Pediatrics

Oral use is not recommended for children under age 12. Dosages for topical use are the same as those for adults.

Bilberry

EFFECTS

The fruit of the bilberry plant (*Vaccinium myrtillus*) contains potent astringent properties and antioxidant flavonoids. More than 15 different flavonoid *anthocyanosides* have been identified and are believed to generate much (if not all) of the plant's medicinal effects. Bilberry fruit has demonstrated the following properties: antiulcer, antineoplastic, antiplatelet, antiatherogenic, wound-healing, and antidiabetic effects. It also has shown an ability to enhance the eye's regenerative capacities.

COMMON USAGE

Accepted uses: Commission E approves of the highly nutritious bilberry fruit as an astringent and for the treatment of acute diarrhea, and topically as a gargle for mild inflammation of throat and mouth mucous membranes.

Unproven uses: Because of its high content of anthocyanins, bilberry fruit has become popular for the prevention and treatment of eye diseases (e.g., cataracts, glaucoma, retinopathy, macular degeneration) in standardized extract form. Its effectiveness for these purposes has been widely tested in Europe and attributed to the plant's antioxidant and collagen-stabilizing actions. Pilots in World War II contended that their visual acuity at night improved after consuming bilberry products, but data for the herb's value in this regard remain inconsistent.

Other uses for bilberry, though not all proven effective, include treatment the following conditions: atherosclerosis, diabetes, hemorrhoids, inflammation, menstrual irregularities, neuralgia and neuropathy, peptic ulcer, peripheral vascular disease, pregnancy-related illnesses, varicose veins, and topically as an eyewash and compress for wounds and ulcers.

CONTRAINDICATIONS

Commission E warns against using the *leaves* of the bilberry plant for medicinal purposes. People with bleeding disorders or taking medications to thin the blood should not take very high doses of bilberry. Breastfeeding is contraindicated given the historical use of bilberries for stopping lactation.

WARNINGS/PRECAUTIONS

Hypersensitivity: Hypersensitivity reactions are possible.

Pregnancy and breastfeeding: No information is available; caution is advised.

DRUG INTERACTIONS

Anticoagulants (including low molecular weight heparins), antiplatelet agents, and thrombolytic agents: Combine with caution; bilberry could add to drugs' blood altering effects and potentially increase the effects of these drugs, promoting bleeding.

ADVERSE REACTIONS

There is potential for excessive bleeding due to decreased platelet aggregation. Nausea is possible and may abate by taking bilberry with food.

ADMINISTRATION AND DOSAGE

Only the berry (fruit, typically dried) is used; do not use the leaf for medicinal purposes. For general use, typical European pharmaceutical formulations are for bilberry fruit extract form standardized for anthocyanidin content (25%): 80-160mg 3 times/day. Another common dosage for general daily use: fluid extract (1:1 concentration), 3-6mL.

Adults

Eye health: tablet/capsule (standardized to 36% anthocyanidin content): 60-160mg three times a day.

Mild inflammation of the mucous membranes of the mouth and throat: Decoction as a gargle (10% bilberry fruit): prepare, swish around for several seconds, and spit out.

Nonspecific acute diarrhea: tablet/capsule: 20-60g/day.

Pediatrics

No information is available.

Black Cohosh

EFFECTS

The chemistry of black cohosh (*Actaea racemosa* or *Cimicifuga racemosa*) has been well studied, with the triterpene glycosides and flavonoids considered to be the herb's active components. How black cohosh works is not known, however. It has demonstrated cardiovascular, circulatory, and anti-inflammatory activities. The possibility that black cohosh exerts estrogenic activity has been examined but the evidence remains contradictory.

COMMON USAGE

Accepted uses: The most common modern use for black cohosh is to lessen the frequency and severity of hot flashes and other symptoms of perimenopause and menopause. Commission E has approved black cohosh for such climacteric complaints, as well as for premenstrual syndrome. Results of clinical trials are mixed. However, open, uncontrolled studies and post-marketing surveillance studies support the evidence in favor of effectiveness and safety for the use of black cohosh for menopausal symptoms. The American College of Obstetricians and Gynecologists stated in 2001 that black cohosh may be helpful in the short-term (6 months or less) for women with vasomotor symptoms of menopause. More definitive research is needed.

Unproven uses: Black cohosh has also been used for intercostal myalgia, sciatica, whooping cough, chorea, tinnitus, dysmenorrhea, uterine colic, and specifically for muscular rheumatism and rheumatoid arthritis.

CONTRAINDICATIONS

There are no known contraindications to the use of black cohosh, aside from pregnancy and breastfeeding.

WARNINGS/PRECAUTIONS

Toxicity: Limit use of black cohosh to no more than three months, as little is known about its toxicity. Long-term safety data are not available.

Estrogenic activity: Because it remains unclear whether black cohosh has estrogenic effects, caution is advised in women with estrogen-dependent tumors. The concern is that herbs with estrogenic activity could stimulate the growth of breast (or endometrial) cancer cells, as well as oppose the effects of competitive estrogen receptor antagonists (such as tamoxifen).

Hypersensitivity: Use of black cohosh should be avoided in people with hypersensitivity to the herb.

Pregnancy and breastfeeding: Black cohosh should not be used during pregnancy or while nursing.

DRUG INTERACTIONS

Immunosuppressants: Avoid concomitant use. Black cohosh could reduce the effects of drugs that suppress the immune system, including drugs such as azathioprine and cyclosporine used to prevent organ rejection.

ADVERSE REACTIONS

Few adverse events have been reported. But even with therapeutic doses, gastroenteritis can occur, as can transient dizziness, headaches, heaviness in the legs, vomiting, mastalgia, weight gain, tremors, and giddiness.

ADMINISTRATION AND DOSAGE

Numerous clinical trials of black cohosh have used a standardized black cohosh extract (Remifemin; each 20mg tablet contains 1mg triterpene glycosides, calculated as 26-deoxyactein) 40mg twice daily for up to 24 weeks.

Adults

Daily dose: Dry rhizome/root: 40-200mg; liquid extract: ethanolic extracts equivalent to 40mg dried rhizome/root; tincture: 0.4-2mL (1:10 in 60% ethanol).

Hot flushes due to tamoxifen therapy: 20mg twice daily, orally.

Menopausal symptoms: specifically, commonly recommended oral daily dosages is as follows: tablet, 1-2mg of 27-deoxyacteine; powdered rhizome: 40 to 200 mg; tincture: 0.4-2mL (1:10 preparation in 60% alcohol); fluid extract, 3-4mL twice daily (1:1 preparation); solid (dry powdered) extract (4:1 preparation), 250-500mg; alcohol-based extracts, 40% to 60% (v/v), dosage should correspond to 40mg black cohosh.

Pediatrics

No information is available.

Chamomile

EFFECTS

The essential oil of chamomile has antibacterial and antifungal properties. The flowers have anti-inflammatory, antispasmodic, and sedative effects. Two species of chamomile—German chamomile (*Matricaria recutita*) and Roman chamomile (*Chamaemelum nobile* or *Anthemis nobilis*)—are commonly used.

COMMON USAGE

Accepted uses: Commission E has approved chamomile for coughs and bronchitis, fevers and colds, inflammation of the skin, mouth, and pharynx, infection, and wounds and burns.

Unproven uses: It is taken orally for tension and anxiety, insomnia, and by many women for discomforts of perimenopausal and menopausal symptoms. Its effectiveness when taken orally for diarrhea is unclear, as the data are inconclusive.

CONTRAINDICATIONS

Chamomile is contraindicated in pregnancy and in people with atopic hay fever or asthma. It also should not be taken by people with a hypersensitivity to chamomile or other members of the *Compositae* family.

WARNINGS/PRECAUTIONS

Pregnancy and breastfeeding: Internal consumption of the whole plant should be avoided during early pregnancy. No data on human teratogenicity are available. *Chamomile anthemis* is contraindicated throughout pregnancy due to its emmenagogic and abortifacient effects. *Chamomile matricaria* is contraindicated in early pregnancy due to its emmenagogic effect; it has been used during pregnancy as a weak tea for insomnia, as a diuretic, and as a carminative, with no apparent adverse effects.

Breastfeeding: Flowers can be safely consumed while breastfeeding.

DRUG INTERACTIONS

Anticoagulants: Caution is advised, as the coumarins present in chamomile could theoretically magnify the effect of anticoagulants, adding to the anticoagulant effect and increasing the risk of bleeding.

ADVERSE REACTIONS

Eczema (facial) has been reported with the tea. Emesis is possible when Roman chamomile is taken in high doses.

Contact dermatitis and eczema are possible with topical use. Conjunctivitis and eyelid angioedema with the use of chamomile tea as an eyewash.

ADMINISTRATION AND DOSAGE

Chamomile is used as a tea, essential oil, liquid extract, or as a topical cream.

Adults

Dermatitis: as a topical cream, applied four times daily.

Tension/anxiety: orally, liquid extract (1:1 in 45 to 70% ethanol) is taken 1-4mL three times daily or as a *tea*, 1-4 times in 8oz cups daily, as needed.

Pediatrics

Dermatitis: a topical cream is applied 4 times daily.

Tension/anxiety: orally 1-4 times daily in 8oz cups as a *tea*, with amount depending on age.

Cranberry

EFFECTS

Cranberry (*Vaccinium macrocarpon*) has antibacterial and antioxidant properties. Among other possible mechanisms, it is believed to inhibit the ability of bacteria to adhere to the urinary tract, thereby protecting against (and possibly resolving) urinary tract infection (UTI).

COMMON USAGE

Unproven uses: For medicinal purposes, cranberry products (primarily juices) have been used for centuries to prevent and treat urinary tract infections. Clinical trials indicate possible effectiveness in adults (and ineffective actions in children) for the use of cranberry for UTIs. It is possibly effective as an antioxidant in humans and in vitro. Used as a urine deodorant in people with incontinence. Evidence for its value in treating nephrolithiasis is inconclusive.

CONTRAINDICATIONS

Cranberry is contraindicated in cases of hypersensitivity to the fruit. It should be used with caution in people with nephrolithiasis (renal colic, blood in the urine, and kidney stones).

WARNINGS/PRECAUTIONS

Pregnancy and breastfeeding: No information is available; caution is advised.

DRUG INTERACTIONS

H_2 blockers: Combine with caution, and avoid regular (daily) use of cranberry juice while taking this medication. Cranberry juice reduces gastric pH, and could theoretically antagonize the effect of H_2 blockers and thereby reduce their effectiveness.

Proton pump inhibitors: Combine with caution, avoid regular (daily) use of cranberry juice while taking this medication. Cranberry juice significantly reduces gastric pH, and could theoretically reduce the effectiveness of proton pump inhibitors.

Warfarin: Avoid excess use of cranberry products while taking this medication due to the increased risk of bleeding.

ADVERSE REACTIONS

Rarely: renal colic, blood in the urine, and kidney stones.

ADMINISTRATION AND DOSAGE

Cranberry is available for oral use as a juice and in capsule and tablet forms. Juice may be hard for women to take daily over very long periods of time. Optimum dosage or method of administration remains to be determined.

Adults

Urinary tract infection, prophylaxis: Cranberry juice: 300mL/day. Cranberry-Lingonberry juice concentrate (7.5g cranberry concentrate and 1.7g lingonberry concentrate in 50mL water): 50mL daily for 6 months. Cranberry juice (unsweetened or saccharin-sweetened): 250mL 3 times/day. Cranberry extract (standardized) in capsule or tablet form: 100-500mg 2-3 times/day.

Urinary tract infection, existing: Cranberry extract (standardized) in capsule or tablet form: 100-500mg 2-3 times daily.

Pediatrics

Dosing information is not available.

Echinacea

EFFECTS

Depending on the type of plant species, echinacea has demonstrated the following properties: antibacterial, anti-inflammatory, antimicrobial, antineoplastic, immunostimulating, infertility effect, radio-protectant, and wound-healing effect.

COMMON USAGE

Commission E approved: When used internally, the aerial (above-ground) parts of *Echinacea purpurea*—but not the root—is approved for treating colds, flu-like symptoms, fever, chronic infections of the respiratory tract (such as bronchitis), urinary tract infections, inflammation of the mouth and pharynx, and recurrent infections. It is also approved for the external treatment of superficial wounds and burns. Additionally, the root of *E pallida* is approved as supportive treatment for fevers and colds.

Unproven uses: A study funded by the National Institutes of Health concluded that extracts of *E angustifolia* root do not have clinically significant effects on rhinovirus infection. Likewise, Commission E has not approved *E angustifolia* herb or root for any indication.

CONTRAINDICATIONS

Parenteral use is contraindicated in patients with allergic tendencies, especially to members of the *Asteraceae* or *Compositae* family (e.g., ragweed, chrysanthemums, marigolds, and daisies). Echinacea extract should not be used intravenously in patients with diabetes, since it could worsen their condition. Due to the possible immunostimulating effects of echinacea, Commission E cites the following contraindications based on theoretical—but not clinical—evidence: progressive systemic diseases such as tuberculosis, leukosis, collagenosis, multiple sclerosis and other autoimmune diseases, AIDS, and HIV infection.

WARNINGS/PRECAUTIONS

Fertility: In lab studies, high concentrations of *E purpurea* interfered with sperm enzymes.

Hypersensitivity: Allergic reactions—including urticaria, angioedema, asthma, and anaphylaxis—have been reported. More than half of the affected patients had a history of asthma, allergic rhinitis, rhinoconjunctivitis, or atopic dermatitis.

Pregnancy and breastfeeding: Safety has not been established; caution is advised.

DRUG INTERACTIONS

Anticancer drugs: Avoid concomitant use. Echinacea could potentially decrease their effectiveness.

Drugs metabolized by cytochrome P450 (CYP): In vitro and in vivo studies found that echinacea inhibited CYP 3A and CYP 1A2; caution is advised when coadministering the herb with drugs dependent on CYP enzymes for their elimination.

Immunosuppressants: Avoid concomitant use. Echinacea could counteract the effects of drugs that suppress the immune system, including corticosteroids and drugs used to prevent organ rejection, such as azathioprine, basiliximab, cyclosporine, daclizumab, muromonab-CD3, mycophenolate, sirolimus, and tacrolimus.

ADVERSE REACTIONS

Oral use: Mainly allergic reactions, including breathing problems, dizziness, headache, itching, and rash. *Topical use*: Rash and other skin reactions. *Parenteral use*: Fever, flu-like symptoms, nausea, and vomiting.

ADMINISTRATION AND DOSAGE

Adults

Therapy should not exceed 8 weeks for prophylactic treatment of recurrent infections and 1-2 weeks for acute infections. When used for extended periods, cycling is advised (e.g., skipping weekend doses or taking weekly drug holidays every 4-6 weeks). Dosing schedule for the following oral forms is 3-4 times daily for short-term treatment and twice daily for long-term treatment.

Dry powdered extract: 150-300mg.

Fluid extract (1:1 preparation): 0.25-1mL.

Freeze-dried whole plant: 325-650mg.

Root extract: 300mg.

Tea: 1-2g of powdered root.

Tincture (1:5 preparation): 1-2mL.

Topical use: Dilute fluid extract in equal amount of water and apply to superficial wounds 2-3 times daily.

Pediatrics

No information is available; caution is advised.

Evening Primrose Oil

EFFECTS

The oil from the wildflower evening primrose (*Oenothera biennis*) contains gamma-linolenic acid, which the body converts to dihomo-gamma-linolenic acid and then to prostaglandins that are believed to have anti-inflammatory effects. Extracts of evening primrose oil have also shown antioxidant actions in the laboratory.

COMMON USAGE

Unproven uses: Evening primrose oil (EPO) is an omega 6 fatty acid that contains approximately 8.9% gamma-linolenic acid. Omega 6 essential fatty acids (EFAs) are generally lacking in the standard American diet. Many chronic illnesses are said to respond to supplementation of EFAs.

Several human placebo-controlled, randomized trials indicate effectiveness for the treatment of rheumatoid arthritis, breast cancer, Raynaud's disease, diabetic neuropathy, and eczema. Several months of use may result in relief from cyclical breast pain (mastalgia), for which evening primrose oil can be considered a first-line treatment; though not all study results are positive. EPO may relieve the physical and psychological symptoms of premenstrual syndrome; however, many of the studies indicating effectiveness are inadequate in dose, length of treatment, or size of treatment/control groups. The North American Menopause Society reports that single clinical trials find no benefit to EPO for menopause-associated hot flashes.

CONTRAINDICATIONS

Contraindicated in people with schizophrenia, epilepsy (plus it may have the potential to manifest temporal lobe epilepsy).

WARNINGS/PRECAUTIONS

Hypersensitivity: Allergic reactions to evening primrose oil have been reported.

Pregnancy and breastfeeding: Scientific evidence for the safe use of evening primrose oil is not available.

DRUG INTERACTIONS

Anticoagulants: Caution is advised when taken concomitantly with EPO due to the theoretical risk of increased bleeding.

Anticonvulsants: Avoid concomitant use due to theoretical potential for EPO to reduce the effectiveness of anticonvulsants by lowering the seizure threshold.

Antiplatelet agents, thrombolytic agents, and low molecular weight heparins: Caution is advised for concomitant use due to the theoretical risk of increased and prolonged bleeding.

Phenothiazines: Avoid concomitant use due to the risk of reduced seizure threshold. Seizures have been reported in people with schizophrenia who started taking evening primrose oil.

ADVERSE REACTIONS

Possible reactions include nausea, diarrhea, flatulence, bloating, mild vomiting.

ADMINISTRATION AND DOSAGE

Adults

Daily Dosage: For effective treatment, EPO must be taken in substantial (gram) doses, typically 3-8g daily in divided doses. Clinical effect is often not seen until 8 to 12 weeks of treatment.

Eczema: 2g-8g daily

Mastalgia: 3g-4g daily

Pediatrics

Eczema: 2g-4g daily.

Flaxseed

EFFECTS

The seed from the flax plant (*Linum usitatissimum*) has demonstrated anti-inflammatory, laxative, demulcent, and cholesterol-lowering properties. The oil from the seeds is the richest known plant source of omega-3 fatty acids (converted from the seeds' alpha-linolenic acid, or ALA). These compounds suppress the production of interleukin-1, tumor necrosis factor, and leukotriene B4 from monocytes and polymorphonuclear leukocytes. Flaxseed is also the richest known source of the phytoestrogen lignans.

COMMON USAGE

Accepted uses: Commission E approves of the use of flaxseed for the treatment of colons damaged by laxative abuse, irritable colon, and diverticulitis. Flaxseed in the diet is nutritional and has medicinal benefits. It traditionally has been used as a gentle bulk laxative. The ground seeds, when presoaked or taken with large quantities of water, are a palatable and valuable for relieving benign and atonic constipation. Flaxseed is also approved for use as a mucilage for gastritis and enteritis. Commission E also approves of flaxseed topically as a cataplasm for local inflammation; the mucilage from the freshly ground flower or boiled seeds is applied directly to mild rashes to pain relief. Boiled seeds also can serve as a base for enemas as part of the treatment for chronic prostatitis.

Unproven uses: Flaxseed can modestly reduce serum total and low-density lipoprotein cholesterol concentrations, reduce postprandial glucose absorption, and decrease certain markers of inflammation. The oil from flaxseed is used for its antiplatelet activity, for which there is documentation of possible effectiveness in adults. Trials indicate that the oil decreases the tendency of platelets to aggregate. Although occasionally used for rheumatoid arthritis, flaxseed products have shown little consistent ability to improve pain, stiffness, and other symptoms.

CONTRAINDICATIONS

Flaxseed should not be taken in cases of ileus (intestinal obstruction), thyroid insufficiency, or hypersensitivity to the seed.

WARNINGS/PRECAUTION

Inflammatory bowel conditions: Flaxseed should be preswollen before use in such cases.

Identification (flaxseed versus linseed): "Flaxseed" refers to products for human consumption while "linseed oil" refers to seed products that have been denatured and are unfit for human consumption. They are used in commercial products, such as paints and varnishes.

Pregnancy and breastfeeding: Scientific evidence for the safe use of flaxseed during pregnancy is not available. Dietary flaxseed oil appears to have no effect on breast milk and is likely safe for use while breastfeeding.

DRUG INTERACTIONS

Drugs of all types: Absorption may be impaired when taken concomitantly due to the mucilage and cellulose in flaxseed.

ADVERSE REACTIONS

There are no known side effects as long as flaxseed products are taken with sufficient amounts of liquid. Allergic reactions with anaphylaxis are possible, however.

ADMINISTRATION AND DOSAGE

Flaxseed is supplied as whole or crushed seeds, powder, or oil. It is administered orally, topically, or rectally.

Adults

Constipation: whole or ground seeds are taken orally 2-3 times daily, 1 tablespoon with 150mL of liquid. Take with large quantities of water, or presoak seeds overnight.

As a demulcent: 1 tablespoon seeds to 1 cup water (about 30g-50g seeds to a liter of water), with liquid poured off after seeds stand in cold water for 20-30 minutes.

Hyperlipidemia: As 35g-50g seeds daily in muffins or breads or 35g-50g seeds daily with adequate water.

Inflammation: 30g-50g flaxseed flour as a moist heat compress.

Prostatitis, chronic: Boiled seeds can serve as a base for enemas as part of the treatment

Pediatrics

Dosing information is not available.

Garlic

EFFECTS

Garlic cloves grow on the plant *Allium sativum L*, and have demonstrated antimicrobial properties as well as positive cardiovascular effects associated with antihyperlipidemic actions.

COMMON USAGE

Accepted uses: Garlic is approved by Commission E for the treatment of hyperlipidemia, arteriosclerosis, and hypertension. Many sources recommend garlic for its ability to reduce mortality from cardiovascular disease, a likely function of its apparent ability to lower cholesterol (including low-density lipoprotein) and high blood pressure, and to prevent and potentially reverse arteriosclerosis. Studies that demonstrate positive cardiovascular risk reduction used products delivering a sufficient dosage of allicin—the ingredient responsible for the easily identifiable odor of garlic.

Unproven uses: Garlic's value for infectious conditions is supported by its antimicrobial and immune-enhancing actions. It is possibly effective in fighting certain cancers. There are inconclusive data on its effectiveness for angina, the common cold, hepatopulmonary syndrome, meningitis, occlusive arterial disease, preeclampsia, and sickle cell anemia.

CONTRAINDICATIONS

Hypersensitivity.

WARNINGS/PRECAUTIONS

Garlic supplements should be discontinued at least 10 days prior to elective surgery.

Hypersensitivity: Contact dermatitis and asthma are possible.

Post-operative bleeding: Exercise caution. Medicinal amounts of garlic have demonstrated an inhibitory effect on blood clotting, which could theoretically cause bleeding problems following surgery.

Pregnancy and breastfeeding: Garlic in greater amounts than found in reasonable consumption through foods should be avoided.

DRUG INTERACTIONS

Anticoagulants: Avoid concomitant use. Garlic may add to the effect of the anticoagulants, increasing the risk for bleeding complications.

Antiplatelet agents, low molecular weight heparins, thrombolytic agents: Avoid concomitant use due to the theoretical risk of increased bleeding risk.

Chlorzoxazone: Avoid concomitant use. Garlic oil significantly reduces the metabolism of chlorzoxazone and may reduce its effectiveness.

Coleus forskolii: Avoid concomitant use due to the risk of excessive bleeding. Regular ingestion of food products containing garlic should not pose a problem. If garlic extract is taken with concomitant use of forskolin, monitor for signs and symptoms of excessive bleeding. Garlic supplements should be discontinued at least 10 days prior to elective surgery.

Drugs induced by CYP450 2E1: Avoid concomitant use. Garlic may reduce the effectiveness of drugs metabolized through this enzyme.

Indomethacin: Avoid concomitant use due to the risk of excessive bleeding. Regular ingestion of food products containing garlic should not pose a problem. If garlic extract is taken with concomitant use of forskolin, monitor for signs and symptoms of excessive bleeding. Garlic supplements should be discontinued at least 10 days prior to elective surgery.

Protease inhibitors: Avoid concomitant use due to the ability of garlic to decreases protease inhibitor concentrations and lead to an increased risk of antiretroviral resistance and treatment failure.

ADVERSE REACTIONS

Smelly breath and body odor are common. Gastrointestinal complaints such as nausea, vomiting, diarrhea, belching, flatulence, and constipation occasionally occur. With garlic powder, headache, myalgia, and fatigue have been reported. Eye tearing may result from crushing garlic. Very high doses may induce anemia and postoperative bleeding. High doses and prolonged use may elevate liver enzymes. Anaphylaxis, asthma, contact dermatitis can occur. Bleeding resulting from anticoagulation has been reported. When used topically, contact dermatitis has been reported. Garlic "burns" have been reported in young children particularly with prolonged contact to garlic cloves.

ADMINISTRATION AND DOSAGE

Garlic is available in raw herb, capsule, and tablet forms. It is taken orally and applied topically. One garlic clove is roughly equal to 4000mcg-1g garlic. Chopping or crushing of fresh garlic cloves releases the medicinal compounds. The composition and concentration of garlic and commercially available garlic powder preparations vary widely and caution must be exercised in determining appropriate dosage regimens. The most common agent of standardization is allicin, but several other components are also active and vary by type of extraction process. "Odorless" garlic products stabilized in enteric-coated tablets provide the benefits of fresh garlic but are more socially acceptable. The products contain sulfur compounds and concentrated allin (relatively odorless) which the body converts into allicin.

Storage Note: Fresh crude garlic extract maintained at room temperature has significantly reduced antiamebic effect after a few days, while frozen or refrigerated garlic extract remains active after 21 days. Commercially available garlic capsules were not inhibitory against the growth of common pathogens (*Endamoeba histolica*).

Adults

Daily dosage: raw herb: 2g-4g, dried powder: 900mg.

Arterial occlusive disease: 600-800mg daily (capsule);

Hyperlipidemia: 900mg-1200mg dried powder daily in divided doses (standardized to 0.5%-1.3% allicin content)

Hypertension (mild): 200mg-300mg three times daily.

Pediatrics

Daily dosage: raw herb: 2g-4g, dried powder: 900mg.

Ginger

EFFECTS

Ginger (*Zingiber officinale*) has antiemetic properties.

COMMON USAGE

Approved uses: Commission E has approved ginger for treating loss of appetite, travel sickness, and dyspeptic complaints. Numerous well-designed clinical trials indicate ginger is effective in relieving and minimizing gastrointestinal distress and related nausea and vomiting due to motion sickness, chemotherapy (in most cases), and pregnancy. Ginger has traditionally been used in China and other countries for gastrointestinal symptoms. Sailors around the world used ginger in times past to alleviate motion sickness.

Unproven uses: Trials exploring the effectiveness of ginger for post-operative nausea and vomiting are inconclusive, as are those for acute chemotherapy-related symptoms. In preliminary trials, outcomes for the treatment of migraine headaches have been positive. It's not clear whether ginger can help in the treatment of osteoarthritis; no significant improvement with ginger was noted in a study that compared hip or knee pain relief with ginger as compared to placebo or ibuprofen.

CONTRAINDICATIONS

Commission E cites the use of ginger for pregnancy morning sickness as a contraindication. Other sources also recommend that ginger not be used in pregnancy or while breastfeeding.

Ginger should not be used by people with bleeding disorders or who are on anticoagulant therapy. Due to its cholagogic effect, people with gallstones should consult a physician before taking ginger. The herb is also contraindicated in people with a hypersensitivity to ginger.

WARNINGS/PRECAUTIONS

Pregnancy and breastfeeding: The American Herbal Products Association recommends against the use of ginger for nausea during pregnancy and the FDA has not evaluated the safety of ginger for use in pregnancy. However, a number of studies found no link to adverse pregnancy outcomes or teratogenicity with the use of ginger during pregnancy. Clearly more definitive research is needed. Many sources recommend that if ginger is to be used, doses be limited to 1g (or less) on a short-term basis only. For lactation, scientific evidence for safety is not available.

DRUG INTERACTIONS

Anticoagulants (including antiplatelet agents, nonsteroidal anti-inflammatory drugs, low molecular weight heparins, thrombo-

lytic agents): Caution is advised with concomitant use, as the combination with ginger could potentially increase the risk of bleeding.

ADVERSE REACTIONS

Mainly gastrointestinal reactions including heartburn, gas, reflux, and bloating. Daily doses of up to 6g ginger cause no apparent side effects. However, administration of 6g or more of dried powdered ginger daily has been shown to cause some gastric distress and could lead to ulcer formation. Allergic reactions have been reported. In addition, the risk of bleeding may increase with the extensive use of ginger; clinical trials have shown a significant effect on platelet aggregation following a single oral dose of 10g powered ginger. Other findings suggest that daily ingestion of more than 4g dried ginger, or 15g raw ginger root, could alter blood coagulation. Smaller daily doses using raw ginger, cooked ginger, and dried ginger, show no significant effect on platelet aggregation.

ADMINISTRATION AND DOSAGE

Ginger is taken orally and is available in capsule, oil, raw root, tablet, tincture, powder, syrup, and other forms. Most clinical research studies have used 1g-2g dry, powdered ginger root. Practically speaking, this is a small dose of ginger considering that it is commonly consumed in India at a daily dose of 8g-10g, albeit typically in other forms such as fresh root. Commercial preparations vary widely in chemical composition and often contain adulterants. Standard dosing regimens for drug-induced and postoperative nausea and vomiting, arthritis, and migraine headache are not available.

Adults

Dyspepsia: 2g-4g

Pregnancy-related nausea and vomiting: 1g capsule/powder daily for up to 4 days

Motion sickness: 0.5g-1g taken 30 minutes before travel or every 4 hours for continuing symptoms

Nausea or vomiting of unknown cause: 0.5g-2g

Pediatrics

No information is available.

Ginkgo

EFFECTS

Ginkgo biloba has antioxidant, anti-inflammatory, and cognition-enhancing properties. It is believed to work in several ways, from increasing blood flow to preventing membrane damage by free radicals, and providing platelet activating factor antagonism. Ginkgo biloba is the world's oldest living tree species. Medicinal use of the leaf can be traced back to ancient Chinese medical texts.

COMMON USAGE

Accepted uses: Commission E approves of ginkgo formulations for the treatment of dementia, peripheral arterial disease (including intermittent claudication), vertigo, and tinnitus. It is widely used (and possibly effective) for cognition problems, acute mountain sickness, ocular disease, premenstrual syndrome, schizophrenia, and vitiligo.

Unproven uses: Data are inconclusive for its use against cancer, as an asthma treatment, and for deafness, erectile dysfunction, hyperlipidemia, exposure to radiation, Raynaud's disease, and drug-induced sexual dysfunction. Use for tinnitus, among other conditions, appears to be inconsistent. Animal or in vitro data

support ginkgo in the treatment of arteriosclerosis, stress, and cardiovascular disease.

Ginkgo leaves have been used in traditional Chinese medicine for their ability to "benefit the brain," or cerebral vascular insufficiency and dementia (including Alzheimer's disease). Modern clinical trials are mixed on the effectiveness and safety for these uses. Ginkgo is popular for treating memory impairment and improving cognitive function, although data similarly are mixed on effectiveness and safety.

CONTRAINDICATIONS

Due to the increased risk for bleeding, ginkgo is contraindicated when using medicines such as aspirin, ticlopidine, and others that alter blood (platelet) counts and coaguability. It should not be used in cases of hypersensitivity to any parts of the plant or its constituents.

WARNINGS/PRECAUTIONS

Chronic use or high dose: Avoid prolonged use, as ginkgo has been associated with an increased bleeding time and heightened risk of spontaneous hemorrhage. The American Herbal Products Association ranks ginkgo seed as class 2d, meaning that recommended dose should not be exceeded and long-term use avoided.

Handling of fruit: Contact dermatitis may occur following handling of ginkgo fruit (or fruit pulp), which is a part of the plant that is not used medicinally. Symptoms include irritation of mucous membranes with itching, edema, and pustule formation. Reaction usually subsides within 7-10 days.

Seizure disorder: Avoid ginkgo leaf and its extracts. People with such a disorder, or who take a drug that lowers the seizure threshold, could develop seizure problems.

Surgery: Consider discontinuing prior to (elective) surgery given the increased risk of postoperative bleeding. Ginkgo can act as a potent inhibitor of platelet-activating factor.

Pregnancy and breastfeeding: Insufficient information is available; extreme caution is advised.

DRUG INTERACTIONS

Anticoagulants, antiplatelet agents, low molecular weight heparins, thrombolytic agents: Avoid concomitant use due to the increased risk of bleeding.

Anticonvulsants: Avoid concomitant use due to reduced anticonvulsant effectiveness.

Buspirone: Avoid concomitant use due to changes in mental status observed.

Insulin: Avoid concomitant use due to the theoretical risk of altered insulin effectiveness.

Monoamine oxidase inhibitors: Avoid concomitant use due to the (theoretically increased) risk of side effects from monoamine oxidase inhibition.

Nicardipine: Avoid concomitant use due to the risk of reduced drug effectiveness.

Nifedipine: Avoid concomitant use due to the increased risk of nifedipine side effects.

Nonsteroidal anti-inflammatory agents: Avoid concomitant use due to the increased risk of bleeding.

Papaverine: Avoid concomitant use due to the risk of potentiation of papaverine therapeutic and adverse effects.

Selective serotonin reuptake inhibitors: Avoid concomitant use due to the (theoretical) increased risk of serotonin syndrome with such possible reactions as hypertension, hyperthermia, mental status changes, and myoclonus.

St. John's wort: Avoid concomitant use due to possible changes in mental status.

Thiazide diuretics: Avoid concomitant use due to the risk of increased blood pressure.

Trazadone: Avoid concomitant use due to the risk of excessive sedation and potential coma.

ADVERSE REACTIONS

Several reports indicate of a risk of bleeding (including cerebrovascular bleeding) and related complications. Also possible are tachycardia and arrhythmia, as well as gastrointestinal upset and nausea, headache, and dizziness. Allergic reactions are rare, although contact dermatitis has been reported following use of ginkgo fruit or pulp (not the leaves). Stevens-Johnson syndrome has occurred. Ginkgo may lower the point (threshold) at which a seizure may occur. Circulatory disturbances and phlebitis may occur if ginkgo is injected.

ADMINISTRATION AND DOSAGE

The part of the ginkgo tree used for medicinal purposes is the leaf. Concentration of ginkgolides and bilobalide vary in relation to the time of year. Commission E restricts ginkgolic acid concentration to 5ppm (parts per million). Most commercial extracts are standardized to contain 24% ginkgo flavonglycosides and 6% terpene lactones. Ginkgo is available to be taken orally as a capsule, extract, powder, tablet, or tea

Adults

Cerebral insufficiency or cognition issues: 120mg-150mg in THREE divided doses.

Dementia: 120mg-240mg in two or three divided doses.

Peripheral vascular disease: 120mg-160mg in two or three divided doses, up to 240mg/day.

Tinnitus: 120mg-160mg in two or three divided doses.

Vertigo: 120mg-160mg in two or three divided doses.

Pediatrics

No information is available.

Ginseng

EFFECTS

Asian ginseng *(Panax ginseng)* is an immune system stimulant. It has demonstrated the following properties: adaptogenic (provides increased resistance to physical, chemical, or biological stress), antineoplastic, antiplatelet, antiviral, gluco-regulatory, and cardiac inotropic. It also has shown the ability to stimulate enzyme reactions, hemostatic actions, hepatoprotective actions, hypoglycemic activity, platelet adhesiveness, radioprotective (radiation-protectant) actions (possible), RNA synthesis, corticotrophin secretion, and protein synthesis. Less information is available on the related American ginseng *(Panax quinquefolium*; also commonly referred to as western ginseng and North American ginseng), which is reported to have antidiabetic, antioxidant and possible hypotensive and liver-protective actions.

COMMON USAGE

Accepted uses: Commission E gives it a positive evaluation for use as a tonic for fatigue, debility, and declining concentration, and for use during convalescence. It has been used medicinally in China for millennia and is in the pharmacopoeia of many countries (Australia, China, France, Germany, Japan, Switzerland). It is used widely to enhance mental and physical well-being. Some trials in humans show positive results for ginseng to improve blood alcohol levels, lower serum cholesterol levels and blood glucose, and control hemoglobin A_{1c} in non-insulin dependent diabetes.

Unproven uses: Ginseng may alleviate post-menopausal symptoms. Some studies show improved endurance, stamina, and mental ability, and possible effectiveness for enhanced cognitive function, immune system stimulation, and male infertility. Possible tumor-preventive properties have been identified. However, numerous analyses in the West fail to consistently find effectiveness of ginseng for most uses. There is no Commission E monograph for American ginseng, which is commonly used for many of the same purposes as *Panax ginseng*. It was long used by Native Americans and others to increase physical and mental endurance, for stress-relief, for its hypoglycemic effects, and to ease menopausal symptoms. A preliminary open-label study indicated some subjective improvement in children with attention deficit hyperactivity disorder (ADHD).

CONTRAINDICATIONS

Ginseng is contraindicated in people with hypersensitivity to the herb, in people with hypertension, diabetes, or those predisposed to hypoglycemia.

WARNINGS/PRECAUTION

Blood pressure: Ginseng may increase blood pressure and alter control in patients with hypertension.

Diabetes: Ginseng may lower blood glucose levels in diabetic as well as nondiabetic individuals; caution is advised in people with diabetes or those predisposed to hypoglycemia.

Ginseng abuse syndrome: A constellation of symptoms consisting of hypertension, nervousness, insomnia, morning diarrhea, and skin eruptions may occur after 1 to 3 weeks of ingestion of 3g/day of *Panax ginseng* root.

Hyperactivity: *Ginseng* should be used with caution in patients who are hyperactive or are taking stimulants like caffeine.

Laboratory modifications: Ginseng may have the potential to generate false increases in digoxin concentrations. Alert clinician to potential for this interaction.

Prior to surgery: Ginseng may interfere with blood coagulation; discontinue use one to two weeks prior to elective surgery.

Pregnancy and breastfeeding: Scientific evidence for the safe use of ginseng during pregnancy or while breastfeeding is not available.

DRUG INTERACTIONS

Albendazole: Exercise caution in combining with ginseng due to reduced intestinal concentration of drug.

Anticoagulants: Avoid concomitant use of ginseng due to risk of decreased drug efficacy. A recent study in health individuals found that American ginseng reduced the effect of the anticoagulant warfarin.

Antidiabetic agents: Exercise caution in concomitant use with ginseng given the (theoretical) risk of increased hypoglycemia.

Drugs metabolized by CYP450 or CYP34A: Herb-mediated modulation of CYP450 activity may underlie interactions with *Panax ginseng* and medications metabolized in this way. CYP activity may decrease in older individuals, many of whom take numerous medications; caution is advised. Also see nifedipine, below.

Estrogen (topical or oral): Avoid concomitant use with any type of ginseng given the (theoretical) risk of additive estrogen effects.

Ethanol: Avoid concomitant use due to (theoretical) risk of additive estrogenic effects.

Loop diuretics: Avoid concomitant use due to increased risk of diuretic resistance.

Monoamine oxidase inhibitors: Avoid concomitant use of ginseng due to increased risk of insomnia, tremor, headache, agitation, and worsening of depression. Separate use by several weeks.

Nifedipine: Exercise caution in combining with ginseng due to increased risk of drug side effects. Other drugs metabolized in a similar way (by CYP34A) may be similarly affected.

Opioid analgesics: Exercise caution in combining with ginseng due to potential for reduced drug effectiveness.

ADVERSE REACTIONS

Possible adverse effects include nervousness, gastrointestinal upset or diarrhea, insomnia, headache, nausea, vomiting, edema, euphoria, vaginal bleeding, skin eruptions and ulcerations, blood pressure problems, and a so-called "Ginseng abuse syndrome." Estrogenic effects have been observed with ginseng products, though the exact type of ginseng (ie, American, Panax, Siberian) was unclear.

ADMINISTRATION AND DOSAGE

Commission E recommends that *Panax ginseng* generally be used for up to 3 months. American ginseng is taken for longer periods of time to generate an effect. For *Panax ginseng,* a two-week break should be observed between all ginseng courses. Dosing can be challenging because commercial ginseng preparations can vary widely in their contents. *Panax ginseng* is available in capsule, powdered root, tablet, tea, and tincture forms for oral use. *American ginseng* is available several forms including in capsule, leaf, powdered root, tablet, tea, and tincture forms for oral use. It is not typically used for its short-term effects but instead for long-term actions.

Adults

Daily dosage (Panax ginseng): 500mg-2g dry root in two divided doses; 200mg-600mg. solid extract; 1 cup tea up to 3 times daily for 3-4 weeks. 3cups/day decoction from powder, to prepare put 0.5 tsp powdered root in a cup of water, bring to a boil, and simmer gently 10 minutes, cool slightly.

Emotional or physical stress (American ginseng): 2oz-4oz cold infusion three times daily; 10-20 drops alcoholic extract three times daily; 20-40 drops cultivated roots three times daily; 30-60 drops leaf preparations three times daily.

Hyperglycemia: 3g/day (capsule).

Pediatrics

No information is available.

Goldenseal

EFFECTS

Goldenseal (*Hydrastis canadensis L*) has demonstrated the following properties in animal and in vitro studies: antibiotic, anti-infective, antineoplastic, anti-diarrheal, anti-inflammatory, antimuscarinic, anticonvulsant, antipyretic, astringent, sedative, hypotensive, uterotonic, carminative, and choloretic actions. Relatively higher doses produce cardiac stimulation, diuretic, muscle relaxant, hemostatic, and central nervous system depressant effects. Key compounds called alkaloids in goldenseal are berberine and hydrastine.

COMMON USAGE

Unproven uses: Once extensively used by Native Americans, goldenseal is commonly used today for treating infections of the gastrointestinal tract (including acute and infectious diarrhea), upper respiratory tract, and genitourinary tract. Several clinical studies indicate effectiveness for the herb for acute infectious diarrhea caused by numerous pathogens including *Escherichia coli* (traveler's diarrhea), *Shigella dysenteriae* (shigellosis), *Salmonella paratyphi* (food poisoning), *Giardia lamblia* (giardiasis), and *Vibrio cholerae* (cholera). In human studies, the berberine in goldenseal was effective in treating trachoma, an infectious eye disease.

Goldenseal has also been shown in clinical trials to stimulate the secretion of bile and bilirubin (thus possibly effective for cholecystitis). Berberine exhibits potent anticancer activity both directly by killing tumor cells and indirectly by stimulating white blood cells. Animal studies demonstrate antispasmodic activity. Goldenseal has been studied in animals for its effects on diabetes, fever, excessive menstrual flow, and muscle relaxation. Also used for cirrhosis of the liver, and as an adjunct to standard cancer therapy.

CONTRAINDICATIONS

Goldenseal is contraindicated in pregnancy, in cases of glucose-6-phosphate-dehydrogenase deficiency, and hypersensitivity to the herb.

WARNINGS/PRECAUTIONS

Labeling problems: Variation in alkaloid (berberine and hydrastine) content in goldenseal products is extreme in some cases. Overuse has depleted much of the goldenseal supply in North America. Other berberine-containing plants (Oregon Grape Root, Barberry, others) may be substituted in some cases.

Infectious diarrhea: Due to the serious health consequences of incompletely treated infectious diarrhea, berberine-containing plants such as goldenseal should only be used as an adjunct—not a replacement for—standard antibiotic therapy.

Pregnancy and breastfeeding: Not to be used during pregnancy. Scientific evidence for its safe use during lactation is not available.

DRUG INTERACTIONS

Drugs metabolized by CYP450: In vitro studies found that goldenseal inhibited CYP450 3A4; caution is advised when co-administered with drugs that metabolize this enzyme.

ADVERSE REACTIONS

At high doses, irritation of the mouth, stomach, and mucous membranes. Extra high doses may be toxic. Jaundice and hemolytic anemia are a risk in people with glucose-6-phosphage-dehydrogenase deficiency.

ADMINISTRATION AND DOSAGE

If using a standardized extract, look for one containing at least 8%-10% alkaloids or 5% hydrastine. Goldenseal is taken orally and is supplied in dried root (powdered or cut), as a bulk tea, tincture, fluid extract, and solid (dried powdered) extract forms, among others.

Adults

Antibacterial effects: 1.25mL-5mL (¼ tsp-1 tsp) fluid extract; 650mg or 10 grains powdered root; 325mg-530mg or 5-8 grains solid extract; 0.25mL-5mL (½ tsp-1 tsp tincture;

Traveler's diarrhea: 500mg-1,000mg root capsule three times daily.

Mouth or throat sores: steep 1 tsp powder for topical use in 8oz boiling water 15 minutes, strain, cool, and swish around mouth or gargle, spit out.

For commercial topical formulations, follow container instructions.

Pediatrics

Information is not available.

Grape Seed Extract

EFFECTS

Grape seed extract has demonstrated powerful antioxidant activity; the membrane of the seed is a rich source of proanthyocyanidins (also known as procyanidins or procyanidolic oligomers, or PCOs), a highly beneficial group of plant flavonoids. Grape seed extract has shown vascular, cytotoxic, chemopreventative, and cytoprotective effects. In experimental models, the antioxidant activity of PCOs from grape seed extract is approximately 50 times greater than that of vitamins C and E.

COMMON USAGE

Unproven uses: Most studies of grape seed extract have been in vitro or in animals. Based on the handful of small but relatively good human trials, there is possible benefit with grape seed extract for venous and capillary disorders such as venous insufficiency and varicose veins. Grape seed extract also is used for eye conditions such as retina disorders, macular degeneration, and diabetic retinopathy.

Excellent antioxidant effects of grape seed extract may also help to protect against chronic degenerative diseases such as atherosclerosis and certain cancers. It may improve resistance to glare and promote recovery from exposure to eye strain such as bright light, and ocular stress, according to data of fair quality. PCOs from grape seeds (and pine bark) have been marketed and promoted in France for decades to improve retinopathies, venous insufficiency, and vascular fragility.

CONTRAINDICATIONS

Grape seed extract is contraindicated in people with hypersensitivity to it.

WARNINGS/PRECAUTIONS

Pregnancy and breastfeeding: Scientific evidence for the safe use of grape seed extract during pregnancy and while breastfeeding is not available.

DRUG INTERACTIONS

No human interaction data are available.

ADVERSE REACTIONS

Information on adverse reactions is not available.

ADMINISTRATION AND DOSAGE

Grape seed extract is taken orally in extract, capsule, or geltab forms. The extract typically contains up to 95% procyanidolic oligomers (PCOs), and PCO content is often indicated on dosing forms.

Adults

Daily dosage: 50mg for preventative antioxidant effect and 150mg-300mg for therapeutic antioxidant effect.

Pediatrics

No information is available.

Green Tea

EFFECTS

Green tea is unfermented and unprocessed tea, and for health effects is considered superior to both oolong (partially fermented tea) and black (fully fermented tea). All varieties are from the same tea plant (*Camellia sinensis*). Green tea specifically has antioxidant, antibacterial, and anticarcinogenic properties. In vitro it decreases DNA damage. Green tea contains six times more antioxidants than black tea.

Green tea polyphenols, which have been investigated for medicinal qualities due to antioxidant and other activities, include epigallocatechin-3-gallate (EGCG; the major constituent, with highest concentration in the leaf bud and first leaves), epigallocatechin (EGC), epicatechin-3-gallate (ECG), epicatechin (EC), and catechin. The usual concentration of total polyphenols in dried green tea leaf is about 8-12%.

COMMON USAGE

Unproven uses: Green tea is used to prevent cancer and heart disease. A 2005 systematic review of clinical trials found that consumption of five or more cups of green tea daily shows a slight trend toward prevention of breast cancer recurrence in early stage (I and II); however, more data are needed to generate definitive findings. A 2004 systematic review of studies found a protective effect for regular green tea consumption on the development of adenomatous polyps and chronic atrophis gastritis formations, but no definitive epidemiological support for a role in preventing stomach and intestinal cancers.

Green tea may be helpful in preventing dental caries and periodontal disease, and in preventing and treating clostridial diarrheal disease. It may help promote the growth of "friendly" bacteria in the gut microflora. The use of green tea for weight loss, beyond the action of its caffeine content, is unclear.

Topical formulas are starting to appear in antioxidant and anti-aging creams and lotions, but their effectiveness remains unclear.

CONTRAINDICATIONS

The use of green tea is contraindicated in people with hypersensitivity to it, and should be used with caution (due to caffeine content) in children and infants.

WARNINGS/PRECAUTIONS

Excessive or prolonged consumption: Not recommended due to caffeine content.

Psychiatric disorders: Excessive consumption of green tea, which does contain some caffeine, has the potential to precipitate or exacerbate psychiatric disorders.

Pregnancy and breastfeeding: Due to caffeine content, minimize consumption during pregnancy. Information on its safety during breastfeeding is unavailable.

DRUG INTERACTIONS

Anticoagulants: Combine with caution. Green tea may interfere with the action of warfarin and other anticoagulants.

ADVERSE REACTIONS

Green tea is not associated with any significant side effects. However, as with any caffeine-containing beverage, high intake of green tea may result in irritability, anxiety, insomnia, and nervousness. Also possible with extremely high intake are diuresis, stomach upset, fast heartbeat, rapid breathing, muscle twitching, arrhythmias, palpitations, and flushing.

ADMINISTRATION AND DOSAGE

Available as dried leaves, capsules, and tea. Increasingly, topical formulations are available. Light steaming of the fresh cut leaf produces green tea. Chemical composition of green tea varies with climate, season, horticultural practices, and age of the leaf. Dosage ranges must be employed as guidelines.

Adults

Daily dosage: 300mg-400mg. Most Japanese and other green tea-drinking cultures consume about 3 cups daily, or 3g soluble components (providing 240mg-320mg polyphenols). Green tea extract (standardized to 80% total polyphenol and 55% epigallo-catechin gallate content) provides equivalent of 300mg-400mg.

Pediatrics

No information is available.

Hawthorn

EFFECTS

Hawthorn (*Crataegus oxyacantha*) is an inotropic agent. It has vasodilator, cardiotonic, and antilipidemic effects. Extracts are useful in treating mild forms of cardiac insufficiency by generating positive inotropy, prolonging the myocardial refractory period, and vasodilating coronary and skeletal muscle vessels.

The compounds in hawthorn are believed to reduce blood cholesterol concentration and lessen myocardial oxygen consumption due in part to antioxidant effects. It is listed as a flavonoid drug in Germany (its flowers and leaves contain up to 2.5% flavonoids). Much of its action on the cardiovascular system is attributed to flavonoid constituents. Certain extracts prevent elevation of such plasma lipids as total cholesterol, triglycerides, and LDL and VLDL fractions, and upregulate LDL receptors in the liver.

COMMON USAGE

Approved uses: Commission E approves of hawthorn leaf with flowers for treatment of heart failure (Stage II NYHA). This herb is well-studied for cardiovascular disease and is commonly used in combination with cardiac glycosides to potentiate their effects and thereby lessen the dose of cardiac glycoside drugs. Clinical trials support its use for mild to moderate congestive heart failure.

Unproven uses: More research is needed to determine hawthorn's value in treating hypertension, atherosclerosis, hyperlipidemia, asthma, arrhythmia in the elderly, and orthostatic hypertension. Due to its high flavonoid content, it may be used to decrease capillary fragility, lessen inflammation, and prevent collagen destruction of joints. The herb been used as coffee substitute and to flavor cigarettes.

CONTRAINDICATIONS

Hawthorn is contraindicated in cases of hypersensitivity or a history of allergic reaction to crataegus or any of its components. It is also contraindicated in children under age 12.

WARNINGS/PRECAUTIONS

Hawthorn is widely considered safe when used appropriately, in usual doses, for most conditions.

Pregnancy and breastfeeding: No information is available; caution is advised both for use in pregnancy and while breastfeeding.

DRUG INTERACTIONS

Antiplatelet agents: Caution is advised when taking hawthorn with antiplatelet agents due to the theoretical risk of increased bleeding. Signs and symptoms of excessive bleeding should be monitored.

Digoxin: Caution is advised in combining hawthorn with digoxin due to the theoretical risk of increased pharmacodynamic effect of digoxin. One trial showed reduced digoxin bioavailability.

ADVERSE REACTIONS

Infrequently, hot flashes and gastrointestinal upset occur. Also possible are palpitations, dyspnea, headache, epistaxis, and dizziness.

ADMINISTRATION AND DOSAGE

Oral forms include capsules, tablets, teas, tinctures, and solutions. Dosage depends upon the preparation used.

Adults

Cardiac insufficiency: 160mg-900mg dried extract in three divided doses daily for at least 6 weeks: *Tincture* (standardized 1:5): 4mL-5mL three times daily.

Pediatrics

Not recommended for children under age 12.

Kava Kava

EFFECTS

Kava kava (*Piper methysticum*) is a perennial shrub from the South Pacific that grows in the wild and has demonstrated anxyiolytic and sedative effects.

COMMON USAGE

Accepted uses: Commission E has approved the use of kava kava for treating nervous anxiety and stress, as well as restlessness, tension, and agitation. The kava kava extract WS 1490, and possibly other extracts, were shown to be effective for anxiety disorders in a 2005 meta-analysis.

Unproven uses: Kava kava is also used to counter insomnia, menopausal symptoms, and muscular aches and pains. Data (animal and in vitro) supports its use for bacterial and fungal infection, muscle tension and pain, cerebral artery occlusion, and seizures.

CONTRAINDICATIONS

Kava kava is contraindicated during pregnancy and while breastfeeding, in people with liver dysfunction or who take medications that affect the liver, and in cases of depression. Due to case reports of kava kava-related dyskinesia, it should not be used by people with neurologic disorders. It is also contraindicated in those with a hypersensitivity to kava or any of its components.

WARNINGS/PRECAUTIONS

Alcohol: Combine with caution. Kava kava and its extracts may intensify the effects of alcohol. Combining the two may result in fatigue, hangover, or drowsiness.

Extended use: Regular use of kava for longer than 3 months is not recommended.

Hepatotoxicity: In 2003, The FDA informed healthcare professionals and issued a consumer advisory noting that products containing herbal extracts of kava kava have been implicated in Europe in at least 25 cases of serious liver toxicity including hepatitis, cirrhosis, and liver failure. These cases of liver damage are rare but serious enough to prompt regulatory agencies in Germany, Switzerland, Canada, and France to either issue warnings or remove kava kava-containing products from the marketplace.

Motor skills: Alteration in motor reflexes and judgment, and a morning "hangover" or fatigue following start of kava kava use.

Pregnancy and breastfeeding: The American Herbal Products Association states that kava kava should not be taken during pregnancy or while nursing.

DRUG INTERACTIONS

Anticoagulant, antiplatelet agents, low molecular weight heparins, thrombolytic agents: Avoid concomitant use due to the (theoretical) risk of increased bleeding.

Barbiturates: Avoid concomitant use. Animal data indicate a potential for increased central nervous system depression.

Benzodiazepines: Avoid concomitant use. A case report indicates risk for increased central nervous system depression.

Centrally acting muscle relaxants: Avoid concomitant use due to (theoretical) risk of increased central nervous system depression.

Dopamine agonists and antagonists: Avoid concomitant use due to (theoretical) risk of reduced drug effectiveness.

Drugs metabolized by CYP450: In vitro studies found that kava kava inhibited CYP450 CYP 1A, 2C9, 2C19, 2D6, 3A4, and 4A9/11. Caution is advised when coadministering the herb with drugs dependent on CYP enzymes for their elimination.

Ethanol: Avoid concomitant use. Animal data indicate risk for increased central nervous system depression and hepatotoxicity.

Hepatotoxic drugs: Avoid concomitant use due to (theoretical) increased risk of liver damage.

Monoamine oxidase inhibitors: Avoid concomitant use due to (theoretical) increased risk of adverse effects from excessive MAO inhibition.

Opioid analgesics: Avoid concomitant use due to (theoretical) risk of increased central nervous system depression.

Phenothiazines: Avoid concomitant use due to (theoretical) additive dopamine antagonist side effects.

ADVERSE REACTIONS

Most cases of adverse reactions are mild, infrequent, transient, and reversible. However, rare but very serious adverse reactions include hepatitis, cirrhosis, jaundice, loss of appetite, and liver failure. Kava kava and its extracts may intensify the effects of alcohol; combining the two may result in fatigue, hangover, or drowsiness. Also reported are mild (and reversible) gastrointestinal complaints, dry mouth, weight loss, various hypersensitivity reactions, and central nervous system complaints (drowsiness, dizziness, headache), as well as near vision abnormalities, pupil dilation, and problems with eye movement coordination. Long-term and high-dosage use of kava kava may result in kava kava "dermopathy," a reversible darkening or yellowing of the skin with scaling and flaking. Erythema of the face and upper body may occur after drinking kava kava.

ADMINISTRATION AND DOSAGE

Kava kava is taken orally in capsule, dried root powder, and tablet forms. Different strengths for kava kava are determined by the variety used, freshness and plant maturity, the soil and climate conditions in which it was grown, and the method of preparing the herb.

Adults

Anxiety: 105mg-210mg kavalactones (extract WS1490, standardized to 70% kavalactone content) daily for 3-4 weeks. However, avoid continuous use of medicinal forms for longer than 3 months.

Pediatrics

No information is available.

Licorice

EFFECTS

The primary medicinal effects of licorice (*Glycyrrhizic glabra*) are anti-ulcer, anti-inflammatory, and expectorant. Licorice also has antiplatelet, antifungal, and antibacterial properties. It has aldolase reductase inhibitor actions as well, and inhibits calcium ions.

COMMON USAGE

Accepted uses: Commission E approves of licorice for the treatment of gastric/duodenal ulcers and catarrhs of the upper respiratory tract. Licorice is a classic sweetener and food flavoring. It is commonly found in cold and flu remedies and is used for bronchitis. Licorice has a long history of use for gastric ulcers, and appears to benefit peptic ulcerations.

Unproven uses: Licorice also is used for symptoms of menopause and premenstrual syndrome, and for stimulating endogenous production of and prolongation of cortical hormones—a quality considered beneficial for numerous conditions. It may reduce dental plaque and treat herpes zoster infections, but more research is needed. An intravenous formula of licorice (glycyrrhizin) has been used in treating hepatitis and in preventing the development of hepatocellular carcinoma.

CONTRAINDICATIONS

The use of licorice is contraindicated in people with hypertension, diabetes, cirrhosis of the liver, hypertonia, hypokalemia, hypertonic neuromuscular disorders, severe renal insufficiency, or hypersensitivity to it or any of its components.

WARNINGS/PRECAUTIONS

Chewing tobacco: Chewing tobacco may contain flavoring agents with derivatives of glycyrrhetinic acid (1.5mg-4.1mg). Avoid excess ingestion, as it may lead to changes in electrolytes and calcium in the body.

Prolonged or excessive ingestion: Do not use licorice for prolonged periods of time unless under the care of a qualified health practitioner. Avoid excess ingestion of licorice chewing gum, which may contain up to 24mg glycyrrhizinic acid in each gum pack and may lead to alterations in electrolytes and calcium.

Drugs metabolized by the enzyme CYP450 3A4: Practice caution, as licorice inhibited this enzyme during in vitro testing.

Pregnancy and breastfeeding: The use of licorice is contraindicated.

DRUG INTERACTIONS

Alpha-1 adrenergic blockers: Avoid concomitant use due to the (theoretical) risk of reduced drug effectiveness.

Angiotensin converting enzyme inhibitors: Avoid concomitant use due to the (theoretical) risk of reduced drug effectiveness.

Angiotensin II receptor antagonists: Avoid concomitant use due to the (theoretical) risk of reduced drug effectiveness.

Antiarrhythmics: Avoid concomitant use due to the (theoretical) increased risk of arrhythmia.

Anticoagulants, antiplatelet agents, low molecular weight heparins, thrombolytic agents: Avoid concomitant use due to the (theoretical) increased risk of bleeding.

Antidiabetic agents: Avoid concomitant use due to the (theoretical) risk of reduced drug effectiveness.

Beta-adrenergic blockers: Avoid concomitant use due to the (theoretical) risk for reduced drug efficacy.

Calcium channel blockers: Avoid concomitant use due to the (theoretical) risk for reduced drug efficacy.

Clonidine: Avoid concomitant use due to the (theoretical) risk for reduced drug efficacy.

Contraceptives (combination): Avoid concomitant use due to the increased risk of fluid retention and elevated blood pressure.

Corticosteroids: Avoid concomitant use due to the (theoretical) increased risk for adverse effects.

Digoxin: Avoid concomitant use due to the increased for drug toxicity.

Diuretics: Avoid concomitant use due to the increased risk of hypokalemia and reduced drug effectiveness.

Estrogens: Avoid concomitant use due to the increased risk of edema and hypertension.

Guanabenz: Avoid concomitant use due to the (theoretical) risk for reduced drug efficacy.

Guanadrel: Avoid concomitant use due to the (theoretical) risk for reduced drug efficacy.

Guanethidine: Avoid concomitant use due to the (theoretical) risk for reduced drug efficacy.

Guanfacine: Avoid concomitant use due to the (theoretical) risk for reduced drug efficacy.

Hyrdralazine: Avoid concomitant use due to the (theoretical risk for reduced drug efficacy.

Insulin: Avoid concomitant use due to the (theoretical) increased risk for hypokalemia and sodium retention.

Laxatives: Avoid concomitant use due to the (theoretical) increased risk of hypokalemia.

Methyldopa: Avoid concomitant use due to the (theoretical) risk of reduced drug efficacy.

Minoxidil: Avoid concomitant use due to the (theoretical) risk of reduced drug efficacy.

Monoamine oxidase inhibitors: Avoid concomitant use due to the (theoretically) increased risk of adverse effects from excessive drug inhibition.

Potassium: Avoid concomitant use as large amounts of licorice may lead to resistance to potassium supplementation.

Reserpine: Avoid concomitant use of licorice and any antihypertensive drug, including reserpine, as it could theoretically reduce reserpine effectiveness.

Testosterone: Avoid concomitant use. In a clinical trial, licorice decreased testosterone effectiveness, resulting in decreased libido and other sexual dysfunction.

ADVERSE REACTIONS

Hypertension, sodium retention, pseudohyperaldosteronism with hypercortisolism.

ADMINISTRATION AND DOSAGE

Licorice is available in several forms, including extracts, root teas, deglycyrrhizinated chews, chewing gum, chewing tobacco, and intravenous solutions. Do note take at medicinal levels for more than 4-6 weeks; simultaneously, consume high-potassium diet.

Adults

Daily dosage: 1g-5g of root three times daily for up to 6 weeks; 2mL-4mL of extract (1:1 preparation): three times daily.

Bronchitis: 1 cup tea following each meal prepared by pouring 150mL of boiling water over 1 teaspoon (2g-4g) licorice root, simmer 5 minutes, and filter.

Chronic gastritis: 1 cup tea (see preparation above) following each meal.

Peptic ulcer: 380mg-760mg 20 minutes before meals.

Gastric/duodenal ulcer: oral Succus liquiritiae 1g-3g daily.

Upper respiratory tract catarrh: oral Succus liquiritae 0.5g-1g daily.

Pediatrics

No dosing information is available.

Milk Thistle

EFFECTS

Milk thistle (*Silybum marianum*) has renal and hepatoprotective properties due to antioxidant effects and free radical elimination. Hepatoprotective actions against chemical, environmental, and infectious toxins have been demonstrated.

COMMON USAGE

Accepted uses: Commission E gives milk thistle seeds a positive evaluation for dyspepsia (when used as a crude drug), toxic liver damage, and hepatic cirrhosis. It is also approved for use as a supportive treatment in chronic inflammatory liver disease when a standardized extract of at least 70% silymarin plus silibinin, silydianin, and silychristin. The active agent in milk thistle is silymarin. It has been used to treat acute and chronic liver problems and bile problems for more than 2,000 years.

Unproven uses: Many but not all clinical studies indicate that it has a positive hepatoprotective effect in the treatment of liver cirrhosis associated with chronic alcohol abuse or viruses (such as hepatitis B or C). Results for treatment of mushroom poisoning with silymarin are positive overall, although its true effectiveness for this purpose is difficult to determine given variations in treatment protocols in studies with adults and animals. It is commonly used for preventing gall stones. Studies are examining effectiveness for protecting against skin cancer.

CONTRAINDICATIONS

Use of milk thistle is contraindicated in people with a known hypersensitivity to it or any of its components.

WARNINGS/PRECAUTIONS

Pregnancy and breastfeeding: Milk thistle has been used safely for as long as three weeks to treat mothers with intrahepatic cholestasis of pregnancy.

DRUG INTERACTIONS

Metronidazole: Concomitant use is not recommended; in a clinical trial of healthy volunteers, the extract silymarin reduced metronidazole and active metabolite exposure. If concomitant use is necessary, metronidazole dose may need to be increased.

ADVERSE REACTIONS

Urticaria and other allergic reactions are rare.

ADMINISTRATION AND DOSAGE

Milk thistle is available in capsule, tablet, and tincture forms for oral use. (Intravenous solutions are not available in the U.S.) Note that silymarin concentrations may vary considerably.

Adults

Hepatoprotection: 420mg/day of extract (standardized to 70%-80% silymarin), divided into three doses for 6-8 weeks, followed by a maintenance dose of 280mg/day.

Cyclopeptide mushroom poisoning: Intravenous solution for parenteral administration (or oral formulation if no intravenous preparation is available) for approximately 33mg/kg/day for a mean duration of 81.67 hours.

Pediatrics

No information is available.

Saw Palmetto

EFFECTS

Saw palmetto (*Serenoa repens*) has demonstrated genitourinary effects due to its testosterone-altering properties (antiandrogenic, antiestrogenic, estrogenic). Also, as demonstrated in animal and tissue studies: anti-inflammatory, antineoplastic, cholesterol-blocking, enzyme inhibition, platelet inhibition, and protein synthesis inhibition actions.

COMMON USAGE

Approved uses: Commission E approves of saw palmetto (typically, the extract *Serenoa repens*) for the treatment of urinary problems of benign prostatic hyperplasia (BPH) stage I (abnormal frequent urination, nocturia, delayed onset of urination, and weak urinary stream) and stage II (urge to urinate and residual urine). Documentation for its use in BPH includes numerous controlled clinical trials. In one study, a Serenoa repens extract of 320mg a day for periods of 30 days to 12 months resulted in significant improvement in urine flow, dysuria, nocturia, residual urine, urgency, prostate volume, and subjective complaints.

Unproven uses: Evidence for saw palmetto's effectiveness in prostate cancer treatment is inconclusive. Other historical uses of the herb include treatment for chronic cystitis and as a mild diuretic, although the main use always has been for a variety of urinary tract conditions. Topically, saw palmetto has been used for androgen-induced acne.

CONTRAINDICATIONS

The use of saw palmetto is contraindicated in cases of hypersensitivity to it or any of its components.

WARNINGS/PRECAUTIONS

Hormone-dependent cancer: Saw palmetto has shown antiandrogenic, antiestrogenic, and estrogenic actions in animals. Caution is warranted, as no information is available about the action of this herb in people with breast cancer, prostate cancer, or other hormone-related diseases.

Pregnancy and breastfeeding: Scientific evidence for the safe use of saw palmetto during pregnancy and lactation is not available.

DRUG INTERACTIONS

Warfarin: Caution is advised due to the increased risk of bleeding likely due to the cyclooxygenase inhibition by saw palmetto.

ADVERSE REACTIONS

Pruritus, headache, dizziness, fatigue, asthenia, dry mouth, postural hypotension, nausea, abdominal pain, and other mild gastrointestinal effects. Rarely: ejaculation disorders, erectile dysfunction, and reduced libido. Estrogenic effects following treatment with the multi-ingredient PC-SPES.

ADMINISTRATION AND DOSAGE

Saw palmetto is available for oral use in capsule and tablet forms, and for topical use in ointment form. For BPH, look for extracts with proven pharmacological activity and clinical efficacy.

Adults

Daily dosage: 320mg of lipophilic extract extracted with lipophilic solvents (90% v/v) or super-critical fluid extraction from carbon dioxide

Pediatrics

No information is available.

Siberian Ginseng

EFFECTS

Siberian ginseng (*Eleutherococcus senticosus*) has demonstrated immunostimulant effects, as well as some antibacterial, antineoplastic, and antioxidant properties. Hormonal effects may occur, but human studies are lacking. Some, but not all, studies demonstrate blood sugar-reducing effects.

COMMON USAGE

Approved uses: Commission E approves of Siberian ginseng as a tonic for invigoration and fortification during times of fatigue, debility, or declining capacity for work and concentration. It is also approved for use during convalescence.

Unproven uses: Siberian ginseng is most often used for its adaptogenic effects-to improve physical stamina and enhance immune states. It is used worldwide to increase endurance, immunity, and resistance to stress. Although not proved in studies, other clinical uses include treatment for cancer, hypotension, immune system depression, and infertility. Its use for Familial Mediterranean Fever is inconclusive. Topically, an extract may slow the manifestation of skin aging, although study results are inconclusive.

CONTRAINDICATIONS

Siberian ginseng is contraindicated in people with hypertension or in those with known hypersensitivity to the herb or any of its extracts. It is also not recommended for use in people with diabetes or those with cardiac conditions such as myocardial infarction.

WARNINGS/PRECAUTIONS

Drug-lab interactions: Possible false increase in digoxin concentrations when Siberian ginseng is taken. The herb has been shown to falsely increase serum digoxin levels using the fluorescence polarization immunoassay (FPIA) and falsely decrease levels using the microparticle enzyme immunoassay (MEIA) ex vivo. Patients should be asked about their use of Siberian ginseng when unanticipated serum digoxin concentrations are obtained.

Pregnancy and breastfeeding: Scientific evidence for the safe use of Siberian ginseng during pregnancy is not available.

Stimulant use: Siberian ginseng is not recommended for patients using stimulants, even mild ones such as caffeine.

DRUG INTERACTIONS

Antidiabetic agents and insulin: the herb may alter the effects of insulin or other medications.

ADVERSE REACTIONS

In rare cases, altered heart rhythm, elevated blood pressure, palpitations, pericardial pain, tachycardia, and neuropathy. Slight drowsiness immediately after taking the extract has been reported, as has insomnia.

ADMINISTRATION AND DOSAGE

Available in capsule, ethanolic extract, powder, tablet, and tincture forms. Therapy should not exceed 3 months, although a repeat course is feasible. When used for extended periods, extract-free periods of 2-3 weeks are recommended between courses of therapy.

Adults

Daily dosage: 2g-3g tea of powdered or cut root daily or aqueous alcoholic extracts (for internal use) daily for up to 3 months; 2g-3g infusion daily in 150mL water. 2mL-3mL fluid extract

(1:1g/mL preparation) daily; 10mL-15mL tincture (1:5g/mL preparation) daily.

Pediatrics

No information is available.

St. John's Wort

EFFECTS

St. John's wort (*Hypericum perforatum*) has demonstrated anti-depressant properties as well as anxiolytic, anti-inflammatory, analgesic, and antimicrobial actions.

COMMON USAGE

Accepted uses: Commission E approves of St. John's wort for oral use to treat depressive moods, postvegetative disturbances, anxiety or nervous unrest, and dyspeptic complaints (oily preparation only). St. John's wort is used primarily for mild to moderate depression. Multiple controlled clinical trials demonstrate the effectiveness of extracts for this use (but not for major depression of moderate severity). It may reduce symptoms of seasonal affective disorder. Commission E approves of its use topically (oily preparations) for acute injuries and bruises, myalgias, and first-degree burns.

Unproven uses: St John's wort is often used as an antiviral, an antibacterial (internally and in eardrops for otitis media), and as a topical analgesic or for wound healing. A cream containing hypericum is used to treat mild to moderate atopic dermatitis. It appears to be ineffective as an antiviral agent for people with AIDS. Primarily positive results have been reported from clinical trials using St. John's wort in the treatment of acute otitis media, menopausal symptoms, obesity, fatigue, premenstrual syndrome, and to improve sleep quality and cognitive function.

CONTRAINDICATIONS

St. John's wort is contraindicated in cases of hypersensitivity or allergy to the herb or any of its constituents, as well as in people with a history of photosensitivity.

WARNINGS/PRECAUTIONS

Drug and herb interactions: St. John's wort interacts with numerous medications (see below). Caution is advised.

Fertility: Genotoxic actions are suggested but not proven. The herb is mutagenic to sperm.

Photosensitivity: Avoid direct sun exposure while taking St. John's wort in cases of previous photosensitization to any chemicals.

Pregnancy and breastfeeding: Contraindicated during pregnancy. Scientific evidence for the safe use of St. John's wort during pregnancy and lactation is not available.

DRUG INTERACTIONS

Acitretin: Avoid concomitant use due to (theoretically) increased risk of unplanned pregnancy and birth defects.

Amiodarone: Avoid concomitant use due to (theoretically) increased risk of reduced drug levels.

Aminolevulinic acid: Avoid concomitant use due to potentially increased risk of phototoxic reaction.

Anesthetics: Avoid concomitant use due to increased risk of cardiovascular collapse or delayed emergence from anesthesia.

Amsacrine: Avoid concomitant use due to possible reduced drug efficacy, as indicated by in vitro studies.

Anticoagulants: Avoid concomitant use due to possible risk of reduced anticoagulant efficacy.

Antidiabetic agents: Avoid concomitant use due to the risk of hypoglycemia.

Barbiturates: Avoid concomitant use due to the risk of decreased central nervous system depressant effect with the drug.

Benzodiazepines: Avoid concomitant use due to the risk for reduced drug efficacy.

Beta-adrenergic blockers: Avoid concomitant use due to the (theoretical) risk of reduced drug efficacy.

Buspirone: Avoid concomitant use due to the increased risk for serotonin syndrome.

Calcium channel blockers: Avoid concomitant use due to the risk of decreased drug efficacy.

Carbamazepine: Avoid concomitant use due to the risk for altered drug blood concentrations.

Chlorzoxazone: Avoid concomitant use due to the risk of reduced drug efficacy.

Clozapine: Avoid concomitant use due to the theoretically increased risk of reduced drug efficacy.

Contraceptives (combination): Avoid concomitant use due to the risk of decreased contraceptive efficacy.

Cyclophosphamide: Avoid concomitant use due to the theoretically increased risk of reduced drug efficacy.

Cyclosporine: Avoid concomitant use due to the risk of decreased drug levels and risk for acute transplant rejection.

Debrisoquin: Avoid concomitant use due the risk of reduced drug efficacy.

Digoxin: Avoid concomitant use due to the risk of reduced drug efficacy.

Drugs metabolized by CYP450 3A4, 1A2, or 2E1: Avoid concomitant use. St. John's wort could potentially decrease drug concentrations and lessen drug effectiveness.

Erlotinib: Avoid concomitant use due to the theoretically increased risk for reduced drug plasma concentrations and clinical efficacy.

Estrogens: Avoid concomitant use due to the theoretically increased risk of reduced drug efficacy.

Etoposide: Avoid concomitant use due to the risk for reduced drug efficacy.

Fenfluramine: Avoid concomitant use due to the increased risk of serotonin syndrome.

Ginkgo biloba: Avoid concomitant use given the increased risk for changes in mental status.

HMG CoA reductase inhibitors: Avoid concomitant use due the risk for reduced drug efficacy.

Imatinib: Avoid concomitant use due to the risk for elevated drug clearance.

Irinotecan: Avoid concomitant use due to the risk for reduced drug effectiveness and treatment failure.

Loperamide: Avoid concomitant use due to the risk for delirium with symptoms of confusion, agitation, and disorientation.

Methadone: Avoid concomitant use due to the risk for reduced drug levels and increased risk for withdrawal symptoms.

Monoamine oxidase inhibitors: Avoid concomitant use due to (theoretically) increased risk for serotonin syndrome or hypertensive crisis.

Nefazodone: Avoid concomitant use due to the increased risk for serotonin syndrome.

Non-nucleoside reverse transcriptase inhibitors: Avoid concomitant use due to the risk for decreased drug concentrations and the increased risk for antiretroviral resistance, and treatment failure.

Opioid analgesics: Avoid concomitant use due to the risk for increased sedation.

Paclitaxel: Avoid concomitant use due to the theoretically increased risk for reduced drug effectiveness.

Phenytoin: Avoid concomitant use due to the theoretically increased risk for reduced drug effectiveness.

Photosensitization drugs: Avoid concomitant use due to the theoretically increased risk for a photosensitivity reaction.

Protease inhibitors: Avoid concomitant use due to the risk for decreased drug concentrations and greater risk for antiretroviral resistance, and treatment failure.

Reserpine: Avoid concomitant use due to the risk for reduced drug effectiveness.

Selective serotonin reuptake inhibitors: Avoid concomitant use due to the increased risk for serotonin syndrome.

Serotonin agonists: Avoid concomitant use due to the theoretically increased risk for additive serotonergic effects and cerebral vasoconstriction disorders.

Sirolimus: Avoid concomitant use due the theoretically increased risk for subtherapeutic drug levels, resulting in possible transplant rejection.

Tacrolimus: Avoid concomitant use due the theoretically increased risk for subtherapeutic drug levels, resulting in possible transplant rejection.

Tamoxifen: Avoid concomitant use due to the theoretically increased risk for reduced drug efficacy.

Theophylline: Avoid concomitant use due to the risk for reduced drug efficacy.

Trazodone: Avoid concomitant use due to the increased risk of serotonin syndrome.

Tricyclic antidepressants: Avoid concomitant use due to the increased risk of serotonin syndrome.

Venlafaxine: Avoid concomitant use due to the theoretically increased risk for serotonin syndrome.

Verapamil: Avoid concomitant use due to the risk for decreased drug bioavailability.

ADVERSE REACTIONS

Common side effects include dry mouth, dizziness, diarrhea, nausea, fatigue, and increased sensitivity to the sun. Also possible: skin rash, frequent urination, edema, anorgasmia, hypersensitivity, neuropathy, anxiety, and hypomania. St. John's wort may elevate thyroid-stimulating hormone levels and precipitate hypothyroidism.

ADMINISTRATION AND DOSAGE

St. John's wort is available in capsule, liquid extract, tablet, and tea forms. Preparations are often standardized to hypericin (0.3%) and/or hyperforin (3%) content; marker compounds may not reflect content of other potentially biologically important compounds.

Adults

Daily dosage: The common dose for most conditions is 300mg of standardized extract (0.3% hypericin content) three times daily, or 200mcg-1,000mcg daily of hypericin.

Depression: 300mg standardized extract (0.3% hypericin content three times daily; 2g-4g dried herb three times daily; 2mL liquid extract (1:1 in 25% ethanol) three times daily; 2g-3g dried herb for tea in boiling water as single dose; 2mL-4mL tincture (1:1 in 45% ethanol) three times daily.

Premenstrual syndrome: 300mg capsule/tablet (standardized to 900mcg hypericin) daily.

Seasonal affective disorder: 300mg three times daily.

Topical use: Various creams and oily preparations are available; use as directed. Note they may only stay stable for a limited time (a few weeks to 6 months).

Pediatrics

Under medical supervision only, oral extract 200mg-400mg in divided doses for children 6-12 years old.

INDEX

Organized alphabetically, this index includes the brand and generic names of each drug listed in the Nonprescription Drug Information section, as well as the therapeutic categories into which the section is divided. If more than one brand name is associated with a generic, each brand can be found under the generic entry. In addition:
• <u>Generic names</u> are underlined; brand names are not.

• *Multi-ingredient products* are shown in italics.
• **Bold and capitalized** entries indicate therapeutic categories (e.g., **ACHES AND PAINS**).
• **Bold and lowercase** entries designate class-specific product dosing tables (e.g., **Acne Products**) or class-specific drug information (e.g., **Topical Corticosteroids**).